Health Promotion

TRANSLATING EVIDENCE INTO PRACTICE

Marilyn Frenn, PhD, RN, CNE, ANEF, FTOS, FAAN
Professor
Marquette University College of Nursing

Diane Whitehead, EdD, DNP, RN, ANEF
Senior Core Faculty
Walden University

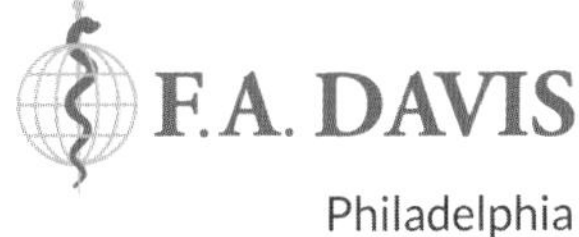

F.A. DAVIS
Philadelphia

F. A. Davis Company
1915 Arch Street
Philadelphia, PA 19103
www.fadavis.com

Printed in the United States of America

Last digit indicates print number: 10 9 8 7 6 5 4 3 2 1

Publisher, Nursing: Susan Rhyner
Manager, Content Development: William W. Welsh
Manager of Project and eProject Management: Catherine H. Carroll
Senior Content Project Manager: Julia L. Curcio
Content Development Specialist: Andrea R. Miller
Program Manager, DavisPlus: Sandra A. Glennie
Design and Illustration Manager: Carolyn O'Brien

As new scientific information becomes available through basic and clinical research, recommended treatments and drug therapies undergo changes. The author(s) and publisher have done everything possible to make this book accurate, up-to-date, and in accord with accepted standards at the time of publication. The author(s), editors, and publisher are not responsible for errors or omissions or for consequences from application of the book, and make no warranty, expressed or implied, in regard to the contents of the book. Any practice described in this book should be applied by the reader in accordance with professional standards of care used in regard to the unique circumstances that may apply in each situation. The reader is advised always to check product information (package inserts) for changes and new information regarding dose and contraindications before administering any drug. Caution is especially urged when using new or infrequently ordered drugs.

Library of Congress Cataloging-in-Publication Data

Names: Frenn, Marilyn, author. | Whitehead, Diane K., 1945- author.
Title: Health promotion : translating evidence to practice / Marilyn Frenn, Diane Whitehead.
Description: Philadelphia : F.A. Davis Company, [2021] | Includes bibliographical references and index.
Identifiers: LCCN 2020035823 (print) | LCCN 2020035824 (ebook) | ISBN 9780803660878 (paperback) | ISBN 9781719645119 (ebook)
Subjects: MESH: Health Promotion | Sociological Factors | Needs Assessment | Evidence-Based Practice
Classification: LCC RC969.H43 (print) | LCC RC969.H43 (ebook) | NLM WA 590 | DDC 362.1--dc23
LC record available at https://lccn.loc.gov/2020035823
LC ebook record available at https://lccn.loc.gov/2020035824

This book is dedicated to all those who seek to improve health. I appreciate the early career mentorship of Nola Pender, PhD, RN, FAAN, and Joanne Harrell, PhD, RN, FAAN, two legends in the world of health promotion. I thank my family and colleagues for their support in the process of bringing this book to fruition. As we add the finishing touches to Health Promotion: Translating Evidence Into Practice, Diane and I are noting many similarities in our lives. One is our gratitude for our granddaughters. In my case, my granddaughter, Lucia, lights up my life, and my daughters, husband, sister, brother—as well as spouses and those we now miss—all help me better understand the many ways to promote health.

Marilyn Frenn PhD, RN, CNE, ANEF, FTOS, FAAN
Professor
Marquette University College of Nursing

To my granddaughter, Julia—your commitment to learning inspires me. Thank you for being part of my life. GD

Diane Whitehead, EdD, DNP, RN, ANEF
Senior Core Faculty
Walden University School of Nursing

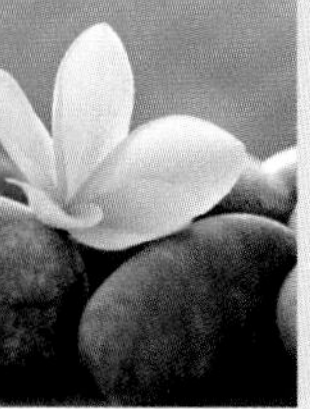

Contributors

Carolyn Baird, DNP, MBA, RN-BC, CARN-AP, CCDPD, FIAAN
Therapist
Counseling and Trauma Services
McMurray, Pennsylvania

April Bigelow, PhD, ANP-BC, AGPCNP-BC
Clinical Assistant Professor Coordinator, AGNP Program
University of Michigan
Ann Arbor, Michigan

Susan Breakwell, DNP, RN, APHN-BC
Clinical, Professor
Marquette University
Milwaukee, Wisconsin

Julia A. Bucher, RN PhD
Contributing Faculty
Walden University

Christine Cassidy, RN, PhD, CIHR
Health System Impact Postdoctoral Fellow
IWK Health Centre & University of Ottawa
Ottawa, Ontario, Canada

Mary Chisholm, BSc, MPA
Senior Policy Advisor
Halifax Regional Municipality
Halifax, Nova Scotia

Margaret R. Colyar, DSN, APRN, C-FNP
Family Nurse Practitioner
Hannibal Clinic
Hannibal, Missouri

Chin Hwa (Gina) Yi Dahlem, PhD, FNP-C, RN
Clinical Assistant Professor
University of Michigan
Ann Arbor, Michigan

Joanne DeSanto Iennaco, PhD, PMHNP-BC, PMHCNS-BC, APRN
Yale University School of Nursing
Orange, Connecticut

Michele J. Eliason, PhD
Professor of Health Education
San Francisco State University
San Francisco, California

Carol Essenmacher, DNP, NCTTP
Certified Tobacco Treatment Specialist, Tobacco Treatment Coordinator
Battle Creek VA Medical Center
Battle Creek, Michigan

Tracie Harrison, PhD, RN, FAAN
Professor Luci Baines Johnson
Fellow in Nursing, Director Center for Excellence in Aging Services & Long Term Care
School of Nursing University of Texas at Austin
Austin, Texas

Diane John, PhD, ARNP, FNP-BC
Family Nurse Practitioner, Informatics;
Associate Faculty, Frontier Nursing University
Hyden, Kentucky

Janet A. Levey, PhD, RN-BC, CNE
Associate Professor
Department of Nursing, Carthage College
Kenosha, Wisconsin

Ruth Martin-Misener, NP, PhD,
Professor and Interim Director
Dalhousie University, School of Nursing
Halifax, Nova Scotia, Canada

Alexandre A. Martins, MI, Ph.D.
College of Nursing and Theology Department Faculty
Marquette University
Milwaukee, Wisconsin

Charmaine McPherson, RN, PhD
Associate Professor
St. Francis Xavier University
Nova Scotia, Canada

Ramona Nelson, PhD, RN-BC, ANEF, FAAN
Professor Emerita Slippery Rock University
Slippery Rock, Pennsylvania
President, Ramona Nelson Consulting
Allison Park, Pennsylvania

Terri Ann Parnell, DNP, MA, RN, FAAN
Clinical Associate Professor in Health Promotion
Stony Brook University
Stony Brook, New York

Denise Saint Arnault, PhD, RN, FAAN
Professor
University of Michigan School of Nursing
Ann Arbor, Michigan

Margaret Sebern, PhD, RN
Associate Professor Emerita
Marquette University College of Nursing
Milwaukee, Wisconsin

Vicky Stone-Gale, DNP, APRN, FNP-C, MSN, FAANP
Family Nurse Practitioner
Associate Professor
Frontier Nursing University
Hyden, Kentucky

Mallory Stonehouse, MSN, APRN, AGPCNP-BC
Marquette University
Master of Science in Nursing Graduate
Nurse Practitioner
Minneapolis, Minnesota

Jane Sumner PhD, RN, PHCM APRN
Professor Emerita
Louisiana State University Health Science Center School of Nursing
New Orleans, Louisiana

Whitney Thurman, RN, PhD
Postdoctoral Fellow
School of Pharmacy
University of Texas at Austin
Austin, Texas

Patricia W. Underwood, PhD, RN, FAAN
Associate Professor (Adjunct)
Case Western Reserve University
Cleveland, Ohio

Adele Vukic, RN, PhD
Assistant Professor
Dalhousie University, School of Nursing
Halifax, Nova Scotia, Canada

Veronica Garcia Walker, RN, PhD
Assistant Professor of Clinical Nursing
School of Nursing
University of Texas at Austin

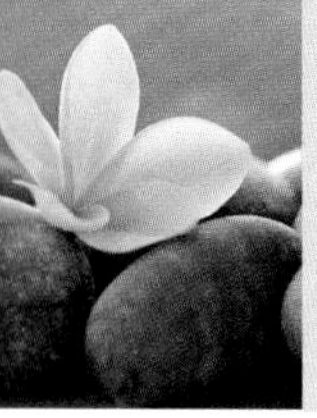

Reviewers

Jo Azzarello, PhD, RN
Associate Professor
College of Nursing
University of Oklahoma
Oklahoma City, Oklahoma

Julie Brandy, PhD, RN, FNP-BC, CNE
Associate Professor
College of Nursing and Health Professions
Valparaiso University
Valparaiso, Indiana

Wilma J. Calvert, PhD, MPE, MS, RN
Associate Professor
St. Louis College of Nursing
University of Missouri
St. Louis, Missouri

Arlene T. Farren, RN, PhD, AOCN, CTN-A, CNE
Associate Professor & Chair
Nursing Department
City University of New York
College of Staten Island
CUNY Graduate Center
Staten Island, New York

Diana Filipek, RN, BSN, MSN, AGACNP-BC
Trauma Nurse Practitioner
Cooper University Hospital
Camden, New Jersey

Teresa Hamilton, PhD, RN
Assistant Professor, NCLEX Specialist
California Baptist University
Riverside, California

Ashley Holen, DNP, MSN, RN, FNP-C
Assistant Professor of Nursing
University of Sioux Falls
Sioux Falls, South Dakota

Cheryl Kruschke, EdD, MS, RN, CNE
Associate Professor
Regis University
Denver, Colorado

Debbie Sheppard LeMoine, PhD, MN, RN, RN
Assistant Professor
St. Francis Xavier University
Antigonish, Nova Scotia, Canada

M. Star Mahara, RN, MSN
Associate Professor,
School of Nursing
Thomson Rivers University
Kamloops, British Columbia, Canada

Dane Menkin, MSN, CRNP, AAHIVM
Clinical Operations Manager
Mazzoni Center Family and Community Medicine
Philadelphia, Pennsylvania

Abigail Mitchell, DHEd, MSN, CNE, FHERDSA
Director of Graduate Nursing, Professor
D'Youville College
Buffalo, New York

Sara Morasch, MSN, RN, BC
Clinical Educator
Providence Health Care
Spokane, Washington

Keith Plowden, PhD, PMHNP-BC
Psychiatric Nurse Practitioner
Greenwood, South Carolina

Lisa Quinn, PhD, CRNP, MSN
Associate Professor of Nursing
Gannon University
Erie, Pennsylvania

Kathryn Wirtz Rugen, PhD, FNP-BC, FAANP, FAAN
National Nurse Practitioner Consultant
Department of Veterans Affairs, Office of Academic Consultant
Chicago, Illinois

Dawn Specht, MSN, PhD, RN, APN
Assistant Professor Nursing
American Sentinel University
Aurora, Colorado

Wendy M. Wheeler, RN, MN,
Instructor
Red Deer College
Red Deer, Alberta, Canada

Robin M. White, PhD, MSN, RN
Associate Professor
University of Tampa
Tampa, Florida

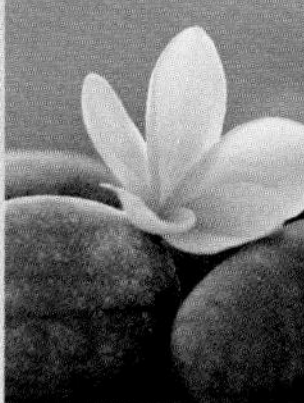

Preface

The research on how best to help people promote their health is constantly changing. Nurses, especially those in advanced practice, need to understand the foundational studies and current evidence to support practice decisions. From the theories of health promotion to the realities of social determinants and special populations, *Health Promotion: Translating Evidence Into Practice* brings together expert insights and knowledge to give you the tools you need to apply evidence-based health promotion strategies to your practice.

In this text, we approach health promotion strategies by focusing on the experience of advanced practice nurses working one-on-one with clients. Nurses must be optimally prepared to approach their clients holistically and evaluate diet, level of physical activity, sleep quality, and mental health concerns. Deficits in many of these areas may manifest as chronic problems later in life. Nurses must be well equipped to help clients tackle the deeper health issues they face, for example, clients who often feel challenged or discouraged, who perhaps have tried and failed repeatedly to address a particular issue, such as smoking cessation or obesity. Clinical evidence changes quickly, and patients presenting with multiple comorbidities (i.e., obesity, high blood pressure, high cholesterol, and diabetes) need help navigating treatment and management decisions in the face of often complex and conflicting evidence.

In Unit 1, we present an overview and the theories of health promotion. We address evidence-based practice and key principles of epidemiology, and we include a chapter devoted to techniques of motivational interviewing. Unit 2 applies these theories to the real-life work with clients, families, and communities. We cover health screening and counseling from birth to age 21, with a separate chapter on health promotion for the adult and older adult. Additional chapters focus on mental health promotion, health literacy, patient education, and informatics in health promotion. Unit 3 explores the current and emerging trends that are shaping the evolution of health promotion, including the need for practitioners to embrace cultural humility, ethical comportment, and interprofessional collaboration, as well as successfully implementing alternative therapies where possible. Unit 4 identifies the special populations and social determinants that affect the health and well-being of patients. We provide guidance on compassionate care and health promotion for clients with disabilities, clients who are homeless and those who are gender diverse, as well as clients struggling with substance use or end-of-life issues.

We know that social determinants play a huge role in health outcomes and the options people have to promote their health successfully. It is vital that all nurses advocate for policies to improve those social determinants. Changing social determinants is a career-long endeavor, so nurses need to be ready to offer the best evidence-based health promotion options to clients, families, and communities as they work toward healthier policies and opportunities on a larger scale.

Health Promotion: Translating Evidence Into Practice provides a variety of special features to enhance user understanding. The book also includes examples of real-life scenarios faced by today's advanced practice nurses.

- **Unfolding case illustrations** present client cases related to chapter content. Follow each client's journey to see how the theories in each chapter apply to practice.
- **PICOT questions** provide a formula for developing answerable, researchable questions, making the process of finding and evaluating evidence much more straightforward, for example:
  P: Population (i.e., age, gender, ethnicity, with a certain health promotion issue or disorder)
  I: Intervention or variable of interest (exposure to a disease, risk behavior, prognostic factor)
  C: Comparison (could be a placebo or "business as usual," as in no disease, absence of risk factor, prognostic factor B)
  O: Outcome (risk of disease, accuracy of a diagnosis, rate of occurrence of adverse outcome)
  T: Time

For an intervention:

In ________ (P), how does ________ (I) compare to ________ (C) affect ________ (O) within ______ (T)?

- **Check Your Understanding questions** close each chapter and assess your grasp of the information covered. Answers to these questions are found in the back of the book.

In addition to the resources in this book, you will find additional material on DavisPlus.

For Students

Case Studies with critical thinking questions

Bonus chapter **"Aggregate Health Promotion and Risk Reduction."**

For Instructors

PowerPoint presentations (one presentation per chapter)

Test Bank

Active Classroom Instructor's Guide

Case Studies with answers to the critical thinking questions

We have made the evidence "practice-ready" for you to align with the values and preferences of clients, families, and communities using your clinical expertise. You can use this book as a starting place to learn the skills you will need throughout your career to review emerging evidence and fine-tune what you offer in practice.

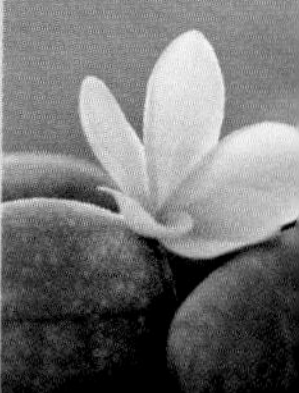

Contents

Unit 1

Overview and Theories

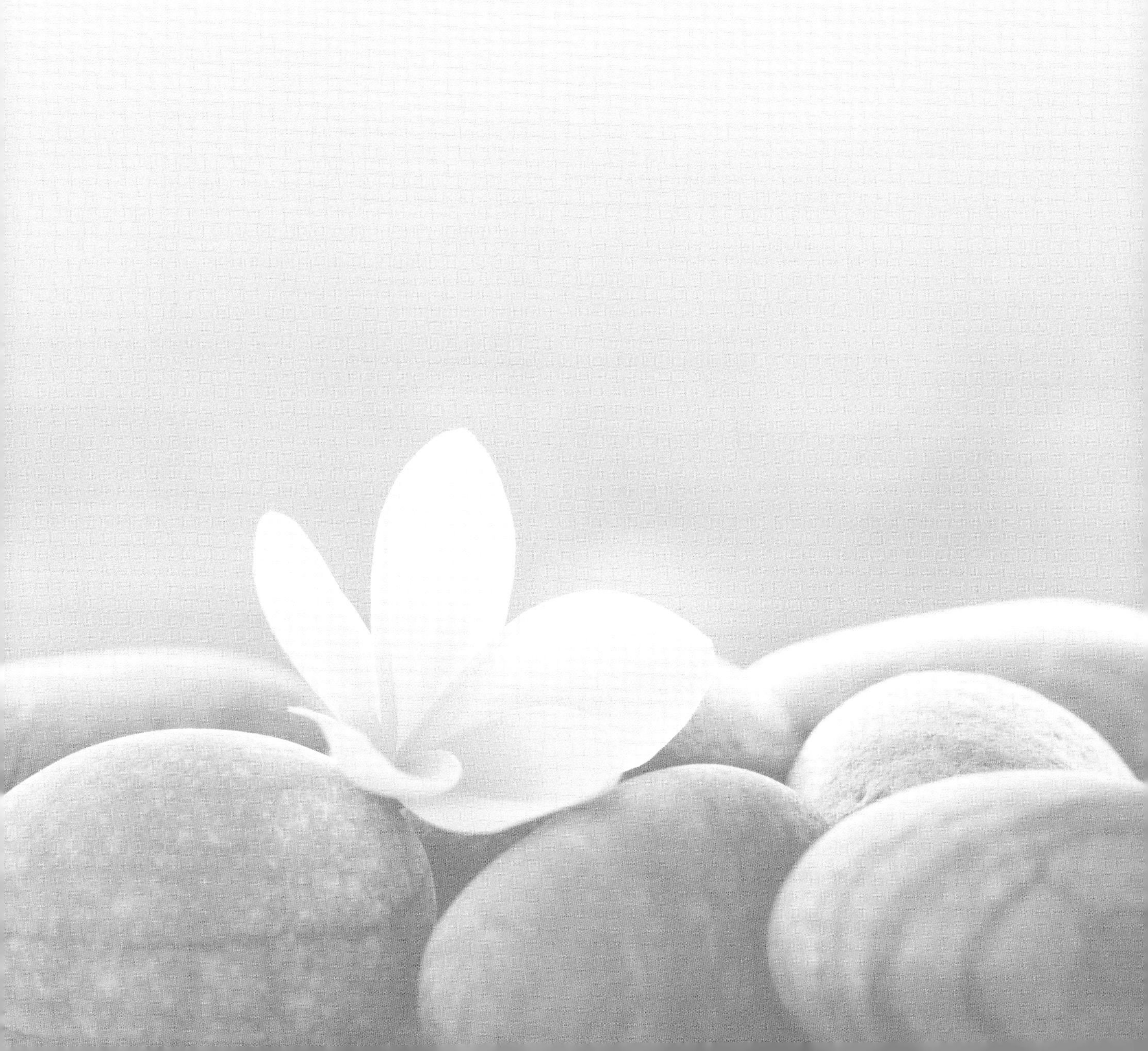

Introduction

Marilyn Frenn

Helping clients promote their health is one of the most exciting and rapidly changing areas of nursing practice. It is critical for nurses to review and weigh the latest evidence to make effective health promotion recommendations. Beyond appraising the evidence, knowing how to help people understand the recommendations and make lasting changes is one of the most challenging endeavors nurses face.

What are the top issues affecting health in the United States and Canada? What can nurses do to improve health outcomes, quality of life, and cost-effective service delivery? This chapter includes an introduction to health promotion and prevention guidelines; resources used for individual, family, and aggregate approaches to health promotion and risk reduction; and approaches for appraisal of evidence. This book addresses health promotion issues included in nursing examinations from NCLEX to certification examinations in advanced practice.

QUALITY OF LIFE AND COST-EFFECTIVE SERVICE DELIVERY

The coronavirus pandemic that started in late 2019 demonstrated the vital importance of promoting health through handwashing and social distancing. It became the largest daily cause of death in the United States (Deese, 2020), with those experiencing chronic illness most at risk of severe illness and death. These chronic illnesses include the longstanding 10 top causes of morbidity and mortality in both the United States and Canada accounting for 75% of deaths in each country (Statistics Canada, 2015). Cardiovascular disease and cancer are the top causes of death in both nations, and many of the remaining eight causes are similarly amenable to effective health promotion.

Health risks that are increasing in incidence include obesity in children and adults, use of e-cigarettes among youth, and diabetes (especially among Hispanic and black adults) (Centers for Disease Control, 2020; National Center for Health Statistics, 2019). A high level of aerobic fitness can ameliorate risks to health such as those related to obesity and hypertension (Clark & Bryan, 2017), which substantiates the need for health promotion throughout the life span to prevent and reduce risks to health. However, only one in five Canadian adults engages in sufficient physical activity to achieve this health benefit (Clarke, Colley, Janssen, & Tremblay, 2019). In the United States, youth and adults are not meeting targets for improvement in physical activity (U.S. Department of Health and Human Services, 2016).

The opioid epidemic is yet another priority area for health promotion. Those with substance use issues and those in treatment have limited access to primary care and prevention resources (Gadbois, Chin, & Dalphonse, 2016). Special skills in promoting health with those dealing with substance use are addressed in Chapter 21.

Health promotion improves quality of life (Fanning et al., 2018) and reduces disease burden that would otherwise occur for the individual (Doran, Resnick, Kim, Lynn, & McCormick, 2017), family, and society through missed days at school or work, reduced productivity, and the need for costly health services (Subramanian, Midha, & Chellapilla, 2017). Health expenditures as a percentage of gross domestic product (GDP) increased from 7.9% to 17.8% in the United States between 1975 and 2015 (National Center for Health Statistics, 2019), so promoting health effectively has important economic benefits. Although there are costs to coach people in undertaking behaviors that reduce their chance of illness such as prediabetes, we have increasing evidence to support feasible cost-effective approaches, such as mobile health (Michaelides et al., 2018).

While nurses work with individuals to promote health, it is also important to engage people using modern media, such as Facebook, Twitter, and YouTube, as well as traditional health message outlets on radio and television pertinent to the subgroup of people to be reached (Vallone et al., 2017). Collaborating with other professions to produce messages that best reach the intended audience for health promotion is crucial (Stanfield & Rogers, 2018).

Just as information systems are essential in acute care, they also save time and foster prioritization of care in settings where health promotion is more usually done, such as in school health settings (Radis, Updegrove, Somsel, & Crowley, 2016). Cutting-edge use of information systems is addressed in Chapter 13.

INDIVIDUAL, FAMILY, AGGREGATE APPROACHES

Nurses work with people as individuals and with their families. Health promotion requires prioritization of those activities that promote health and examination of barriers to that action. For example, women face lifelong social disparities in staying physically active (Coen, Rosenberg, & Davidson, 2018). Effective health promotion requires a deeper understanding of these barriers and engaged, creative discovery of workable options, not just a list of recommendations. Avoiding stigmatizing messages is also incredibly important because such messages may actually reduce people's willingness to take health-promoting action, such as smoking cessation (Kim, Cao, & Meczkowski, 2018).

As a nurse who realizes the importance of immunizations, for example, it may be difficult to understand some parents' unwillingness to immunize their children. Seeking evidence to understand parents' perspectives (Attwell, Ward, Meyer, Rokkas, & Leask, 2018), working with them by listening to their perspectives, and explaining how vaccines are created and help the body build resources to prevent illness likely will be more effective than a stigmatizing approach for noncompliance with vaccines.

Promoting health is often more difficult for individuals and families experiencing disparities based on race and ethnicity (Lai, Alfaifi, & Althemery, 2017); income; neighborhood resources; access to food (Gosliner, Brown, Sun, Woodward-Lopez, & Crawford, 2018); safe places to engage in physical activity (Hong et al., 2018); and access to health-care services for prevention, early detection, and screening. For these reasons, it is important for nurses to work with community advocates to address these disparities, which in themselves create risk to health beyond those of lifestyle behaviors (Lachance, Kelly, Wilkin, Burke, & Waddell, 2018).

Nurses must also work to promote health policy that reduces risk to health for aggregates. For example, an overall plan involving government and private groups to improve physical activity (Spence, Faulkner, Costas Bradstreet, Duggan, & Tremblay, 2015) has a higher likelihood for improving physical activity than when nurses work only with individuals and families.

Promoting one's own health is vital for nurses and other health professionals (Lobelo & de Quevedo, 2016). People are more likely to listen to nurses engaged in healthy behaviors, and professionals who engage in healthy behaviors are more likely to prioritize addressing these health promotion issues with clients (Doran et al., 2017; Kelly, Wills, & Sykes, 2017). Developing resilience through personal health promotion reduces burnout (Klein, Riggenbach-Hays, Sollenberger, Harney, & McGarvey, 2018) and the consequences of job-related stress, such as obesity (Geiker et al., 2018), suicide (Davidson, Zisook, Kirby, DeMichele, & Norcross, 2018), poor patient outcomes (Linzer et al., 2015), and intent to leave the profession (Farinaz, MacPhee, & Dahinten, 2016). Engaging in health-promoting behaviors was associated with lower perceived work stress and higher job satisfaction for nurses in acute-care settings (Williams, Costley, Bellury, & Moobed, 2018). Supporting health professionals to prevent burnout through more effective teamwork has now become part of the quadruple aim along with improving patient experience and health outcomes and reducing costs (Farrell, Luptak, Supiano, Pacala, & De Lisser, 2018). Learning how to promote health, including your own, is thus one of the most important things you can do as a nurse, regardless of the area in which you practice. However, sometimes those preparing to be nurses or advanced practice nurses have not been taught how to help people engage effectively in healthier behaviors (Wills & Kelly, 2017).

APPRAISAL OF EVIDENCE: GREATEST IMPROVEMENT AT THE LOWEST COST

A large, rapidly growing body of evidence exists about how to promote health effectively, so much so that many people have difficulty understanding what actions are most important, let alone have the necessary skills and resources to engage in and sustain the health-promoting behaviors. Chapter 5 includes approaches to evaluating and synthesizing evidence pertinent to health promotion at the individual, family, and aggregate levels. Evidence-based practice means integrating the best evidence from high-quality research; clinical judgment; and individual, family, and/or community preferences to develop and implement effective interventions. Many chapters include an example **P**atient, **I**ntervention, **C**ontrol, **O**bservation, and **T**ime (PICOT) question showing how evidence is evaluated and organized to translate health promotion into practice.

While 80% to 90% of people seeing a physician might benefit from taking steps to improve their health, only 35% to 45% are counseled during doctors appointments and even fewer are referred for support (Maners, Bakow, Parkinson, Fischer, & Camp, 2018). It is important to examine the patient characteristics for which nurse-led health promotion produces significant improvement, such as sustaining the oldest old in the community (Bleijenberg et al., 2017), so that practice changes produce measurable results.

Systematic reviews are an excellent resource to deal with the large body of evidence in health promotion because the quality of studies is examined, and important findings across studies are synthesized. For example, choosing culturally congruent interventions acceptable to students, parents, and school personnel through a systematic review can help school nurses seeking to prevent type 2 diabetes (Brackney & Cutshall, 2015).

Reaching people at each nursing encounter we have with them is essential. For example, one-third of adolescents enrolled in a health plan for at least 4 years had no preventive visits, and 40% had only one visit during that period. This lack of care is unfortunate because half of sexually transmitted illnesses occur in this age group, costing $16 billion (Santa Maria, Guilamo-Ramos, Jemmott, Derouin, & Villarruel, 2017). Only 10% of Americans receive the benefits of evidence-based practice, particularly in health promotion, so it is important that nurses intervene to promote health even in acute-care settings (FitzGerald, Rorie, & Salem, 2015). When intervening with patients, use of effective behavior change approaches, such as motivational interviewing, is essential. (See Chapter 6 for more information on motivational interviewing.) Simply warning people of dangers associated with their behavior rarely helps them to change (Lomba, Kroll, Apostólo, Gameiro, & Apostólo, 2016). People often know they have risks, but they do not know how to make and sustain changes because of the barriers they encounter. Understanding the complex interrelationships of physiologic as well as motivational aspects of integrated behavior change is critical (Outland, 2018).

Nurses must also stay aware of changes in risk patterns. For example, cardiovascular disease is now the leading cause of death in Canadian women, so screening and addressing risks early as well as raising awareness can improve treatment outcomes (Gujral & Sawatzky, 2017). Outreach may be especially important in rural areas, and nurse practitioner interventions have been effective in increasing awareness of risk (Pearson, 2017).

Incorporating the views of those who we seek to help is crucial in ethical health promotion. An action research approach can be a useful way to integrate the views of community members in choosing the most pressing issues and examining acceptable solution options (Kyoon-Achan et al., 2018). Ethical comportment is important whenever and wherever we seek to help others, and it is a topic discussed more thoroughly in Chapter 16.

Once the evidence has been evaluated, using a systematic process to integrate the evidence in practice is essential. Useful theories are described in Chapter 4. Using a theoretical framework to guide health promotion efforts aids in effectiveness (Doran et al., 2017). One example is the social ecological model in which the environment and policies are assessed; education is provided, including approaches to address barriers and build self-efficacy; and technology-enhanced motivational messages and booster sessions are used to sustain positive changes. Another approach commonly used is Plan-Do-Study-Act (PDSA), which was helpful in improving children's oral health (Okah, Williams, Talib, & Mann, 2018).

Sustaining systematic changes must also be addressed to translate evidence successfully. The reach, effectiveness, adoption, implementation, maintenance (RE-AIM) framework is an approach to ensure that evidence-based interventions reach the intended populations in sufficient numbers, that they are implemented with fidelity to the evidence, and that they become institutionalized as part of organizational policies and procedures. Incorporating charismatic champions in the community is one way to ensure that interventions are sustained (Miyawaki, Belza, Kohn, & Petrescu-Prahova, 2018).

HEALTH PROMOTION GUIDELINES AND RESOURCES

Implementing practice changes using international, national, regional, and topic-specific guidelines and resources is an excellent way to improve health outcomes. The World Health Organization (WHO) is part of the United Nations system and promotes health throughout the world (http://www.who.int/about-us). It provides leadership, directs research priorities, and sets norms and standards for ethical and evidence-based initiatives. WHO also provides technical support and monitors health issues and trends around the world.

Canada's publicly funded health system sets standards for 13 provincial and territorial health plans (https://www.canada.ca/en/health-canada/services/canada-health-care-system.html). Federal regulations are in place for issues such as environmental and workplace health, food, pesticides, and devices such as cell phones that emit radiation. Research, health promotion, monitoring, and disease prevention as well as services for special groups such as the elderly, disabled, and children are also provided nationally. Healthy living resources and information on disease prevention are available online (https://www.canada.ca/en/health-canada.html).

In the United States, health objectives based on population data are developed every decade. Work is underway for Healthy People 2030 (https://www.healthypeople.gov/2020/About-Healthy-People/Development-Healthy-People-2030) as we complete evaluation of Healthy People 2020 objectives. Specific objectives are set based on the overall burden, preventable burden, ability to reduce health inequities and disparities, as well as cost and prevention effectiveness. Specific Healthy People objectives are provided in many chapters in this book.

The Million Hearts initiative was led by the U.S. Department of Health and Human Services and more than 100 collaborating organizations with a five-year goal of preventing 1 million heart attacks and strokes (https://millionhearts.hhs.gov/index.html). Four evidence-based initiatives deliverable by advanced practice nurses form the basis of a Million Hearts: appropriate aspirin therapy, blood pressure control, cholesterol control, and smoking cessation (Melnyk et al., 2016).

Similarly, the Community Preventive Services Task Force offers guidelines to promote health and prevent illness (Campos-Outcalt, 2017). The Community Guide is available at www.thecommunityguide.org/index.html. Webinars, implementation stories of practice changes, approaches to improve immunizations, ways to reach Latinx members of the community, and ideas to address environmental support for health promotion are examples of concrete information on this Web site that could help promote health.

The U.S. Preventive Services Task Force is composed of multidisciplinary volunteer experts who identify areas where research is needed and examine evidence to grade recommendations for clinicians and patients/clients to consider. Guidelines are searchable at https://epss.ahrq.gov/ePSS/search.jsp by client characteristics, topic, and evidence grade.

HEALTH PROMOTION IN NURSING LICENSING AND CERTIFICATION

Health promotion is part of initial licensure for nurses in both the United States and Canada, with 6% to 12% of the National Council Licensure Exam for Registered Nursing (NCLEX-RN) under the heading Health Promotion and Risk Reduction. In addition, components of other headings in the NCLEX test plan include areas considered health promotion, such as mobility, sleep and rest, and injury prevention.

For those working with children in the United States, the Pediatric Nursing Certification Board offers a certification exam. Fourteen percent of this exam is specifically focused on health promotion, while other parts of the exam address risk reduction.

The American Academy of Nurse Practitioners offers certification examinations for adult/gerontology, family, and emergency nurse practitioner. Health promotion, harm reduction, disease prevention, and anticipatory guidance are among the knowledge areas covered in the exams.

Certification examinations are offered in a variety of clinical nurse and nurse practitioner specializations by the American Nurses Credentialing Center. These exams include population health, risk identification, health promotion and prevention of illness, considerations for diverse populations, ethics, and standards integrated in several sections of the test plan.

REFERENCES

Attwell, K., Ward, P. R., Meyer, S. B., Rokkas, P. J., & Leask, J. (2018). "Do-it-yourself": Vaccine rejection and complementary and alternative medicine (CAM). *Social Science & Medicine, 196*, 106–114. doi:10.1016/j.socscimed.2017.11.022

Bleijenberg, N., Imhof, L., Mahrer-Imhof, R., Wallhagen, M. I., Wit, N. J., & Schuurmans, M. J. (2017). Patient characteristics associated with a successful response to nurse-led care programs targeting the oldest-old: A comparison of two RCTs. *Worldviews on Evidence-Based Nursing, 14*(3), 210–222. doi:10.1111/wvn.12235

Brackney, D. E., & Cutshall, M. (2015). Prevention of Type 2 diabetes among youth: A systematic review, implications for the school nurse. *Journal of School Nursing, 31*(1), 6–21. doi:10.1177/1059840514535445

Campos-Outcalt, D. (2017). CPSTF: A lesser known, but valuable, resource for FPs. *Journal of Family Practice, 66*(1), 34–37.

Centers for Disease Control and Prevention. (2020). *National Diabetes Statistics Report, 2020*. Atlanta, GA: Centers for Disease Control and Prevention, U.S. Dept of Health and Human Services. Available at: https://www.cdc.gov/diabetes/pdfs/data/statistics/national-diabetes-statistics-report.pdf

Clark, J., & Bryan, S. (2017). *Aerobic fitness, body mass index, and health-related risk factors*. Statistics Canada. Retrieved from http://www.statcan.gc.ca/pub/82-624-x/2017001/article/14783-eng.pdf

Clarke, J., Colley, R., Janssen, I., & Tremblay, M. S. (2019). *Accelerometer-measured moderate-to-vigorous physical activity of Canadian adults, 2007 to 2017*. Retrieved from: https://www150.statcan.gc.ca/n1/pub/82-003-x/2019008/article/00001-eng.htm

Coen, S. E., Rosenberg, M. W., & Davidson, J. (2018). "It's gym, like g-y-m not J-i-m": Exploring the role of place in the gendering of physical activity. *Social Science & Medicine*, *196*, 29–36. doi:https://doi.org/10.1016/j.socscimed.2017.10.036

Davidson, J. E., Zisook, S., Kirby, B., DeMichele, G., & Norcross, W. (2018). Suicide prevention: A healer education and referral program for nurses. *Journal of Nursing Administration*, *48*(2), 85–92. doi:10.1097/nna.0000000000000582

Deese, K. (April 15, 2020). Coronavirus now leading cause of death in US. *MSN News*. Retrieved from https://www.msn.com/en-ca/news/world/coronavirus-now-leading-cause-of-death-in-us/ar-BB12oOuT

Doran, K., Resnick, B., Kim, N., Lynn, D., & McCormick, T. (2017). Applying the social ecological model and theory of self-efficacy in the Worksite Heart Health Improvement Project-PLUS. *Research and Theory for Nursing Practice*, *31*(1), 8–27. doi:10.1891/1541-6577.31.1.8

Fanning, J., Walkup, M. P., Ambrosius, W. T., Brawley, L. R., Ip, E. H., Marsh, A. P., & Rejeski, W. J. (2018). Change in health-related quality of life and social cognitive outcomes in obese, older adults in a randomized controlled weight loss trial: Does physical activity behavior matter? *Journal of Behavioral Medicine*, *41*(3), 299–308. doi:10.1007/s10865-017-9903-6

Farinaz, H., MacPhee, M., & Dahinten, V. S. (2016). RNs and LPNs: Emotional exhaustion and intention to leave. *Journal of Nursing Management*, *24*(3), 393–399. doi:10.1111/jonm.12334

Farrell, T. W., Luptak, M. K., Supiano, K. P., Pacala, J. T., & De Lisser, R. (2018). State of the science: Interprofessional approaches to aging, dementia, and mental health. *Journal of the American Geriatrics Society*, *66*, S40–S47. doi:10.1111/jgs.15309

FitzGerald, L. Z., Rorie, A., & Salem, B. E. (2015). Improving secondary prevention screening in clinical encounters using mHealth among prelicensure master's entry clinical nursing students. *Worldviews on Evidence-Based Nursing*, *12*(2), 79–87. doi:10.1111/wvn.12081

Gadbois, C., Chin, E. D., & Dalphonse, L. (2016). Health promotion in an opioid treatment program. *Journal of Addictions Nursing (Lippincott Williams & Wilkins)*, *27*(2), 127–142. doi:10.1097/JAN.0000000000000124

Geiker N. R. W., Astrup A., Hjorth M. F., Sjödin A., Pijls L., & Rob, M. C. (2018). Does stress influence sleep patterns, food intake, weight gain, abdominal obesity and weight loss interventions, and vice versa? *Obesity Reviews*, *19*(1), 81–97. doi:10.1111/obr.12603

Gosliner, W., Brown, D. M., Sun, B. C., Woodward-Lopez, G., & Crawford, P. B. (2018). Availability, quality and price of produce in low-income neighbourhood food stores in California raise equity issues. *Public Health Nutrition*, *21*(9), 1639–1648. http://dx.doi.org/10.1017/S1368980018000058

Gujral, G., & Sawatzky, J.-A. V. (2017). Cardiovascular disease risk: A focus on women. *Canadian Journal of Cardiovascular Nursing*, *27*(1), 22–30.

Hong, A., Sallis, J. F., King, A. C., Conway, T. L., Saelens, B., Cain, K. L., . . . Frank, L. D. (2018). Linking green space to neighborhood social capital in older adults: The role of perceived safety. *Social Science & Medicine*, *207*, 38–45. doi:10.1016/j.socscimed.2018.04.051

Kelly, M., Wills, J., & Sykes, S. (2017). Do nurses' personal health behaviours impact on their health promotion practice? A systematic review. *International Journal of Nursing Studies*, *76*, 62–77. https://doi.org/10.1016/j.ijnurstu.2017.08.008

Kim, J., Cao, X., & Meczkowski, E. (2018). Does stigmatization motivate people to quit smoking? Examining the effect of stigmatizing anti-smoking campaigns on cessation intention. *Health Communication*, *33*(6), 681–689. doi:10.1080/10410236.2017.1299275

Klein, C. J., Riggenbach-Hays, J. J., Sollenberger, L. M., Harney, D. M., & McGarvey, J. S. (2018). Quality of life and compassion satisfaction in clinicians: A pilot intervention study for reducing compassion fatigue. *American Journal of Hospice & Palliative Medicine*, *35*(6), 882–888. doi:10.1177/1049909117740848

Kyoon-Achan, G., Lavoie, J., Kinew, K. A., Phillips-Beck, W., Ibrahim, N., Sinclair, S., & Katz, A. (2018). Innovating for transformation in First Nations health using community-based participatory research. *Qualitative Health Research*, *28*(7), 1036–1049. doi:10.1177/1049732318756056

Lachance, L., Kelly, R. P., Wilkin, M., Burke, J., & Waddell, S. (2018). Community-based efforts to prevent and manage diabetes in women living in vulnerable communities. *Journal of Community Health*, *43*(3), 508–517. doi:10.1007/s10900-017-0444-2

Lai, L., Alfaifi, A., & Althemery, A. (2017). Healthcare disparities in Hispanic diabetes care: A propensity score-matched study. *Journal of Immigrant & Minority Health*, *19*(5), 1001–1008. doi:10.1007/s10903-016-0505-0

Linzer, M., Poplau, S., Grossman, E., Varkey, A., Yale, S., Williams, E., . . . Barbouche, M. (2015). A cluster randomized trial of interventions to improve work conditions and clinician burnout in primary care: Results from the Healthy Work Place (HWP) study. *Journal of General Internal Medicine*, *30*(8), 1105–1111. doi:10.1007/s11606-015-3235-4

Lobelo, F., & de Quevedo, I. G. (2016). The evidence in support of physicians and health care providers as physical activity role models. *American Journal of Lifestyle Medicine*, *10*(1), 36–52. doi:10.1177/1559827613520120

Lomba, L., Kroll, T., Apostólo, J., Gameiro, M., & Apostólo, J. (2016). The use of motivational interviews by nurses to promote health behaviors in adolescents: A scoping review protocol. *JBI Database of Systematic Reviews & Implementation Reports*, *14*(5), 27–37. doi:10.11124/JBISRIR-2016-002564

Maners, R. J., Bakow, E., Parkinson, M. D., Fischer, G. S., & Camp, G. R. (2018). UPMC Prescription for Wellness: A quality improvement case study for supporting patient engagement and health behavior change. *American Journal of Medical Quality*, *33*(3), 274–282. doi:10.1177/1062860617741670

Melnyk, B. M., Orsolini, L., Gawlik, K., Braun, L. T., Chyun, D. A., Conn, V. S., . . . Olin, A. R. (2016). The Million Hearts initiative: Guidelines and best practices. *Nurse Practitioner, 41*(2), 46–54. doi:10.1097/01.NPR.0000476372.04620.7a

Michaelides, A., Major, J., Pienkosz Jr., E., Wood, M., Kim, Y., & Toro-Ramos, T. (2018). Usefulness of a novel mobile diabetes prevention program delivery platform with human coaching: 65-week observational follow-up. *JMIR Mhealth Uhealth, 6*(5), e93. doi:10.2196/mhealth.9161

Miyawaki, C. E., Belza, B., Kohn, M. J., & Petrescu-Prahova, M. (2018). Champions of an older adult exercise program: Believers, promoters, and recruiters. *Journal of Applied Gerontology, 37*(6), 728–744. doi:10.1177/0733464816645921

National Center for Health Statistics. (2019). *Health, United States, 2018*. Hyattsville, MD.

Okah, A., Williams, K., Talib, N., & Mann, K. (2018). Promoting oral health in childhood: A quality improvement project. *Pediatrics, 141*(6), 1–8. doi:10.1542/peds.2017-2396

Outland, L. (2018). Evidence-based ways to promote metabolic health. *Journal for Nurse Practitioners, 14*(6), 456–462. doi:10.1016/j.nurpra.2018.02.010

Pearson, J. T. (2017). *Implementation and evaluation of coronary heart disease outreach community education: Improvement in evidence based screening for nurse practitioner clinical office follow up ProQuest Dissertations Publishing (Order No. 10248068).*

Radis, M. E., Updegrove, S. C., Somsel, A., & Crowley, A. A. (2016). Negotiating access to health information to promote students' health. *Journal of School Nursing, 32*(2), 81–85. doi:10.1177/1059840515615676

Santa Maria, D., Guilamo-Ramos, V., Jemmott, L. S., Derouin, A., & Villarruel, A. (2017). Nurses on the front lines: Improving adolescent sexual and reproductive health across health care settings. *American Journal of Nursing, 117*(1), 42–51.

Spence, J. C., Faulkner, G., Costas Bradstreet, C., Duggan, M., & Tremblay, M. S. (2015). Active Canada 20/20: A physical activity plan for Canada. *Canadian Journal of Public Health, 106*(8), e470–e473. doi:10.17269/cjph.106.5041

Stanfield, K., & Rodgers, S. (2018). A multi-year study of tobacco control in newspaper editorials using community characteristic data and content analysis findings. *Health Communication, 33*(7), 842–850. doi:10.1080/10410236.2017.1315679

Statistics Canada. (2015). *Leading causes of death in Canada, 2009*. Retrieved from http://www.statcan.gc.ca/pub/84-215-x/2012001/hl-fs-eng.htm

Subramanian, K., Midha, I., & Chellapilla, V. (2017). Overcoming the challenges in implementing Type 2 diabetes mellitus prevention programs can decrease the burden on healthcare costs in the United States. *Journal of Diabetes Research, 2017*. doi:10.1155/2017/2615681

U.S. Department of Health and Human Services. (2016). *Physical activity*. Retrieved from https://www.healthypeople.gov/2020/topics-objectives/topic/physical-activity/national-snapshot

Vallone, D., Greenberg, M., Xiao, H., Bennett, M., Cantrell, J., Rath, J., & Hair, E. (2017). The effect of branding to promote healthy behavior: Reducing tobacco use among youth and young adults. *International Journal of Environmental Research and Public Health, 14*(12), 1517. doi:http://dx.doi.org/10.3390/ijerph14121517

Williams, H. L., Costley, T., Bellury, L. M., & Moobed, J. (2018). Do health promotion behaviors affect levels of job satisfaction and job stress for nurses in an acute care hospital? *Journal of Nursing Administration, 48*(6), 342–348. doi:10.1097/NNA.0000000000000625

Wills, J., & Kelly, M. (2017). What works to encourage student nurses to adopt healthier lifestyles? Findings from an intervention study. *Nurse Education Today, 48*, 180–184. https://doi.org/10.1016/j.nedt.2016.10.011

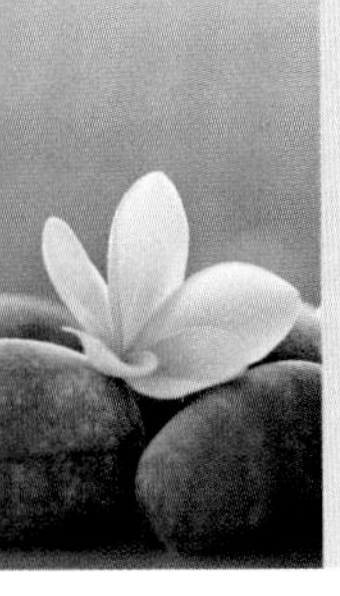

Chapter 2

The Social Determinants of Health, Health Equity, and Social Justice

Translating the Evidence for Advanced Nursing Health Promotion Practice

Charmaine McPherson and Mary Chisholm

LEARNING OBJECTIVES

After completing this chapter, the student will be able to:

1. Analyze the relationships among concepts of social determinants of health, health equity, social justice, and health-promoting public policy.
2. Discuss the conditions that contribute to health inequalities.
3. Discuss issues important to applying social determinants of health evidence in practice.
4. Differentiate between traditional models of health promotion that raise the overall health of a population and the social determinants of health approach.
5. Apply evidence to promote health equity.
6. Integrate the social determinants of health care into assessments and interventions to promote health equity.

INTRODUCTION

The social determinants of health are a key concept in health promotion. We know interdependence exists between health and social conditions. The World Health Organization (WHO), in its final report by the Commission on Social Determinants of Health (2008), pointed to the burdens of illness and premature loss of life that stem from the conditions in which people are born, grow, live, work, and age. Inequalities in the distribution of the social determinants of health are widely recognized as a public policy problem requiring immediate and substantial action.

Framing health as a social phenomenon emphasizes health in relation to social justice. Thus, consideration of the social determinants of health is necessarily a dialogue concerning health equity and social justice. Working toward health equity requires certain antecedents, such as systemwide changes that include cross-sectoral policy designed to promote public health. The nursing profession, and public health nursing in particular, are well-positioned to lead interdisciplinary and cross-sectoral dialogue and policy action on these known antecedents to ameliorate health inequities.

This chapter encourages you to reflect on the conditions that make health inequalities unjust and consider the merits of policies and practices that prioritize the elimination of health disparities versus those that focus on raising the overall standard of health in a population. We will consider key concepts important for this discussion; review the historical development of the social determinants of health approach; and examine three related and interconnected themes: health equity, social justice, and public policy. As a health promotion practitioner, in-depth knowledge of these concepts and related systems issues is paramount to providing the leadership required to shift policy, programming, and ultimately health outcomes, especially across the life span of particularly vulnerable populations.

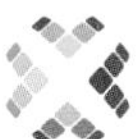

Case Illustration

Throughout this chapter, we consider these issues through the case of Erin Walzak, an advanced practice public health nurse of 20 years working for the provincial health authority in Nova Scotia, Canada. She has been asked by a colleague from municipal government to work with her local urban community to examine the issue of affordable housing. Erin's unit director does not believe, however, that this is an appropriate use of her time as a public health practitioner.

KEY CONCEPTS FOR UNDERSTANDING SOCIAL DETERMINANTS OF HEALTH

In the design of policy for health, a broader understanding of risk factors for disease across the life span and an increasing awareness of the social determinants of health have led to the development of more comprehensive, cross-sectoral strategies to tackle complex problems. A growing and compelling body of research has made it increasingly clear that material contexts—access to food, safe housing, adequate income, a supportive workplace, and so forth—have a major impact on health (Anderson et al., 2009). Although some groups are particularly vulnerable to ill health, we know that health status diminishes continually along this social gradient (Marmot, Friel, Bell, Houweling, & Taylor, 2008). These differences relate to the social determinants of health (SDHs): the conditions of daily life, which in turn are shaped by the unequal distributions of power, money, and resources (Commission on Social Determinants of Health, 2008). These circumstances are shaped by the different distributions at global, national, and local levels, which themselves are influenced by policy choices. The social determinants mantra is necessarily focused away from health services to help people understand that health is more about social factors rather than entirely about provision of adequate health services (McGibbon, 2016). This is why we consider "policy *for* health" rather than "health policy" alone—policy that is the chief responsibility of other sectors, such as social services, education, and justice, is known to have a major impact on health status through SDHs. At a local practice level, it is critical for nurses to understand the impact that SDHs have on the individuals and groups they care for and to integrate these factors in plans of care.

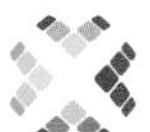

Case Illustration

Erin Walzak must have a strong knowledge and understanding of the SDHs to be able to educate her director and hopefully influence the director's position on Erin's strategies. One tool Erin could use to help prepare her for the discussion with her director is the Canadian Nurses Association (2010) Social Justice Gauge at https://www.cna-aiic.ca/on-the-issues/better-health. The tool will guide Erin through three key questions about the policy issue she is investigating.

SDHs have a significant impact on susceptibility to illness and on how people experience and recover from illness. This information may affect our understanding of a family's support system, intervention selection, and decision making regarding the need for other service resources. At a broader systems level, nurses need to know how the health of their patients can be improved by advancing progressive policies that address SDHs (Canadian Nurses Association, 2015).

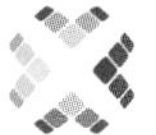

Case Illustration

How might Erin use her knowledge of social justice, SDHs, and health equity to shift her director's position on the matter?

Some suggest that recent approaches to population health have encouraged public health practitioners and policy makers to consider the broader determinants of health as part of a more comprehensive approach to improving health, addressing health inequalities, and accelerating health impact (Dean, Williams, & Fenton, 2013; McPherson, Ndumbe-Eyoh, Betker, Oickle, & Peroff-Johnston, 2016). We could argue that the notion of systematic differences in health has been recognized since at least the 19th century. Our own profession has witnessed early evidence-informed public health action in areas such as public sanitation through nursing pioneers like Florence Nightingale (1820–1910). Lavinia Dock (1858–1956), a feminist, suffragist, and social and union activist, believed that nurses should be politically active, especially regarding Victorian-era social evils such as poverty, malnutrition, housing overcrowding, and health disparities. In the 20th century, links were made between widespread economic inequalities and health inequalities primarily in Europe thanks to the emergence of studies such as the 1977 Black Report (Whitehead, 1998). Since we entered the 21st century, increased attention has been paid to health inequalities with the United Nations' Millennium Development Goals (MDGs) (United Nations, 2000) and the 2008 WHO Commission on Social Determinants of Health. These initiatives are discussed in more detail throughout this chapter.

Different sources cite variations on the actual components of SDHs (McGibbon, 2012). For the purpose of this discussion, the following sections outline a list of 10 determinants compiled from four sources: WHO (Commission on Social Determinants of Health, 2008; World Health Organization, 2017; World Health Organization & Alliance for Health Policy and Systems Research, 2014), the Canadian Nurses Association (2010, 2015), the Public Health Agency of Canada (2015), and the Toronto Charter (Raphael, Brassolotto, & Baldeo, 2014). All lists focus on the WHO (2008) SDH definition outlined in this chapter because they are concerned with the conditions in which people are born, grow, live, work, and age.

Many excellent sources offer a more detailed review of the elements presented later in Table 2-1 (Canadian Nurses Association, 2015; D. Raphael, 2010; Raphael, 2016; World Health Organization, 2017). Each element is briefly described here, and the discussion is adapted from Table 2-2 in McGibbon and Etowa (2009) and Canadian Nurses Association (2015).

Early Childhood Development

This determinant includes elements such as a nurturing and abuse-free environment, financial and geographic access to appropriate child-care support, and access to early childhood education. Substantial evidence indicates that these factors have a great impact on health outcomes in the early years. When families have enough annual income to provide quality child care and opportunities for community participation, children have much better health and social outcomes (Ryan, Johnson, Rigby, & Brooks-Gunn, 2002; Chung et al., 2016). A notable mismatch exists between the proven opportunities provided by early childhood education and public investment in these programs (McPherson, Popp, & Lindstrom, 2006; Campbell et al., 2014).

Education

This category includes access to culturally appropriate education throughout the life course and opportunities for postsecondary education. Recent reports continue to highlight the growing unaffordability of higher education for North American students (Canadian Federation of Students, 2013; Poutré, Rorison, & Voight, 2017). This situation is of great concern because we know that education is linked to health and well-being.

Employment and Working Conditions

This determinant includes issues such as meaningful employment, work safety, dependable and consistent full-time work, and workplaces that provide strong health and social benefits. The lack of meaningful employment is linked to health and health disparities for individuals, communities, and societies. We know that key positive and negative exposures can generate health disparities among the employed. These include psychosocial factors, such as the benefits of a high-status job or the burden of perceived job insecurity, and physical exposures to dangerous working conditions, such as asbestos or rotating shift work (Burgard & Lin, 2013). Continued empirical research is needed to examine the impact of unemployment and precarious employment on individual health outcomes. However, most studies support the proposition that higher socioeconomic positions and thus better working conditions are generally beneficial to health (Benach, Vives, Tarafa, Delclos, & Muntaner, 2016; Vancea & Utzet, 2017).

Food Security

Food security is defined as "a situation in which all community residents obtain a safe, culturally acceptable, nutritionally adequate diet through a sustainable food system that maximizes community self-reliance and social justice" (Hamm & Bellows, 2003, p. 37). Community food security is a fundamental component of enabling people and communities to enjoy health and well-being, and includes availability, consumption, source, quality, and cost dimensions of nutritious food, among other factors (Haering & Syed, 2009).

Health-Care Services and Access

This social determinant of health includes elements such as culturally safe access to community-based collaborative primary health-care teams and specialist services. Access to comprehensive, high-quality health-care services is critical for promoting and maintaining health, preventing and managing disease, reducing unnecessary disability and premature death, and achieving health equity (Office of Disease Prevention and Health Promotion, 2017a). Although health care is essential to health, research demonstrates that it is a relatively weak health determinant (Marmot et al., 2008). Improving population health and achieving health equity require broader approaches that address social, economic, and environmental factors that influence health. For example, people living in rural areas have less access to health services and subsequently tend to have poorer health than those who live in urban areas (Douthit, Kiv, Dwolatzky, & Biswas, 2015; McGibbon & Etowa, 2009).

Housing Security

This determinant includes a consistent, stable, safe shelter and green space for play. As more North Americans spend an increasingly higher proportion of their income on shelter, housing security is threatened. Millions of people develop chronic diseases such as asthma or die annually due to largely preventable environmental risks; eliminating such risks as a leading cause of chronic disease is a major public health concern (Centers for Disease Control and Prevention, 2017). Calls to address children's environmental health over the past decade have been gaining momentum because more is known about how adverse environments, such as exposure to household lead paint, can put children's growth, development, well-being, and very survival at risk (Drisse & Goldizen, 2017; World Health Organization, 2010).

Equitable Distribution of Income

This term refers to annual income that is adequate for an individual, family, or community to meet basic needs. A body of evidence strongly suggests that income inequality affects population health and well-being. Further, the evidence that large income differences, or disparities, have damaging health and social consequences is strong, and in most countries, inequality is increasing. It is well established that narrowing the gap between the rich and the poor will improve the health and well-being of populations (Pickett & Wilkinson, 2015).

Self-Determination

Self-determination is the right of all to determine their own economic, social, and cultural development. Although this determinant applies to all, it is especially relevant to consider and understand historically marginalized populations such as indigenous peoples. For example, the right of self-determination is a fundamental principle enshrined in international law and is a basic expectation that indigenous peoples have of their governments. By virtue of that right, they freely determine their political status and freely pursue their economic, social, and cultural development (International Work Group for Indigenous Affairs, 2017). Given how the interplay of racism, paternalism, and disempowerment have inflicted a serious toll in terms of social, health, economic, and cultural costs (Ladner, 2009), self-determination must be a key SDH consideration in public health and health promotion practice with indigenous communities as well as other marginalized populations.

Social Exclusion and Social Inclusion

This determinant considers issues such as access to social supports and community participation. Groups experiencing social exclusion tend to sustain higher health risks and have lower health status. These groups include indigenous peoples, immigrants, refugees, people of color, people with disabilities, single parents, children, youth in disadvantaged circumstances, women, elderly people, unpaid caregivers, gays, lesbians, bisexuals, and transgendered people (Galabuzi, 2009). We sometimes see this determinant of health explained only in terms of social inclusion. However, using a health equity and social justice lens means that it is important to name exclusion because it is linked to societal discrimination (Canadian Nurses Association, 2015).

Social Safety Nets

This term refers to a range of government-provided benefits, programs, and supports that protect a nation's citizens during life changes that affect their health and well-being. These changes include routine life transitions such as having and raising children, seeking housing, or entering or retiring from the labor force, as well as unexpected life events, such as being involved in an accident, experiencing family breakups, becoming unemployed, and developing a physical or mental illness or disability. These events threaten health by substantially increasing economic insecurity. If there are no effective social safety nets in place to mitigate the increased economic insecurity, significant psychological and physiological stress can develop (McGibbon, Waldron, & Jackson, 2013). Ensuring that social safety nets and supports are in place can increase the resilience of communities to economic shock and mitigate the mental health impacts of fear of job loss, unemployment, loss of social status, and the stress-related consequences of economic downturns (Stuckler, Basu, Suhrcke, Coutts, & McKee, 2009).

Health Inequality and Health Inequity

Two other concepts integral to this discussion are health inequality and health inequity. Health inequality, a term sometimes used interchangeably with health disparities, refers to measurable differences in health between individuals, groups, or communities (National Collaborating Centre for Determinants of Health, 2017). Absent from this definition of health inequality is moral judgment regarding whether observed differences are fair or just (Arcaya, Arcaya, & Subramanian, 2015).

Health inequity is a subset of health inequality and refers to differences in health associated with social disadvantages that are modifiable and thus considered unfair. Health equity means that all people (individuals, groups, and communities) have a fair chance to reach their full health potential and are not disadvantaged by social, economic, and environmental conditions (National Collaborating Centre for Determinants of Health, 2017). Thus, health inequity points to *unjust* differences in health. Whitehead (1992) has long since argued that when health differences are preventable and unnecessary, allowing them to persist is unjust. The key distinction between the terms *inequality* and *inequity* is that "the former is simply a dimensional description employed whenever quantities are unequal, while the latter requires passing a moral judgment that the inequality is wrong" (Arcaya et al., 2015).

Some authors distinguish between unavoidable health inequalities and unjust and preventable health inequities. For example, the term *health inequality* can be used to describe the differences (or disparities) in 2011–2013 infant mortality rates in Wisconsin for non-Hispanic black (14.0) and non-Hispanic white (5.0) infants (Henry J. Kaiser Family Foundation, 2017). In Canada, the First Nations infant mortality rate reported in 2010 remains twice as high as the rest of the country, and for Inuit infants, the rate is four times higher (Smylie, Fell, Ohlsson, & Joint, 2010).

We can also discuss these differences as health inequities because the root of the disparity is along racial and ethnic lines. The United States–based infant mortality disparities are partially attributable to preventable differences in education and access to health and prenatal care (Centers for Disease Control and Prevention, 2011). Although some First Nations' reserves have physicians and good-quality health services for mothers and babies, many others are plagued by inadequate housing, poor food quality, and contaminated water supplies, among other primarily socially determined issues (Douglas, 2013; National Collaborating Centre for Aboriginal Health, 2010; Richmond & Cook, 2016). Research also shows that health inequities are prevalent among indigenous people worldwide (Hunt, 2015). Such inequities in health outcomes are avoidable; they can be prevented or at least ameliorated with policies and programs that improve appropriate access to the goods and services necessary for health.

Along this same line of argument, evidence suggests that poor and minority children in the United States are less likely to wear a bike helmet than white children in higher-income families (Gulack et al., 2015). Children on Medicaid had 67% lower odds of helmet use than children with private health insurance, suggesting that poor children who actually had access to a bike are more likely to skip the helmet. This example connects income, race, and inequities in health outcomes and in this case traumatic brain and bodily injuries.

An example of an unavoidable health inequality is the fact that people in their 20s typically enjoy better health than those in their 60s (Arcaya et al., 2015). Health differences based on age are generally seen as largely unavoidable and as such are inequalities but not inequities. When health differences are observed, a primary question of interest is whether the inequality in question is also inequitable.

Health inequalities remain persistent and in some instances are increasing within and between countries despite action to reduce them. Experts in the field have been warning for over 15 years that this situation is often due to deeply embedded structural barriers to change (Kickbusch, 2003; McPherson et al., 2016; Raphael, 2010). For example, data from low- and middle-income countries show that inequalities persist for reproductive, maternal, newborn, and child health despite having narrowed over the past decade. In a review of the health inequality concept, Arcaya and colleagues (2015) reported that striking differences in health still exist among and within countries today:

> . . . [I]n 2010, for example, Haitian men had a healthy life expectancy of 27.8 years, while men in Japan could expect 70.6 years, over twice as long, in full health. Social group differences within countries are also often substantial. In India, for example, individuals from the poorest quintile of families are 86% more likely to die than are those from the wealthiest fifth of families, even after accounting for the influence of age, gender, and other factors likely to influence the risk of death. (p. 1)

Action through equity-oriented policies, programs, and practices is needed to ameliorate this global state of inequality (World Health Organization, 2015, 2017). A well-known position is that political attention to health inequalities is more likely when the political left is in power (Whitehead, 1998). Economic concerns may also move a country to action because there is a growing realization that health inequalities have considerable economic impacts when left unresolved (Mackenbach, Meerding, & Kunst, 2011). Beyond the economic imperative, health inequities raise moral questions of justice and fairness; they are an ethical concern and a human rights issue (McPherson, 2012).

Social justice refers to "the fair distribution of society's benefits, responsibilities, and their consequences" (Canadian Nurses Association, 2010, p. 10). In addition to the concept of fairness, social justice focuses on the advantage that some groups or individuals have relative to others, the need to understand root causes of inequities, and the need to take responsible action to eliminate inequities (p. 13). The Canadian Nurses Association social justice policy discussion paper presents a Social Justice Gauge designed to spark discussion and to support the development of more equitable programs, policies, and products.

A chief purpose of this chapter is to encourage reflection about which conditions make health inequalities unjust and about the merits of nursing practice focusing on targeting policies and practices that prioritize the elimination of health disparities compared to those that focus on raising the overall standard of health in a population.

BOX 2-1 The Canadian Nurses Association SDH e-Learning Course

In 2015, the Canadian Nurses Association (CNA) released a social determinants of health e-learning course that is freely available to the public online. Developed by Dr. Charmaine McPherson, Dr. Elizabeth McGibbon, and Joyce Douglas with the support of CNA staff, the open-access, self-paced course consists of four interconnected modules that consider concepts such as SDHs, health equity, and social justice in application to nursing practice. This resource is intended as an introduction for nurses practicing in any context, and it is a good starting resource for any professional nurse, regardless of level of educational preparation and role. Walking through the course modules will provide you with additional opportunities for in-depth nursing practice reflection.

Source: https://www.cna-aiic.ca/en/on-the-issues/better-health/social-determinants-of-health/social-determinants-of-health-e-learning-course.

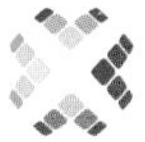

Case Illustration

Once Erin has her director's support, she should consider these factors in preparing for her first cross-sectoral meeting of public health services branch of the provincial health authority, municipal government, and the provincial department of community services. To prepare for the first meeting, Erin may consider completing the Canadian Nurses Association SDH e-Learning course so that she can bring her knowledge of SDHs and health equity to the discussion (Box 2-1).

BRIEF HISTORY OF SDHS

The SDH concept has been around for a long time (Labonté, 1986), but we have only just begun to embrace this idea in the health sector over the past 20 years. Raphael (2009) traced the history of SDHs as far back as the 19th century when political economist Friedrich Engels and physician and politician Rudolf Virchow both linked social conditions and health. The social dimensions of health were strongly affirmed in the original World Health Organization (1946) constitution. However, the ensuing technology-based era that affected all of health care, including public health, diverted global attention from the connection between SDHs and health outcomes for decades.

The 1978 Alma-Ata conference on Primary Health Care, co-organized by WHO and UNICEF, created a new focal point for SDH consideration in the *Health for All* movement and conversations linking health promotion, comprehensive primary health care, and cross-sectoral action on SDH (Rootman, Dupéré, Pederson, & O'Neill, 2012). There were some early successes reported in low-income countries during that time (Irwin & Scali, 2005). However, a subsequent shift toward cost-cutting primary health-care interventions by global agencies (e.g., UNICEF's growth monitoring, oral rehydration, breastfeeding and immunization [GOBI] strategy) downplayed the social dimension in what became known as *selective primary health care*, which minimized the broader social change ambitions of the original vision by emphasizing responses to diseases and narrowly defined health outcomes at the expense of preventive and promotive actions (Baum, Freeman,

Lawless, Labonte, & Sanders, 2017; Solar & Irwin, 2006; Walsh & Warren, 1979).

More recently, significant contributions to the field have been made by Canadian politicians (Epp, 1986; Lalonde, 1974) and British politicians and researchers (Wilkinson & Marmot, 1998). Blane, Brunner and Wilkinson (1996) are credited with coining the term *social determinants of health* and thus expanding the environmental determinants of health outlined in the earlier Lalonde report.

During the 1990s, we gained a better scientific understanding of SDHs, and in the late 1990s, several countries, particularly in Europe, began to design and implement innovative health policies to improve health and reduce health inequalities through action on SDHs. Some programs embraced redistributive principles, while others were more palliative, protecting vulnerable groups against SDH-related exposures (Solar & Irwin, 2010).

Global attention was again drawn to SDHs by the WHO Commission on Social Determinants of Health (CSDH) (2008). To support the work of the commission, the WHO Secretariat examined the history, successes, and failures on SDH action. Its report noted:

> Like other aspects of comprehensive primary health care, action on determinants was weakened by the neoliberal economic and political consensus dominant in the 1980s and beyond, with its focus on privatization, deregulation, shrinking states and freeing markets. Under the prolonged ascendancy of variants of neoliberalism, state-led action to improve health by addressing underlying social inequities appeared unfeasible in many contexts. (Irwin & Scali, 2005, p. 44)

The 21st century has seen incredible global growth in the recognition of the social roots of health outcomes. This acknowledgment was evident in the adoption of the MDGs (United Nations, 2000) by 189 countries at the United Nations Millennium Summit in 2000. These MDGs targeted many SDHs and called for cross-sectoral action on issues such as poverty and hunger reduction, women's empowerment, maternal health, child health, and environmental protection. In September 2015, UN member nations adopted a set of 17 sustainable development goals (SDGs) to end poverty, protect the planet, and ensure prosperity for all as part of a new 15-year sustainable development agenda.

Today, the existence and deep impact of SDHs are generally accepted globally. However, even powerful countries such as Canada, Australia, and the United States struggle with truly embedding an SDH approach in country- and local-level health and public system ideology, policies, and programs (Baum et al., 2017; Office of Disease Prevention and Health Promotion, 2017b; Public Health Agency of Canada, 2015). Deciding how best to act on SDHs and health inequities at national, regional, and local practice levels should be a policy, practice, and research priority that raises deep ethical and political contextual questions (McPherson et al., 2016).

CURRENT THEORIES AND RELATED EVIDENCE

Many frameworks exist for understanding the social determinants of health as a guide for health promotion. International health agendas have historically shifted between a focus on technology-based medical care and public health interventions, and an understanding of health as a social phenomenon that requires more complex forms of cross-sectoral policy action. A chief purpose of the WHO's CSDH was to revive the latter understanding and thus reinvigorate WHO's constitutional commitment to health equity and social justice (Solar & Irwin, 2010).

Framing health as a social phenomenon highlights the association with health equity—the absence of unfair and unavoidable or remediable differences in health among social groups (Solar & Irwin, 2010)—and the search for social justice. This social and equity frame points to the use of human rights frameworks to broker health equity for individuals and social groups (McPherson, 2012).

The authors of the theoretical framework supporting WHO's CSDH examined theories on the social production of health and disease. Table 2-1 summarizes key aspects of the theoretical underpinnings framing SDHs.

In developing the theoretical framework used by the CSDH, Solar and Irwin (2010) considered three main theoretical explanations, which they viewed as not mutually exclusive. Each theoretical approach is examined here in brief:

1. Psychosocial approaches: The primary emphasis is on psychosocial factors. Stress from the social environment alters a person's susceptibility, which affects neuroendocrine function and can thus make the person more vulnerable to disease. These approaches include the notion that living in social settings of inequality forces people constantly to compare their status, possessions, and life circumstances with those of others, engendering feelings of shame and worthlessness in the disadvantaged along with chronic stress that undermines health (p. 15–17).

Table 2-1 Theoretical Underpinnings of Social Determinants of Health Concept

1. Three Main Theoretical Explanations (Not Mutually Exclusive)	2. Three Pathways and Mechanisms to Explain Causation (Social Position)	3. Diderichsen's Model: The Mechanisms of Health Inequality (1998)	4. Social Position
Psychosocial approaches	Social selection or social mobility	Social contexts	Central role of power in understanding social pathways and mechanisms
Social production of disease/political economy of health	Social causation	Social stratification → differential exposure → differential vulnerability	Distinction between the social *causes* of health and the social *factors determining the distribution* of these causes
Ecosocial frameworks	Life-span perspectives	Differential consequences	

Source: Solar, O., & Irwin, A. (2010). *A conceptual framework for action on the social determinants of health. Social Determinants of Health Discussion Paper 2 (Policy and Practice).*

2. Social production of disease/political economy of health: This approach explicitly addresses economic and political determinants of health. Interpretation of the links between income inequality and health must begin with the structural causes of inequities and not just focus on the perceptions of that inequality. The effect of income inequality on health is related to both lack of resources and systematic underinvestment across community infrastructure (p. 17).
3. Ecosocial frameworks: Multilevel frameworks integrating social and biological factors and a dynamic historical and ecological perspective seek to analyze current and changing population patterns of health, disease, and well-being in relation to these multiple levels. These frameworks assume that no aspect of our biology can be divorced from knowledge of history and individual and societal ways of living (p. 18).

Integral to the CSDH theoretical framework is that each of these theories and associated pathways and mechanisms strongly emphasizes the concept of social position, which plays a central role in the social determinants of health inequities. Solar and Irwin (2010) highlighted Diderichsen's (1998) model of the mechanisms of health inequality to explain how differences in social position account for health inequities. Diderichsen considered how the following mechanisms stratify health outcomes:

- Social contexts, including the ways that societal structure creates stratification, assign individuals to different social positions.
- Social stratification engenders differential exposure to health-damaging conditions and differential vulnerability in terms of health conditions and material resource availability.
- Social stratification also determines differential consequences of ill health for different social levels, including economic and social consequences as well as differential health outcomes.

Solar and Irwin (2010) also explained that the role of social position in generating health inequities necessitates an understanding of the central role of power in alleviating social determinants of health; they noted that it's a "political process that engages both the agency of disadvantaged communities and the responsibility of the state" (p. 5). The authors caution that conflating the social determinants of health and the social processes that shape the unequal distribution of these determinants can seriously mislead policy. For example, social and economic policies associated with educational attainment, a positive aggregate trend in a health-determining social factor, have also been associated with persistent inequalities in the distribution of this factor across population groups. Policy objectives are defined quite differently depending on whether the aim is to address determinants of health or determinants of health inequities (Solar & Irwin, 2010).

CONNECTING SOCIAL DETERMINANTS OF HEALTH WITH SOCIAL JUSTICE

The connection between social justice and SDHs has been a focus in nursing professional literature for some time (McGibbon, Etowa, & McPherson, 2008). Notions of justice and social justice have long been embedded as values in the nursing profession. Indeed, our nursing code of ethics guides us to equity and fairness. Professional and regulatory nursing organizations have developed position statements on the role of social justice in our practice (ANA Center for Ethics and Human Rights, 2016; Canadian Nurses Association, 2010). Individual nurses and the nursing profession overall need to be concerned about human rights and achieving societal equity and equality; nurses must be key contributors and essential partners in formulating and implementing public policy, systems design, and service delivery (International Council of Nurses, 2015). Nursing leaders must contribute to the advancement of global health and equity. The Commission on Social Determinants of Health (2008) from WHO argued that:

> Social justice is a matter of life and death. It affects the way people live, their consequent chance of illness, and their risk of premature death. We watch in wonder as life expectancy and good health continue to increase in parts of the world and in alarm as they fail to improve in others . . . within countries there are dramatic differences in health that are closely linked with degrees of social disadvantage. Differences of this magnitude, within and between countries, simply should never happen. (p. 3)

A girl born today can expect to live more than 80 years in some countries and fewer than 45 years in others (Commission on Social Determinants of Health, 2008). "These inequalities in health, avoidable health inequalities, arise because of the circumstances in which people grow, live, work, and age, and the systems put in place to deal with illness. The conditions in which people live and die are, in turn, shaped by political, social, and economic forces" (Commission on Social Determinants of Health, 2008, p. iii).

The nursing profession should be concerned with SDHs if we hope to lead in health promotion and to prevent chronic disease and unnecessary death. SDHs and the associated underlying pathways and mechanisms are often at the root of health inequities, connecting diminishing health status to a social gradient in health (Marmot et al., 2008). SDHs also intersect to deepen disadvantage and/or increase advantage (McGibbon, 2012; McGibbon & McPherson, 2011; McPherson & McGibbon, 2010, 2014). Some experts argue that there are particular prerequisites or antecedents for health, often provided for (or not) in the form of health-promoting public policy (Kickbusch & Cassar Szabo, 2014). A deep understanding of SDHs and their link to innovation in healthy public policy is clearly necessary for advanced practice nursing to engage in this space in the health promotion policy field.

Discussion in the nursing profession questions how we can learn about and enact social justice (Fahrenwald, Taylor, Kneipp, & Canales, 2007; Paquin, 2011) and in public health nursing practice, in particular (McPherson et al., 2016). Remarkably, deliberate connections between social justice and health equity in the nursing literature are mainly addressed in discussion type or concept analysis papers (Braveman et al., 2011; Buettner-Schmidt & Lobo, 2012; Roush, 2011) rather than with empirical research (McPherson et al., 2016), and little discussion exists in advanced practice nursing fields (Phillips & Malone, 2014). Public health nursing literature has discussed the notion of the waning and resurgence of social justice in practice (Drevdahl, Kneipp, Canales, & Dorcy, 2011), arguing that nurses' work as social activists has largely diminished over the past century. Some argue that we need more clarity in terms of how to translate and integrate social activism into practice, especially in advanced practice situations (Bell & Hulbert, 2008; Browne & Tarlier, 2008; McPherson et al., 2016), and we continue to examine how best to teach and learn the concept of social justice (Vliem, 2015). Nevertheless, we continue to call for action around social justice (Yanicki, Kuschner, Kaysi, & Reutter, 2015).

Anderson and colleagues (2009) argued that the concept of critical social justice is a powerful ethical lens through which to view inequities in health and in health-care access. They examined the kind of knowledge needed to move toward the ideal of social justice and pointed to strategies for engaging in dialogue about knowledge and actions to promote more equitable health and health care from the local to the global level. To date, social justice action strategies have largely been developed outside the nursing profession by pioneers such as Raphael (2016) and Marmot and colleagues (2008). Understanding and working with SDHs offer nurses a clear and practical way to apply the social and political contexts of people's lives in everyday nursing care. This helps nurses get to the root causes of health inequities, which, in turn, helps nurses determine the best intervention points. Coupling social justice and human rights provides a strong ethical lens through which to view nursing practice.

A recent study of the implementation of SDH public health nursing roles in Ontario, Canada, highlighted many structural reasons why this work is difficult for public health nurses (McPherson et al., 2016). Findings pointed to lack of understanding of the key concepts surrounding health equity and an array of contextual structural barriers to diffusion of health equity and social justice into public health practice as key elements in the difficulty in moving from theory to effective practice. This knowledge-to-action gap to improve health equity has been identified by others (Davison, Ndumbe-Eyoh, & Clement, 2015), as has a call for more robust equity supporting models and frameworks to encourage knowledge uptake and guide health equity practice in public health.

Nursing social justice action in advocating for health equity is highly contextual and politically charged, so understanding our context is critical (International Council of Nurses, 2010). As advanced practice nurses and nursing leaders, do we understand the public policy development and change process? Do we know where we stand politically? Do we have the skill set to engage politically? These are key questions for health policy and system change aimed at health equity.

PICOT QUESTION AND EVIDENCE TABLE

In stating your patient, intervention, control, observation, and time (PICOT) question, consider the client circumstances you see frequently in your practice setting, where understanding and intervening for SDHs could make an important contribution to health equity for some populations. Your work may or may not relate directly to our example PICOT question. However, the importance of understanding and integrating an approach to practice that systematically factors in SDHs, health equity, and social justice cannot be understated. The remainder of this chapter considers a PICOT question related to SDHs. Several ways of examining the evidence related to the questions are presented and discussed.

Poor housing is strongly linked to poor health, but this does not necessarily mean that better housing leads to improved health. We need to consider the degree to which housing improvements may generate improvements in physical and mental health. The association between housing and health is complex (Thomson, Thomas, Sellström, & Petticrew, 2013), and causal relationships can be hidden or otherwise influenced by a host of confounding variables and effect modifiers (Jacobs & Baeder, 2009).

A PICOT question related to this might be:

Is housing improvement a potential health improvement strategy for those living in poverty?

The evidence related to this question was retrieved and synthesized in 2005 by the European Health Evidence Network (HEN) (www.euro.who.int/HEN) (Health Evidence Network, 2005). WHO/Europe started HEN in 2003 in recognition that public health, health care, and health systems policy makers need access to timely, independent, and reliable health information. This network continues to act as a platform, providing evidence in multiple formats to help decision making.

The issue outlined in this PICOT question recognizes the well-established links among poor health, poor housing, and poverty. Because people living in poverty and poor housing are likely touched by several other SDHs, it is safe to say that this question broadly considers those affected by issues related to housing, income, social safety nets, food security, and working conditions, among other SDHs. If we maintain the evidence question on the outlined PICOT, we learn that evidence supports that housing improvements in disadvantaged areas or social housing may provide a population-based strategy to improve health and reduce health inequalities. Housing improvements that reduce exposure to specific hazards have potential to lead to health improvements for current residents and to prevent harmful exposure by future generations.

The evidence outlined in the HEN evidence review (Health Evidence Network, 2005) remains relevant today. Since 2005, several other evidence reviews related to the initial PICOT question have been completed within the WHO European region, representing a refinement of the original question to examine aspects of the original evidence base.

Table 2-2 provides an overview of the systematic review studies resulting from a search on the topic covering the period from 2009 to 2016. The search yielded five systematic reviews, four of which were meta-syntheses. An overview of the five reviews follows, with an emphasis on particular SDHs involved in this housing issue as well as consideration of intervention evidence for some populations differentially affected by housing shortfalls.

Thomson, Thomas, Sellström, and Petticrew (2009) conducted a systematic review of the health impacts of housing improvement. Of the 45 relevant and included studies, evidence supported improvements in general, respiratory, and mental health following warmth improvement measures, but these health improvements varied across studies. Varied health impacts were reported following housing-led neighborhood renewal. Studies from the low- and middle-income countries suggest that provision of basic housing amenities may lead to reduced illness. There were few reports of adverse health impacts following housing improvement. Some studies reported that the housing improvement was associated with positive impacts on socioeconomic determinants of health. These findings have implications for advanced practice nurses in the area of health promotion as they consider appropriate targets for policy levers in housing for health improvement.

Table 2-2 Systematic Reviews Focusing on Health Impacts of Housing Improvement

Reference	Study Purpose	Study Design and Methods	Intervention(s)	Number of Articles Included in Review	Impact of Housing Interventions	Limitations
Thomson et al., 2009	To conduct a systematic review of the health impacts of housing improvement through housing intervention studies from 1887 to 2007	Narrative literature review of meta-analyses of randomized control trials (RCTs), prospective, controlled, and qualitative studies	Warmth improvement measures, housing-led neighborhood renewal, provision of basic housing amenities	45 primary studies	Improvements in general, respiratory and mental health were reported following warmth improvement measures. Varied health impacts were reported following housing-led neighborhood renewal. Studies from low- and middle-income countries suggest that provision of basic housing amenities may lead to reduced illness. Some studies reported that the housing improvement was associated with positive impacts on socioeconomic determinants of health.	Not identified

Table 2-2 Systematic Reviews Focusing on Health Impacts of Housing Improvement—cont'd

Reference	Study Purpose	Study Design and Methods	Intervention(s)	Number of Articles Included in Review	Impact of Housing Interventions	Limitations
Jacobs et al., 2010	To conduct a systematic review to assess the effectiveness of housing interventions on improving health	Expert panel used to review evidence systematically. Initial database search covered the period between 1990 and 2007. Used *Guide to Community Preventive Services* to frame reviews.	Interior biological agents (toxins) interventions, interior chemical agents (toxics) interventions, structural deficiency (injury) interventions, community-level housing interventions	170 studies reviewed	Sufficient evidence now shows that specific housing interventions can improve certain health outcomes in the following areas: • Interior biological agents (toxins) interventions—multifaceted in-home tailored interventions for asthma; cockroach control through integrated pest management; combined elimination of moisture intrusion and leaks and removal of moldy items • Interior chemical agents (toxics) interventions—active radon air mitigation strategies; integrated pest management; smoke-free policies; residential lead hazard controls • Structural deficiency (injury) interventions—installed working smoke detectors; four-sided pool fencing; preset safe temperature hot water heaters • Community-level housing interventions—rental voucher systems	Not identified

(continued)

Table 2-2 Systematic Reviews Focusing on Health Impacts of Housing Improvement—cont'd

Reference	Study Purpose	Study Design and Methods	Intervention(s)	Number of Articles Included in Review	Impact of Housing Interventions	Limitations
Fitzpatrick-Lewis et al., 2011	To identify new research examining interventions to increase access to health and health care for people who are homeless or at risk of homelessness, published since the 2005 systematic review by Hwang et al. (2005), with an additional focus on the effect of these interventions on housing status from January 2004 to December 2009	Rapid systematic review; narrative review using the Effective Public Health Practice Project (EPHPP) tool for assessing methodological quality of primary studies in public health	• Provision of housing at discharge for homeless people with mental illness, or homeless people with substance use issues/ concurrent disorders • Abstinence-dependent housing	84	For homeless people with mental illness, provision of housing at hospital discharge was effective in improving sustained housing. For homeless people with substance abuse issues or concurrent disorders, provision of housing was associated with decreased substance use, fewer relapses from periods of substance abstinence, increased health services utilization, and increased housing tenure. Abstinence-dependent housing was more effective in supporting housing status, substance abstinence, and improved psychiatric outcomes than non-abstinence-dependent housing or no housing. Provision of housing also improved health outcomes among homeless populations with HIV. Integrated models appear to be most effective in achieving and sustaining long-term housing as well as increasing utilization of health-care services for chronically ill homeless populations. These services can range from case management to the provision of meals. There is some evidence that a relatively simple intervention such as rental assistance increases time housed.	No studies were of strong quality, and 10 were rated moderate quality, so weak studies were not discussed in detail.; short time lines determined by contracting agency to conduct review created limitations; for example, grey literature searching was limited in its scope, conference proceedings and trial registers were excluded, and a limited number of relevant Web sites were selected for searching. Authors couldn't be contacted to clarify data and citation tracking for subsequently published studies.

Table 2-2 Systematic Reviews Focusing on Health Impacts of Housing Improvement—cont'd

Reference	Study Purpose	Study Design and Methods	Intervention(s)	Number of Articles Included in Review	Impact of Housing Interventions	Limitations
Gibson et al., 2011	To conduct a systematic overview of systematic reviews of housing and community interventions published and unpublished between 2002 and 2007; sought reviews of housing interventions focused on health outcomes and particularly on health inequalities	Systematic review of systematic reviews; each systematic review was critically appraised using a checklist adapted from the Database of Abstracts of Reviews of Effects (DARE)	The impact of area characteristic. United States: reducing the concentration of poverty by using various means to relocate families living in high-poverty areas to more affluent areas. United Kingdom: area-based urban regeneration); internal housing conditions such as warmth and energy efficiency interventions, housing improvement, refurbishment, or relocation; range of interventions, for example, rehousing, injury prevention and behaviour change interventions.	Five reviews met the criteria for inclusion, containing total of 130 studies of relevance. The number of unique studies is smaller because there was some overlap between the reviews.	Lack of systematic reviews of the health impact of housing interventions aimed at altering housing tenure represents a significant gap in the systematic review evidence based on pathways linking housing and health. Attempting to address area characteristics by moving disadvantaged people to lower-poverty areas appears to have some success in improving health outcomes for those who move, but it does not help to improve conditions in these areas, thus leaving the remaining residents to contend with the existing problems. Warmth and energy efficiency interventions targeted at those in most need deliver at least short-term improvements in health, suggesting that interventions to improve internal housing conditions that are targeted at the most vulnerable individuals within a disadvantaged area may yield the best results. Improved evaluation of area-level interventions may demonstrate that these also have the potential to improve health.	Not clear how data were tabulated and synthesized. Acknowledged loss of detail in the progress of information from primary studies to systematic reviews and then to systematic overview, limited by the level of detail reported in the original reviews; for example, reporting of intervention information is often limited, and few review authors discuss implementation issues.

(continued)

Table 2-2 Systematic Reviews Focusing on Health Impacts of Housing Improvement—cont'd

Reference	Study Purpose	Study Design and Methods	Intervention(s)	Number of Articles Included in Review	Impact of Housing Interventions	Limitations
Thomson et al., 2013	Campbell Collaboration review to assess the health and social impacts on residents following improvements to the physical infrastructure of housing	Narrative literature review of meta-analyses of quantitative studies (RCTs, nonexperimental designs) qualitative, and mixed methods study designs. Hamilton tool used to accommodate nonexperimental and uncontrolled studies. Qualitative data were summarized using a logic model to map reported impacts and links to health impacts; quantitative data were incorporated into the model.	• Warmth improvements • Rehousing or retrofitting • Provision of basic improvements in low- or middle-income countries	39 studies included (33 quantitative, 6 qualitative)	Data from studies of warmth and energy efficiency interventions suggested that improvements in general health, respiratory health, and mental health are possible. Studies targeting those with inadequate warmth and existing chronic respiratory disease were most likely to report health improvement. Impacts following housing-led neighborhood renewal were less clear; these interventions targeted areas rather than individual households in most need. There were few reports of adverse health impacts following housing improvement. A small number of studies gathered data on social and socioeconomic impacts associated with housing improvement. Warmth improvements were associated with increased usable space, increased privacy, and improved social relationships; absences from work or school due to illness were also reduced. Very few studies reported differential impacts relevant to equity issues, and what data were reported were not amenable to synthesis.	Very little quantitative synthesis was possible because the data were not amenable to meta-analysis

In a 2010 study, subject matter experts conducted a systematic review of the evidence on the effectiveness of specific housing interventions in improving health (Jacobs et al., 2010). Panelists reviewed housing interventions associated with exposure to biological and chemical agents, structural injury hazards, and community-level interventions.

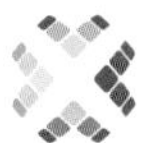

Case Illustration

At Erin's first meeting with her director, the issue of reducing emphasis on winter heating rebates as a cost-saving measure is brought forward by the municipal government and provincial department of community services representatives. The 2010 review found that, although many housing conditions are associated with adverse health outcomes, sufficient evidence shows that specific housing interventions such as warmth interventions can improve certain health outcomes. During Erin's meeting, she will need to inject the known evidence on warmth interventions in housing and the impact on health outcomes into the discussion.

Fitzpatrick-Lewis and colleagues (2011) conducted a rapid systematic literature review to examine research on interventions that have a positive impact on the health and housing status of people who are homeless. This study examined the literature since a previous systematic review by Hwang, Tolomiczenko, Kouyoumdjian, and Garner (2005) and covered the period from January 2004 to December 2009. Evidence indicated that provision of housing at hospital discharge was effective in improving sustained housing for homeless people with mental illness. For homeless people with substance abuse issues or concurrent disorders, provision of housing was associated with decreased substance use, fewer relapses from periods of substance abstinence, increased health services utilization, and increased housing tenure. Abstinence-dependent housing was more effective in supporting housing status, substance abstinence, and improved psychiatric outcomes than non-abstinence-dependent housing or no housing. Provision of housing also improved health outcomes among homeless populations with HIV. Evidence from this review indicated that integrated models appear to be most effective in achieving and sustaining long-term housing, as well as increasing utilization of health-care services for chronically ill homeless populations. These services can range from case management to the provision of meals. Some evidence shows that a relatively simple intervention such as rental assistance increases time housed.

In a systematic overview of systematic reviews, Gibson and colleagues (2011) examined reviews of housing interventions focused on health outcomes and particularly on health inequalities between 2002 and 2007. They only found five reviews that met the inclusion and screening criteria, representing 130 studies (the unique number of studies is smaller because there is some overlap across studies). They reported that attempting to address area characteristics by moving disadvantaged people to lower-poverty areas appears to have some success in improving health outcomes for those who move, but it does not help to improve conditions in these areas, thus leaving the remaining residents to contend with the existing problems. Warmth and energy efficiency interventions targeted at those in most need deliver at least short-term improvements in health, suggesting that interventions to improve internal housing conditions that are targeted at the most vulnerable individuals within a disadvantaged area may yield the best results. They concluded that the lack of systematic reviews of the health impact of housing interventions aimed at altering housing tenure represents a significant gap in the systematic review evidence based on pathways linking housing and health.

Finally, Thomson et al. (2013) completed a meta-synthesis under a Campbell Collaboration review to assess the health and social impacts on residents following improvements to the physical infrastructure of housing. Interventions focused on warmth improvements, rehousing or retrofitting, and provision of basic improvements in low- and middle-income countries. Data from studies of warmth and energy efficiency interventions suggested that improvements in general health, respiratory health, and mental health are possible. Studies targeting those with inadequate warmth and existing chronic respiratory disease were most likely to report health improvement. Warmth improvements were associated with increased usable space, increased privacy, and improved social relationships; absences from work or school due to illness were also reduced. Impacts following housing-led neighborhood renewal were less clear; these interventions targeted areas rather than individual households in most need. There were few reports of adverse health impacts following housing improvement. A small number of studies gathered data on social and socioeconomic impacts associated with housing improvement.

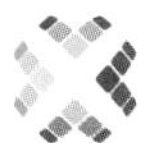

Case Illustration

Throughout Erin's meeting with her director, she will need to bring evidence into the discussion to challenge the policy option dialogue. She will also need to highlight other aspects of housing evidence that should be brought forward for consideration. She will need to pay attention to this evidence vis-à-vis particular populations such as those with mental illness and housing difficulties.

APPLYING THE EVIDENCE IN PRACTICE: ACTION ON SDHS

Leaders in the field (Marmot et al., 2008; Raphael, 2010; Raphael et al., 2014) have argued that addressing SDHs helps us to begin to ameliorate the root causes of health inequities. The WHO CSDH (2008) clarified that policies for health equity involve very different sectors with very different core tasks and scientific traditions. Policies for education, economic growth, immigration, and transportation, for example, are not put in place primarily for health purposes (Solar & Irwin, 2010). This points to the need for complex forms of cross-sectoral action. You can see why global initiatives such as the aforementioned UN MDGs and SDGs are relevant to this discussion. This also explains why the WHO CSDH, with its global network of policy makers, researchers, and civil society organizations, took a cross-sectoral approach to examining the policy-related social causes of poor health and avoidable health disparities and inequities worldwide. The commission ultimately recommended improvements in the conditions of daily life, including tackling the inequitable distribution of power, money, and resources.

Powerful system intervention points are currently underutilized in public health when it comes to action on SDHs. Efforts targeting government policy can have only limited effectiveness if they are aimed at changing relatively weak leverage points, such as those we see with many individual-level interventions. A recent analysis of recommendations from major SDH reports found several major changes over time in the types of recommendations made to ameliorate inequalities in the distribution of SDHs, including a shift toward paradigmatic change and away from individual interventions (Carey & Crammond, 2015). Powerful and effective action on SDHs increasingly targets government action on non-health issues that drive health outcomes, such as sound housing standards and real living wages, education, and transportation infrastructure. The change is targeted at the system level with a public policy goal of equitably distributing SDHs.

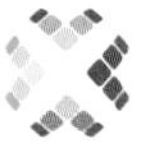

Case Illustration

Advanced practice nurses like Erin working in the health promotion field must connect the elements of social justice, health equity, and public policy to improve health outcomes. The distribution of SDHs is shaped by public policies that reflect the influence of prevailing political ideologies of those governing a jurisdiction (Mikkonen & Raphael, 2010). The political nature of this work must be an explicit part of any strategy to tackle the pathways and mechanisms associated with SDHs and resultant health inequities.

Let us return to the earlier chapter section on "Is housing improvement a potential health improvement strategy for those living in poverty?". Consider how an advanced practice nurse might integrate elements of social justice, health equity, and public policy in a plan to improve health outcomes of those living in poverty and struggling with inadequate housing.

KEY POINTS

- The social determinants of health (SDHs) are a key concept in health promotion that describe the interdependencies between health and social conditions. SDHs have a significant impact on susceptibility to illness and on how people experience and recover from illness.
- Inequalities in the distribution of SDHs are widely recognized as a public policy problem requiring immediate and substantial action.
- Linking the concepts of SDHs, health equity, and social justice is necessary for effective health-promoting public policy or *policy for health*.
- Working toward health equity requires certain antecedents, such as systemwide changes that include cross-sectoral policy designed to promote public health.
- The nursing profession is well positioned to lead interdisciplinary and cross-sectoral dialogue and policy action on these known antecedents to ameliorate health inequities.
- A key difference between traditional models of health promotion that raise the overall health of a population and an SDH approach is that the latter pays attention to the processes by which the social determinants act.

Check Your Understanding

1. A community receives a grant for a health promotion program in a local school. The community health department plans to appoint one representative from its nursing division to serve on the

implementation planning committee. Who is the most appropriate representative?

A. An advanced public health nurse from the health department clinic whose own children attend the school

B. An advanced public health nurse who is the nursing supervisor for the school's geographic area

C. An advanced public health nurse who is a preceptor for nursing students in providing school-based health care

D. The school nurse who is responsible for one census tract in the geographic area

2. The primary role of an advisory board for a community-based health organization is to:

A. Advocate for the community

B. Determine services to be provided

C. Develop policies and regulations

D. Provide funding advice to the health director

3. Which type of power is associated with the role of the advanced public health nurse?

A. Expert

B. Legitimate

C. Referent

D. Reward

4. In planning a telehealth consultation system for a rural community, an advanced public health nurse first focuses on the:

A. Distances between the hub and the spoke servers

B. Needs of the community's residents and providers

C. Number of anticipated contacts per week

D. Sources of funding for capital and operating expenses

5. A grant proposal for a domestic violence prevention program addresses which characteristic of the target population?

A. Current health-care needs

B. Prevalent risk factors

C. Specific health conditions

D. Utilization of health-care service

See "Reflections on Check Your Understanding" at the end of the book for answers.

REFERENCES

ANA Center for Ethics and Human Rights. (2016). *The Nurse's Role in Ethics and Human Rights: Protecting and Promoting Individual Worth, Dignity, and Human Rights in Practice Settings*. Retrieved from http://www.nursingworld.org/MainMenuCategories/EthicsStandards/Resources/Ethics-Position-Statements/NursesRole-EthicsHumanRights-PositionStatement.pdf

Anderson, J., Rodney, P., Reimer-Kirkham, S., Browne, A., Khna, K., & Lynam, M. (2009). Inequities in health and healthcare viewed through the ethical lens of critical social justice: Contextual knowledge for the global priorities ahead. *Advances in Nursing Science, 32*(4), 282–294. doi:10.1097/ANS.0b013e3181bd6955

Arcaya, M. C., Arcaya, A. L., & Subramanian, S. V. (2015). Inequalities in health: Definitions, concepts, and theories. *Global Health Action, 8*(27106), 1–12. doi:doi.org/10.3402/gha.v8.27106

Baum, F., Freeman, T., Lawless, A., Labonte, R., & Sanders, D. (2017). What is the difference between comprehensive and selective primary health care? Evidence from a five-year longitudinal realist case study in South Australia. *BMJ Open*, 7(4), 1–8. doi:10.1136/bmjopen-2016-015271

Bell, S. E., & Hulbert, J. R. (2008). Translating social justice into clinical nurse specialist practice. *Clinical Nurse Specialist, 22*(6), 293–299. doi:10.1097/01NUR.0000325387.22589.d7

Benach, J., Vives, A., Tarafa, G., Delclos, C., & Muntaner, C. (2016). What should we know about precarious employment and health in 2025? Framing the agenda for the next decade of research. *International Journal of Epidemiology, 45*(1), 232–238.

Blane, D., Brunner, E., & Wilkinson, R. (1996). *Health and social organization* (D. Blane, E. Brunner, & R. Wilkinson, Eds.). London, UK: Routledge.

Braveman, P. A., Kumanyika, S., Fielding, J., Laveist, T., Borrell, L. N., Manderscheid, R., et al. (2011). Health disparities and health equity: the issue is justice. *American Journal of Public Health, 101*(S1): S149–S155. doi: 10.2105/ajph.2010.300062

Browne, A. J., & Tarlier, D. S. (2008). Examining the potential of nurse practitioners from a critical social justice perspective. *Nursing Inquiry, 15*(2), 83–93. doi:10.1111/j.1440-1800.2008.00411.x

Buettner-Schmidt, K., & Lobo, M. L. (2012). Social justice: A concept analysis. *Journal of Advanced Nursing, 68*(4), 948–958. doi:10.1111/j.1365-2648.2011.05856.x

Burgard, S., & Lin, K. L. (2013). Bad jobs, bad health? How work and working conditions contribute to health disparities. *American Journal of Behavioral Science, 57*(8), 1105-1127. doi:10.1177/0002764213487347

Campbell, F., Conti, G., Heckman, J. J., Moon, S. H., Pinto, R., Pungello, E., & Pan, Y. (2014). Early childhood investments substantially boost adult health. *Science, 343*(6178), 1478–1485.

Canadian Federation of Students. (2013). Findings in new report point to increasingly unaffordable higher education. Retrieved from https://cfs-fcee.ca/findings-in-new-report-point-to-increasingly-unaffordable-higher-education/

Canadian Nurses Association. (2010). *Social justice: A means to an end . . . an end in itself*. Retrieved from https://www.cna-aiic.ca/~/media/cna/page-content/pdf-en/social_justice_2010_e.pdf

Canadian Nurses Association. (2015). *Online social determinants of health e-learning course*. Retrieved from https://www.cna-aiic.ca/en/on-the-issues/better-health

/social-determinants-of-health/social-determinants-of-health-e-learning-course

Carey, G., & Crammond, B. (2015). Systems change for the social determinants of health. *BMC Public Health, 15*, 662–672. doi:10.1186/s12889-015-1979-8

Centers for Disease Control and Prevention. (2011). CDC health disparities and inequalities report United States. *Morbidity and Mortality Weekly Report, 60*, 49–51.

Centers for Disease Control and Prevention. (2017). *Preventing chronic disease: Eliminating the leading preventable causes of premature death and disability in the United States*. Retrieved from https://www.cdc.gov/chronicdisease/pdf/preventing-chronic-disease-508.pdf

Chung, E. K., Siegel, B. S., Garg, A., Conroy, K., Gross, R. S., Long, D. A., . . . Yin, H. S. (2016). Screening for social determinants of health among children and families living in poverty: A guide for clinicians. *Current Problems in Pediatric and Adolescent Health Care, 46*(5), 135–153.

Commission on Social Determinants of Health. (2008). *Closing the gap in a generation: Health equity through action on the social determinants of health*. Retrieved from http://www.who.int/social_determinants/thecommission/finalreport/en/

Davison, C. M., Ndumbe-Eyoh, S., & Clement, C. (2015). Critical examination of knowledge to action models and implications for promoting health equity. *International Journal for Equity in Health, 14*(49), 1–11. doi:10.1186/s12939-015-0178-7

Dean, D., Williams, K., & Fenton, K. (2013). From theory to action: Applying social determinants of health to public health practice. *Public Health Reports, 128*(Supplement 3), 1–4.

Diderichsen, F. (1998). Understanding Health Equity in Populations—Some Theoretical and Methodological Considerations. In *Promoting Research on Inequality in Health*. Stockholm: Swedish Council for Social Research.

Douglas, V. (2013). *Introduction to aboriginal health and health care in Canada: Bridging health and healing*. New York, NY: Springer Publishing Company.

Douthit, N., Kiv, S., Dwolatzky, T., & Biswas, S. (2015). Exposing some important barriers to health care access in the rural USA. *Public Health, 129*(6), 611–620.

Drevdahl, D., Kneipp, S. M., Canales, M. K., & Dorcy, K. S. (2011). Reinvesting in social justice: A capital idea for public health nursing. *Advances in Nursing Science, 24*(2), 19–31.

Drisse, M. N., & Goldizen, F. (2017). Inheriting a sustainable world? Atlas on children's health and the enviroment. Retrieved from https://www.who.int/ceh/publications/inheriting-a-sustainable-world/en/

Epp, J. (1986). *Achieving health for all: A framework for health promotion*. Ottawa, ON: Government of Canada.

Fahrenwald, N. L., Taylor, J. Y., Kneipp, S. M., & Canales, M. K. (2007). Academic freedom and academic duty to teach social justice: A perspective and pedagogy for public health nursing faculty. *Public Health Nursing, 24*(2), 190–197. doi:10.1111/j.1525-1446.2007.00624.x

Fitzpatrick-Lewis, D., Ganann, R., Krishnaratne, S., Ciliska, D., Kouyoumdjian, F., & Hwang, S. (2011). Effectiveness of interventions to improve the health and housing status of homeless people: A rapid systematic review. *BMC Public Health, 11*. doi:https://doi.org/10.1186/1471-2458-11-638

Galabuzi, G. E. (2009). Social exclusion. In L. S. G. E. G. M. A. Wallis (Ed.), *Colonialism and Racism in Canada: Historical Traces and Contemporary Issues*. Toronto, ON: Nelson Education.

Gibson, M., Petticrew, M., Bambra, C., Sowden, A., Wright, K., & Whitehead, M. (2011). Housing and health inequaities: A synthesis of systematic reviews of interventions aimed at different pathways linking housing and health. *House & Place, 17*(1), 175–184. doi:https://doi.org/10.1016/j.healthplace.2010.09.011

Gulack, B. C., Englum, B. R., Rialon, K. L., Talbot, L. J., Keenan, J. E., Rice, H. E., . . . Adibe, O. O. (2015). Inequalities in the use of helmets by race and payer status among pediatric cyclists. *Surgery, 158*(2), 556–561. doi:https://doi.org/10.1016/j.surg.2015.02.025

Haering, S. A., & Syed, S. B. (2009). *Community food security in United States cities: A survey of the relevant scientific literature*. Retrieved from http://www.jhsph.edu/research/centers-and-institutes/johns-hopkins-center-for-a-livable-future/research/clf_publications/pub_rep_desc/CFS_USA.html

Hamm, M. W., & Bellows, A. C. (2003). Community food security: Background and future directions. *Journal of Nutrition Education and Behaviour, 35*(1), 37–43.

Health Evidence Network. (2005). *Is housing improvement a potential health improvement strategy?* Retrieved from http://www.euro.who.int/__data/assets/pdf_file/0007/74680/E85725.pdf

Henry J. Kaiser Family Foundation. (2017). Infant mortality rate (deaths per 1,000 live births) by race/ethnicity. Retrieved from http://kff.org/other/state-indicator/infant-mortality-rate-by-race-ethnicity/

Hunt, S. (2015). *A review of core competencies for public health: An aboriginal public health perspective*. Retrieved from http://www.nccah-ccnsa.ca/Publications/Lists/Publications/Attachments/145/2015-06-04-RPT-CoreCompentenciesHealth-Hunt-EN-Web.pdf

Hwang, S., Tolomiczenko, G., Kouyoumdjian, F., & Garner, R. (2005). Interventions to improve the health of the homeless: A systematic review. *American Journal of Preventive Medicine, 29*(4), 311. doi:https://doi.org/10.1016/j.amepre.2005.06.017

International Council of Nurses. (2010). *Promoting health: Advocacy guide for health professionals*. Retrieved from http://www.icn.ch/images/stories/documents/publications/free_publications/ICN-NEW-28%203%202010.pdf

International Council of Nurses. (2015). *Our mission, strategic intent, core values and priorities.* Retrieved from http://www.icn.ch/who-we-are/our-mission-strategic-intent-core-values-and-priorities/

International Work Group for Indigenous Affairs. (2017). Self-determination of Indigenous peoples. Retrieved from http://www.iwgia.org/human-rights/self-determination

Irwin, A., & Scali, E. (2005). *Action on the social determinants of health: Learning from previous experiences: A background paper prepared for the Commission on Social Determinants of Health*. Retrieved from http://www.who.int/social_determinants/resources/action_sd.pdf

Jacobs, D., & Baeder, A. (2009). *Housing interventions and health: A review of the evidence*. Retrieved from http://www.nchh.org/LinkClick.aspx?fileticket=2lvaEDNBIdU%3D&tabid=229

Jacobs, D., Brown, M., Baeder, A., Sucosky, J., Scalia, M., Margolis, S., . . . Morley, R. (2010). A systematic review of housing interventions and health: Introduction, methods and summary findings. *Journal of Public Health Management & Practice, 16*(5), S5–S10. doi:10.1097/PHH.0b013e3181e31d09

Kickbusch, I. (2003). The contribution of the World Health Organization to a new public health and health promotion. *American Journal of Public Health, 93*(3), 383.

Kickbusch, I., & Cassar Szabo, M. (2014). A new governance space for health. *Global Action Health*, 7, 1–7. doi:10.3402/gha.v7.23507

Labonté, R. (1986). Social inequality and healthy public policy. *Health Promotion, 1*(3), 341–351.

Ladner, K. (2009). Understanding the impact of self-determination on communities in crisis. *Journal of Aboriginal Health, 5*(2), 88–101.

Lalonde, M. (1974). *A new perspective on the health of Canadians*. Ottawa, ON: Government of Canada.

Mackenbach, J. P., Meerding, W. J., & Kunst, A. E. (2011). Economic costs of health inequalities in the European Union. *Journal of Epidemiology and Community Health, 65*(5), 412–419.

Marmot, M., Friel, S., Bell, R., Houweling, T. A., & Taylor, S. (2008). Closing the gap in a generation: Health equity through action on the social determinants of health. *Lancet, 372*(9650), 1661–1669.

McGibbon, E. (Ed.) (2012). *Oppression as a determinant of health*. Toronto, ON: Brunswick Books.

McGibbon, E. (2016). Oppressions and access to health care: Deepening the conversation. In D. Raphael (Ed.), *Social determinants of health, Canadian perspectives* (3rd ed., pp. 491–520). Toronto, ON: Canadian Scholars' Press.

McGibbon, E., & Etowa, J. (2009). *Anti-racist health care practice*. Toronto, ON: Canadian Scholars' Press.

McGibbon, E., Etowa, J., & McPherson, C. (2008). Health care as a social determinant of health. *Canadian Nurse, 104*(7), 22–27.

McGibbon, E., & McPherson, C. (2011). Applying intersectionality and complexity theory to address the social determinants of women's health. *Women's Health Urban Life (Special Issue Focusing on Women's Health & Public Policy), 10*(1), 59–86.

McGibbon, E., Waldron, I., & Jackson, J. (2013). The social determinants of cardiovascular disease: Time for a focus on racism. *Diversity and Equality in Health and Care, 10*, 139–142.

McPherson, C. (2012). A rights-based approach to primary health care: Increasing accountability for health inequities within health systems strengthening. In E. McGibbon (Ed.), *Oppression as a determinant of health* (pp. 150–166). Halifax, NS: Fernwood Publishing.

McPherson, C., & McGibbon, E. (2010). Addressing the determinants of child mental health: Intersectionality as a guide to primary health care renewal. *Canadian Journal of Nursing Research, 42*(3), 50–64.

McPherson, C., & McGibbon, E. (2014). Intersecting contexts of oppression within complex public systems: A criminal justice application. In A. P. C. Bartollas (Ed.), *Applying complexity theory: A whole systems approach to criminal justice and social work* (pp. 159–180). Bristol, UK: Policy Press.

McPherson, C., Ndumbe-Eyoh, S., Betker, C., Oickle, D., & Peroff-Johnston, N. (2016). Swimming against the tide: A Canadian qualitative study examining the implementation of a province-wide public health initiative to address health equity. *International Journal for Equity in Health, 15*(1), 129. doi:10.1186/s12939-016-0419-4

McPherson, C., Popp, J., & Lindstrom, R. (2006). Re-examining the paradox of structure: A child health network perspective. *Healthc Pap*, 7(2), 46–52.

Mikkonen, J., & Raphael, D. (2010). *Social determinants of health: The Canadian facts*. Toronto, ON: York University School of Health Policy and Public Management.

National Collaborating Centre for Aboriginal Health. (2010). *Housing as a social determinant of First Nations, Inuit and Métis health*. Retrieved from http://www.nccah-ccnsa.ca/docs/fact%20sheets/social%20determinates/NCCAH_fs_housing_EN.pdf

National Collaborating Centre for Determinant of Health. (2017). Glossary of essential health equity terms. Retrieved from http://nccdh.ca/resources/glossary/

Office of Disease Prevention and Health Promotion. (2017a). Healthy People 2020: Access to health services. Retrieved from https://www.healthypeople.gov/2020/topics-objectives/topic/Access-to-Health-Services

Office of Disease Prevention and Health Promotion. (2017b). Social determinants of health. Retrieved from https://www.healthypeople.gov/2020/topics-objectives/topic/social-determinants-of-health

Paquin, S. (2011). Social justice advocacy in nursing: What is it? How do we get there? *Creative Nursing, 17*(2), 63–67.

Phillips, J. M., & Malone, B. (2014). Increasing racial/ethnic diversity in nursing to reduce health disparities and achieve health equity. *Public Health Rep, 129*(Suppl 2): 45–50. doi:10.1177/00333549141291S209

Pickett, K. E., & Wilkinson, R. G. (2015). *Income inequality and health: A causal review*. Retrieved from http://www.ahrq.gov/professionals/education/curriculum-tools/population-health/pickett.html

Poutré, A., Rorison, J., & Voight, M. (2017). *Limited means, limited options: College remains unaffordable for many Americans*. Retrieved from http://www.ihep.org/sites/default/files/uploads/docs/pubs/limited_means_limited_options_report_final.pdf

Public Health Agency of Canada. (2015). *Rio political declaration on social determinants of health: A snapshot of Canadian actions 2015*.Retrieved from http://www.healthycanadians.gc.ca/publications/science-research-sciences- researches/rio/alt/rio2015-eng.pdf

Raphael, D. (Ed.) (2009). *Social determinants of health: Canadian perspectives* (2nd ed.). Toronto, ON: Canadian Scholars' Press.

Raphael, D. (2010). The health of Canada's children. Part III: Public policy and the social determinants of children's health. *Paediatrics & Child Health, 15*(3), 143–149. doi:PMC2865950

Raphael, D. (Ed.) (2016). *Social determinants of health: Canadian perspectives* (3rd ed.). Toronto, ON: Canadian Scholars' Press.

Raphael, D., Brassolotto, J., & Baldeo, N. (2014). Ideological and organizational components of differing public health strategies for addressing the social determinants of health. *Health Promotion International, 30*(4), 855–867. doi:10.1093/heapro/dau022

Richmond, C. A., & Cook, C. (2016). Creating conditions for Canadian aboriginal health equity: The promise of healthy public policy. *Public Health Reviews, 37*(1), 2.

Rootman, I., Dupéré, S., Pederson, A., & O'Neill, M. (2012). *Health promotion in Canada: critical perspectives on practice* (3rd ed.). Toronto, ON: Canadian Scholars' Press.

Roush, K. (2011). Speaking out on social justice. *American Journal of Nursing, 111*(8), 11.

Ryan, R. M., Johnson, A., Rigby, E., & Brooks-Gunn, J. (2002). The impact of child care subsidy use on child care quality. *Early Child Research Quarterly, 26*(3), 320–331. doi:10.1016/j.ecresq.2010.11.004

Smylie, J., Fell, D., Ohlsson, A., & Joint Working Group on First Nations Indian Inuit., (2010). A review of aboriginal infant mortality rates in Canada: Striking and persistent aboriginal/non-aboriginal inequities. *Canadian Journal of Public Health, 101*(2), 143–148.

Solar, O., & Irwin, A. (2006). Social determinants, political contexts and civil society action: A historical perspective on the Commission on Social Determinants of Health. *Health Promotion Journal of Australia, 17*(3), 180–185.

Solar, O., & Irwin, A. (2010). *A conceptual framework for action on the social determinants of health. Social Determinants of Health Discussion Paper 2 (Policy and Practice).* Retrieved from http://www.who.int/sdhconference/resources/ConceptualframeworkforactiononSDH_eng.pdf

Stuckler, D., Basu, S., Suhrcke, M., Coutts, A., & McKee, M. (2009). The public health effect of economic crises and alternative policy responses in Europe: An empirical analysis. *Lancet, 374*(9686), 315–323. doi:10.1016/S0140-6736(09)61124-7

Thomson, H., Thomas, S., Sellström, E., & Petticrew, W. (2009). The health impacts of housing improvement: A systematic review of intervention studies from 1887 to 2007. *American Journal of Public Health, 99*(Supplement 3), S681–S692. doi:10.2105/AJPH.2008.143909

Thomson, H., Thomas, S., Sellström, E., & Petticrew, W. (2013). *Housing improvements for health and associated socio-economic outcomes: A systematic review.* Retrieved from https://www.campbellcollaboration.org/media/k2/attachments/Thomson_Housing_Improvements_Review.pdf

United Nations. (2000). *Millennium Development Goals.* Retrieved from http://www.un.org/millenniumgoals/

Vancea, M., & Utzet, M. (2017). How unemployment and precarious employment affect the health of young people: A scoping study on social determinants. *Scandinavian Journal of Public Health, 45*(1), 73–84.

Vliem, S. (2015). Nursing students' attitudes toward poverty: Does experiential learning make a difference? *Nursing Education, 40*(6), 308–312. doi:10.1097/NNE.0000000000000168

Walsh, J. A., & Warren, K. S. (1979). Selective primary health care: An interim strategy for disease control in developing countries. *New England Journal of Medicine, 301*(18), 967–974.

Whitehead, M. (1992). The concepts and principles of equity and health. *International Journal of Health Services, 22*(3), 523–524.

Whitehead, M. (1998). Diffusion of ideas on social inequalities in health: A European perspective. *Millbank Quarterly, 76*(3), 469–492.

Wilkinson, R., & Marmot, M. (1998). *Social determinants of health: The solid facts.* Copenhagen, Denmark: WHO Regional Office for Europe. Retrieved from http://apps.who.int/iris/bitstream/10665/108082/1/e59555.pdf

World Health Organization. (1946). Constitution of the World Health Organization. *American Journal of Public Health, 36*(11), 1315–1323.

World Health Organization. (2010). *Healthy environments for healthy children: Key messages for action*. Retrieved from http://www.who.int/ceh/publications/hehc_booklet_en.pdf

World Health Organization. (2015). *State of inequality: Reproductive, maternal, newborn and child health*. Retrieved from http://apps.who.int/iris/bitstream/10665/170970/1/WHO_HIS_HSI_2015.2_eng.pdf?ua=1

World Health Organization. (2017). Social determinants of health. Retrieved from http://www.who.int/social_determinants/en/

World Health Organization & Alliance for Health Policy and Systems Research. (2014). *Building momentum and community: Annual report 2014*. Retrieved from http://www.who.int/alliance-hpsr/resources/alliancehpsr_annualreport2014.pdf?ua=1&ua=1

Yanicki, S., Kuschner, M., Kaysi, E., & Reutter, L. (2015). Social inclusion/exclusion as matters of social (in)justice: A call for nursing action *Nursing Inquiry, 22*(2), 121–133. doi:10.1111/nin.12076

Chapter 3

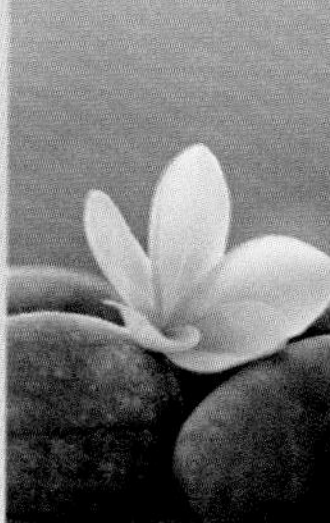

Utilization-Focused Epidemiology (UFE)

Julia A. Bucher

LEARNING OBJECTIVES

After completing this chapter, students will be able to:

1. Define epidemiology.
2. Describe why epidemiology data must be understood according to demographic groups and person, place, and time.
3. Apply utilization-focused evaluation to epidemiologic data.
4. Designate major sources of publicly available epidemiological data.
5. Describe strategies to read and communicate epidemiological data accurately.
6. Interpret confidence intervals to determine statistical differences in data.
7. Identify uses of epidemiology data in health promotion initiatives to reduce health disparities.
8. Apply a modified method of synthetic estimation to plan and evaluate population size for health promotion activities.

INTRODUCTION

Public health nurses and public health/community health nurse educators are the main users of epidemiological data in the nursing profession (Association of Public Health Nurses, 2016). However, other nurses also benefit from knowing how to use this type of data, especially as health-care systems are incentivized to become more involved in and responsible for community health status (Centers for Medicare and Medicaid, 2016). Hospital nurses serve on publicly sponsored collaborative groups that plan, implement, and/or evaluate large-scale health promotion initiatives. Nurses also gather and contribute information to community health assessments, report assessment data from community health assessments generated by outside data consultants, and serve as volunteers or board members in nonprofit organizations involved in health promotion initiatives, such as the American Cancer Society and the American Heart Association.

Epidemiological reports are part of assessment data used to prioritize health promotion initiatives as staff members in health-care systems adopt what is known as a culture of health (Robert Wood Johnson Foundation, 2015). At the very least, as nurses obtain higher educational degrees, epidemiology concepts are embedded in one of the **American Association of Colleges Essentials** (AACN, 2011) indicating that this field is not just the domain of public health nurses.

This chapter introduces the use of epidemiological data as a skill in information literacy. It will describe how volumes of data can be harnessed and abstract epidemiological rates can be changed to actual numbers to estimate the number of people who need to be reached. It will define epidemiology and describe why epidemiology data must be understood according to demographic groups and according to person, place, and time in an approach called utilization-focused epidemiology (UFE). The chapter will designate major sources of publicly available epidemiological data and describe strategies to read and communicate this data accurately and to interpret confidence intervals to determine statistical differences in measures. These information literacy skills can aid health promotion initiatives, and a specific skill will be described that is useful to planning and evaluating health promotion initiatives: a modified method of synthetic estimation to plan and evaluate population sizes needed to reduce health disparities and improve health.

EPIDEMIOLOGY AS A HEALTH SCIENCES FIELD

Epidemiology centers on health statistics about groups or populations. It is defined as "the study (scientific, systematic, and data-driven) of the distribution (frequency, pattern) and determinants (causes, risk factors) of health-related states and events (not just diseases) in specified populations (neighborhood, school, city, state, country, global). It is also the application of this study to the control of health problems" (Centers for Disease Control and Prevention [CDC], 2012).

As a field of study, descriptive epidemiology furnishes assessment data to investigate patterns and causes of disease and injury in humans. Descriptive epidemiological data are derived from surveillance methods: the processes that collect and make data available. Surveillance efforts may be ongoing or episodic. For example, cancer registrars collect and register information on cancers every day across the country. This stream of data is aggregated and organized by state departments of health into reports for public use (Pennsylvania Department of Health, 2015). Infectious disease surveillance, by contrast, may require collection of more in-depth data about locations of problems or transmissions during outbreaks of illnesses such as mumps. These investigations are episodic. Thus, analytical epidemiology contributes inferences about risk factors and causations. Health professionals use both types of reports when seeking to reduce the risk of negative health outcomes through research, community education, and health policy.

Descriptive data are examined first in total numbers, such as all lung cancer deaths in a certain year, but examination according to demographic characteristics reveals a more detailed story about disease or behavior trends (CDC, 2016a, 2016b). Classically, data are sorted by age, sex, race/ethnicity, and socioeconomic and educational status, and this sorting tells us about the persons or population of interest in a geographical location and in a specified time, such as one year, several years, or several years averaged over time. Examining and comparing data according to demographic characteristics can unearth differences in which groups have specific diseases or conditions (or undergo specific events) and reveal patterns or distributions and trends over time and place. Any differences found are referred to as data disparities. For example, when lung cancer mortality rates are compared, older people contract the disease more often than younger people do, and more males than females contract and die from lung cancer (Pennsylvania Department of Health, 2015; U.S. Cancer Statistics Working Group, 2016).

Health professionals and nurses learn the methods of epidemiology in online courses (CDC, 2012), textbooks (Friis & Sellars, 2014; Merrill, 2016), certificate programs, and continuing education courses. However, most of this education concentrates on complex variables and calculations, such as absolute or relative risk ratios and standardized incidence rates. The educational programs also focus on epidemiological study designs to analyze outbreaks or assess major public health problems. Calculations in real life and research studies are conducted by biostatisticians and epidemiologists on government datasets. Many health professionals and nurses do not need to learn these complex skills to discover and use what epidemiological reports reveal. This is where the importance of learning UFE emerges.

The Role of UFE

UFE borrows a term from Patton (2008), who promoted its use. The main purposes of UFE are to locate, read, and understand trends in behavior and disease distribution and communicate these trends so that problems, especially those that are preventable or inequitable in distribution, can be assessed and addressed. Because epidemiologists collect and analyze health data in aggregated forms, they supply information at a higher level than public health/community health nurses and other health promotion planners and evaluators need to understand trends in health statistics in the communities that they serve. Finding, reading, and understanding reports about behavior and disease trends is a high-level information literacy skill. Health professionals who adopt these skills and use epidemiological reports for health promotion and disease prevention efforts can be called consumers of epidemiology; they need to learn less about the specific calculations and study designs used by epidemiologists and more about how to use the information and data. Consumers of epidemiology need to master three main skills of information literacy: locating, reading and understanding, and communicating health statistics data.

Locating Health Statistics Data

Government Web sites such as CDC Wonder (2016) and nonprofit Web sites such as the Kaiser Family Foundation and state hospital associations are usually the best source for trend data and health statistics. These data resources are accessible to the public at no cost and are available on the internet. These Web sites provide updated demographic information and many forms of epidemiological information—both of which are critical to UFE.

The major public database for epidemiology at the national level is the CDC, which lists infectious and chronic disease patterns and trends for the nation and each state. The CDC Web site also posts summary reports and plans to change patterns or trends that are problematic. Particular datasets important to health promotion activities are generated by the Behavioral Risk Factor Surveillance Survey (BRFSS) for the nation and for each state. Adults ages 18 and older receive phone calls and are asked about healthy and unhealthy behaviors as well as if they have been diagnosed with certain conditions, such as hypertension or osteoporosis. They also report if they have a regular source of health care. Healthy People 2020 (HP2020), the U.S.' main health document, sets ideal goals for percentages of these reported behaviors, and state government officials fund action plans to collaborative groups to improve health promotion behaviors and lower risk of disease if possible. HP2020 is also on the CDC Web site, where many disease and behavior trends for each state are compared to the nation's goals.

In addition, the National Health and Nutrition Examination Survey (NHANES), now in its third iteration, presents data obtained through interview and by physical examination. NHANES III data (CDC, 2010) include "demographic, socioeconomic, dietary, and health-related questions as well as medical, dental, and physiological measures and laboratory tests" to determine epidemiological prevalence and trends.

Epidemiological data are often listed with demographic data in easy-to-read state and county health status profiles or county health assessments often available on state department of health Web sites, commonly within Vital Statistics sections. Hospitals and health systems are required to compile community health assessments every three years. These assessments are posted on hospital and health system Web sites in text format for the public that incorporates shorter paragraphs with pie charts or graphs. The assessments include recommended priorities to improve population health.

Another worthwhile Web site to explore for general or specific knowledge is the CMS Community Indicators Web site at http://www.healthindicators.gov/Indicators/Initiative_CMS-Community-Indicators_5/Selection, which presents Medicare data at the levels of the nation, state, county, and hospital referral region. The Healthcare Effectiveness Data and Information Set (HEDIS) is used by a majority of health plans, and its measures and report cards provide information to compare performance across settings and organizations. The HEDIS Web site includes data from the National Committee on Quality Assurance (NCQA), at http://www.ncqa.org/tabid/59/default.aspx, with several roadmaps to help health-care organizations become what are called accountable health communities (Centers for Medicare and Medicaid, 2016). Most large nonprofit health organizations also publish report cards, assessment data, and future goals. Examples include the American Lung Association, which records air quality and posts tobacco cessation resources and improvements in smoke-free air, and the National Alliance for the Mentally Ill, which posts data about severe mental health disorders and data.

Major public databases for demographic data are driven by the U.S. Census. Census data are housed at the census Web site and in the Vital Statistics sections of state government Web sites. In addition, the Kaiser Family Foundation houses census data in general, with particular datasets related to poverty and a link to the American Community Survey, which contains data on population, housing, and work derived from the census.

Reading and Understanding Health Statistics Data

The ability to locate health statistics online is a foundational skill of UFE; understanding what these datasets reveal is the next step. Public databases report epidemiological or demographic data precisely, so providers must read the numbers precisely to understand their meaning.

Terms

Start by understanding the basic language and definitions used in health datasets. The three most commonly reported measures are incidence, prevalence, and mortality data.

- **Incidence:** New cases, numbers, or rates in a specific time period
- **Prevalence:** New cases, numbers, or rates of people living with the disease or condition
- **Mortality:** Death number or rates

Two other common terms are *cases* and *rates*. Cases are actual numbers (or counts) of diseases, conditions, events, or behaviors. Counts (cases) and rates can also be averaged (often over 3 or 5 years), and the titles of tables displayed in reports or documents identify what years are averaged by using a dash between the years.

Rates are calculated with a numerator or denominator. They are not percentages and should not be reported as percentages except in certain cases. An example is a rate of 6.5 for infant mortality, which is infant deaths per 1,000 live births. Biostatisticians and epidemiologists calculate many types of rates. The most useful rates in UFE are age-adjusted rates, which factor population size and likelihood of contracting a disease for each age group (calculated at either 5- or 10-year intervals) into calculations of rates using the number of cases reported for each age group.

- **Cases:** Individual or unique numbers (or counts) in a defined population
- **Rates:** Frequency with which an event occurs in a defined population in a defined time
- **Age-adjusted rates:** Frequency with which an event occurs that can be compared among different event distributions across different age groups

Trends over time

Data consumers must realize that time elapses between data collection, analysis, and publication. Carefully note the years of data collection listed in the titles of tables or charts and narrative reports. Another critical use of data is to observe and compare different years to assess distribution trends or patterns over time. Looking at trends or patterns over years is considered more accurate than snapshots or reports just for one year. This type of data provides more information about progress toward meeting goals or desired direction.

Graphic elements

Tables, graphs, and images are found in summary reports or are posted in health plans for health systems, regions, states, or the nation. These data are accompanied by precise narratives, and authors of these reports and health plans provide text to quote, citations to copy, and statistical inferences about health statistics trends. These data comparisons are about persons, but place and time are also very important and may identify differences or disparities across geographic locations and time spans.

Communicating Health Statistics Data

When reading, summarizing, or paraphrasing data, use the following tips to avoid common mistakes in reporting:

1. Report rates given and do not calculate rates independently.
2. Read table titles closely and report data the way the title presents data, especially the population and years for which the data were collected.
3. Note when a hyphen or dash is placed between years in a table title (or other image) because this represents an average of years. For example, "2003–2005" means that 3 years of data for 2003, 2004, and 2005 were averaged to create the cases, rates, or numbers presented; "2003–2007" means that 5 years of data were averaged to create the cases, rates, or numbers presented.
4. If cases, rates, or numbers are reported, then they will be formally named as such in titles. Sometimes tables are titled with different types of data, so table columns specify the data type.
5. Do not add percentage signs to numbers or counts unless they are used in tables or images and titled as percentages.
6. Read the definition of the data type by checking the technical notes at the end of reports, footnotes, or written passages.
7. If a case, rate, or number is followed by "per" and a population number, then it should be reported this way. Examples are (a rate) per 1,000 live births, a (rate) per 10,000 population, or a (rate) per 100,000 population. When comparing data, compare the same rate derivation.

Communicating statistical significance with confidence intervals

The confidence interval, sometimes called the "uncertainty interval," is abbreviated in many reports and tables as CI. CIs are calculated by statisticians to inform readers about the probability that the sampling rate or statistic contains the population rate or statistic. A CI is defined by the "sample statistic plus or minus the margin of error" (Friis & Sellars, 2014). It contains numbers set within a confidence level of probability such as 90%, 95%, or 99%, and these describe the uncertainty associated with a sampling method. The margin of error "expresses the maximum expected difference between the true population parameter and a sample estimate of that parameter" (Salazar, Crosby, & DiClemente, 2015), and the CI equals the sample statistic plus or minus (±) the margin of error. The interval indicates an upper and lower number that surrounds the true population parameter and not just the sample parameter most of the time. In other words, if the same population is sampled repeatedly and CIs are also calculated, then these intervals surround the true population parameter at the level of confidence set, such as 95% of the time.

Epidemiological data is communicated more precisely when they are taken from written reports that not only present data but also interpret that data, especially when indicating which data trends are statistically significant. In addition to narrative sentences and paragraphs that explain such differences, reports may also portray statistical differences with asterisks directly after numbers or rates that are compared. If CIs do *not* overlap between rates, then an asterisk is placed by the rates or a sentence is written to note that their differences are statistically significant. When CIs do overlap, then numbers or rates are not statistically significant; therefore, no differences are noted, even if the numbers or rates are different from each other in a raw numbers sense. An example of two means with nonoverlapping CIs is:

40.5 (CI 38.2–42.8) and 43.8 (CI 43.0–44.6)

Another, more complex example of a statistically significant difference in two comparisons is noted in Table 3-1.

USE OF EPIDEMIOLOGY DATA IN HEALTH PROMOTION INITIATIVES

Health promotion initiatives aimed at certain populations or communities are planned by collaborative partners after assessing "where we are now." This common phrase in public health circles means that health statistics, community assessments, and data trends are collected, examined, and summarized first before action plans are created. Committee members search library databases to find articles that analyze local or regional health problems. For example, they may examine scholarly manuscripts about what population types "carry the burden" of disease in a state by having the highest rates of diseases or unhealthy behaviors (Easley, Petersen, & Holmes, 2010). After discussion, collaborators choose the most realistic level of prevention to influence either knowledge or behavioral change among population types or systems changes in communities and institutions in the hope of changing health status in the long run (Auerbach, 2013).

Epidemiological data supply important assessment information for discussion and review before evidence-based health promotion activities are planned and implemented. Using this data can reveal the magnitude of a problem so planners can judge whether resources are sufficient for an effective health promotion initiative or if more resources need to be recruited either through proposal writing or staff recruiting. A lesser-known method of UFE is to calculate the population size that must be reached by the initiative to change the health status in the specified community. Turning percentage goals into actual numbers can be accomplished by a simplified version of synthetic estimation (Data Resource Center, 2011; Pickering, Sholes, & Bajekal, 2005) called rates to numbers (Berumen et al., 2002).

Calculating Rates to Numbers in Planning and Evaluation

Health promotion projects often set goals in terms of percentages of people to be reached to improve a health outcome, such as: "Increase the number of women screened for breast cancer by 2% from 2015 to 2020 in Franklin County." Note the use of the word *by*, which implies a percentage increase from a starting number. Another way to state this example is to set a percentage goal: "Increase the percent of women screened for breast cancer in Franklin County from 70% in 2015 to 72% in 2020." Note the word *to*, which implies the end goal. Regardless of how planners and collaborators agree on goals as percentages, they will need to interpret what these percentages mean in *actual numbers* to influence

Table 3-1 Number of Female Breast Cancer Cases, Age-Adjusted Incidence Rates, and 95% Confidence Intervals by Race and Year, Pennsylvania Female Residents

Year	Number	Rate	Confidence Interval (CI)	CI Overlap
2010	10,206	124.9	CI 122.5-127.3	Statistically significant difference in rate/CIs do not overlap
2009	10,421	131.0	CI 128.5-133.5	
2010	10,206	124.9	CI 122.5-127.3	No statistically significant difference in rate/CI overlap
2011	10,561	128.1	CI 125.7-130.5	

Notes: Age-adjusted rates are per 100,000 and are computed by the direct method using the 2000 U.S. standard million population. CI = 95% confidence interval based on a formula for estimating the standard error (SE). Cancer primary site/type groupings follow the definitions used by the National Cancer Institute's Surveillance, Epidemiology, and End Results (SEER) program. Pennsylvania Department of Health. (2015). Pennsylvania Cancer Incidence and Mortality 2013, p. 95.

their activities and help them judge if the resource capacity is in place to carry out these goals.

Demographic data specify the size of the target population for a health promotion or social program. Epidemiological data are then used to estimate the number of this population that currently reports the positive or negative health condition or behavior the planned intervention targets. Next, estimate the size of the population that must change the specified condition or behavior for the project goal to be met. Illustrating these steps reveals the usefulness of size estimates to positive health or social change efforts. In the following example, we calculate the number of adult smokers who must quit within a specific county over a four-year period for a project goal to be met. County data are presented about the size of the county population age 18 years and older; epidemiological data about adults smoking cigarettes are presented from the BRFSS.

> How many adults age 18 or older will need to change their behavior annually over 4 years from 23% adults smoking cigarettes (from 2004 BRFSS data) starting in 2014 to reach 12% of adults smoking cigarettes by 2020 (HP2020 goal)?

County adults 18+ population	10,000
Current smokers (23%) × 10,000 =	2,300 adults
HP2020 goal (12%) × 10,000 =	– 1,200 adults
County annual goal to change	1,100 adults
County annual goal (divide by 4 yrs)	275 adults/year need not to smoke or to stop smoking

The above example demonstrates that an additional 275 adults in the county need to report not smoking cigarettes each year for the county goal to be met by 2020. This does not account for the number that needs to sustain cessation and report not smoking from the previous years.

This modified estimation method has several advantages. First, stakeholders and program leaders are able to understand the size of the population to be reached. Second, an estimate helps stakeholders set common goals among partners and plan the capacity needed for program implementation. Third, output calculations as actual numbers allow project leaders to discuss contributions to HP2020 objectives. For example, if a statewide planning group sets an annual goal of 3,000 women and reaches 2,000 new participants in the National Breast and Cervical Cancer Early Detection Program (NBCCEDP), then they can calculate the percentage of those reached in two ways: what percentage of their own goal did they reach (2,000/3,000, or 67%), or they can calculate and report what percentage they contributed to the numerical goal through their outreach efforts when 10,000 new women needed to be added to the statewide BCCEDP. They added 2,000/10,000, or they made a 20% contribution, to the actual outreach goal. This approach is very useful for both planning and evaluation, and many government-sponsored health promotion proposals require use of this model (Bucher, 2009).

In summary, knowing the actual numerical size implied by goals set by health promotion projects improves the likelihood of buy-in from partners and community members, such as funders and volunteers. Having clear numeric goals also allows periodic formative evaluation that could suggest adjustments to implementation or resource capacity.

In addition, in nursing research terms, this simplified estimation method could be applied to a patient, intervention, control, observation, and time (PICOT) format. For example, related to the above example, a health promotion nurse could ask about the effectiveness (as a percentage of the agreed-upon numerical goal to be reached) of two different methods to inform women of the availability of the National Council of Certified Dementia Practitioners (NCCDP) and enroll them in the health promotion program, which includes a full physical exam, mammogram, cervical exam and Pap smear, and assessment of Medicaid eligibility. The PICOT question would be written this way:

P: new eligible women served by NCCDP
I: those who identified the reason as one-on-one education by health providers
C: those who identified the reason as a statewide public media campaign
O: percentage of annual goal
T: year 2020

KEY POINTS

- Nurses and other health professionals and community health educators can use health statistics from epidemiological databases when they master how to locate, read, understand, and communicate this information to undergird health promotion initiatives.
- The methods of UFE are those of advanced information literacy. These methods provide health statistics that can be used to plan effective health promotion activities and evaluation (Keyes & Galea, 2015). Teaching nurses and graduate students in many fields about how to locate, read, understand, and use data in calculations enhances activities to reduce health disparities and advance health promotion, no matter the stage of disease

or the level of implementation—a goal to which we all aspire.

- These data help professionals understand health status needs and problems in local communities and also identify what types of populations carry the burden of the problem by having the highest rates of diseases or unhealthy behaviors.
- When members of health promotion collaboratives know more about the burden of disease or the unhealthy behaviors of disparate populations, they can focus evidence-based approaches to promote health in a tailored and culturally sensitive fashion.
- Applying modified methods of epidemiological analysis also helps planning and evaluation collaboratives calculate the size of populations who need to change behaviors or health status to meet the actual goals set by health promotion stakeholder partners.
- Both planners and evaluators of health promotion activities can use the skills of UFE to help achieve the goals of health promotion across settings and in all stages of disease.

Check Your Understanding

1. Which three key terms are essential to the definition of epidemiology?
   A. Distribution, population, and health status
   B. Place, location, and time
   C. Descriptive study, analytical study, and inferential statistics
   D. Biostatisticians, public health officials, and disease detectives

2. Which of the following is one practical use of epidemiology data by county public health/community health nurses and other county health officials?
   A. Tracking school enrollments over the last 20 years
   B. Comparing infant mortality rates from 1930 to today for the nation
   C. Calculating how many adults need to stop smoking before a countywide tobacco cessation initiative is planned
   D. Setting goals to reach without assessing current or recent health statistics data

3. New cases of a disease or condition are referred to as:
   A. Incidence data
   B. Prevalence data
   C. Mortality data
   D. Morbidity data

4. Epidemiological rates that can be compared across age groups are called:
   A. Crude rates
   B. Cause-specific rates
   C. Age-specific rates
   D. Age-adjusted rates

5. Which of the following is the major public source of epidemiological data?
   A. County government Web sites
   B. Hospital Web sites
   C. State government Web sites
   D. U.S. Census

6. When reading a title and table of incidence rates, which three characteristics are important to identify?
   A. Number, percentage, and confidence interval
   B. Persons, place, and time
   C. Disease, condition, and time
   D. Location, years, and time

7. Which set of confidence intervals confirms a statistical difference between mortality rates?
   A. 45.5 (CI 42.2–47.8) and 43.5 (CI 40.2–45.5)
   B. 45.5 (CI 42.2–47.8) and 49.5 (CI 48.2–50.8)
   C. 42.2 (CI 38.5–45.9) and 45.2 (44.0–46.4)
   D. 42.2 (CI 40.2–44.4) and 44.1 (CI 42.2–45)

8. What is the formula for the size of the population who needs to change from 15% in 2015 to achieve the HP2020 goal of 25% adults aged 18 years of age or older eating five fruits and vegetables daily in any defined geographic area?
   A. Fifteen percent reporting this healthy behavior in 2015 minus an ideal 25% reporting this healthy behavior in 2018 added to the population size of adults aged 18 years or older for a defined geography
   B. Data are not available for a defined geography to calculate this population size needed to change behavior
   C. The population size of adults aged 18 years or older is multiplied by how many reported eating five fruits and vegetables daily for a defined geography
   D. Twenty-five percent to report this healthy behavior in 2020 minus 15% reporting this healthy behavior in 2015 multiplied by the population size of adults aged 18 years or older for a defined geography

See "Reflections on Check Your Understanding" at the end of the book for answers.

REFERENCES

American Association of Colleges of Nursing. (2011). *The essentials of master's education in nursing*. Washington DC: American Association of Colleges of Nursing.

Association of Public Health Nurses. (2016). *The public health nurse: Necessary partner for the future of healthy communities*. Retrieved from http://www.quadcouncilphn.org/documents-3/2016-the-public-health-nurse-necessary-partner-for-the-future-of-healthy-communities

Auerbach, J. (2016). The three buckets of prevention. *Journal of Public Health Management and Practice, 22*(3), 1–4. doi:10.1097/PHH.0000000000000381

Berumen, A., Black, B., Bucher, J., Cowans, R., Gates, C., Goodman, J., et al. (2002). *Community action planning: A model for cancer control planning: A handbook for American Cancer Society volunteers and staff.* Atlanta, GA: American Cancer Society.

Bucher, J. (2009). Using the logic model for planning and evaluation: Examples for new users. *Home Health Care Management and Practice, 22*(5), 325–333. Retrieved from http://journals.sagepub.com/doi/abs/10.1177/1084822309353154

CDC Wonder. (2016). Health and Nutrition. Retrieved from https://wonder.cdc.gov

Centers for Disease Control and Prevention. (2010). National Center for Health Statistics (NCHS). National Health and Nutrition Examination Survey data. Hyattsville, MD: U.S. Department of Health and Human Services, Centers for Disease Control and Prevention. Retrieved from https://accelerate.ucsf.edu/research/celdac/3748

Centers for Disease Control and Prevention. (2012). *Principles of epidemiology* (3rd ed.). Atlanta GA: Centers for Disease Control and Prevention. Retrieved from https://www.cdc.gov/ophss/csels/dsepd/ss1978/ss1978.pdf

Centers for Disease Control and Prevention. (2016a). Lung Cancer Statistics. Retrieved from https://www.cdc.gov/cancer/lung/statistics/index.htm

Centers for Disease Control and Prevention. (2016b). *1999–2013 Cancer incidence and mortality data.* Retrieved from https://nccd.cdc.gov/uscs

Centers for Medicare and Medicaid. (2016). *Accountable health communities model.* Retrieved from https://innovation.cms.gov/initiatives/ahcn

Data Resource Center. (2011). *Local uses of national and state data*. Retrieved from https://www.childhealthdata.org/docs/nsch-docs/local-use-of-state-data-and-synthetic-estimates.pdf

Easley, C., Petersen, R., & Holmes, M. (2010). The health and economic burden of chronic diseases in North Carolina. *North Carolina Medical Journal, 71*(1), 92–95.

Friis, R. H., & Sellers, T. A. (2014). *Epidemiology for public health practice* (5th ed.). Sudbury, MA: Jones & Bartlett.

Healthy People 2020. Washington, DC: U.S. Department of Health and Human Services, Office of Disease Prevention and Health Promotion. Retrieved from https://www.healthypeople.gov/2020

Keyes, K. M., & Galea, S. (2014). Current practices in teaching introductory epidemiology: How we got here, where to go. *American Journal of Epidemiology, 180*(7), 661–668. doi:10.1093/aje/kwu219

Merrill, R. M. (2016). *Introduction to epidemiology* (7th ed.). Burlington, MA: Jones & Bartlett Learning.

Nash, D. B., Fabius, R. J., Skoufalos, A., Clarke, J. L., & Horowitz, M. R. (2016). *Population health: Creating a culture of wellness* (2nd ed.). Burlington, MA: Jones & Bartlett Learning.

Patton, M. Q. (2008). *Utilization-focused evaluation* (4th ed.). Los Angeles, CA: Sage.

Pennsylvania Department of Health. (2015). *Pennsylvania cancer incidence and mortality 2013*. Harrisburg, PA: Author.

Pickering, K., Sholes, S., & Bajekal, M. (2005). *Synthetic Estimation of Healthy Lifestyles Indicators: Stage 3 Report.* London UK: National Centre for Social Research.

Robert Wood Johnson Foundation. (2015). The value of nursing in building a culture of health (Part 1): Reaching beyond traditional care settings to promote health where people live, learn, and play. *Charting Nursing's Future* (25). Retrieved from http://rwjf.org/en/library/research/2015/04/the-value-of-nursing-in-building-a-culture-of-health—part-1.html?cid=xtw_rwjf

Salazar, R. F., Crosby, R. J., & DiClemente, R. J. (2015). *Research methods in health promotion*. (2nd ed.). San Francisco, CA: Jossey-Bass.

U.S. Cancer Statistics Working Group. (2016). *United States cancer statistics: 1999–2013.* Atlanta, GA: U.S. Department of Health and Human Services, Centers for Disease Control and Prevention and National Cancer Institute. Retrieved from www.cdc.gov/uscs

Chapter 4

Theories Guiding Health Promotion and Risk Reduction:

Concepts and Applications

Marilyn Frenn, Margaret Sebern, and Mallory Stonehouse

LEARNING OBJECTIVES

After completing this chapter, the student will be able to:

1. Describe similarities and differences in theories and models used in health promotion research and practice.
2. Evaluate evidence for a theory or model(s) pertinent to a health promotion need(s) of people with whom the student commonly works.
3. Describe how health promotion evidence is synthesized and applied for use with a given group of people.
4. Discuss the merits of various Web sites and assessment tools for theory-based health promotion.
5. Discuss the merits of evidence that is theory-based for promoting the health of individuals, families, and aggregates.

INTRODUCTION

Theories guide practice and research. They help us organize what we know so that we can use that knowledge more effectively in nursing practice. The theories most utilized by nurses doing health promotion research are summarized to guide translation into practice. For example, in a review of 86 skin cancer prevention studies (Taber et al., 2018) with a randomized controlled or quasi-experimental design that targeted behavioral intervention in skin cancer for children and/or adults, 65.8% of the studies included theory-based interventions. The most common theories were social cognitive theory (SCT) (n = 20; 25.3%), health belief model (HBM) (n = 17; 21.5%), and the theory of planned behavior/reasoned action (n = 12; 15.2%). Despite an extensive search in eight databases from inception to 2015, older adult polypharmacy medication adherence was found to be directed by theory in only five studies, including SCT, HBM, transtheoretical model (TTM), and self-regulation model (Cadogan, Ryan, Patton, & Hughes, 2017). Consumption of fruit and vegetables by older adults was found to be better accomplished with theory-based interventions (Hazavehei & Afshari, 2016).

Knowledge of theory-based interventions becomes especially important when new threats to health emerge, such as the coronavirus pandemic (Garg et al., 2020). Because whole nations needed to change behavior to protect those most vulnerable to COVID-19, understanding what factors are effective in changing behavior before there is time to get sufficient evidence is essential.

When searching for evidence to guide nursing practice, the Cumulative Index to Nursing and Allied Health Literature (CINAHL) may have the most related studies, but other indices, such as Medline, PsychINFO, and Web of Science, provide studies from a variety of disciplines that can guide practice change decisions. When searching for evidence on a given topic, the number of years to include varies. Generally, the most recent evidence should be examined, but early seminal studies, systematic reviews, meta-analyses, and meta-syntheses are useful to consider. Working with a librarian helps ensure all relevant work is included.

As theories are examined for evidence that can be translated into practice, systematic reviews are helpful because a careful attempt to find all studies is made and the studies are carefully examined in terms of rigor. Meta-analyses, where a systematic review of the literature is conducted before the data from these studies are combined and statistically analyzed to determine overall results, are wonderful sources of information for translation into practice. Meta-syntheses are qualitative analyses of qualitative studies on a similar topic. Theories used by nurses for research and practice are reviewed citing recent evidence, meta-analyses, meta-syntheses, and systematic reviews. The theories are organized moving from individual and interpersonal aspects toward greater integration of environmental and policy components affecting health.

HEALTH PROMOTION MODEL (HPM)

First among the theories used by nurses studying better ways to improve health is the health promotion model (HPM) developed by Nola Pender, PhD, RN, FAAN (Figure 4–1). HPM was first published in 1982 and modified based on evolving research and conceptualizations

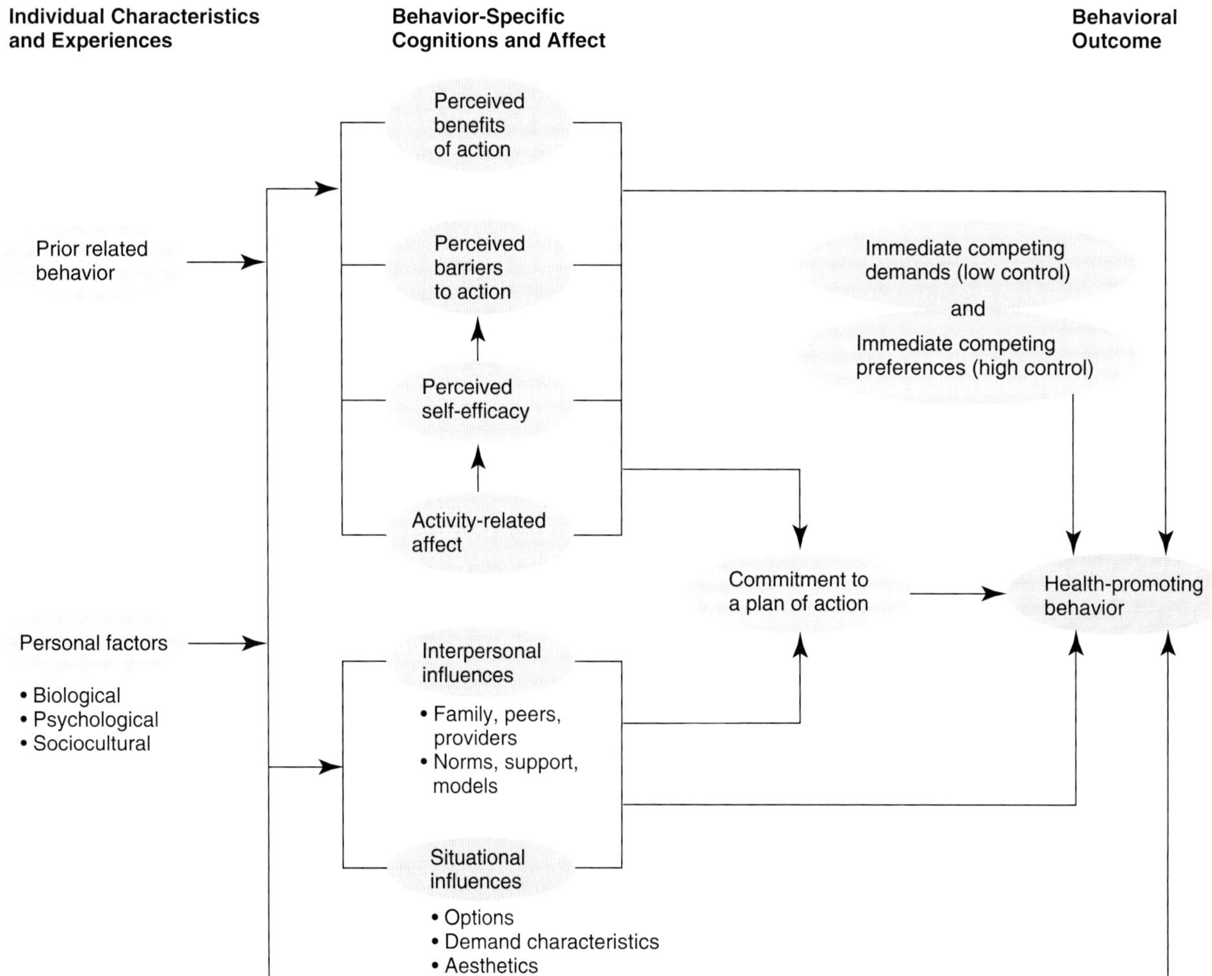

FIGURE 4–1 Health Promotion Model (HPM) *Source: From Pender, N. J., Murdaugh, C. L., & Parsons, M. A. (2011).* Health promotion in nursing practice *(6th ed.). Upper Saddle River, NJ: Pearson Prentice Hall. Reprinted with permission.*

of it in 1996 (Pender, 2011). Major constructs in HPM include: (1) individual characteristics and experiences, (2) behavior-specific cognitions and affect, and (3) behavioral outcomes. HPM focus is on health promotion, not just disease prevention, although it includes constructs developed in other disciplines. See Chapter 17 for examples of how HPM can be used.

Among the 357 studies indexed in CINAHL in the last five years, HPM has been recently used to examine Korean nursing student behaviors related to obesity and osteoporosis (Park, Choi-Kwon, & Han, 2015), home exercise training for people using hemodialysis in China (Xingjuan, Ka Yee Chow, & Kam Yuet Wong, 2015), social support and adherence to healthy lifestyle among Jordanian people with coronary artery disease (Tawalbeh, Tubaishat, Batiha, Al-Azzam, & AlBashtawy, 2015), and along with the diffusion of innovation model (DIM) for an evidence-based practice implementation of an epilepsy self-management protocol in the United States (Cole & Gaspar, 2015).

One meta-analysis (Tilokskulchai, Sitthimongkol, Prasopkiitikun, & Klainin, 2004) demonstrating effect sizes for model components and one meta-synthesis (Ho, Berggren, & Dahlborg-Lyckhage, 2010) were retrieved using the CINAHL publication type function. Fourteen systematic reviews were found, four of which were within the last 4 years. HPM was found to be most helpful in tailoring multiple behavior changes among those who smoke, in comparison to HBM, theory of reasoned action (TRA), and TTM because the latter models were focused on one behavior (Seung Hee & Duffy, 2017). Gacheru (2017) examined diabetes prevention best practices among young adult Hispanic Americans with prediabetes in order to develop an evidence-based intervention. Lewis (2014) examined the effects of stretching on preventing athletic injuries and concluded that a warmup session specific to the activity demonstrated effective outcomes. Dada (2014) examined health-care worker influenza vaccination using both HPM and HBM.

In a comparison of three theories, HPM was found to be most applicable to Hispanic women's health promotion needs (Garcia, 2016). The other two models (HBM and SCT) provide constructs used in many health behavior theories.

HEALTH BELIEF MODEL (HBM)

HBM (Figure 4–2) is based in social psychology and behavioral science, and was developed in the 1950s to understand preventive health behavior (Rosenstock, 1974). It was then expanded to apply to behavior related to illness symptoms and disease treatment (Becker, 1974; Kirscht, 1974). Major concepts of HBM include perceived susceptibility to illness and severity of the illness, along with perceived benefits and barriers to preventive or treatment actions. Cues to action, which can be internal or external, are factors that prompt and modify behavior change. Perceived susceptibility and severity affect the motivation for behavior change, and benefits and barriers shape the action taken to change behavior (Janz & Becker, 1984).

Recent examples of research done with HBM include examination of a stress management program to increase readiness for substance use treatment (Moeini et al., 2018), where HBM constructs improved with the intervention. Breast cancer screening beliefs were examined among Native American women and barriers to screening from HBM were related to less screening (Roh et al., 2018). HBM was used to develop a motion comic (wherein sound effects, voice-overs, and a musical score are added with animation to digital comics) to reach

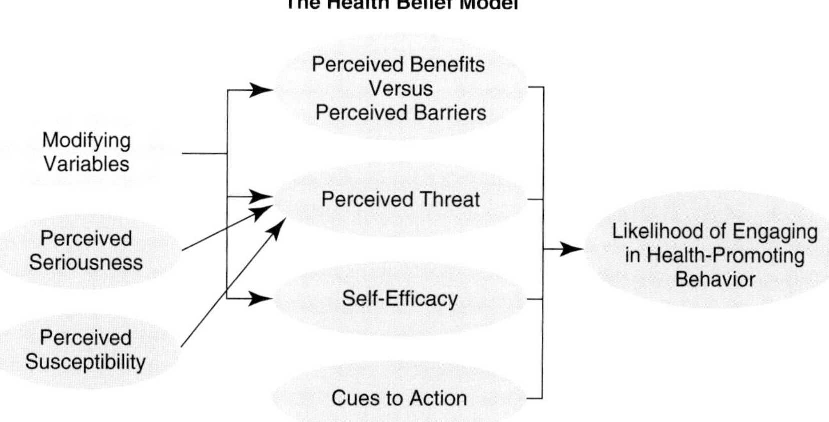

FIGURE 4–2 Health Belief Model (HBM) *Source: Original model created by United States Public Health Service.*

those 15 to 24 years old for sexually transmitted disease prevention (Willis et al., 2018). Treatment adherence in children with cystic fibrosis and their parents were found related to HBM, but children and parents had significantly different health beliefs (Dempster, Wildman, Masterson, & Omlor, 2018). HBM may also be helpful in designing messages to increase vaccination in pandemics by increasing benefits while decreasing barriers (Scherr, Jensen, & Christy, 2017). When combined with black feminist theory, HBM was also helpful in understanding women's perception of susceptibility of risk and severity of risk as well as the perceived benefit of the intervention to prevent HIV (Dyson, Davis, Counts-Spriggs, & Smith-Bankhead, 2017). An HBM-guided intervention to prevent burn injuries from electronic cigarettes can also be utilized (Smith, Smith, Cheatham, & Smith, 2017). Fewer barriers to mammography were found to be the most salient factor increasing frequency among Appalachian women (VanDyke & Shell, 2017) and among Asian immigrant women in Canada (Nguyen, Kornman, & Baur, 2011), which is consistent with HBM.

One meta-analysis using HBM was found in CINAHL. Carpenter (2010) found benefits and barriers to be the strongest predictors of behavior, but those were moderated by length of time before the behavior was measured as well as whether preventive or treatment behavior was measured. One meta-synthesis was also found (Lorenc, Jamal, & Cooper, 2013) showing that the risk and severity of skin cancer is not of concern in high-income countries and that unintentional tanning is seen as less dangerous.

Thirty-one systematic reviews guided by HBM were found in CINAHL, including three within the last 4 years. Factors influencing influenza vaccination among older adults included all components of HBM and some components of the TRA (Kan & Zhang, 2018). Use of an electronic health record in childhood obesity identification and management was reviewed using HBM and the chronic care model (Yabut & Rosenblum, 2017). The relationship between breast cancer risk perception and health-protective behavior in women with a family history of breast cancer was reviewed showing links with mammography and chemoprevention but not with self-breast exam and lifestyle change prevention (Paalosalo-Harris & Skirton, 2017).

SOCIAL COGNITIVE THEORY (SCT)

SCT was developed by Albert Bandura from the concept of self-efficacy, the perceived capability to perform behavior needed to produce expected outcomes (Bandura, 1977). SCT also includes the concepts of knowledge, outcome expectations, goals, facilitators, and impediments (Figure 4–3) (Bandura, 2004). Knowledge of the risks and benefits of the behavior is a precursor to change. Outcome expectations can include physical pleasure or discomfort, social approval or disapproval, and self-satisfaction or self-dissatisfaction. Goals provide a guide for behavior change and contain specific plans and strategies. Facilitators and impediments include sociostructural factors existing in the social, political, economic, and environmental systems (Bandura, 2004).

To build self-efficacy, the most important approach is to help clients check prior behavior consistent with their goals. Even if they make a small step in the right direction, this helps to build confidence that they can do this and more again. Seeing others accomplish similar goals can often be effective; this is called vicarious

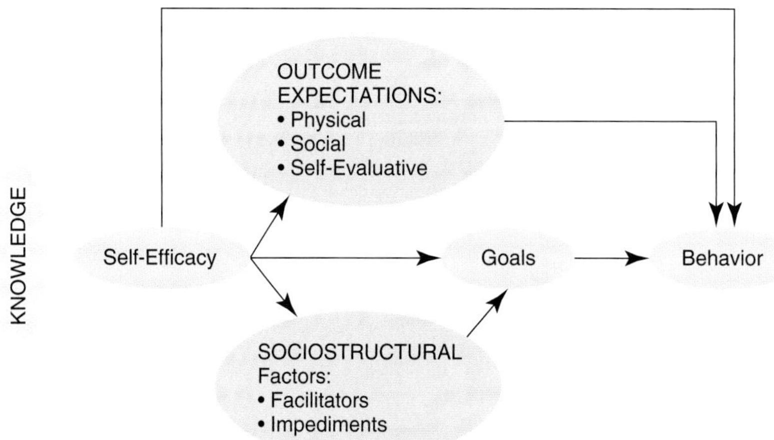

FIGURE 4–3 Social Cognitive Theory (SCT) *Source: From Bandura, A. (2004). Health promotion by social cognitive means.* Health Education and Behavior, *31, 143–164. Reprinted with permission.*

experience or modeling. Nurses can encourage clients to reflect on others who have been successful in the specific health promotion endeavor. Verbally persuading clients may be helpful, but this is a weaker form of support for self-efficacy. Helping clients reflect on their feelings and reactions may foster self-efficacy. Were they excited by their success? Did they feel better after taking even a small step toward improving their health?

Among recent studies using SCT, prelicensure employment was related to senior nursing student self-efficacy in caring for three to four patients (Grimm, 2018). Self-efficacy was associated with health literacy and was the strongest predictor of physical health status among those with chronic heart failure (Como, 2018). White-collar workers' diet and physical activity improved with a self-efficacy-based minimal contact intervention (Gretebeck, Bailey, & Gretebeck, 2017).

Two meta-analyses using the SCT were found in CINAHL. E-Health interventions were found to improve physical activity in young people, and theory-based interventions were successful, with the SCT-based interventions showing the most success and with mixed results for the theory of planned behavior (TPB) (McIntosh, Jay, Hadden, & Whittaker, 2017). Franklin and Lee (2014) found that simulation was effective in increasing nursing student self-efficacy.

One meta-synthesis was found in CINAHL for SCT describing self-efficacy instrumentation studies (Sheer, 2014). Twenty-eight systematic reviews were found, five in the last 4 years. SCT was the third most frequent theory used to guide nursing student simulation studies, after the National League for Nursing/Jeffries Simulation Framework and Kolb's theory of experiential learning (Lavoie et al., 2018). Few studies were found in a systematic review using SCT to examine parents with substance use disorder (Raynor & Pope, 2016). A systematic review of youth physical activity self-efficacy informed a concept analysis consistent with SCT (Voskuil & Robbins, 2015). SCT and Benner's novice to expert model guided a systematic review of new graduate transition programs and clinical leadership skills, finding that programs 24 or more weeks in length were associated with continued nurse employment compared with programs that were 12 weeks or less, yielding significant organizational cost savings (Chappell, Richards, & Barnett, 2014). Compassion fatigue in military health-care teams was examined using SCT (Peterson Owen & Wanzer, 2014).

THEORY OF PLANNED BEHAVIOR (TPB)

TPB was developed by the psychologist Icek Ajzen in the 1980s to explain human social behavior (Ajzen, 1991). TPB extends from TRA, which was previously developed by Ajzen along with Martin Fishbein (Fishbein & Ajzen, 1975). According to TPB (Figure 4–4), behavior change is influenced by intention to perform the behavior (Ajzen, 1991, 2016).

Nine meta-analyses for TPB were found in CINAHL (eight in the last 4 years), showing that most elements of the theory explained sun-protective behaviors (Starfelt Sutton, 2016), condom use in men who have sex with men (Andrew et al., 2016), breastfeeding (Guo, Wang, Liao, & Huang, 2016), unplanned pregnancy and sexually transmitted diseases in heterosexuals (Tyson,

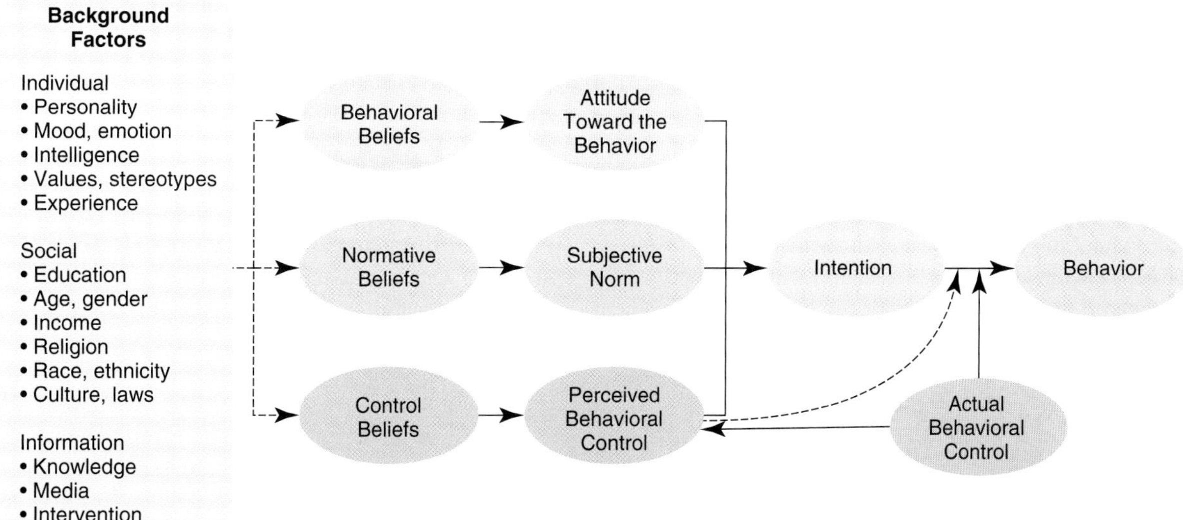

FIGURE 4–4 Theory of Planned Behavior *Source: Copyright © Icek Ajzen. Reprinted with permission.*

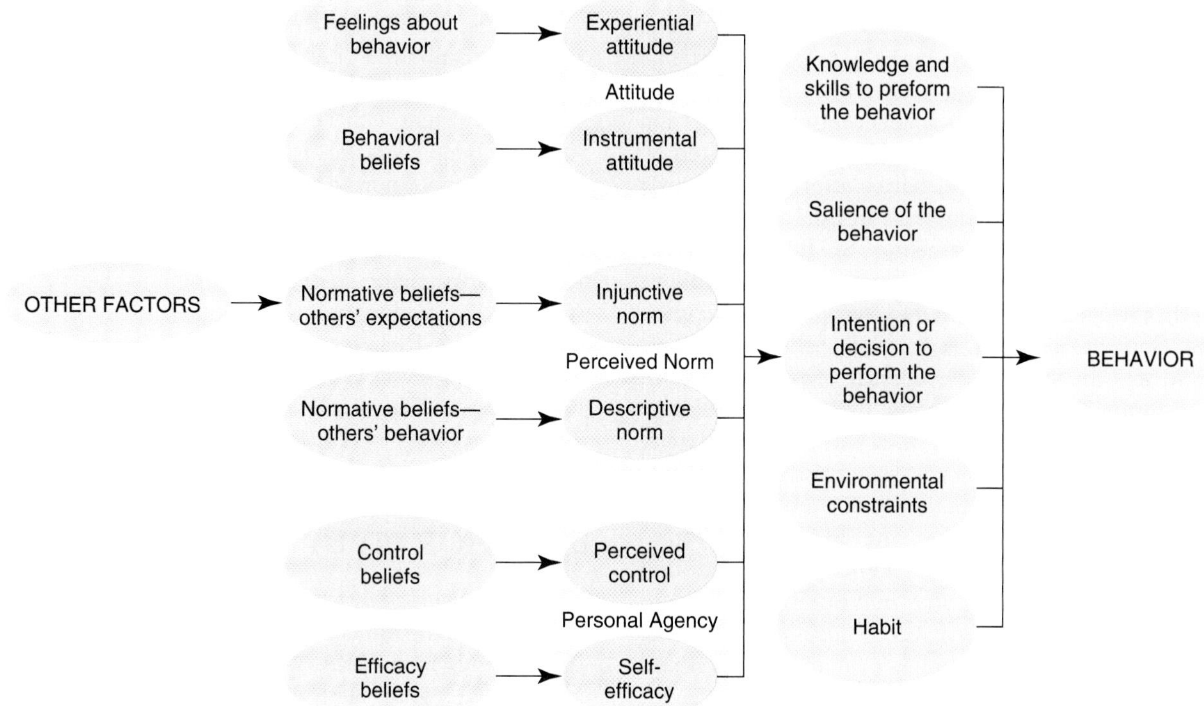

FIGURE 4–5 Integrated Behavior Model *Source: Montano, D., & Kasprzyk, D. (2015).* Theory of reasoned action, theory of planned behavior, and the integrated behavioral model. *In K. Glanz, B. K. Rimer, & B. Viswanath (Eds.),* Health behavior theory, research, and practice *(5th ed., pp. 95–124). San Francisco, CA: Jossey-Bass. Reprinted with permission.*

Covey, & Rosenthal, 2014), and steroid use among athletes to enhance physical performance (Ntoumanis, Ng, Barkoukis, & Backhouse, 2014). TPB relationships between concepts were supported for chronic illness adherence, although effect sizes were small, especially for the relationship between intention and behavior (Rich, Brandes, Mullan, & Hagger, 2015). Affective attitude predicted intention and behavior across a number of health behaviors, while anticipated affective reaction predicted behavior, but not intention while controlling for other TPB variables (Conner, McEachan, Taylor, O'Hara, & Lawton, 2015). As previously mentioned, TPB had mixed results for e-health physical activity interventions in young people, with one study showing positive results and one showing none (McIntosh et al., 2017). TPB was further developed into the integrated behavioral model.

INTEGRATED BEHAVIORAL MODEL (IBM)

In 2002, the Institute of Medicine called for an integration of theoretical models used to develop communication strategies that target health behavior change (Institute of Medicine, 2002). Fishbein, Ajzen, and colleagues responded by expanding TRA and TPB to incorporate constructs from SCT (i.e., self-efficacy and perceived control) (Montano & Kasprzyk, 2015). The expanded model was called the integrated behavioral model (IBM) (Figure 4–5) and focused on individual motivational factors that predict the likelihood of performing specific behaviors. According to IBM, behavior is likely to occur when the person has intention to perform it and necessary knowledge and skills, perceived control, and self-efficacy.

Similar to TRA and TPB, IBM proposed that the most important determinant of behavior is intention to perform the behavior. Behavioral intention is determined by three constructs: attitude, perceived norm, and personal agency. First, attitude toward the behavior includes experiential attitude or the person's emotional response to performing the behavior. A strong positive emotional response to performing the behavior increases the likelihood of performing the behavior. Perceived norms reflect the social pressures one feels to perform or not perform a specific behavior. Subjective norms are defined as a belief about what others think one should do. Perceptions about what others actually do (descriptive norm) may also be part of subjective norms. Subjective norms vary across cultures based on the importance of social identity in various cultures (Fishbein & Ajzen, 2010).

Finally, personal agency, which consists of self-efficacy and perceived control, is a major factor influencing behavior. Perceived control is determined by one's perception of the degree to which various environmental factors make it easy or difficult to perform the behavior. Self-efficacy is one's confidence in performing the behavior in situations that make it easy or difficult to perform the behavior. The degree to which each of these three constructs (attitude, perceived norm, and personal agency) determine intention vary by demographic, social, and cultural factors (Fishbein & Ajzen, 2010).

TRA, TPB, and IBM have been used to understand and predict a variety of health behaviors (e.g., condom use, immunizations, screening for diseases, diet, and physical activity) (Montano & Kasprzyk, 2015). IBM is not indexed in CINAHL. A Web of Science search conducted to identify interventions studies that applied TRA/TPB or IBM from 2014 to 2018 resulted in 211 national and international intervention studies. These publications applied the models to health behaviors such as substance abuse, dental checkups, hand washing, traffic violations, physical activity, and sexual function. Reviewing these publications is beyond the scope of this chapter.

When the Web of Science search was limited to systematic reviews or meta-analyses of interventions from 2014 to 2018, 20 publications resulted. Seven of these did not include studies that applied the model to health behavior change. Of the 13 meta-analyses that did apply TRA/TPB or IBM to health behavior change interventions, all studies supported the relationships between attitude, perceived norm, and personal agency and intention. Behaviors targeted in these reviews included advanced-care planning, safe food handling, physical activity, oral health, immunizations, dietary intake, sexual behavior, and self-care in chronic illnesses (Table 4–1).

Meta-analysis studies provide strong support for the relationships between attitudes, perceived norms, personal agency beliefs, and intention to engage in specific health behaviors (Steinmetz, Knappstein, Aizin, Schmidt, & Kabst, 2016). The theoretical constructs are relevant across cultures. TRA, TPB, and IBM were studied in over 50 developed and developing countries (Fishbein & Ajzen, 2010). In applying the theories in research, it is critical to investigate and understand the behavior from the perspective of the clinical populations' attitudes, perceived norms, and personal agency to perform the specific behavior. The elicitation process makes the model applicable across cultures (Montano & Kasprzyk, 2015).

Thus, when applying the models in health behavior research, it is important to conduct qualitative interviews to assess individual beliefs in a formative stage. The qualitative interviews inform development of interventions used to target behavior change. In this formative stage, people should be asked to provide the following four types of information:

1. Positive and negative feelings about preforming the behavior (attitude toward the behavior)
2. Positive and negative attributes or outcomes of performing the behavior (behavioral beliefs)
3. Individuals or groups to whom they might listen who are in favor or opposed to their performing the behaviors (norms)
4. Situational or other facilitators and barriers that make the behavior easy or difficult to perform (personal agency) (Montano & Kasprzyk, 2015, p. 108).

In applying TRA, TPB, and IBM in practice, it is important to ask the client about his or her attitudes, social norms, and personal agency toward the specific behavior being targeted for change. For example, the practitioner can ask the client about her emotional response to engaging in the behavior and to the outcomes, beliefs about personal gain resulting from the behavior, what people close to her think about the behavior, if people close to her engage in the behavior, and finally her confidence to engage in the behavior in a variety of settings that may facilitate or act as barriers to performing the behavior.

TRANSTHEORETICAL MODEL (TTM)

James Prochaska and Carlo DiClemente integrated processes and principles of change theories to develop TTM (Prochaska & DiClemente, 1983). TTM is composed of six stages of change that occur over time: precontemplation, contemplation, preparation, action, maintenance, and termination (Figure 4–6) (Prochaska & Velicer, 1997). In the precontemplation stage, the client does not intend to change in the foreseeable future, generally within the next six months; in the contemplation stage, he or she has intention to change in the foreseeable future. The preparation stage is characterized by intention to change in the immediate future, generally within one month. The action stage is when overt, specific activities are carried out to make a change. Maintenance is the stage in which the change has been made and work is done to prevent relapse, although less work is required than in the action stage. Termination is a stage

Table 4–1 Meta-Analysis and Systematic Review Behavior Change Interventions, 2014–2018

Author	Nation	Theory	Behavioral Intervention Target	Results
Scherrens et al. (2018)	Belgium and Europe	TPB (9/31) TRA (4/31)	Advanced care planning	Need more use of theory to understand end of life (EOL)
Young et al. (2018)	Canada	TPB most commonly used 45%	Consumer food-handling safety	Many theories explain behavior
Durks et al. (2018)	Australia and Europe	TPB most commonly used	Health-care professional training	Used in developing practice change interventions. Did not include studies that applied the models to health behavior change.
Fleming et al. (2017)	England	TPB	Unlawful file sharing	Social approval influence. Did not include studies that applied the models to health behavior change.
Schüz et al. (2017)	England	TPB	Physical activity	Education moderated association between variable and physical activity
Scalco et al. (2017)	Italy and Europe	TPB	Organic food consumption	Meta-analysis confirms attitude in shaping buying intention, followed by subjective norms and perceived behavioral control. Intention-behavior shows a large effect size.
Polk (2017)	United States	TRA/TPB	Oral self-care behaviors in children	Support attitude, norms effect intention
Schmid et al. (2017)	Germany	TPB	Influenza vaccine	Attitudes supported
Hagger et al. (2017)	Australia, China, and Europe	TPB	Alcohol and diet	Support SCT
Tebb et al. (2016)	United States	TPB and other models	Computer interventions, no behavior	Did not include studies that applied the models to health behavior change
Corace et al. (2016)	Canada	Several models included TPB	Immunization	Did not include studies that applied the models to health behavior change
Steinmetz et al. (2016)	Germany and United States	TPB meta-analysis	Health behaviors	Confirmed the effectiveness of TPB-based interventions, with a mean effect size of .50 for changes in behavior and effect sizes ranging from .14 to .68 for changes in antecedent variables (behavioral, normative, and control beliefs; attitude; subjective norm; perceived behavioral control; and intention)

Table 4–1 Meta-Analysis and Systematic Review Behavior Change Interventions, 2014–2018—cont'd

Author	Nation	Theory	Behavioral Intervention Target	Results
McDermott et al. (2015)	Australia	TRA/TPB	Discrete food choices	Attitudes had the strongest association with intention (r(+) = 0.54) followed by perceived behavioral control (PBC, r(+) = 0.42) and subjective norm (SN, r(+) = 0.37)
Thompson-Leduc (2015)	Canada and United States	TRA	Shared decision making	Did not include studies that applied the models to health behavior change
Asarnow et al. (2015)	United States	IBM	Mental health behaviors in children in primary care	Did not include studies that applied the models to health behavior change
Cooper et al. (2015)	United States		Post-concussion treatment	Did not include studies that applied the models to health behavior change
Riebl et al. (2015)	United States	TPB	Dietary behavior	Attitude had the strongest relationship with dietary behavioral intention (mean r = 0.52), while intention was the most common predictor of behavior performance (mean r = 0.38; both $p < 0.001$)
Rich et al. (2015)	Australia and Netherlands	TPB	Adherence in chronic illness	The theory explained 33% and 9% of the variance in intention and adherence behavior, respectively.
Tyson et al. (2014)	England	TPB	Heterosexual risk behavior	Larger effects were found for interventions that provided opportunities for social comparison. TPB provides a valuable framework for designing interventions to change heterosexual risk behaviors. However, effect sizes varied between studies, and further research is needed to explore the reasons.
Hackman et al. (2014)	United States	TPB	Dietary interventions in adolescents and young adults	Interventions directed toward changing dietary behaviors in adolescents should aim to incorporate multifaceted, theory-based approaches. More research is needed to identify the optimal TPB and TRA modalities to modify dietary behaviors.

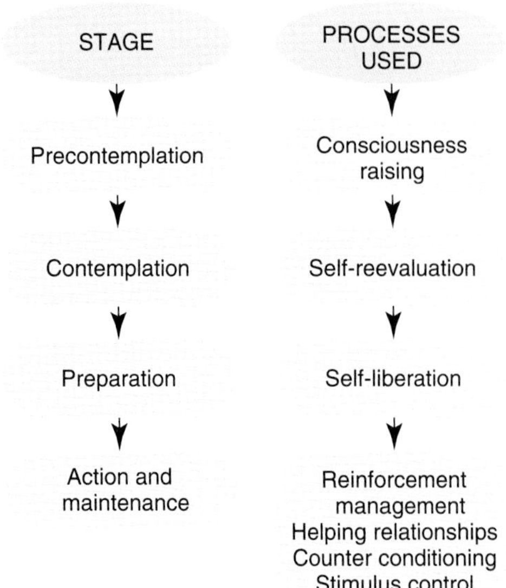

FIGURE 4–6 Transtheoretical Model (TTM)

in which 100% self-efficacy is achieved with no temptation to revert to the previous behavior. Termination is the part of the framework that is not always included because it is more realistic to expect behavior change to require ongoing effort, which necessitates remaining in the maintenance stage (Prochaska, 2008; Prochaska & Velicer, 1997).

During each stage in TTM, processes of change are used (Table 4–2). Experiential processes include feelings and thoughts about the behavior: consciousness raising, dramatic relief, self-reevaluation, environmental reevaluation, and social liberation. Behavioral processes of change entail observable changes in the situation or social interactions: self-liberation, helping relationships, counterconditioning, reinforcement management, and stimulus control (Romain, Horwath, & Bernard, 2018). Assessing an individual's, a family's, or a community's stage of change helps in recommending effective interventions utilizing processes associated with that stage.

As people move from precontemplation through the stages, the pros of the health behavior change increase and the cons decrease, self-efficacy is likely to improve, and use of the processes associated with action increase (Scruggs et al., 2018). No differences for in-person compared to computer-generated brief alcohol counseling using TTM were found (Freyer-Adam et al., 2018), although meta-analyses have shown improved results for in-person counseling. It may be that all components of TTM were included in the computer-generated feedback, whereas at least two were used in the in-person motivational interviewing sessions. TTM was effectively used to guide a household disaster preparedness program (Thomas et al., 2018) and sun protection programs (Yusufov, Rossi, et al., 2016). Mammography among Chinese American women was examined with TTM (Lee-Lin, Nguyen, Pedhiqala, Diedkmann, & Menon, 2016). TTM was used to assess Appalachian (Krok-Schoen et al., 2016), Latina (Tung, Smith-Gagen, Lu, & Warfield, 2016), Chinese American (Tung, Granner, Lu, & Qiu, 2017) and Korean American women's cervical cancer screening (Tung, Lu, Granner, & Sohn, 2017).

The TTM processes of change were integrated into over half of 100 mobile applications for smoking cessation (Paige, Alber, Stellefson, & Krieger, 2018). TTM was found to be more effective than HBM for smoking cessation among nurses in Turkey (Bakan & Erci, 2018). Hypnosis was helpful in helping people quit smoking using TTM (Munson, Barabasz, & Barabasz, 2018).

Both total and vigorous physical activity were predicted by behavioral processes of change within TTM (Romain et al., 2018). The use of a greater number of processes of change indicated greater success in reducing dietary fat, even among those who relapsed (Yusufov, Paiva, et al., 2016). Family nutrition and physical activity was improved with a TTM-based intervention (Dinkel et al., 2017), as was physical activity among obese college students (Ickes, McMullen, Pflug, & Westgate, 2016). SCT and TTM were the most reported in a systematic review of rural physical activity interventions (Walsh, Umstattd Meyer, Gamble, Patterson, & Moore, 2017).

One meta-analysis and no meta-syntheses were listed for TTM in CINAHL. Adult diet and physical activity studies published between 1990 and 2008 were included in the meta-analysis. The interventions were delivered by non-health-care professionals (46.8%) directly to individuals (51.1%) in community-based settings (54.2%) over 8 months, with follow-up at 10 months, and did not show differences for inclusion of theory, specifically TTM or SCT (Prestwich et al., 2014). Because many other meta-analyses have shown improved results with theory-based interventions, it could be that individually delivered, community-based interventions by non-health-care professionals included in this meta-analysis did not have fidelity to the theories tested, although the investigators carefully examined the degree of intended theoretical integration.

Twenty-six systematic reviews were located in CINAHL for TTM, three in the last 4 years. TTM and TRA were the most frequently used theories guiding end-of-life care planning found in a systematic review (Scherrens et al., 2018). TTM and SCT were found to be the most frequently used behavioral models for helping cancer survivors return to work (Duijts, Bleiker,

Table 4–2 Processes of Change in TTM

Process		Description
Experiential Processes	Consciousness raising	Increasing awareness about pros and cons of behavior
	Dramatic relief	Emotional response to the behavior
	Self-reevaluation	Examining oneself with and without the behavior
	Environmental reevaluation	Examining how the behavior affects social relationships
	Social liberation	Social opportunities supporting changing the behavior
Behavioral Processes	Self-liberation	Believing one can change the behavior
	Helping relationships	Being open and trusting with someone who cares, self-help groups, social support
	Counterconditioning	Substituting alternatives for problem behaviors
	Reinforcement management	Rewarding oneself or being rewarded for making changes
	Stimulus control	Avoiding stimuli that elicit problem behaviors, adding stimuli that encourage alternative behaviors, restructuring one's environment

Paalman, & Beek, 2017). SCT and TTM were found to be the most frequently used to examine rural physical activity interventions (Walsh et al., 2017).

PATIENT ACTIVATION/ EMPOWERMENT

Patient activation is defined as an "individual's knowledge, skill, and confidence for managing his/her own health and health care" (Hibbard & Mahoney, 2010). Experiencing success leads to positive emotion and further success, so clinicians are urged to ask people to do what they can accomplish and then build on that success with more complex action (Figure 4–7). Patient activation is associated with most health behaviors (Hibbard, 2017), better health-care outcomes, reduced hospital admissions, and reduced costs because people feel more in control (Greene, Hibbard, Sacks, Overton, & Parrotta, 2015). Patient engagement is "a broader concept that includes activation; the interventions designed to increase activation; and patients' resulting behavior, such as obtaining preventive care or engaging in regular physical exercise" (Hibbard & Greene, 2013, p. 203). In ambulatory care, patient engagement is a nurse-sensitive indicator (Esposito, 2016) because nurses elicit people's self-determined goals of care and follow up to keep them involved in their care. This approach is useful in promoting health among patients and caregivers of those experiencing illness.

No meta-analyses and one meta-synthesis were found in CINAHL for patient activation. The meta-synthesis concerned caregiver activation for those caring for someone with dementia (Sadak, Souza, & Borson, 2016). Three systematic reviews related to health promotion were found in the last 4 years. Further support of parent activation in caring for children with special needs by navigating the systems available and further research including those with socioeconomic disadvantage emerged from the review (Mirza, Krischer, Stolley, Magaña, & Martin, 2018). The need for better understanding the activation needs of older adults with cancer was found (Ee, Hagedoorn, Slaets, & Smits, 2017). Consumer involvement in activation of emergency response systems was found to work without overwhelming the systems (Vorwerk & King, 2016).

One meta-analysis was found in CINAHL showing patient empowerment in those with metabolic disease had improved hemoglobin A1c, waist circumference, and empowerment levels (Kuo, Lin, & Tsai, 2014). Three meta-syntheses were found for patient empowerment in the last 4 years dealing with the role of concierge medicine in primary care for one study (Palumbo, 2017), with health and social care professionals self-management support of people with chronic health issues (Morgan et al., 2017), and nurses' attitudes toward complementary therapies (Hall, Leach, Brosnan, & Collins, 2017). Sixteen systematic reviews were found in CINAHL for patient empowerment in the last 4 years. The importance of nurse involvement in health literacy with immigrant groups was identified (Fernández-Gutiérrez, Bas-Sarmiento, Albar-Marín, & Paloma-Castro, 2018). The remainder dealt with patient empowerment in coping with illness.

Level 1	Level 2	Level 3	Level 4
Disengaged and overwhelmed	**Becoming aware, but still struggling**	**Taking action**	**Maintaining behaviors and pushing further**
Individuals are passive and lack confidence. Knowledge is low, goal-orientation is weak, and adherence is poor. Their perspective: "My doctor is in charge of my health."	Individuals have some knowledge, but large gaps remain. They believe health is largely out of their control, but can set simple goals. Their perspective: "I could be doing more."	Individuals have the key facts and are building self-management skills. They strive for best practice behaviors, and are goal-oriented. Their perspective: "I'm part of my health care team."	Individuals have adopted new behaviors, but may struggle in times of stress or change. Maintaining a healthy lifestyle is a key focus. Their perspective: "I'm my own advocate."

Increasing Levels of Activation

FIGURE 4–7 Patient Activation Measure *Source: © Insignia Health. Patient Activation Measure® (PAM®) Survey Levels. All rights reserved.*

DIFFUSION OF INNOVATION MODEL (DIM)

DIM was developed by Everett Rogers in the 1960s to enhance communication from innovation development to integration (Rogers, 1962, 2003). The model is comprised of four main elements: innovation, communication channels, time, and social system (Figure 4–8). The innovation is a new idea, practice, or object that is diffused or communicated through certain channels over time. A quality innovation is compatible with the values and needs of the target population, is not overly complex, can be trialed, is more advantageous than previous ideas, and produces observable results. The communication channels are the routes in which messages are passed within a social system, and the social system is a set of connected entities working together to accomplish a common goal. A series of stages is included in DIM: knowledge or learning of the innovation's existence, persuasion or forming an opinion about the innovation, decision or choosing to adopt or reject the innovation, implementation or completing activities to apply the innovation, and confirmation or evaluation of the success of the innovation in use (Rogers, 2003).

DIM has been used infrequently recently to guide health promotion research but was used to examine how information about the Zika virus was disseminated. News media, public health agencies, and grassroots users were the most frequent sources of Tweets about Zika, with the latter suggesting conspiracy theories (Vijaykumar, Nowak, Himelboim, & Jin, 2018). Understanding how clients, families, and communities get information can

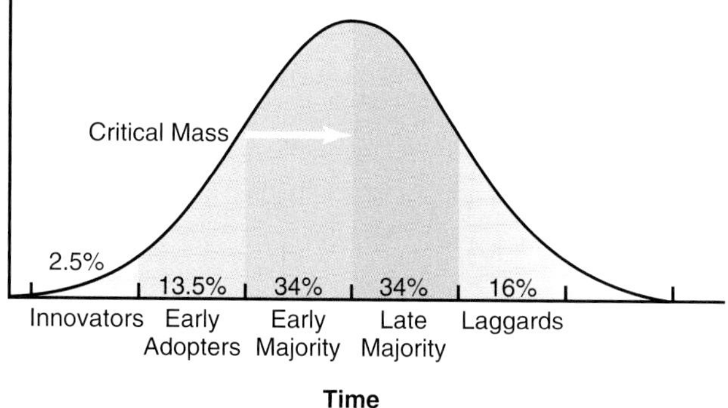

FIGURE 4–8 Diffusion of Innovation Model (DIM) *Source: Kaminski, J. (Spring 2011). Diffusion of innovation theory.* Canadian Journal of Nursing Informatics, *6(2). Theory in nursing informatics column. http://cjni.net/journal/?p=1444. Reprinted with permission.*

be helpful in promoting health and in understanding impediments to evidence-based approaches. However, DIM is considered the most influential of theories guiding translational or implementation science, which is focused on understanding "uptake and use of evidence to improve patient outcomes and population health" as well as how evidence is used, where, and by whom (Titler, 2018).

Three meta-analyses were found in CINAHL for DIM, and none are related to health promotion. Two meta-syntheses were found, one dealing with interprofessional teamwork related to health promotion and all areas of practice (Sims, Heewitt, & Harrais, 2015). Four central themes were found essential to teamwork: a shared purpose, critical reflection, innovation, and leadership. Eighty-four systematic reviews were found for DIM in CINAHL, one in the last 4 years related to health promotion in that implementation of school health policy was examined (Harriger, Lu, McKyer, Pruitt, & Goodson, 2014).

SOCIAL ECOLOGICAL MODEL (SEM)

SEM was developed based upon the concept of the ecosystem and focused on the interaction between the individual and the environment (Bronfenbrenner, 1979, 1994; McLeroy, Bibeau, Steckler, & Glanz, 1988). Building on this, SEM (Figure 4–9) includes five levels of influence: intrapersonal, interpersonal, institutional, community, and public policy factors (McDaniel, 2018; McLeroy et al., 1988). Examining where populations are at risk can help to develop interventions where they are most needed, in the context of the other levels of influence.

For example, SEM recently was useful in discovering that the incidence of chronic obstructive pulmonary disease rose nationally between 2012 and 2014 and that prevalence was highest in Appalachian counties of Virginia. Racial composition, ethnic composition, poverty rates, altitude, air pollution, and smoking policies were all significant contributors to the increased prevalence (McDaniel, 2018). SEM was also helpful in evaluating whether a population-based program to reduce cardiovascular disease risk factors had better outcomes than a comparison community (Sidebottom et al., 2018). SEM was used to explore the multi-level factors influencing black college women's HIV testing behavior (Dyson et al., 2018).

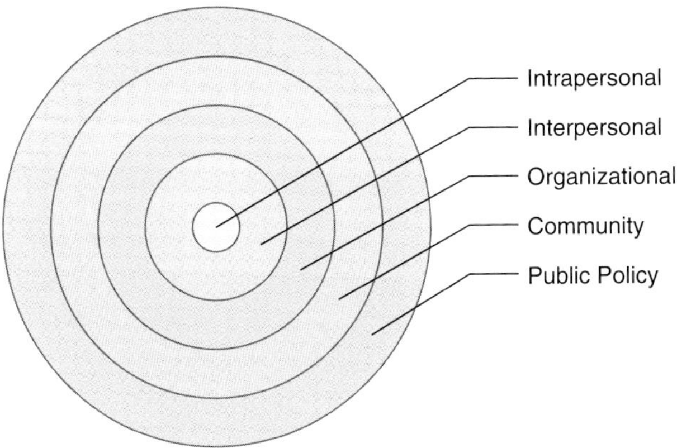

FIGURE 4–9 Social Ecological Model (SEM) *Source: King, J. L., Merten, J. W., Wong, T.-J., & Pomeranz, J. L. (2018). Applying a social-ecological framework to factors related to nicotine replacement therapy for adolescent smoking cessation.* American Journal of Health Promotion, *32(5), 1291–1303. doi:10.1177/0890117117718422. Reprinted with permission.*

Nurses' eating habits in acute care were examined in a qualitative study using SEM, which showed that "nurses' perceived inability to take breaks was due to patient load, unpredictability of patient needs, reluctance to burden other nurses, a tendency to prioritize patient care over self-care, and the repercussions of working longer hours to complete work. Other influential factors included the presence of unhealthy food options, regulations restricting nurses' ability to eat and drink in the workplace, and the need for more staff" (Monaghan, Dinour, Liou, & Shefchik, 2018).

One meta-analysis was found in CINAHL for SEM, and it described the correlates of gross motor competence in children and adolescents (Barnett et al., 2016). A combined meta-analysis and meta-synthesis using SEM examined physical activity in pregnant women (Harrison, Taylor, Shields, & Frawley, 2018). A meta-synthesis described the challenging barriers faced by socially marginalized adults with type 2 diabetes (Vanstone et al., 2017). A meta-ethnography using SEM listed in CINAHL described resilience in young refugees to Western countries (Sleijpen, Boeije, Kleber, & Mooren, 2016).

Seventeen systematic reviews were found for SEM in CINAHL, eight related to health promotion in the last 4 years. A systematic review of studies related to nicotine replacement therapy for adolescents guided by SEM examined evidence at each level (King, Merten, Wong, & Pomeranz, 2018). Physical activity, nutrition, and screen time of adolescents were primarily mediated by factors at the individual level of SEM (Kelly et al., 2017), whereas physical activity and sedentary behavior of young children were influenced by all levels of SEM (Lindsay, Greaney, Wallington, Mesa, & Salas, 2017). Because physical activity can slow cognitive decline, a systematic review described ways providers can facilitate physical activity among those with dementia (van Alphen, Hortobágyi, & van Heuvelen, 2016). Barriers to healthy eating for adults in rural areas are comparatively underexamined compared to urban areas, including lack of grocery stores and social support, cost, and work issues (Reed et al., 2016). Physical activity and sports among culturally and linguistically diverse migrants were found to be related to social support and safety, but further study better incorporating measures of acculturation is needed (O'Driscoll, Banting, Borkoles, Eime, & Polman, 2014).

Factors influencing breastfeeding decisions incorporating multiple levels of SEM were reviewed (Roll & Cheater, 2016). HIV testing in U.S. youth was examined, yielding implications for research, practice, and policy (Adebayo & Gonzalez-Guarda, 2017). Social media use for sexual health promotion yielded evidence at the individual level, but mainly at the societal level, to support long-lasting improvements (Condran, Gahagan, & Isfeld-Kiely, 2017). Case management and brief intervention were found to help youth violence prevention (Mikhail & Nemeth, 2016). Facilitators and barriers for culturally diverse nursing students' progression and graduation were examined in a systematic review using SEM (Clary Muronda, 2016).

PRECEDE-PROCEED

The PRECEDE-PROCEED model was developed by Green and Kreuter (1991, 2005) as a guide for health program planning and evaluation (Figure 4–10). PRECEDE is an acronym for predisposing, reinforcing, and enabling constructs in educational diagnosis and evaluation; PROCEED is an acronym for policy, regulatory, and organizational constructs in educational and environmental development (Gielen, McDonald, & Gary, 2008; Porter, 2016). The model contains eight phases: PRECEDE is composed of the assessment and planning Phases 1–4, while PROCEED is composed of the implementation and evaluation Phases 5–8. Phase 1 (PRECEDE) is social assessment and situational analysis, Phase 2 is an epidemiological assessment, Phase 3 is an educational and ecological assessment, and Phase 4 is development of an action plan and selection of interventions to address problems identified during assessment. Phase 5 (PROCEED) is implementation, Phase 6 is process evaluation, Phase 7 is impact evaluation, and Phase 8 is outcome evaluation. Active participation by the target population is fundamental to developing and implementing behavior change using the PRECEDE-PROCEED model (Gielen et al., 2008; Porter, 2016).

Recent studies using the PRECEDE-PROCEED model showed it to be effective in increasing exercise while decreasing pain and ergonomic risk among intensive-care nurses (Sezgin & Esin, 2018). The model was used to transform a shopping mall in Montreal, Canada, while incorporating community feedback to create accessibility for a diverse population (Ahmed et al., 2017). A college chef program was also developed by incorporating focus groups using the PRECEDE-PROCEED model (McMullen, Ickes, Noland, Erwin, & Helme, 2017). A cardiovascular disease prevention and acculturation approach for West

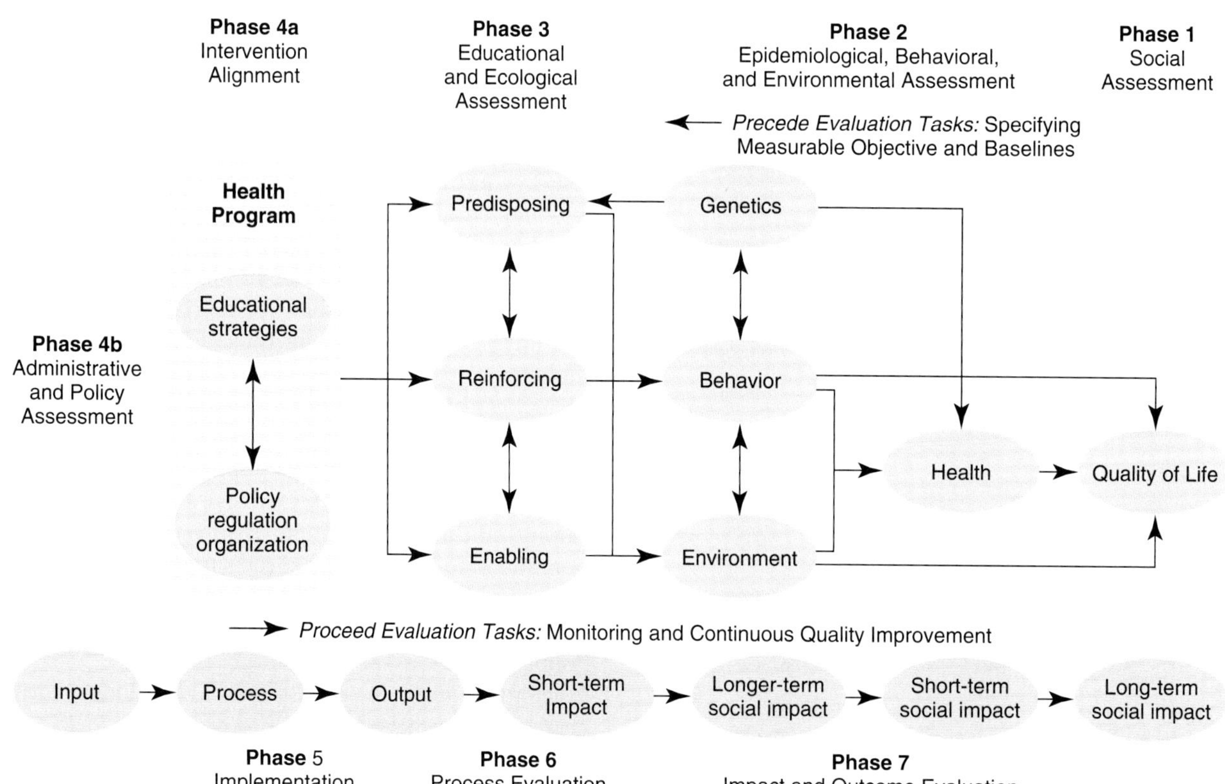

FIGURE 4–10 PRECEDE-PROCEED Model *Source: Green, L.W., & Kreuter, M.W. (2005).* Health program planning: An educational and ecological approach *(4th ed.). New York, NY: McGraw-Hill. Reprinted with permission.*

African immigrants to the United States was developed using the model (Commodore-Mensah et al., 2016).

No meta-analysis or meta-synthesis were found for the PRECEDE-PROCEED model in CINAHL. Six systematic reviews were found, two in the last 4 years. Inclusion of parents and children in home-visit protocols were examined, and most elements of PRECEDE were found in assessment, but few elements incorporating parents and children were found for the PROCEED component of the model (Lam, Dawson, & Fowler, 2017). Clinical behavior of home-care providers working with transgender clients was examined, finding multifactorial barriers to provision of mental health care (MacKinnon, Tarasoff, & Kia, 2016).

COMBINED THEORETICAL APPROACHES

Sometimes research is conducted by combining theoretical approaches. For example, both HBM and commonsense self-regulation models were used to examine college students' self-management behaviors for food allergies (Duncan & Annunziato, 2018). Both HBM and TTM were used to improve Vietnamese American immigrant women's stage of change, benefits, and intention to use mammography (Nguyen-Truong et al., 2017). Health promotion at the ballpark was facilitated by a combined PRECEDE-PROCEED, social cognitive, social marketing, and diffusion of innovation approach to incorporate healthy events, foods, and activities for players and spectators (Hodges, 2017).

PICOT QUESTION, EVIDENCE TABLE, BRIEF REPORT

To provide an example of how theories would be used to examine the evidence for a client health promotion issue, consider the case of a school nurse working in a school district serving a largely African American group of students where a high percentage are overweight or obese, presenting risks to their current and future health. A literature review was conducted to identify which conceptual frameworks have been used among African American children at risk for obesity to reduce successfully body mass index (BMI) percentile or percentage of body fat, improve nutrition, or increase physical activity. Often reviews of evidence are organized in a patient, intervention, control, observation, and time (PICOT) format as described in Chapter 5 (time is not always included). To support population health initiatives best, it is useful to examine Healthy People 2020 objectives that relate to the health promotion topic. The PICO format for this example is shown below and the related Healthy People 2020 Objectives are shown in Box 4–1.

BOX 4–1 Healthy People 2020 Objectives

NWS-10.4 Reduce the proportion of children and adolescents aged 2 to 19 years who are considered obese.

NWS-14 Increase the contribution of fruits to the diets of the population aged 2 years and older.

NWS-15 Increase the variety and contribution of vegetables to the diets of the population aged 2 years and older.

NWS-16 Increase the contribution of whole grains to the diets of the population aged 2 years and older.

NWS-17 Reduce consumption of calories from solid fats and added sugars in the population aged 2 years and older.

PA-13.2 Increase the proportion of trips of 1 mile or less made to school by walking by children and adolescents aged 5 to 15 years.

PA-14.2 Increase the proportion of trips of 2 miles or less made to school by bicycling by children and adolescents aged 5 to 15 years.

Source: Retrieved from https://www.healthypeople.gov/2020/topics-objectives/topic/nutrition-and-weight-status/objectives#4928.

P: African American children at risk for obesity
I: Conceptually based interventions
C: Usual care or attention control group, interventions without a conceptual basis
O: Reduce BMI percentile or percentage of body fat, improve nutrition, or increase physical activity.

Discussion of the Evidence

One meta-analysis was found for this topic (Annesi, 2010) where interventions using SCT resulted in decreased BMI, increased self-efficacy, and increased physical activity in predominately African American preadolescents. One systematic review was found examining obesity prevention in adolescents using the SCT, but race was not addressed (Bagherniya et al., 2018). In addition, 388 articles published after 2007 were indexed in CINAHL, Medline, or PsycINFO, of which 18 clearly referred to a conceptual framework and were targeted toward African American children (Table 4–3).

Programs were evaluated (Burnet et al., 2011; Choudhry et al., 2011) based on a combination of behavior change theories that included HBM, social learning

Table 4–3 What Conceptual Frameworks Guide Effective Childhood Obesity Prevention/Amelioration?

Citation	Subjects	Method*	Theory	Setting	Results	Rigor of Evidence
Burnet et al. (2011)	18 African American children aged 9–12 years and parents	2.d	Behavior change theories	Community setting	Participants decreased BMI, increased waist-to-hip ratio, increased walking; no difference in other measures.	No masking. Poor instrument reliability for diet.
Choudhry et al. (2011)	40 African American children aged 5–12 years	2.d	Behavior change theories	After-school setting	Participants decreased BMI, increased physical activity intentions, and improved diet intentions.	No masking. Long-term effects not measured.
Annesi (2010)	200 African American children aged 7–12 years	2.a	SCT (social cognitive theory; Bandura, 1997)	After-school setting	Participants decreased BMI and increased physical activity.	No masking. Long-term effects not measured.
Annesi et al. (2013)	885–1,154 (based on measure) final-year preschoolers (mean age 4.4 ± 0.5 y), 86% African American	1.c	SCT	YMCA-affiliated preschool setting	Intervention group increased physical activity time and decreased BMI.	No masking
Black et al. (2010)	179 African American children aged 11–16 years	1.c	SCT, motivational interviewing	Home and community setting	Intervention group decreased BMI, decreased percentage body fat, decreased fruit/juice and snacks/desserts; no difference in other measures.	Not applicable
Cullen (2008)	55 African American girls aged 9–12 years and mothers	2.d	SCT	Home setting	Following intervention, girls reported increased parent modeling of eating fruit and vegetables.	No masking. Moderate instrument reliability. Long-term effects not measured.
Fitzgibbon et al. (2011)	618 children aged 3–5 years, 94% African American, and parents	1.c	SCT, self-determination theory	School setting	Intervention group increased moderate-to-vigorous physical activity; no difference in other measures.	No masking. Long-term effects not measured.

Table 4–3 What Conceptual Frameworks Guide Effective Childhood Obesity Prevention/ Amelioration?—cont'd

Citation	Subjects	Method*	Theory	Setting	Results	Rigor of Evidence
Klesges et al. (2010)	243 African American girls aged 8–10 years	1.c	SCT	Community setting	Intervention group increased water consumption, increased sweetened beverage intake less than control, decreased vegetable intake less than control; no difference in other measures.	No masking.
Leung et al. (2014)	57 children aged 8–16 years, 74% African American	1.c	SCT, transportation-imagery model	After-school setting	Intervention group more likely to choose a healthy snack.	No masking. Limited power. Long-term effects not measured.
Raman et al. (2010)	109 overweight African American children aged 9–11 years	2.c	SCT	Community setting	No difference between intervention and control group.	No masking.
Robinson et al. (2010)	225 African American girls aged 8–10 years	1.c	SCT	Community setting	No difference between intervention and control group.	Not applicable
Shin et al. (2015)	152 African American children aged 10–14 years	1.c	SCT	City recreation center and food outlet (corner stores, carryout) settings	Intervention group decreased BMI; no difference in food purchase or preparation.	No masking. Insufficient power (planned on 300 participants, but did get statistically significant results). Diffusion to control group not prevented.
Wilson et al. (2011)	1,422 children in 6th grade, 73% African American	1.c	SCT, self-determination theory	After-school setting	Intervention group increased moderate to vigorous physical activity at midintervention but not at postintervention.	Institutional Review Board (IRB) approval not stated. Masking only at baseline.

(*continued*)

Table 4–3 What Conceptual Frameworks Guide Effective Childhood Obesity Prevention/ Amelioration?—cont'd

Citation	Subjects	Method*	Theory	Setting	Results	Rigor of Evidence
Wright et al. (2013)	43 children aged 9–12 years and parents, 72% African American	1.c	SCT	Home setting	Intervention group decreased BMI, no difference in diet.	Insufficient power. No masking. Long-term effects not measured.
Moore (2009)	126 children aged 9–11 years, 93% African American	2.d	Self-care deficit nursing theory	School setting	Participants improved nutrition self-care practice, increased physical activity, decreased systolic blood pressure (SBP); no difference in nutrition knowledge or body mass percentile.	Pretest, post-test no control group.
Chomitz (2010)	1,858 children K-5, 37% African American	2.d	SEM, community-based participatory research over 3 years	Community, schools, families, individuals	BMI z-score decreased, physical activity increased in all race/ethnic groups, though African American and Latin had greater obesity at start.	Pretest, post-test no control group except prior obesity rates
Bibeau et al. (2008)	2 African American children age 10 and 12	2.c	TTM	Home (intervention) and primary care clinic (control)	Intervention child decreased BMI and waist circumference, increased total skinfold, decreased sedentary time, increased moderate physical activity time. No diet results due to underreporting.	Insufficient power. No masking. Long-term effects not measured.
Di Noia and Prochaska (2010)	549 African American adolescents aged 11–14 years	1.d	TTM	Community setting	Intervention group increased fruit and vegetable consumption.	No masking. Long-term effects not measured.

Table 4-3 What Conceptual Frameworks Guide Effective Childhood Obesity Prevention/Amelioration?—cont'd

Citation	Subjects	Method*	Theory	Setting	Results	Rigor of Evidence
Topp et al. (2009)	49 children in grades K–5, 92% African American; 33 children completed dietary analysis.	2.d	TTM	After-school setting	Participants improved cardiovascular fitness score, increased vegetable intake, decreased fruit juice intake; no difference in other measures.	No masking. Long-term effects not measured.

*Methods above according to Joanna Briggs Institute. (2014).
Level 1: Experimental Designs
Level 1.a: Systematic review of randomized controlled trials (RCTs)
Level 1.b: Systematic review of RCTs and other study designs
Level 1.c: RCT
Level 1.d: Pseudo-RCTs
Level 2: Quasi-Experimental Designs
Level 2.a: Systematic review of quasi-experimental studies
Level 2.b: Systematic review of quasi-experimental and other lower study designs
Level 2.c: Quasi-experimental prospectively controlled study
Level 2.d: Pretest and posttest or historic/retrospective control group study
Level 3: Observational and Analytic Designs
Level 3.a: Systematic review of comparable cohort studies
Level 3.b: Systematic review of comparable cohort and other lower study designs
Level 3.c: Cohort study with control group
Level 3.d: Case-controlled study
Level 3.e: Observational study without a control group
Level 4: Observational and Descriptive Studies
Level 4.a: Systematic review of descriptive studies
Level 4.b: Cross-sectional study
Level 4.c: Case series
Level 4.d: Case study
Level 5: Expert Opinion and Bench Research
Level 5.a: Systematic review of expert opinion
Level 5.b: Expert consensus
Level 5.c: Bench research/single expert opinion

theory, TPB, and SEM. Both studies found that participants decreased BMI, and Burnet et al. (2011) found that, while participants increased waist-to-hip ratio, amount of walking also increased.

SCT was the most frequently used theory, with 12 studies utilizing the framework to develop interventions targeting obesity among African American children. Of these studies, five found a decrease in BMI among participants (Annesi, 2010; Annesi, Smith, & Tennant, 2013; Black et al., 2010; Shin et al., 2015; Wright, Giger, Norris, & Suro, 2013), five found an improvement in diet outcomes (Black et al., 2010; Cullen & Thompson, 2008; Fitzgibbon et al., 2011; Klesges et al., 2010; Leung, Tripicchio, Agaronov, & Hou, 2014), four found an increase in physical activity (Annesi, 2010; Annesi et al., 2013; Fitzgibbon et al., 2011; Wilson et al., 2011), and one found a decrease in percent body fat (Black et al., 2010). However, Raman et al. (2010) and Robinson et al. (2010) did not find any significant results among participants following interventions based on SCT.

TTM was utilized to develop interventions in three studies (Bibeau, Moore, Caudill, & Topp, 2008; Di Noia & Prochaska, 2010; Topp et al., 2009). Bibeau et al. (2008) found a decrease in BMI and waist circumference, and an increase in physical activity. Topp et al. (2009) found an improvement in cardiovascular fitness and diet outcomes, and Di Noia and Prochaska (2010) found an increase in fruit and vegetable consumption.

Strengths and Limitations of the Body of Evidence

The meta-analysis and systematic review cited the need for further research, and the individual studies in Table 4–3 did not employ masking, which could bias the results in favor of the interventions. However, the preponderance of evidence suggests that theory-based interventions help to decrease BMI and increase physical activity and diet outcomes in African American youth.

Important Client Differences to Consider in Applying the Evidence in Practice

Having high fidelity to the interventions in practice would be very important, starting with assessing the students in each school with questions relevant to the given theory. Interventions were found for youth in elementary, middle, and high schools, so developmentally appropriate applications would also be important. Acceptability of the intervention to students, parents, and school personnel is essential. Because multiple theory-based interventions were effective, options can be presented for discussion and the intervention tailored for the needs of students in a particular school.

Areas Where Further Research Is Needed

For preadolescents, the meta-analysis-indicated replication is needed across age groups, ethnicities, and administration conditions (Annesi et al., 2013). For adolescents, the systematic review demonstrated that further research with more rigorous designs, better measures, and larger samples is needed (Bagherniya et al., 2018). The individual studies with African American youth indicated the need for masking of intervention status and longitudinal follow-up.

Recommendations for Practice

A systematic review of obesity interventions in elementary schools indicated that multicomponent interventions including environment, education, and physical approaches lasting 6 to 12 months seemed to be the most effective (Brown et al., 2016), so these elements should also be considered. It is important to realize that obesity occurs for many reasons beyond diet and physical activity. Children are exposed to toxic levels of stress that lead to obesity (Condon, Sadler, & Mayes, 2018), so working with parents to care for these children is very important.

Risks, Costs, and Benefits of Applying the Evidence

Lifestyle interventions of at least 26 hours were effective in reducing BMI without evidence of harm, so screening of children and adolescents and this type of intervention were recommended by a U.S. Preventive Services systematic review (O'Connor et al., 2017). Encouraging parents to focus on health and be involved, rather than urging weight control or criticizing the child's weight, was recommended in a meta-analysis to avoid child disordered eating (Gillison, Lorenc, Sleddens, Williams, & Atkinson, 2016).

Feasibility and System Issues to Consider in Applying the Evidence

Involving parents in obesity prevention and treatment for children is essential for success (Youfa et al., 2017). Schools have been effective environments, especially when multicomponent interventions have been implemented for 6 to 12 months (Brown et al., 2016). Getting parents involved can be challenging, so it is important to include them from the start in planning interventions. Schools also have academic outcomes that may supersede interest in health promotion, so it is also important to share the importance and likelihood of success with teachers and administrators in planning effective programs.

Key Stakeholders in Making Evidence-Based Practice Changes

Including children, parents, school staff members, school board members, and other policy makers is important to addressing the childhood obesity epidemic. For example, involvement in sports, along with a diet intervention, was found to be effective in reducing body weight for children and adolescents in a meta-analysis (Kim, Ok, Jeon, Kang, & Lee, 2017). When budgets at the federal, state, and local area are considered, sports and nutrition programs are often cut as groups strive to improve academic outcomes. It is important for nurses to participate regularly in policy forums and work with all stakeholders so that relevant evidence can inform policy decisions.

Safe and Effective Care Planning Implications

Childhood obesity is widely known to be a problem, and sometimes adults and children emphasize weight in a way that stigmatizes those affected and makes attaining and sustaining a healthy weight even more difficult. Nurses need to identify weight stigma clearly as a problem early in planning processes and throughout interventions. Comments about another person's weight are not helpful. Disordered eating, fad diets, unsafe diet pills, and other ineffective approaches are often tried by those whose weight is higher than they might perceive to be socially desirable. As many as 25% of individuals who are overweight or obese may be affected by disordered eating (He, Cai, & Fan, 2017).

Health promotion efforts need to focus on health and emphasize healthy eating and physical activity, regardless of weight status, which is the evidence-based approach. Physical activity interventions in meta-analyses have been found to improve aspects of disordered eating (Ruotsalainen, Kyngäs, Tammelin, & Kääriäinen, 2015) as well as reduce body fat (Stoner et al., 2016). The effects of diet interventions require further study (Vissers, Hens, Hansen, & Taeymans, 2016).

Interprofessional Health Education Implications

Schools were found to be an effective venue for obesity prevention in a meta-analysis of randomized controlled trials (Tidwell, Hung, & Hall, 2016). Involving stakeholders requires a multidisciplinary approach. Physical activity interventions have been found to improve math performance and memory in one meta-analysis, but effects on academic performance need to be studied further (Martin, Saunders, Shenkin, & Sproule, 2014). Routine surveillance and counseling in clinic settings has been found only marginally effective in addressing the childhood obesity epidemic (Shaughnessy, 2017; Sim, Lebow, Zhen, Koball, & Murad, 2016), so interprofessional efforts including parents and a wide range of professionals (Kitzmann et al., 2010) continue to be needed.

USEFUL RESOURCES

These resources can help nurses understand and implement various HPMs.

Assessment Tools

- A 52-item instrument is available to measure HPM constructs at https://deepblue.lib.umich.edu/bitstream/handle/2027.42/85349/HPLP_II-English_Version.pdf?sequence=3&isAllowed=y. Clinical questions based on the model (Pender, 2011), which aids translation to practice, can also be found at this site.
- The Breast Cancer Belief Scale (Champion, 1999) has 38 questions based on HBM constructs: perceived susceptibility to breast cancer, perceived seriousness of breast cancer, perceived benefits of mammograms, and perceived barriers to mammograms. A five-point Likert scale ranges from 1 (strongly disagree) to 5 (strongly agree). Reliability and validity among white women and African American women demonstrated Cronbach's alpha for the subscales from .75 to .93 and test-retest reliability from .45 to .70. Exploratory factor analysis yielded three factors: perceived susceptibility, perceived benefits, and perceived barriers to mammography accounting for 54% of the variance. Champion's Health Belief scale was translated and back-translated, and culturally appropriate times were added for use with 250 Thai American women to form the Thai Breast Cancer Belief Scale (Kumsuk et al., 2012). Cronbach's alpha ranged from .77 to .90, and 45.8% of the variance was explained in four factors based in HBM of this 41-item scale.
- Applications for IBM elicitation and interventions are available at http://www.med.upenn.edu/hbhe4/part2-ch4-application-non-intervent.shtml
- The University of Rhode Island Change Assessment (URICA) scale is an effective tool for TTM that has been used to measure change for a variety of health and addictive behaviors such as alcohol treatment and smoking cessation. It can be found at https://pubs.niaaa.nih.gov/publications/AssessingAlcohol/InstrumentPDFs/75_URICA.pdf

Client Education Materials

Web sites can be useful for client education; however, it is important to ensure that the links provided remain active. In choosing Web sites, review the content for currency and accuracy. A few Web sites that the authors believe are useful have been listed below. The links were current at the time of submission.

- Several theories and applications are provided at https://www.ruralhealthinfo.org/toolkits/health-promotion/2/theories-and-models
- Theory of planned behavior: https://people.umass.edu/aizen/tpb.html
- Nursing theories: http://currentnursing.com/nursing_theory/
- Health promotion model manual: https://deepblue.lib.umich.edu/handle/2027.42/85350

- Transtheoretical model: https://web.uri.edu/cprc/about-ttm/
- National Institutes of Health, Office of Behavioral & Social Sciences Research: http://www.esourceresearch.org/tabid/724/default.aspx

KEY POINTS

- Several meta-analyses and studies indicate that theory-based interventions are more effective than those without a theoretical basis; however, many interventions are tested without mention of a guiding theory.
- Studies have been done in a wide range of health promotion areas for the theories included in this chapter. When clinical practice changes are based on the evidence, notions (also known as individual theories) that providers have that may not be supported by evidence have a better chance of being changed.
- Theories help direct clinical translation of the evidence. Interview guides for individuals, families, and communities can be developed based on major components of the theory. As with other assessment formats, this helps to avoid missing important areas for assessment.
- Theories also guide intervention so that fidelity to the evidence is sustained. Improvements in theory components can be measured following the intervention.

Check Your Understanding

1. HPM:
   A. Is similar to HBM because benefits, barriers, and self-efficacy are included in both
   B. Differs from HBM because its focus is on promoting health rather than mainly prevention of illness
   C. Is the only model discussed that was developed by a nurse
   D. All of the above
   E. B and C only
2. The constructs in HBM that are associated most often with outcomes are:
   A. Benefits and barriers
   B. Perceived susceptibility
   C. Perceived seriousness
   D. Cues to action
   E. C and D only
3. The most effective way to build self-efficacy for a walking program is:
   A. Telling clients sternly that they must walk or they will be in serious trouble
   B. Asking about walking the client has already engaged in
   C. Providing contact information for a walking group
   D. Asking how the client felt the last time she or he walked
4. When using TTM to help with smoking cessation:
   A. Instruct the person in the precontemplation stage to stop smoking tomorrow.
   B. Help the person in the precontemplation stage become aware of the pros and cons of stopping.
   C. Help people in the preparation stage to develop a contract for quitting.
   D. A and B only
   E. B and C only
5. When using the PRECEDE-PROCEED model, a nurse would:
   A. Inform the group of the action plan determined from assessment and implement it.
   B. Involve members of the group in doing the assessment, creating the plan, and implementing and evaluating it.
   C. Use data to inform the group of important health risks they face and evidence regarding options.
   D. A and B only
   E. B and C only

See "Reflections on Check Your Understanding" at the end of the book for answers.

REFERENCES

Adebayo, O. W., & Gonzalez-Guarda, R. M. (2017). Factors associated with HIV testing in youth in the United States: An integrative review. *Journal of the Association of Nurses in AIDS Care, 28*(3), 342–362. doi:10.1016/j.jana.2016.11.006

Ahmed, S., Swaine, B., Milot, M., Gaudet, C., Poldma, T., Bartlett, G., . . . Kehayia, E. (2017). Creating an inclusive mall environment with the PRECEDE-PROCEED model: A living lab case study. *Disability & Rehabilitation, 39*(21), 2198–2206. doi:10.1080/09638288.2016.1219401

Ajzen, I. (1991). The theory of planned behavior. *Organizational Behavior and Human Decision Processes, 50*, 179–211.

Ajzen, I. (2016). Theory of planned behavior. Retrieved from https://people.umass.edu/aizen/tpb.html

Andrew, B., Mullan, B., Wit, J., Monds, L., Todd, J., & Kothe, E. (2016). Does the theory of planned behaviour explain condom use behavior among men who have sex with men? A meta-analytic review of the literature. *AIDS & Behavior, 20*(12), 2834–2844. doi:10.1007/s10461-016-1314-0

Annesi, J. J. (2010). Initial body mass index and free-time physical activity moderate effects of the youth fit for life treatment in African-American pre-adolescents. *Perceptual & Motor Skills, 110*(3), 789–800. doi:10.2466/PMS.110.3.789-800

Annesi, J. J., Smith, A. E., & Tennant, G. A. (2013). Effects of a cognitive-behaviorally based physical activity treatment for 4- and 5-year-old children attending US preschools. *International Journal of Behavioral Medicine, 20*(4), 562–566.

Asarnow, J. R., Rozenman, M., Wiblin, J., & Zeltzer, L. (2015). Integrated medical-behavioral care compared with usual primary care for child and adolescent behavioral health: A meta-analysis. *Journal of the American Medical Association Pediatrics, 169*(10), 929–937. doi:10.1001/jamapediatrics.2015.1141

Bagherniya, M., Taghipour, A., Sharma, M., Sahebkar, A., Contento, I. R., Keshavarz, S. A., . . . Safarian, M. (2018). Obesity intervention programs among adolescents using social cognitive theory: A systematic literature review. *Health Education Research, 33*(1), 26–39. doi:10.1093/her/cyx079

Bakan, A. B., & Erci, B. (2018). Comparison of the effect of trainings based on the transtheoretical model and the health belief model on nurses' smoking cessation. *International Journal of Caring Sciences*, 213–224.

Bandura, A. (1977). Self-efficacy: Toward a unifying theory of behavior change. *Psychological Review, 84*(2), 191–215.

Bandura, A. (2004). Health promotion by social cognitive means. *Health Education and Behavior, 31*, 143–164.

Barnett, L., Lai, S., Veldman, S., Hardy, L., Cliff, D., Morgan, P., . . . Okely, A. (2016). Correlates of gross motor competence in children and adolescents: A systematic review and meta-analysis. *Sports Medicine, 46*(11), 1663–1688. doi:10.1007/s40279-016-0495-z

Becker, M. H. (1974). The health belief model and sick role behavior. *Health Education Monographs, 2*(4), 409–419.

Bibeau, W. S., Moore, J. B., Caudill, P., & Topp, R. (2008). Case study of a transtheoretical case management approach to addressing childhood obesity. *Journal of Pediatric Nursing, 23*(2), 92–100. doi:10.1016/j.pedn.2007.08.006

Black, M. M., Hager, E. R., Le, K., Anliker, J., Arteaga, S. S., DiClemente, C., . . . Wang, Y. (2010). Challenge! Health promotion/obesity prevention mentorship model among urban, Black adolescents. *Pediatrics, 126*(2), 280–288. doi:10.1542/peds.2009-1832

Bronfenbrenner, U. (1979). *The ecology of human development: Experiments by nature and design* (1st ed.). Cambridge, MA: Harvard University Press.

Bronfenbrenner, U. (1994). Ecological models of human development. In T. Husen & T. N. Postlethwaite (Eds.), *The international encyclopedia of education* (Vol. 2, pp. 1643–1647). New York: Elsevier Science.

Brown, E. C., Buchan, D. S., Baker, J. S., Wyatt, F. B., Bocalini, D. S., & Kilgore, L. (2016). A systematized review of primary school whole class child obesity interventions: Effectiveness, characteristics, and strategies. *BioMed Research International, 2016*, 1–15. doi:10.1155/2016/4902714

Burnet, D. L., Plaut, A. J., Wolf, S. A., Huo, D., Solomon, M. C., Dekayie, G., . . . Chin, M. H. (2011). Reach-out: A family-based diabetes prevention program for African American youth. *Journal of the National Medical Association, 103*(3), 269–277.

Cadogan, C., Ryan, C. A., Patton, D., & Hughes, C. (2017). Theory-based interventions to improve medication adherence in older adults prescribed polypharmacy: A systematic review. *Drugs & Aging, 34*(2), 97–113. doi:10.1007/s40266-016-0426-6

Carpenter, C. J. (2010). A meta-analysis of the effectiveness of health belief model variables in predicting behavior. *Health Communication, 25*(8), 661–669. doi:10.1080/10410236.2010.521906

Champion, V. (1999). Revised susceptibility, benefits, and barriers scale for mammography screening. *Research in Nursing and Health, 22*, 341–348.

Chappell, K. B., Richards, K. C., & Barnett, S. D. (2014). New graduate nurse transition programs and clinical leadership skills in novice RNs. *Journal of Nursing Administration, 44*(12), 659–668. doi:10.1097/NNA.0000000000000144

Chomitz, V. R., McGowan, R. J., Wendel, J. M., Williams, S. A., Cabral, H. J., King, S. E., . . . Hacker, K. A. (2010). Healthy Living Cambridge Kids: A community-based participatory effort to promote healthy weight and fitness. *Obesity* (19307381), 18, S45–53. doi:10.1038/oby.2009.431

Choudhry, S., McClinton-Powell, L., Solomon, M., Davis, D., Lipton, R., Darukhanavala, A., . . . Burnet, D. L. (2011). Power-up: A collaborative after-school program to prevent obesity in African American children. *Progress in Community Health Partnerships, 5*(4), 363–373.

Clary Muronda, V. (2016). The culturally diverse nursing student. *Journal of Transcultural Nursing, 27*(4), 400–412. doi:10.1177/1043659615595867

Cole, K. A., & Gaspar, P. M. (2015). Implementation of an epilepsy self-management protocol. *Journal of Neuroscience Nursing, 47*(1), 3–9. doi:10.1097/JNN.0000000000000105

Commodore-Mensah, Y., Sampah, M., Berko, C., Cudjoe, J., Abu-Bonsrah, N., Obisesan, O., . . . Himmelfarb, C. (2016). The Afro-Cardiac study: Cardiovascular disease risk and acculturation in West African immigrants in the United States: Rationale and study design. *Journal of Immigrant & Minority Health, 18*(6), 1301–1308. doi:10.1007/s10903-015-0291-0

Como, J. M. (2018). Health literacy and health status in people with chronic heart failure. *Clinical Nurse Specialist: The Journal for Advanced Nursing Practice, 32*(1), 29–42. doi:10.1097/NUR.0000000000000346

Condon, E. M., Sadler, L. S., & Mayes, L. C. (2018). Toxic stress and protective factors in multi-ethnic school age children: A research protocol. *Research in Nursing & Health, 41*(2), 97–106. doi:10.1002/nur.21851

Condran, B., Gahagan, C., & Isfeld-Kiely, H. (2017). A scoping review of social media as a platform for multi-level sexual health promotion interventions. *Canadian Journal of Human Sexuality, 26*(1), 26–37. doi:10.3138/cjhs.261-A1

Conner, M., McEachan, R., Taylor, N., O'Hara, J., & Lawton, R. (2015). Role of affective attitudes and anticipated affective reactions in predicting health behaviors. *Health Psychology, 34*(6), 642–652. doi:10.1037/hea0000143

Cooper, D. B., Bunner, A. E., Kennedy, J. E., Ballin, V., Tate, D. F., Eapen, B. C., & Jaramillo, C. A. (2015). Treatment of persistent post-concussive symptoms after mild traumatic brain injury: A systematic review of cognitive rehabilitation and behavioral health interventions in military service members and veterans. *Brain Imaging and Behavior, 9*, 403-420. doi:10.1007/s11682-015-9440-2

Corace, K. M., Srigley, J. A., Hargadon, D. P., Yu, D., MacDonald, T. K., Fabrigar, L. R., & Garber, G. E. (2016). Using behavior change frameworks to improve healthcare worker influenza vaccination rates: A systematic review. *Vaccine, 34*(28), 3235–3242. doi:10.1016/j.vaccine.2016.04.071

Cullen, K. W., & Thompson, D. (2008). Feasibility of an 8-week African American Web-based pilot program promoting healthy eating behaviors: Family eats. *American Journal of Health Behavior, 32*(1), 40–51.

Dada, Y. M. (2014). *Evidence-based health care worker influenza vaccination program.* (D.N.P.), Walden University. Retrieved from http://0-search.ebscohost.com.libus.csd.mu.edu/login.aspx?direct=true&db=c8h&AN=109751733&site=ehost-live

Dempster, N. R., Wildman, B. G., Masterson, T. L., & Omlor, G. J. (2018). Understanding treatment adherence with the health belief model in children with cystic fibrosis. *Health Education & Behavior, 45*(3), 435–443. doi:10.1177/1090198117736346

Dinkel, D., Tibbits, M., Hanigan, E., Nielsen, K., Jorgensen, L., & Grant, K. (2017). Healthy families: A family-based community intervention to address childhood obesity. *Journal of Community Health Nursing, 34*(4), 109–202. doi:10.1080/07370016.2017.1369808

Di Noia, J., & Prochaska, J. O. (2010). Mediating variables in a transtheoretical model dietary intervention program. *Health Education & Behavior, 37*(5), 753–762.

Duijts, S. F. A., Bleiker, E. M. A., Paalman, C. H., & Beek, A. J. (2017). A behavioural approach in the development of work-related interventions for cancer survivors: An exploratory review. *European Journal of Cancer Care, 26*(5). doi:10.1111/ecc.12545

Duncan, S. E., & Annunziato, R. A. (2018). Barriers to self-management behaviors in college students with food allergies. *Journal of American College Health, 66*(5), 331–339. doi:10.1080/07448481.2018.1431898

Durks, D., Fernandez-Llimos, F., Hossain, L. N., Franco-Trigo, L., Benrimoj, S. I., & Sabater-Hernández, D. (2017). Use of intervention mapping to enhance health care professional practice: A systematic review. *Health Education & Behavior, 44*(4), 524–535. doi:10.1177/1090198117709885

Dyson, Y. D., Davis, S. K., Counts-Spriggs, M., & Smith-Bankhead, N. (2017). Gender, race, class, and health: Interrogating the intersection of substance abuse and HIV through a cultural lens. *Affilia: Journal of Women & Social Work, 32*(4), 531–542. doi:10.1177/0886109917713975

Ee, I. B., Hagedoorn, M., Slaets, J. P. J., & Smits, C. H. M. (2017). Patient navigation and activation interventions for elderly patients with cancer: A systematic review. *European Journal of Cancer Care, 26*(2). doi:10.1111/ecc.12621

Esposito, E. M. (2016). Ambulatory care nurse-sensitive indicators series: Patient engagement as a nurse-sensitive indicator in ambulatory care. *Nursing Economic$, 34*(6), 303–306.

Fernández-Gutiérrez, M., Bas-Sarmiento, P., Albar-Marín, M. J., Paloma-Castro, O., & Romero-Sánchez, J. M. (2018). Health literacy interventions for immigrant populations: A systematic review. *International Nursing Review, 65*(1), 54–64. doi:10.1111/inr.12373

Fishbein, M., & Ajzen, I. (1975). *Belief, attitude, intention, and behavior: An introduction to theory and research.* Reading, MA: Addison-Wesley.

Fishbein, M., & Ajzen, I. (2010). *Predicting and changing behavior: The Reasoned Action approach.* New York: Psychology Press (Taylor & Francis).

Fitzgibbon, M., Stolley, M., Schiffer, L., Braunschweig, C., Gomez, S., Van Horn, L., & Dyer, A. (2011). Hip-hop to health jr. obesity prevention effectiveness trial: Postintervention results. *Obesity, 19*(5), 994–1003.

Fleming, P., Watson, S. J., Patouris, E., Bartholomew, K. J., & Zizzo, D. J. (2017). Why do people file share unlawfully? A systematic review, meta-analysis and panel study. *Computers in Human Behavior, 72*, 535–548. doi:10.1016/j.chb.2017.02.014

Franklin, A. E., & Lee, C. S. (2014). Effectiveness of simulation for improvement in self-efficacy among novice nurses: A meta-analysis. *Journal of Nursing Education, 53*(11), 607–614. doi:10.3928/01484834-20141023-03

Freyer-Adam, J., Baumann, S., Haberecht, K., Tobschall, S., Bischof, G., John, U., & Gaertner, B. (2018). In-person alcohol counseling versus computer-generated feedback: Results from a randomized controlled trial. *Health Psychology, 37*(1), 70–80. doi:10.1037/hea0000556

Gacheru, T. G. (2017). *A developmental project focusing on young adult Hispanic-Americans.* (D.N.P.), Walden University. Retrieved from http://0-search.ebscohost.com.libus.csd.mu.edu/login.aspx?direct=true&db=c8h&AN=124664856&site=ehost-live

Garcia, D. S. (2016). Evaluation of 3 behavioral theories for application in health promotion strategies for Hispanic women. *Advances in Nursing Science, 39*(2), 165–180. doi:10.1097/ANS.0000000000000116

Garg, S., Kim, L., Whitaker, M., O'Halloran, A., Cummings, C., Holstein, R., . . . Sue, K. (2020). Hospitalization rates and characteristics of patients hospitalized with laboratory-confirmed coronavirus disease 2019 - COVID-NET, 14 States, March 1-30, 2020. *MMWR Morbidity and Mortality Weekly Report, 69*, 458–464.

Gielen, A. C., McDonald, E. M., & Gary, T. (2008). Using the PRECEDE-PROCEED planning model to apply health behavior theories. In K. Glanz, B. K. Rimer, & F. M. Lewis (Eds.), *Health behavior and health education: Theory, research, and practice* (4th ed., pp. 407–433). San Francisco, CA: Jossey-Bass.

Gillison, F. B., Lorenc, A. B., Sleddens, E. F. C., Williams, S. L., & Atkinson, L. (2016). Can it be harmful for parents to talk to their child about their weight? A meta-analysis. *Preventive Medicine, 93*, 135–146. doi:10.1016/j.ypmed.2016.10.010

Green, L. W., & Kreuter, M. W. (1991). *Health promotion planning: An educational and environmental approach.* Mountain View, CA: Mayfield Publishing.

Green, L. W., & Kreuter, M. W. (2005). *Health program planning: An educational and ecological approach* (4th ed.). New York, NY: McGraw-Hill.

Greene, J., Hibbard, J. H., Sacks, R., Overton, V., & Parrotta, C. D. (2015). When patient activation levels change, health outcomes and costs change, too. *Health Affairs, 34*(3), 430–437. doi:10.1377/hlthaff.2014.0452

Gretebeck, K. A., Bailey, T., & Gretebeck, R. J. (2017). A minimal contact diet and physical activity intervention for white-collar workers. *Workplace Health & Safety, 65*(9), 417–423. doi:10.1177/2165079916674483

Grimm, K. L. (2018). Prelicensure employment and student nurse self-efficacy. *Journal for Nurses in Professional Development, 34*(2), 60–66. doi:10.1097/NND.0000000000000431

Guo, J. L., Wang, T. F., Liao, J. Y., & Huang, C. M. (2016). Efficacy of the theory of planned behavior in predicting breastfeeding: Meta-analysis and structural equation modeling. *Applied Nursing Research, 29*(1), 37–42. doi:10.1016/j.apnr.2015.03.016

Hackman, C. L., & Knowlden, A. P. (2014). Theory of reasoned action and theory of planned behavior-based dietary interventions in adolescents and young adults: A systematic review. *Adolescent Health, Medicine and Therapeutics, 5*, 101–114. doi:10.2147/AHMT.S56207

Hagger, M. S., Polet, J., & Lintunen, T. (2018). The reasoned action approach applied to health behavior: Role of past behavior and tests of some key moderators using meta-analytic structural equation modeling. *Social Science & Medicine, 213*, 85–94. doi:10.1016/j.socscimed.2018.07.038

Hall, H., Leach, M., Brosnan, C., & Collins, M. (2017). Nurses' attitudes towards complementary therapies: A systematic review and meta-synthesis. *International Journal of Nursing Studies, 69*, 47–56. doi:10.1016/j.ijnurstu.2017.01.008

Harriger, D., Lu, W., McKyer, E. L. J., Pruitt, B. E., & Goodson, P. (2014). Assessment of school wellness policies implementation by benchmarking against diffusion of innovation framework. *Journal of School Health, 84*(4), 275–283. doi:10.1111/josh.12145

Harrison, A. L., Taylor, N. F., Shields, N., & Frawley, H. C. (2018). Attitudes, barriers and enablers to physical activity in pregnant women: A systematic review. *Journal of Physiotherapy, 64*(1), 24–32. doi:10.1016/j.jphys.2017.11.012

Hazavehei, S., & Afshari, M. (2016). The role of nutritional interventions in increasing fruit and vegetable intake in the elderlies: A systematic review. *Aging Clinical & Experimental Research, 28*(4), 583–598. doi:10.1007/s40520-015-0454-9

He, J., Cai, Z., & Fan, X. (2017). Prevalence of binge and loss of control eating among children and adolescents with overweight and obesity: An exploratory meta-analysis. *International Journal of Eating Disorders, 50*(2), 91–103. doi:10.1002/eat.22661

Hibbard, J. H. (2017). Patient activation and the use of information to support informed health decisions. *Patient Education & Counseling, 100*(1), 5–7. doi:10.1016/j.pec.2016.07.006

Hibbard, J. H., & Greene, J. (2013). What the evidence shows about patient activation: Better health outcomes and care experiences; fewer data on costs. *Health Affairs, 32*(2), 207–214. doi:10.1377/hlthaff.2012.1061

Hibbard, J. H., & Mahoney, E. (2010). Toward a theory of patient and consumer activation. *Patient Education and Counseling, 78*(3), 377–381. doi:10.1016/j.pec.2009.12.015

Ho, A. Y. K., Berggren, I., & Dahlborg-Lyckhage, E. (2010). Diabetes empowerment related to Pender's health promotion model: A meta-synthesis. *Nursing & Health Sciences, 12*(2), 259–267. doi:10.1111/j.1442-2018.2010.00517.x

Hodges, B. C. (2017). Health promotion at the ballpark. *Health Promotion Practice, 18*(2), 229–237. doi:10.1177/1524839916663684

Ickes, M. J., McMullen, J., Pflug, C., & Westgate, P. M. (2016). Impact of a university-based program on obese college students' physical activity behaviors, attitudes, and self-efficacy. *American Journal of Health Education, 47*(1), 47–55. doi:10.1080/19325037.2015.1111178

Institute of Medicine. (2002). *Speaking of health: Assessing health communication strategies for diverse populations.* Washington, DC: National Academies Press.

Janz, N. K., & Becker, M. H. (1984). The health belief model: A decade later. *Health Education Quarterly, 11*, 1–47. doi:10.1177/109019818401100101

Joanna Briggs Institute. (2014). *Levels of evidence for effectiveness.* Retrieved from https://joannabriggs.org/sites/default/files/2019-05/JBI-Levels-of-evidence_2014_0.pdf

Kan, T., & Zhang, J. (2018). Factors influencing seasonal influenza vaccination behaviour among elderly people: A systematic review. *Public Health, 156*, 67–78. doi:10.1016/j.puhe.2017.12.007

Kelly, S., Stephens, J., Hoying, J., McGovern, C., Melnyk, B. M., & Militello, L. (2017). A systematic review of mediators of physical activity, nutrition, and screen time in adolescents: Implications for future research and clinical practice. *Nursing Outlook, 65*(5), 530–548. doi:10.1016/j.outlook.2017.07.011

Kim, K., Ok, G., Jeon, S., Kang, M., & Lee, S. (2017). Sport-based physical activity intervention on body weight in children and adolescents: A meta-analysis. *Journal of Sports Sciences, 35*(4), 369–376. doi:10.1080/02640414.2016.1166389

King, J. L., Merten, J. W., Wong, T.-J., & Pomeranz, J. L. (2018). Applying a social-ecological framework to factors related to nicotine replacement therapy for adolescent smoking cessation. *American Journal of Health Promotion, 32*(5), 1291–1303. doi:10.1177/0890117117718422

Kirscht, J. P. (1974). The health belief model and illness behavior. *Health Education & Behavior, 2*(4), 387–408. doi:10.1177/109019817400200406

Kitzmann, K. M., Dalton, W. T., III, Stanley, C. M., Beech, B. M., Reeves, T. P., Buscemi, J., . . . Midgett, E. L. (2010). Lifestyle interventions for youth who are overweight: A meta-analytic review. *Health Psychology, 29*(1), 91–101. doi:10.1037/a0017437

Klesges, R. C., Obarzanek, E., Kumanyika, S., Murray, D. M., Klesges, L. M., Relyea, G. E., . . . Slawson, D. L. (2010). The Memphis girls' health enrichment multi-site studies (GEMS): An evaluation of the efficacy of a 2-year obesity prevention program in African American girls. *Archives of Pediatrics & Adolescent Medicine, 164*(11), 1007–1014.

Krok-Schoen, J. L., Oliveri, J. M., Young, G. S., Katz, M. L., Tatum, C. M., & Paskett, E. D. (2016). Evaluating the stage of change model to a cervical cancer screening intervention among Ohio Appalachian women. *Women & Health, 56*(4), 468–486. doi:10.1080/03630242.2015.1101736

Kumsuk, S., Flick, L. H., & Schneider, J. K. (2012). Development of the Thai Breast Cancer Belief Scale for Thai immigrants in the United States. *Journal of Nursing Measurement, 20*(2), 123–141.

Kuo, C.-C., Lin, C.-C., & Tsai, F.-M. (2014). Effectiveness of empowerment-based self-management interventions on patients with chronic metabolic diseases: A systematic review and meta-analysis. *Worldviews on Evidence-Based Nursing, 11*(5), 301–315. doi:10.1111/wvn.12066

Lam, W., Dawson, A., & Fowler, C. (2017). Approaches to better engage parent-child in health home-visiting programmes: A content analysis. *Journal of Child Health Care, 21*(1), 94–102. doi:10.1177/1367493516653260

Lavoie, P., Michaud, C., Bélisle, M., Boyer, L., Gosselin, É., Grondin, M., . . . Pepin, J. (2018). Learning theories and tools for the assessment of core nursing competencies in simulation: A theoretical review. *Journal of Advanced Nursing, 74*(2), 239–250. doi:10.1111/jan.13416

Lee-Lin, F., Nguyen, T., Pedhiwala, N., Dieckmann, N. F., & Menon, U. (2016). A longitudinal examination of stages of change model applied to mammography screening. *Western Journal of Nursing Research, 38*(4), 441–458. doi:10.1177/0193945915618398

Leung, M. M., Tripicchio, G., Agaronov, A., & Hou, N. (2014). Manga comic influences snack selection in Black and Hispanic New York City youth. *Journal of Nutrition Education and Behavior, 46*(2), 142–147.

Lewis, J. (2014). A systematic literature review of the relationship between stretching and athletic injury prevention. *Orthopaedic Nursing, 33*(6), 312–322. doi:10.1097/NOR.0000000000000097

Lindsay, A. C., Greaney, M. L., Wallington, S. F., Mesa, T., & Salas, C. F. (2017). A review of early influences on physical activity and sedentary behaviors of preschool-age children in high-income countries. *Journal for Specialists in Pediatric Nursing, 22*(3). doi:10.1111/jspn.12182

Lorenc, T., Jamal, F., & Cooper, C. (2013). Resource provision and environmental change for the prevention of skin cancer: Systematic review of qualitative evidence from high-income countries. *Health Promotion International, 28*(3), 345–356. doi:heapro/das015

MacKinnon, K. R., Tarasoff, L. A., & Kia, H. (2016). Predisposing, reinforcing, and enabling factors of trans-positive clinical behavior change: A summary of the literature. *International Journal of Transgenderism, 17*(2), 83–92. doi:10.1080/15532739.2016.1179156

Martin, A., Saunders, D. H., Shenkin, S. D., & Sproule, J. (2014). Lifestyle intervention for improving school achievement in overweight or obese children and adolescents. *Cochrane Database of Systematic Reviews* (3) (1469-493X [Electronic])

McDaniel, J. T. (2018). Prevalence of chronic obstructive pulmonary disease: County-level risk factors based on the social ecological model. *Perspectives in Public Health, 1398*(4), 200–208. doi:10.1177/1757913918772598

McDermott, M. S., Oliver, M., Svenson, A., Simnadis, T., Beck, E. J., Coltman, T., . . . Sharma, R. (2015). The theory of planned behaviour and discrete food choices: A systematic review and meta-analysis. *International Journal of Behavioral Nutrition and Physical Activity, 12*(162). doi:10.1186/s12966-015-0324-z

McIntosh, J. R. D., Jay, S., Hadden, N., & Whittaker, P. J. (2017). Do e-health interventions improve physical activity in young people: A systematic review. *Public Health, 148*, 140–148. doi:10.1016/j.puhe.2017.04.001

McLeroy, K. R., Bibeau, D., Steckler, A., & Glanz, K. (1988). An ecological perspective on health promotion programs. *Health Education Quarterly, 15*(4), 351–377.

McMullen, J., Ickes, M., Noland, M., Erwin, H., & Helme, D. (2017). Development of "College CHEF," a campus-based culinary nutrition program. *American Journal of Health Education, 48*(1), 22–31. doi:10.1080/19325037.2016.1250016

Mikhail, J. N., & Nemeth, L. S. (2016). Trauma center based youth violence prevention programs. *Trauma, Violence & Abuse, 17*(5), 500–519. doi:10.1177/1524838015584373

Mirza, M., Krischer, A., Stolley, M., Magaña, S., & Martin, M. (2018). Review of parental activation interventions for parents of children with special health care needs. *Child: Care, Health & Development, 44*(3), 401–426. doi:10.1111/cch.12554

Moeini, B., Hazavehei, S. M. M., Shahrabadi, R., Faradmal, J., Ahmadpanah, M., Dashti, S., . . . Mehri, A. (2018). The effectiveness of cognitive-behavioral stress-management training on the readiness for substance use treatment in Iran. *Journal of Substance Use, 23*(4), 371–376. doi:10.1080/14659891.2018.1436597

Monaghan, T., Dinour, L., Liou, D., & Shefchik, M. (2018). Factors influencing the eating practices of hospital nurses during their shifts. *Workplace Health & Safety, 66*(7), 331–342. doi:10.1177/2165079917737557

Montano, D., & Kasprzyk, D. (2015). Theory of reasoned action, theory of planned behavior, and the integrated behavioral model. In K. Glanz, B. K. Rimer, & B. Viswanath (Eds.), *Health behavior theory, research, and practice* (5th ed., pp. 95–124). San Francisco, CA: Jossey-Bass.

Moore, J. B., Pawloski, L. R., Goldberg, P., Oh, K. M., Stoehr, A., & Baghi, H. (2009). Childhood obesity study: A pilot study of the effect of the nutrition education program Color My Pyramid. *Journal of School Nursing, 25*(3), 230–239. doi:10.1177/1059840509333325

Morgan, H. M., Entwistle, V. A., Cribb, A., Christmas, S., Owens, J., Skea, Z. C., & Watt, I. S. (2017). We need to talk about purpose: A critical interpretive synthesis of health and social care professionals' approaches to self-management support for people with long-term conditions. *Health Expectations, 20*(2), 243–259. doi:10.1111/hex.12453

Munson, S. O., Barabasz, A. F., & Barabasz, M. (2018). Ability of hypnosis to facilitate movement through stages of change for smoking cessation. *International Journal of Clinical & Experimental Hypnosis, 66*(1), 56–82. doi:10.1080/00207144.2018.1396115

Nguyen, B., Kornman, K., & Baur, L. (2011). A review of electronic interventions for prevention and treatment of overweight and obesity in young people. *Obesity Reviews, 12*(5), e298–e314.

Nguyen-Truong, C. K. Y., Pedhiwala, N., Nguyen, V., Le, C., Le, T. V., Lau, C., . . . Lee-Lin, F. (2017). Feasibility of a multicomponent breast health education intervention for

Vietnamese American immigrant women. *Oncology Nursing Forum, 44*(5), 615–625. doi:10.1188/17.ONF.615-625

Ntoumanis, N., Ng, J., Barkoukis, V., & Backhouse, S. (2014). Personal and psychosocial predictors of doping use in physical activity settings: A meta-analysis. *Sports Medicine, 44*(11), 1603–1624. doi:10.1007/s40279-014-0240-4

O'Connor, E. A., Evans, C. V., Burda, B. U., Walsh, E. S., Eder, M., Lozano, P., & O'Connor, E. A. (2017). Screening for obesity and intervention for weight management in children and adolescents: Evidence report and systematic review for the US Preventive Services Task Force. *JAMA, 317*(23), 2427–2444. doi:10.1001/jama.2017.0332

O'Driscoll, T., Banting, L., Borkoles, E., Eime, R., & Polman, R. (2014). A systematic literature review of sport and physical activity participation in culturally and linguistically diverse (CALD) migrant populations. *Journal of Immigrant & Minority Health, 16*(3), 515–530. doi:10.1007/s10903-013-9857-x

Paalosalo-Harris, K., & Skirton, H. (2017). Mixed method systematic review: The relationship between breast cancer risk perception and health-protective behaviour in women with family history of breast cancer. *Journal of Advanced Nursing, 73*(4), 760–774. doi:10.1111/jan.13158

Paige, S. R., Alber, J. M., Stellefson, M. L., & Krieger, J. L. (2018). Missing the mark for patient engagement: mHealth literacy strategies and behavior change processes in smoking cessation apps. *Patient Education & Counseling, 101*(5), 951–955. doi:10.1016/j.pec.2017.11.006

Palumbo, R. (2017). Keeping candles lit: The role of concierge medicine in the future of primary care. *Health Services Management Research, 30*(2), 121–128. doi:10.1177/0951484816682397

Park, D.-I., Choi-Kwon, S., & Han, K. (2015). Health behaviors of Korean female nursing students in relation to obesity and osteoporosis. *Nursing Outlook, 63*(4), 504–511. doi:10.1016/j.outlook.2015.02.001

Pender, N. J. (2011). Health promotion model manual. Retrieved from https://deepblue.lib.umich.edu/bitstream/handle/2027.42/85350/HEALTH_PROMOTION_MANUAL_Rev_5-2011.pdf?sequence=1&isAllowed=y

Peterson Owen, R., & Wanzer, L. (2014). Compassion fatigue in military healthcare teams. *Archives of Psychiatric Nursing, 28*(1), 2–9. doi:10.1016/j.apnu.2013.09.007

Polk, D. E. (2017). Some but not all psychosocial factors are correlated with oral hygiene behavior among children age 9 to 19 years. *Journal of Evidence Based Dental Practice, 17*(1), 53–55. doi:10.1016/j.jebdp.2017.01.011

Porter, C. M. (2016). Revisiting precede-proceed: A leading model for ecological and ethical health promotion. *Health Education Journal, 75*(6), 753–764. doi:10.1177/0017896915619645

Prestwich, A., Whittington, C., Rogers, L., Sniehotta, F. F., Dombrowski, S. U., & Michie, S. (2014). Does theory influence the effectiveness of health behavior interventions? Meta-analysis. *Health Psychology, 33*(5), 465–474. doi:10.1037/a0032853

Prochaska, J. O. (2008). Decision making in the transtheoretical model of behavior change. *Medical Decision Making, 28*(6), 845–849. doi:10.1177/0272989X08327068

Prochaska, J. O., & DiClemente, C. C. (1983). Stages and processes of self-change of smoking: Toward an integrative model of change. *Journal of Consulting and Clinical Psychology, 51*(3), 390.

Prochaska, J. O., & Velicer, W. F. (1997). The transtheoretical model of health behavior change. *American Journal of Health Promotion, 12*, 38–48.

Raman, A., Ritchie, L. D., Lustig, R. H., Fitch, M. D., Hudes, M. L., & Fleming, S. E. (2010). Insulin resistance is improved in overweight African American boys but not in girls following a one-year multidisciplinary community intervention program. *Journal of Pediatric Endocrinology and Metabolism, 23*(1–2), 109–120.

Raynor, P., & Pope, C. (2016). The role of self-care for parents in recovery from substance use disorders. *Journal of Addictions Nursing, 27*(3), 180–189. doi:10.1097/JAN.0000000000000133

Reed, J. R., Yates, B. C., Houfek, J., Briner, W., Schmid, K. K., & Pullen, C. (2016). A review of barriers to healthy eating in rural and urban adults. *Online Journal of Rural Nursing & Health Care, 16*(1), 122–153. doi:10.14574/ojrnhc.v16i1.379

Rich, A., Brandes, K., Mullan, B., & Hagger, M. S. (2015). Theory of planned behavior and adherence in chronic illness: A meta-analysis. *Journal of Behavioral Medicine, 38*(4), 673–688. doi:10.1007/s10865-015-9644-3

Riebl, S. K., Estabrooks, P. A., Dunsmore, J. C., Savla, J., Frisard, M. I., Dietrich, A. M., . . . Davy, B. M. (2015). A systematic literature review and meta-analysis: The Theory of Planned Behavior's application to understand and predict nutrition-related behaviors in youth. *Eating Behaviors, 18*, 160–178. doi:10.1016/j.eatbeh.2015.05.016

Robinson, T. N., Matheson, D. M., Kraemer, H. C., Wilson, D. M., Obarzanek, E., Thompson, N. S., . . . Killen, J. D. (2010). A randomized controlled trial of culturally tailored dance and reducing screen time to prevent weight gain in low-income African American girls: Stanford GEMS. *Archives of Pediatrics & Adolescent Medicine, 164*(11), 995–1004. doi:10.1001/archpediatrics.2010.197

Rogers, E. M. (1962). *Diffusion of innovations* (1st ed.). Glencoe, IL: Free Press.

Rogers, E. M. (2003). *Diffusion of innovations* (5th ed.). New York, NY: Free Press.

Roh, S., Burnette, C. E., Lee, Y.-S., Jun, J. S., Lee, H. Y., & Lee, K. H. (2018). Breast cancer literacy and health beliefs related to breast cancer screening among American Indian women. *Social Work in Health Care, 57*(7), 465–482. doi:10.1080/00981389.2018.1455789

Roll, C. L., & Cheater, F. (2016). Expectant parents' views of factors influencing infant feeding decisions in the antenatal period: A systematic review. *International Journal of Nursing Studies, 60*, 145–155. doi:10.1016/j.ijnurstu.2016.04.011

Romain, A. J., Horwath, C., & Bernard, P. (2018). Prediction of physical activity level using processes of change from the transtheoretical model: Experiential, behavioral, or an interaction effect? *American Journal of Health Promotion, 32*(1), 16–23. doi:10.1177/0890117116686900

Rosenstock, I. M. (1974). The health belief model and preventative health behavior. *Health Education Monographs, 2*(4), 354–386. doi:10.1177/109019817400200405

Ruotsalainen, H., Kyngäs, H., Tammelin, T., & Kääriäinen, M. (2015). Systematic review of physical activity and exercise interventions on body mass indices, subsequent physical activity and psychological symptoms in overweight and obese adolescents. *Journal of Advanced Nursing*, *71*(11), 2461–2477. doi:10.1111/jan.12696

Sadak, T., Souza, A., & Borson, S. (2016). Toward assessment of dementia caregiver activation for health care. *Research in Gerontological Nursing*, *9*(3), 145–155. doi:10.3928/19404921-20151019-02

Scalco, A., Noventa, S., Sartori, R., & Ceschi, A. (2017). Predicting organic food consumption: A meta-analytic structural equation model based on the theory of planned behavior. *Appetite*, *112*, 235-248. doi:10.1016/j.appet.2017.02.007

Scherr, C. L., Jensen, J. D., & Christy, K. (2017). Dispositional pandemic worry and the health belief model: Promoting vaccination during pandemic events. *Journal of Public Health*, *39*(4), e242–e250. doi:10.1093/pubmed/fdw101

Scherrens, A. L., Beernaert, K., Robijn, L., Deliens, L., Pauwels, N. S., Cohen, J., & Deforche, B. (2018). The use of behavioural theories in end-of-life care research: A systematic review. *Palliative Medicine*, *32*(6), 1055–1077. doi:10.1177/0269216318758212

Schmid, P., Rauber, D., Betsch, C., Lidolt, G., & Denker, M. (2017). Barriers of influenza vaccination intention and behavior – A systematic review of influenza vaccine hesitancy, 2005 – 2016. *PloS one*, *12*(1). doi:10.1371/journal.pone.0170550

Schüz, B., Li, A. S.-W., Hardinge, A., McEachan, R. R. C., & Conner, M. (2017). Socioeconomic status as a moderator between social cognitions and physical activity: Systematic review and meta-analysis based on the Theory of Planned Behavior. *Psychology of Sport and Exercise*, *30*, 186–195. doi:10.1016/j.psychsport.2017.03.004

Scruggs, S., Mama, S. K., Carmack, C. L., Douglas, T., Diamond, P., & Basen-Engquist, K. (2018). Randomized trial of a lifestyle physical activity intervention for breast cancer survivors: Effects on transtheoretical model variables. *Health Promotion Practice*, *19*(1), 134–144. doi:10.1177/1524839917709781

Seung Hee, C., & Duffy, S. A. (2017). Analysis of health behavior theories for clustering of health behaviors. *Journal of Addictions Nursing*, *28*(4), 203–209. doi:10.1097/JAN.0000000000000195

Sezgin, D., & Esin, M. N. (2018). Effects of a PRECEDE-PROCEED model based ergonomic risk management programme to reduce musculoskeletal symptoms of ICU nurses. *Intensive & Critical Care Nursing*, *47*, 89–97. doi:10.1016/j.iccn.2018.02.007

Shaughnessy, A. F. (2017). Brief interventions for weight management in kids are not effective. *American Family Physician*, *95*(3), 194–196.

Sheer, V. C. (2014). A meta-synthesis of health-related self-efficacy instrumentation: Problems and suggestions. *Journal of Nursing Measurement*, *22*(1), 77–93. doi:10.1891/1061-3749.22.1.77

Shin, A., Surkan, P. J., Coutinho, A. J., Suratkar, S. R., Campbell, R. K., Rowan, M., . . . Gittelsohn, J. (2015). Impact of Baltimore healthy eating zones: An environmental intervention to improve diet among African American youth. *Health Education & Behavior*, *42*(1 Suppl), 97S–105S. doi:10.1177/1090198115571362

Sidebottom, A. C., Sillah, A., Vock, D. M., Miedema, M. D., Pereira, R., Benson, G., . . . Vanwormer, J. J. (2018). Assessing the impact of the heart of New Ulm Project on cardiovascular disease risk factors: A population-based program to reduce cardiovascular disease. *Preventive Medicine*, *112*, 216–221. doi:10.1016/j.ypmed.2018.04.016

Sim, L. A., Lebow, J., Zhen, W., Koball, A., & Murad, M. H. (2016). Brief primary care obesity interventions: A meta-analysis. *Pediatrics*, *138*(4), 1–11. doi:10.1542/peds.2016-0149

Sims, S., Hewitt, G., & Harris, R. (2015). Evidence of a shared purpose, critical reflection, innovation and leadership in interprofessional healthcare teams: A realist synthesis. *Journal of Interprofessional Care*, *29*(3), 209–215. doi:10.3109/13561820.2014.941459

Sleijpen, M., Boeije, H. R., Kleber, R. J., & Mooren, T. (2016). Between power and powerlessness: A meta-ethnography of sources of resilience in young refugees. *Ethnicity & Health*, *21*(2), 158–180. doi:10.1080/13557858.2015.1044946

Smith, S. L., Smith, C., Cheatham, M., & Smith, H. G. (2017). Electronic cigarettes: A burn case series. *Journal for Nurse Practitioners*, *13*(10), 693–699. doi:10.1016/j.nurpra.2017.09.003

Starfelt Sutton, L. C., & White, K. M. (2016). Predicting sun-protective intentions and behaviours using the theory of planned behaviour: A systematic review and meta-analysis. *Psychology & Health*, *31*(11), 1272–1292. doi:10.1080/08870446.2016.1204449

Steinmetz, H., Knappstein, M., Aizin, I., Schmidt, P., & Kabst, R. (2016). How effective are behavior change interventions based on the theory of planned behavior? *Zeitschrift für Psychologie*, *224*(3), 216–233. doi:10.1027/2151-2604/a000255

Stoner, L., Rowlands, D., Morrison, A., Credeur, D., Hamlin, M., Gaffney, K., . . . Matheson, A. (2016). Efficacy of exercise intervention for weight loss in overweight and obese adolescents: Meta-analysis and implications. *Sports Medicine*, *46*(11), 1737–1751. doi:10.1007/s40279-016-0537-6

Taber, J. M., Dickerman, B. A., Okhovat, J.-P., Geller, A. C., Dwyer, L. A., Hartman, A. M., & Perna, F. M. (2018). Skin cancer interventions across the cancer control continuum: Review of technology, environment, and theory. *Preventive Medicine*, *111*, 451–458. doi:10.1016/j.ypmed.2017.12.019

Tawalbeh, L. I., Tubaishat, A., Batiha, A.-M., Al-Azzam, M., & AlBashtawy, M. (2015). The relationship between social support and adherence to healthy lifestyle among patients with coronary artery disease in the north of Jordan. *Clinical Nursing Research*, *24*(2), 121–138. doi:10.1177/1054773813501194

Tebb, K. P., Erenrich, R. K., Jasick, C. B., Berna, M. S., Lester, J. C., & Ozer, E. M. (2016). Use of theory in computer-based interventions to reduce alcohol use among adolescents and young adults: A systematic review. *BMC Public Health*, *16*(517). doi:10.1186/s12889-016-3183-x

Thomas, T. N., Sobelson, R. K., Wigington, C. J., Davis, A. L., Harp, V. H., Leander-Griffith, M., & Cioffi, J. P. (2018). Applying instructional design strategies and behavior theory to household disaster preparedness training. *Journal of Public Health Management & Practice*, *24*(1), e16–e25. doi:10.1097/PHH.0000000000000511

Thompson-Leduc, P., Clayman, M. L., Turcotte, S., & Légaré, F. (2015). Shared decision-making behaviours in health professionals: A systematic review of studies based on the Theory of Planned Behaviour. *Health Expect*, *18*, 754–774. doi:10.1111/hex.12176

Tidwell, D., Hung, L. S., & Hall, M. (2016). A meta-analysis of randomized controlled school-based programs demonstrates improvement in childhood obesity prevention. *Journal of the Academy of Nutrition & Dietetics, 116*, A42–A42. doi:10.1016/j.jand.2016.06.133

Tilokskulchai, F., Sitthimongkol, Y., Prasopkiitikun, T., & Klainin, P. (2004). Meta-analysis of health promotion research in Thailand. *Asian Journal of Nursing Studies, 7*(2), 18–32.

Titler, M. G. (2018). Translation research in practice: An introduction. *Online Journal of Issues in Nursing, 23*(2), 1–1. doi:10.3912/OJIN.Vol23No02Man01

Topp, R., Jacks, D. E., Wedig, R. T., Newman, J. L., Tobe, L., & Hollingsworth, A. (2009). Reducing risk factors for childhood obesity: The Tommie Smith Youth Athletic Initiative. *Western Journal of Nursing Research, 31*(6), 715–730. doi:10.1177/0193945909336356

Tung, W. C., Granner, M., Lu, M., & Qiu, X. (2017). Predictors of cervical cancer screening for Chinese American women. *European Journal of Cancer Care, 26*(4). e12552 doi:10.1111/ecc.12552

Tung, W. C., Lu, M., Granner, M., & Sohn, J. (2017). Assessing perceived benefits/barriers and self-efficacy for cervical cancer screening among Korean American women. *Health Care for Women International, 38*(9), 945–955. doi:10.1080/07399332.2017.1326495

Tung, W. C., Smith-Gagen, J., Lu, M., & Warfield, M. (2016). Application of the transtheoretical model to cervical cancer screening in Latina women. *Journal of Immigrant & Minority Health, 18*(5), 1168–1174. doi:10.1007/s10903-015-0183-3

Tyson, M., Covey, J., & Rosenthal, H. E. S. (2014). Theory of planned behavior interventions for reducing heterosexual risk behaviors: A meta-analysis. *Health Psychology, 33*(12), 1454–1467. doi:10.1037/hea0000047

van Alphen, H. J. M., Hortobágyi, T., & van Heuvelen, M. J. G. (2016). Barriers, motivators, and facilitators of physical activity in dementia patients: A systematic review. *Archives of Gerontology & Geriatrics, 66*, 109–118. doi:10.1016/j.archger.2016.05.008

VanDyke, S. D., & Shell, M. D. (2017). Health beliefs and breast cancer screening in rural Appalachia: An evaluation of the health belief model. *Journal of Rural Health, 33*(4), 350–360. doi:10.1111/jrh.12204

Vanstone, M., Rewegan, A., Brundisini, F., Giacomini, M., Kandasamy, S., & DeJean, D. (2017). Diet modification challenges faced by marginalized and nonmarginalized adults with type 2 diabetes: A systematic review and qualitative meta-synthesis. *Chronic Illness, 13*(3), 217–235. doi:10.1177/1742395316675024

Vijaykumar, S., Nowak, G., Himelboim, I., & Jin, Y. (2018). Virtual Zika transmission after the first U.S. case: Who said what and how it spread on Twitter. *American Journal of Infection Control, 46*(5), 549–557. doi:10.1016/j.ajic.2017.10.015

Vissers, D., Hens, W., Hansen, D., & Taeymans, J. A. N. (2016). The effect of diet or exercise on visceral adipose tissue in overweight youth. *Medicine & Science in Sports & Exercise, 48*(7), 1415–1424. doi:10.1249/MSS.0000000000000888

Vorwerk, J., & King, L. (2016). Consumer participation in early detection of the deteriorating patient and call activation to rapid response systems: A literature review. *Journal of Clinical Nursing, 25*(1/2), 38–52. doi:10.1111/jocn.12977

Voskuil, V. R., & Robbins, L. B. (2015). Youth physical activity self-efficacy: A concept analysis. *Journal of Advanced Nursing, 71*(9), 2002–2019. doi:10.1111/jan.12658

Walsh, S. M., Umstattd Meyer, M. R., Gamble, A., Patterson, M. S., & Moore, J. B. (2017). A systematic review of rural, theory-based physical activity interventions. *American Journal of Health Behavior, 41*(3), 248–258. doi:10.5993/AJHB.41.3.4

Willis, L. A., Kachur, R., Castellanos, T. J., Spikes, P., Gaul, Z. J., Gamayo, A. C., . . . Sutton, M. Y. (2018). Developing a motion comic for HIV/STD prevention for young people ages 15–24, part 1: Listening to your target audience. *Health Communication, 33*(2), 212–221. doi:10.1080/10410236.2016.1255840

Wilson, D. K., Van Horn, M. L., Kitzman-Ulrich, H., Saunders, R., Pate, R., Lawman, H. G., . . . Brown, P. V. (2011). Results of the "Active by Choice Today" (ACT) randomized trial for increasing physical activity in low-income and minority adolescents. *Health Psychology, 30*(4), 463–471. doi:10.1037/a0023390

Wright, K., Giger, J. N., Norris, K., & Suro, Z. (2013). Impact of a nurse-directed, coordinated school health program to enhance physical activity behaviors and reduce body mass index among minority children: A parallel-group, randomized control trial. *International Journal of Nursing Studies, 50*(6), 727–737. doi:10.1016/j.ijnurstu.2012.09.004

Xingjuan, T., Ka Yee Chow, S., & Kam Yuet Wong, F. (2015). A nurse-led case management program on home exercise training for hemodialysis patients: A randomized controlled trial. *International Journal of Nursing Studies, 52*(6), 1029–1041. doi:10.1016/j.ijnurstu.2015.03.013

Yabut, L., & Rosenblum, R. (2017). An integrative review of the use of EHR in childhood obesity identification and management. *Online Journal of Nursing Informatics, 21*(3). Available at http://www.himss.org/ojni

Youfa, W., Jungwon, M., Khuri, J., Miao, L., Wang, Y., Min, J., & Li, M. (2017). A systematic examination of the association between parental and child obesity across countries. *Advances in Nutrition, 8*(3), 436–448. doi:10.3945/an.116.013235

Young, I., Thaivalappil, A., Greig, J., Meldrum, R., & Waddell, L. (2018). Explaining the food safety behaviours of food handlers using theories of behaviour change: A systematic review. *International Journal of Environmental Health Research, 28*(3), 323-340. doi:10.1080/09603123.2018.1476846

Yusufov, M., Paiva, A. L., Redding, C. A., Lipschitz, J. M., Gokbayrak, N. S., Greene, G., . . . Prochaska, J. O. (2016). Fat reduction efforts. *Health Promotion Practice, 17*(1), 116–126. doi:10.1177/1524839915606423

Yusufov, M., Rossi, J., Redding, C., Yin, H.-Q., Paiva, A., Velicer, W., . . . Prochaska, J. (2016). Transtheoretical model constructs' longitudinal prediction of sun protection over 24 months. *International Journal of Behavioral Medicine, 23*(1), 71–83. doi:10.1007/s12529-015-9498-7

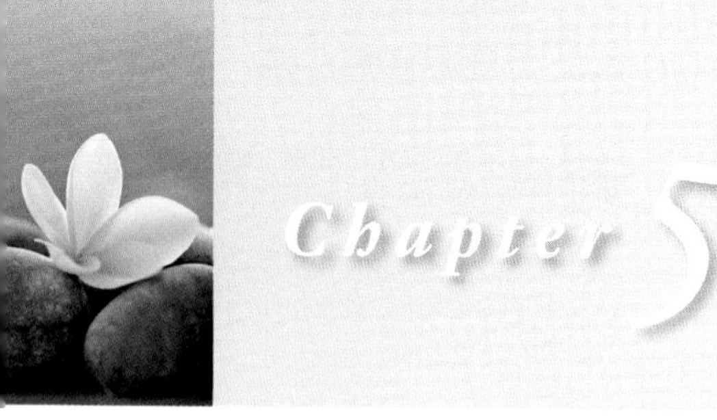

Evidence-Based Health Promotion

Marilyn Frenn

LEARNING OBJECTIVES

After completing this chapter, the student will be able to:

1. Develop a PICOT question for health promotion.
2. Differentiate the best sources of evidence.
3. Discuss issues important to applying evidence in practice.
4. Discuss importance of policy change in health promotion.

INTRODUCTION

There is substantial, constantly changing evidence on promoting health as well as diverse consumer expectations and values to consider when applying evidence to practice. In this chapter, concepts of evidence-based practice will be applied to guide decisions, including appraisal of existing evidence; examining goodness of fit, cost, and feasibility; gaining support and resources; using information systems in assessment and evaluation; promoting healthy public policies; and presenting the evidence with impact.

APPRAISAL OF EVIDENCE

Health consumers have the benefit of a rich and rigorously developed body of evidence in the area of health promotion. Despite this, consumers may be confused when they hear of a study indicating an action that would promote their health, only to hear of another study indicating the opposite advice.

By preparing to appraise the quality of health promotion evidence, nurses can help consumers learn to evaluate evidence and take appropriate action. Reading the texts referenced at the end of this chapter and conducting coursework on the appraisal of evidence can provide the nurse with a deep understanding of the methods used to critique research as well as the ability to apply these methods in practice.

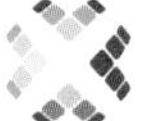

Case Illustration

Consider the publications presented in Table 5-1. Which of these studies provides the best quality evidence to guide recommendations for Sheena, an 11-year-old African American female client? Sheena weighs 115 pounds at 4 feet 3 inches tall, with a body mass index of 31.2. She is categorized as obese and is in the 95th weight percentile for her age and gender.

To engage in evidence-based practice, first develop a patient, intervention, control, observation, and time (PICOT) question to examine all the evidence that might guide care decisions for a specific situation. An example PICOT question for Sheena might be:

Table 5-1 Publications to Consider for Evidence-Based Practice

Citation	Type of Report
Anguita, M. (2013). Local measures to tackle childhood obesity. *Nurse Prescribing, 11*(12), 578–580.	Health-care writer provides case examples and resources for working with potentially overweight youth; includes seven references.
Hilton, L. (2013). Weighty matters. *Contemporary Pediatrics, 30*(9), 37–41. http://contemporarypediatrics.modernmedicine.com/contemporary-pediatrics/news/overview-childhood-overweight-obesity-diagnosis-treatment	Medical writer discusses resources for childhood obesity treatment; includes billing codes and 14 references.
Hoelscher, D. M., Kirk, S., Ritchie, L., & Cunningham-Sabo, L. (2013). Position of the Academy of Nutrition and Dietetics: Interventions for the prevention and treatment of pediatric overweight and obesity. *Journal of the Academy of Nutrition & Dietetics, 113*(10), 1375–1394. doi: 10.1016/j.jand.2013.08.004	Systematic review by doctorally prepared dieticians; includes 150 references.
Sorg, M. J., Yehle, K. S., Coddington, J. A., & Ahmed, A. H. (2013). Implementing family-based childhood obesity interventions. *Nurse Practitioner, 38*(9), 14–22. doi: 10.1097/01.NPR.0000433074.22398.e2	Masters and doctorally prepared nurses discuss family-based obesity prevention; includes relevant guidelines and 43 references.
The Community Preventive Services Taskforce. (2019). The Community Guide: CPSTF findings for obesity. Retrieved from https://www.thecommunityguide.org/content/task-force-findings-obesity	Systematic reviews conducted by expert panels; references vary by topic.

P: For African American females (10 to 15 years old) does
I: brief counseling in the clinic
C: compared to a multicomponent intervention program
O: reduce body mass index
T: over a two-year period?

In stating your PICOT question, consider the client conditions you see frequently in your practice. For these conditions, providing the best available evidence could mean improved health outcomes for many of your clients.

Once you have formulated your PICOT question, consult with a reference librarian to find studies that are relevant to your PICOT question. Librarians may also be aware of reliable sources for practice guidelines. Considering individual studies that may guide care recommendations is often called "using evidence in practice" (Brown, 2018). Although this approach may prove helpful for some clients, making recommendations based on only one or two studies can be confusing and may not provide the best evidence to improve clients' health. The coronavirus pandemic created a situation where one or two studies might be the only ones that are pertinent. For example, African Americans experienced higher rates of the virus and higher death rates than other groups. This could well be because of long-standing racial disparities in 1) access to health care; 2) African Americans having low wage jobs without sick pay, but requiring ongoing work on site with risk to health when others worked from home; or 3) that even though they may have known of the risk to health, it didn't rise high enough on the priority list when trying to deal with food, rent, and basic necessities (Center for Economic Development College of Letters and Science University of Wisconsin-Milwaukee April 2020). Racial disparities also create higher incidence of toxic stress, which may worsen health problems (Barnes, Anthony, Karatekin, Lingras, Mercado, & Thompson, 2020; Warren, 2020).

Usually a better option when searching for evidence to help clients, is a comprehensive meta-analysis, in which data from many quantitative studies are critiqued and analyzed, or a meta-synthesis, in which qualitative findings across studies are analyzed. In some cases, however, findings from an individual study may best address client characteristics and values, in which case it would be appropriate to use those findings. For example, findings from Simen-Kapeu and Veugelers (2010) published in the *Canadian Journal of Health* indicated that parents of lower socioeconomic status were more likely to engage

Table 5-2 Evidence-Based Health Promotion Appraisal

What is your PICOT question?

What data base(s), years and key words will be searched?

Can you enlist a research librarian to help?

Data Base (s)	Years	Key Words

Citation	Subjects	Method(s)	Results	Rigor of Evidence	Applicable?

Strength of *overall* evidence:

Recommendation:

BOX 5-1 Elements for Consideration in Appraising Qualitative Health Promotion Research

Was the design appropriate for the research question(s)?

Was an intensive examination of the questions presented?

Were the rights of study participants protected, including review by an institutional review board?

Were rich data presented based on sufficient time spent?

Was the qualitative method applied with sufficient reflexivity to prevent bias?

Do the themes capture the meaning of the narratives?

Does the report give you a meaningful understanding of how to promote health?

BOX 5-2 Elements for Consideration in Appraising Quantitative Health Promotion Research

Were the selection criteria reasonable and the sample size sufficient for statistical power?

Did the research question guide selection of the strongest design?

Did a conceptual framework guide the choice of variables and health promotion interventions?

Were reliability and validity estimates for instruments acceptable?

Were the rights of study participants protected, including review by an institutional review board?

Was diffusion to the control group prevented (if applicable) and fidelity to the intervention assured?

Were data collected at appropriate times to address research questions?

Was masking/blinding used for intervention and control groups (if applicable)?

Were statistics appropriate for the level of measurement, that is, nominal, ordinal, interval, or ratio levels?

Were conclusions based on the data?

in physical activity with their children, whereas parents with higher socioeconomic status provided healthier nutrition. Guidance for Canadian parents might be tailored based on these findings. Evaluation of risk in the United States might be based on Balistreri and Van

BOX 5-3 Elements to Include in Your Brief Report of the Evidence

1. Strengths and limitations of the body of evidence
2. Important client differences to consider in applying the evidence in practice
3. Areas where further research is needed
4. Recommendations for practice
   a. Risk, costs, and benefits of applying the evidence
   b. Feasibility and system issues to consider in applying the evidence
   c. Key stakeholders in making evidence-based practice changes
   d. Safe and effective care planning implications
   e. Interprofessional health education implications
5. Relevance to Healthy People 2030 and national guidelines
6. Useful resources may be helpful to include to facilitate implementation, such as:
   a. Assessment tools
   b. Client education materials
   c. Web sites

Hook's (2011) findings that low socioeconomic status raised obesity risk for girls, while low parental education was associated with greater risk of obesity in boys.

You may be fortunate enough to find a recent rigorous systematic review with appropriate recommendations for your client, such as the Hoelscher, Kirk, Ritchie, and Cunningham-Sabo (2013) report. But in some cases, you and your colleagues will have to conduct an independent review or search for additional studies that have been performed after the most recent systematic review. Use online databases such as the Cumulative Index of Nursing and Allied Health Literature (CINAHL) and Medline to find relevant studies and those that cite relevant studies. Depending on your PICOT question, PsycINFO and Education Resources Information Center (ERIC) may also be helpful resources. As you review the research, check each reference list for key studies that you might not have discovered otherwise.

As you locate useful studies, prepare an evidence table, as shown in Table 5-2. This should include the author(s), year, sample characteristics, method, major findings, and your critique as to the rigor of the study and its applicability to your PICOT question. Refer to the critique guides found in Box 5-1 and Box 5-2 for guidance in evaluating each study. For PICOT questions that have been addressed in extensive studies, separate tables for quantitative and qualitative studies, guidelines, and general reports may be useful.

Once you have completed your review, distill your evidence table into a "best studies" version, limited to high-quality studies with the most relevance to your PICOT question. Based on your appraisal of all the evidence, create a brief report summarizing the best practices for the client issue at hand. Your appraisal of evidence may also provide information to modify best practices based on client characteristics. See Box 5-3 for aspects to include in your brief report.

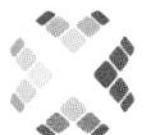

Case Illustration

Fortunately, a careful review of the evidence relevant to the care of Sheena, our 11-year-old client whose BMI percentile indicates obesity, has been conducted (U.S. Preventive Services Taskforce [USPST], 2017). Measuring her height and weight and discussing her BMI percentile with her and her parent or guardian is the first step. More than two of five parents misperceive their child's weight, and this was the strongest predictor of child obesity in multiyear surveys of public school children's parents (*N* = 14,808) (McKee, Long, Southward, Walker, & McCown, 2016).

Next, the evidence shows that high-intensity multicomponent treatment programs have been effective in reducing childhood obesity (USPST, 2017).

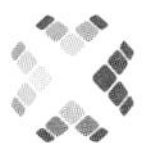

Case Illustration

Prepare information for Sheena and her parents about available treatment programs, distance, cost, and coverage with their insurance. Assess Sheena and her family members' readiness to consider an obesity treatment program, along with their understanding of the risks ongoing obesity presents for Sheena. Chapter 6 provides essential information on motivational interviewing and patient activation.

EXAMINING FIT, COST, AND FEASIBILITY

Tailoring your recommendation to client values and preferences is the next step in evidence-based health promotion.

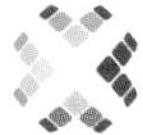

Case illustration

Use your assessment of readiness to inform your work with Sheena and her family. If they do not consider her weight to be a problem, reflect your understanding of their perspectives: "I understand many of Sheena's classmates are as heavy as she is, so you do not think it is necessary to start a treatment program now. Would you be willing to consider this information (USPST, 2017) and talk with me again in one month?"

Keep in mind the major findings of the best-quality studies. This will help you discuss recommendations for health promotion based on what the client is most willing to consider. Keep the best studies evidence table close at hand while you assess how well the evidence fits your client, which may be an individual, family, group, or community depending on the focus of your practice. The theories guiding health promotion discussed in Chapter 4 can help you assess the factors necessary for changes in health behavior to make the evidence most useful for the client. Throughout this book, the word *client* may refer to individuals, families, groups, or communities, so choose a model congruent with your practice focus.

Well before meeting with the client, determine which of the evidence-based recommendations you will make. Then create a list of resources that can help the client make healthy changes as recommended and the cost to access these resources. For example, your resource list for your 11-year-old overweight African American client may include a free child-focused nutrition class, information about area farmer's markets and other sources for fresh produce, and a list of neighborhood recreation programs and teams. Keeping this list in an electronic file makes it easy to update as availability and cost changes and to tailor the recommendations to other clients as needed.

When you meet with the client, discuss the feasibility of your health promotion recommendations. Involve significant others and family members in this conversation whenever possible and use the techniques of motivational interviewing.

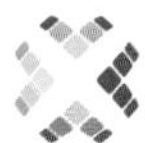

Case Illustration

Let's try this process with the 11-year-old client, Sheena, whose mother has accompanied her to her next appointment. You might say, "I understand you're interested in eating more vegetables for a healthier diet. Studies show that this can be beneficial in losing weight and preventing disease. Here are a few farmer's markets and produce stands within a few miles of your home. Mom, are you able to dedicate part of the household budget to fresh produce? Can your daughter walk to these locations safely, or are you able to go with her? What do you need help with before getting started? Are there things that you think may get in your way?"

When you have determined the feasibility of the recommended options, create a contract with the client, in this case, Sheena, that includes his or her feedback. For example, Sheena's mother may agree to walk to the produce stand with her at least once a week or involve Sheena in preparing two new healthy foods for the family each week. Sheena might agree to play basketball or kickball with friends twice a week. You can contact them in two weeks to check on their progress, modify the plan as needed, and congratulate their success. By building on successes, Sheena and her family may begin making small changes and be ready to consider an obesity treatment program that the evidence shows has the best chance of helping her stabilize or reduce her weight as she grows taller, reducing her BMI percentile.

GAINING SUPPORT AND RESOURCES

Support for evidence-based health promotion and resources to implement them in practice is essential. Do you have up-to-date resources to support health promotion? For example, to prepare for your visit with Sheena and her mother, can an administrative assistant download the consumer information from the USPST and prepare a handout? Can an assistant prepare a list of community resources for healthy foods; produce stands; and safe and free walking, biking, and other options for physical activity? If you have chosen a PICOT question important to a substantial proportion of the clients in your setting, locating or preparing resource materials will be important to making a successful practice change. Assessment tools, client education materials, and Web sites all help professionals to implement practice change effectively.

Do you have time to appraise the evidence on major health promotion issues for clients in your practice setting where there isn't a recent USPST guideline? Appraising the evidence can take weeks. Working with colleagues to identify crucial PICOT questions, identifying who will do the initial appraisal of evidence on each question, and establishing a time line for the work to be completed are essential.

Build on initial successes in implementing evidence-based practice for one or more important client health promotion issues. As you work with the literature, you may discover effective ways to begin evidence tables on related PICOT questions. For example, the USPST guideline we used included not only information for African American girls but also for other demographic groups.

Schaffer, Sandau, and Diedrick (2012) examined six models for evidence-based practice change. It may be helpful to examine these and implement change using elements that best fit your practice setting. Consider how information is usually shared in your practice setting and what methods have been most effective when introducing new ideas, equipment, or protocols. Be sure to include managers, informal leaders, and members of various disciplines affected by a practice change indicated by your review of evidence. Bringing people into the discussion as soon as possible and asking how they might like to be involved will help them engage in the process rather than creating roadblocks to practice change. Present evidence indicating that change is needed in areas that your colleagues already care about and understand. By thoroughly evaluating the rigor of study findings, you can clearly state results in an accessible way for colleagues who may not understand complex data or specialized jargon, and you can provide citations for those who want to examine complex statistical analyses.

Getting evidence into practice takes time and the help of many people. Do you have multicomponent obesity treatment programs in your geographic area? The most effective programs from the systematic review conducted for the USPST included: 26 hours or more, with those greater than 52 hours of contact having the greatest effect; both the parent and child (separately, together, or both); individual and group family sessions; healthy lifestyle choice information; encouraged limiting access to obesity risks like screen time and tempting foods, and other behavioral strategies like setting goals, self-monitoring, problem-solving and rewards; as well as supervised physical activity (USPST, 2017).

If these programs exist in your area, does insurance cover them? Are the local schools and community engaged in obesity prevention through provision of safe, walkable routes to school, community gardens, and coalitions to mobilize parents? These resources have been found to be effective agents of child obesity prevention and treatment.

Working with coalitions; professional groups; and health promotion organizations such as the American Heart Association, Diabetes Association, Lung Association, Cancer Society, and the Obesity Society may be necessary to get evidence-based health promotion programs started in a community. These organizations may also generate up-to-date, evidence-based health education materials with attention to cultural congruence and client literacy levels. Such organizations also help inform nurses and other members of the community about needed policy changes, upcoming legislation, and how people can help. Should your practice change require funding for items such as training, equipment, and client education materials, linking your evidence to Healthy People 2030 and/or state and local health priorities may generate greater commitment from existing coalitions and demonstrate greater need to those who may provide funding.

USING INFORMATION SYSTEMS IN ASSESSMENT AND EVALUATION

As you collect studies on a topic, study information can be downloaded to a reference manager such as RefWorks, Endnote, or Mendeley. This will enable you to search your study information and create reference lists without retyping. See Chapter 12 for online practice guidelines, information on electronic health records and personal health records, and guidelines for using eHealth and mHealth for health promotion. You may also want to consult helpful resources on evidence-based practice (Melnyk & Fineout-Overholt, 2018), using statistics (Kim & Mallory, 2014), evaluating outcomes (Kleinpell, 2017), and improving quality (Duncan, Montalvo, & Dunton, 2011).

PROMOTING HEALTHY POLICIES

Changes in overall health policies tend to have a larger impact in less time and with less cost than individual and family-based health promotion efforts. Providers can use public health approaches, working with others at the community, professional, and systemic levels, to advocate for policies that support improved health outcomes (Foltz, Belay, & Blackburn, 2013; Sommers & Heiser, 2013). For example, we can advocate to improve evidence-based health promotion at the state and federal level so that resources and programs address areas of highest need and impact (Stamatakis et al., 2012). When advocating policy alternatives, it is especially important that we consider the evidence and the viewpoints of various stakeholders likely to have an impact on the likelihood of policy adoption and effectiveness (Franck, Grandi, & Eisenberg, 2013). We must also examine the evidence carefully for possible differential effects of policies on certain subpopulations; for example, school-based policies have shown greater effectiveness for boys than for girls (Ling & Thomas, 2013).

Once you have invested in preparing a brief report on an important health promotion PICOT question, consider submitting a manuscript for publication. This will provide a starting place for others to begin. We know that the practices of individual clinicians vary dramatically (Shaikh, Nettiksimmons, Joseph, Tancredi, & Romano, 2012), so if more of our colleagues have the best evidence readily available, this can help improve health for many more people.

PRESENTING THE EVIDENCE WITH IMPACT

It is particularly important in advocating for healthy policies that we reach those who need to use the evidence. We can best accomplish this by considering how we present the information. Gollust, Niederdeppe, and Barry (2013) found that obesity prevention messages were best understood by conservatives as indicating government action was needed when the information was framed in terms of promoting the health of youth so youth could pass military fitness requirements. It is important to acknowledge that people have different perspectives on how the obesity epidemic might be addressed best. Some think responsibility belongs with individuals and parents rather than with schools, tax policy, or government programs. Consider those perspectives when presenting evidence to individuals, families, professional, and/or community groups.

The Locate the evidence, Evaluate the evidence, Assemble the evidence, and inform Decisions (LEAD) framework provides a useful approach to gathering, evaluating, and presenting evidence to various audiences (Chatterji, Green, & Kumanyika, 2014). The expert committee convened by the Institute of Medicine recommended LEAD as a systems approach for presenting evidence by answering the following questions: Why is it important that we consider this issue? What should be done? How do we implement this for our particular client group?

SUMMARY

Evidence-based health promotion includes appraisal of evidence; examining the fit, cost, and feasibility of implementing an evidence-based practice change; and gaining support and resources for a necessary practice change. Using information systems in assessment and evaluation is also important and will be discussed further in Chapter 13. As well as working with individual clients and families, we may best help everyone improve their health by advocating for healthy institutional and public policies. Whether our audience is peers, an interprofessional team in our practice setting, policy makers, or consumers, it is important to understand the perspectives of those we are working with to present the evidence with impact.

Web sites that may be helpful for evidence-based practice are listed in Box 5-4. Key points for this chapter to consider include consideration of health promotion and evidence-based practice in certification examinations. Web sites for content blueprints for these examinations are also included in Box 5-4.

BOX 5-4 Online Resources for Certification Exam Content and Evidence-Based Practice

CERTIFICATION

American Nurses Credentialing Center (ANCC): http://nursecredentialing.org/certification.aspx#specialty

American Academy of Nurse Practitioners Certification Program Candidate Handbook: https://www.aanpcert.org/resource/documents/2016%20Certificant_Candidate_Handbook%20(Final)%2001%2004%2016.pdf

Pediatric Nursing Certification Board (PNCB) http://www.pncb.org/ptistore/resource/content/exams/pn/2012_CPN_Content_Outline.pdf

EVIDENCE-BASED PRACTICE

Agency for Healthcare Research and Quality: https://www.guideline.gov/

Canadian Nurses Association NurseOne.CA: https://www.nurseone.ca/tools/evidence-based-practice

Joanna Briggs Institute. *Evidence-based practice resources and publications*. Retrieved from: https://joannabriggs.org/ebp

Johns Hopkins Nursing Evidence-Based Practice Model and Tools: https://www.ijhn-education.org/content/johns-hopkins-nursing-evidence-based-practice-model-and-tools

U.S. National Library of Medicine: https://www.nlm.nih.gov/hsrinfo/evidence_based_practice.html

KEY POINTS

- Develop a PICOT question for health promotion based on client issues frequently encountered in your practice setting.
- Differentiate best sources of evidence using an evidence table with appraisal relating to the quality of the evidence.
- Distill your evidence table into a "best studies" version that is limited to high-quality studies with the most relevance to your PICOT question.
- Issues important to applying evidence in practice include:
  - Examine goodness of fit, cost, and feasibility.
  - Gain support and resources.
  - Use information systems in assessment and evaluation.
  - Importance of policy change in health promotion: Changes in overall health policies tend to have a larger impact in less time and with less cost than individual and family-based health promotion efforts.

Check Your Understanding

1. Which of the following provide the best evidence on which to base health promotion practice?
   A. A study you found related to the client health issue
   B. Systematic review of randomized controlled trials
   C. Review published in a practice journal
   D. Opinions of authorities and expert committees

2. Which of the following are barriers to evidence-based health promotion?
   A. Staff members lecture clients on what they should do to improve their health rather than incorporating evidence to improve practice.
   B. The practice group attends the presentation but does not ask questions about a brief report summarizing evidence due to research jargon and complex statistical information.
   C. The job description and staffing pattern do not provide time for review of the evidence.
   D. All of these may be barriers to evidence-based health promotion.

3. When critically appraising evidence, which of the following questions are appropriate to consider when evaluating a study?
   A. Will these study results help me improve health with my clients?
   B. Did the results show a significant change?
   C. Was the study conducted using the best research method possible?
   D. All of these are important.

4. Which of the following is the least important to evidence-based health promotion?
   A. Use of knowledge from a single study
   B. Presenting evidence using clinical expertise
   C. Systematic examination of research findings
   D. Client preferences and values

5. In critiquing qualitative findings for improving health, which of the following would provide the strongest evidence?
   A. A grounded theory study using a constant comparative method
   B. A phenomenological study using theoretical sampling
   C. A meta-synthesis of several qualitative studies related to the PICOT question
   D. A meta-analysis of findings from several studies

See "Reflections on Check Your Understanding" at the end of the book for answers.

REFERENCES

Anguita, M. (2013). Local measures to tackle childhood obesity. *Nurse Prescribing, 11*(12), 578–580.

Balistreri, K., & Hook, J. (2011). Trajectories of overweight among US school children: A focus on social and economic characteristics. *Maternal & Child Health Journal, 15*(5), 610–619. doi:10.1007/s10995-010-0622-7

Barnes, A. J., Anthony, B. J., Karatekin, C., Lingras, K. A., Mercado, R., & Thompson, L. A. (2020). Identifying adverse childhood experiences in pediatrics to prevent chronic health conditions. *Pediatric Research, 87*(2), 362–370. doi:10.1038/s41390-019-0613-3

Brown, S. J. (2018). *Evidence-based nursing: The research-practice connection* (4th ed.). Burlington, MA: Jones & Bartlett Publishers.

Center for Economic Development College of Letters and Science University of Wisconsin-Milwaukee. (April 2020). Milwaukee's coronavirus racial divide: A report on the early stages of COVID-19 spread in Milwaukee County. Retrieved from: https://uwm.edu/ced/wp-content/uploads/sites/431/2020/04/COVID-report-final-version.pdf

Chatterji, M., Green, L. W., & Kumanyika, S. (2014). L.E.A.D.: A framework for evidence gathering and use for the prevention of obesity and other complex public health problems. *Health Education & Behavior, 41*(1), 85–99. doi:10.1177/1090198113490726

The Community Preventive Services Taskforce. (2019). *The Community Guide: CPSTF findings for obesity.* Retrieved from https://www.thecommunityguide.org/content/task-force-findings-obesity

Duncan, J., Montalvo, I., & Dunton, N. (2011). *NDNQI case studies in nursing quality improvement*. Silver Spring, MD: American Nurses Association.

Foltz, J. L., Belay, B., & Blackburn, G. L. (2013). Improving the weight of the nation by engaging the medical setting in obesity prevention and control. *Journal of Law, Medicine & Ethics, 41*, 19–26. doi:10.1111/jlme.12105

Franck, C., Grandi, S. M., & Eisenberg, M. J. (2013). Taxing junk food to counter obesity. *American Journal of Public Health, 103*(11), 1949–1953. doi:10.2105/AJPH.2013.301279

Gollust, S. E., Niederdeppe, J., & Barry, C. L. (2013). Framing the consequences of childhood obesity to increase public support for obesity prevention policy. *American Journal of Public Health, 103*(11), e96–e102. doi:10.2105/AJPH.2013.301271

Hilton, L. (2013). Weighty matters. *Contemporary Pediatrics, 30*(9), 37–41. Retrieved from http://contemporarypediatrics.modernmedicine.com/contemporary-pediatrics/news/overview-childhood-overweight-obesity-diagnosis-treatment

Hoelscher, D. M., Kirk, S., Ritchie, L., & Cunningham-Sabo, L. (2013). Position of the Academy of Nutrition and Dietetics: Interventions for the prevention and treatment of pediatric overweight and obesity. *Journal of the Academy of Nutrition & Dietetics, 113*(10), 1375–1394. doi:10.1016/j.jand.2013.08.004

Kim, M. J., & Mallory, C. (2014). *Statistics for evidence-based practice in nursing*. Burlington, MA: Jones and Bartlett Learning.

Kleinpell, R. M. (2017). *Outcomes assessment in advanced practice nursing* (4th ed.). New York: Springer.

Ling, Z., & Thomas, B. (2013). School-based obesity policy, social capital, and gender differences in weight control behaviors. *American Journal of Public Health, 103*(6), 1067–1073. doi:10.2105/AJPH. 2012.301033

McKee, C., Long, L., Southward, L. H., Walker, B., & McCown, J. (2016). The role of parental misperception of child's body weight in childhood obesity. *Journal of Pediatric Nursing, 31*, 196–203. doi:http://dx.doi.org/10.1016/j.pedn.2015.10.003

Melnyk, B. M., & Fineout-Overholt, E. (2018). *Evidence-based practice in nursing & healthcare: A guide to best practice* (4th ed.). Philadelphia, PA: Lippincott.

Schaffer, M. A., Sandau, K. E., & Diedrick, L. (2013). Evidence-based practice models for organizational change: Overview and practical applications. *Journal of Advanced Nursing, 69*(5), 1197–1209. doi:10.1111/j.1365-2648.2012.06122.x

Shaikh, U., Nettiksimmons, J., Joseph, J. G., Tancredi, D. J., & Romano, P. S. (2012). Clinical practice and variation in care for childhood obesity at seven clinics in California. *Quality in Primary Care, 20*(5), 335–344.

Simen-Kapeu, A., & Veugelers, P. J. (2010). Socio-economic gradients in health behaviours and overweight among children in distinct economic settings. *Canadian Journal of Public Health, 101*, S32–S36.

Sommers, J. K., & Heiser, C. (2013). The role of community, state, territorial, and tribal public health in obesity prevention. *Journal of Law, Medicine & Ethics, 41*, 35–39. doi:10.1111/jlme.12107

Sorg, M. J., Yehle, K. S., Coddington, J. A., & Ahmed, A. H. (2013). Implementing family-based childhood obesity interventions. *Nurse Practitioner, 38*(9), 14–22. doi:10.1097/01.NPR.0000433074.22398.e2

Stamatakis, K. A., Leatherdale, S. T., Marx, C. M., Yan, Y., Colditz, G. A., & Brownson, R. C. (2012). Where is obesity prevention on the map? Distribution and predictors of local health department prevention activities in relation to county-level obesity prevalence in the United States. *Journal of Public Health Management & Practice, 18*(5), 402–411.

U.S. Preventive Services Taskforce. (2017). Screening for obesity in children and adolescents: Consumer guide (draft recommendation). Retrieved from https://www.uspreventiveservicestaskforce.org/Page/Document/draft-recommendation-statement165/obesity-in-children-and-adolescents-screening1

Warren, B. J. (2020). The synergistic influence of life experiences and cultural nuances on development of depression: A cognitive behavioral perspective. *Issues in Mental Health Nursing, 41*(1), 3–6. doi:10.1080/01612840.2019.1675828

Unit 2

Working with Clients, Families, and Communities

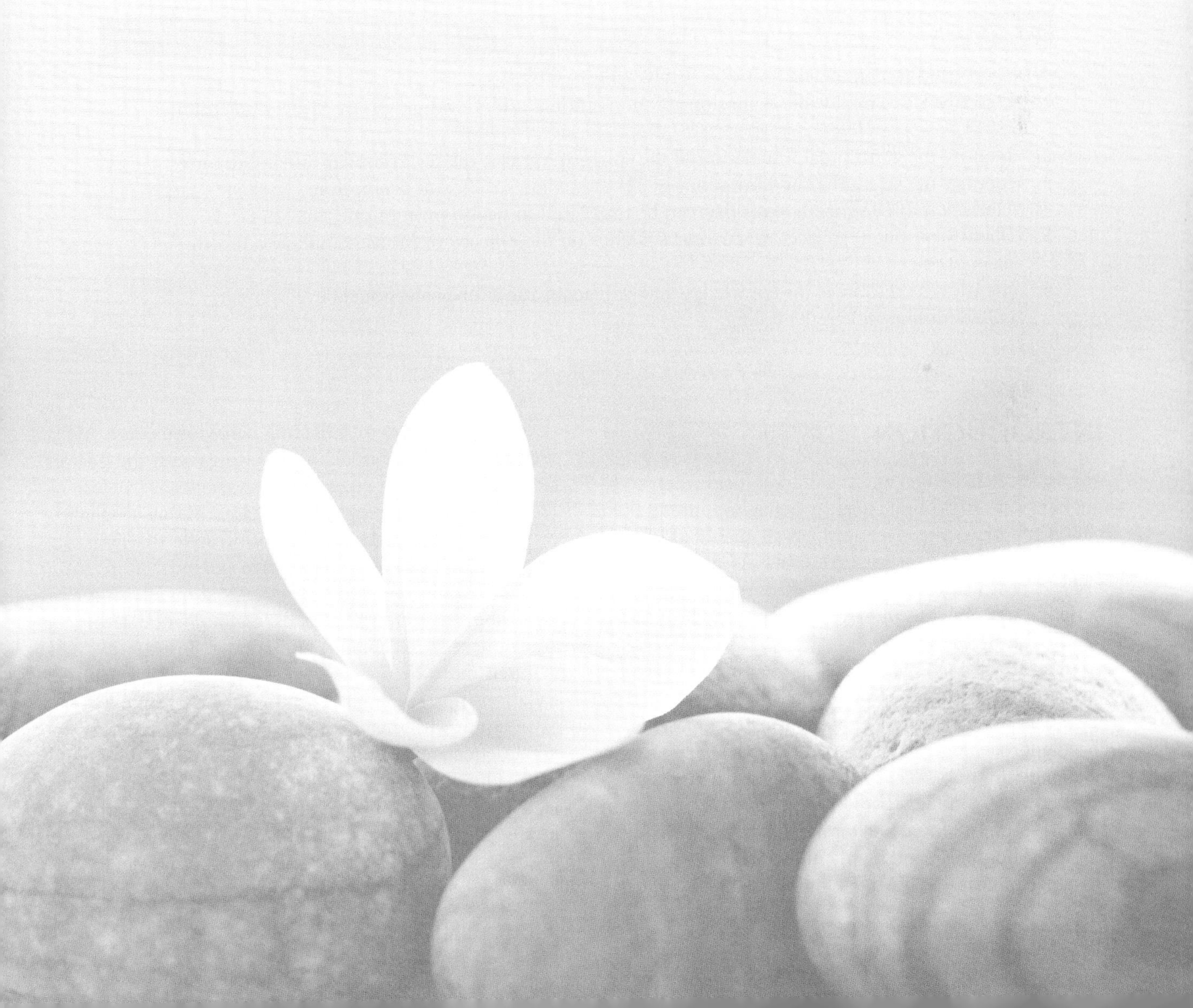

Motivational Interviewing (MI) and Patient Activation

Carol Essenmacher and Alexandre A. Martins

LEARNING OBJECTIVES

After completing this chapter, the student will be able to:

1. Describe three applicable definitions of motivational interviewing (MI) by Miller and Rollnick (2013).
2. Identify the conceptual foundation of the spirit of MI as it relates to similar nursing theories.
3. Identify the strengths and limitations of MI as it applies to health promotion.
4. Understand relevant MI skills that can be translated to health promotion.
5. Identify pertinent sources for current evidence on the efficacy of MI as it applies to health promotion.
6. Identify MI resources for knowledge and skill acquisition for professional development, collaboration, and credentialing.

INTRODUCTION

Nurses face challenges and conflicting ideas when seeking new ways to promote healthy behaviors among their patients, both to improve their overall quality of life and to reduce systemic health-care costs. As professionals, nurses are learning to shift focus from a disease-based patient-care model to disease prevention by promoting healthy lifestyles.

In all areas of practice, nurses are required to perform new and increasingly complex interventions that they have little time to learn, let alone learn and perform at levels approaching effectiveness. This presents significant challenges for nurses charged with helping patients identify and change unhealthy behaviors in a wide variety of clinical settings. Motivation for human behavior change is complex, nonlinear, and highly individualized. Abundant evidence indicates that MI is a highly useful and effective skill when it comes to activating behavior change. MI is used in clinical and nonclinical settings with the goal of facilitating behavior change among clients.

Miller and Rollnick (2013) define MI as a collaborative, goal-oriented communication style that uses the language of change "to strengthen personal motivation for and commitment to a specific goal by eliciting and exploring the person's own reasons for change within an atmosphere of acceptance and compassion" (p. 29). MI is much more than a set of techniques to be mastered. Relationships are at the core of MI, which make it an excellent fit with the nursing profession, where establishing an effective relationship is critical to providing good care. The absence of a relationship with one's patient leads to poor treatment adherence, which is costly and ineffective. For example, a nurse may deliver excellent information about a new medication or treatment, but unless he or she understands what it means for a patient to adhere consistently to the medication or treatment, the patient is unlikely to follow the recommendations fully.

When observing a session using MI, MI may appear deceptively easy to perform. Resnicow and McMaster (2012) describe it as "an egalitarian, empathetic way of being" (p. 1). However, it requires the clinician to have a significant understanding of what is called the underlying spirit of MI and to demonstrate skills that adhere to core MI principles. Although MI had its start in psychology, many other health-care disciplines are advocating that their clinicians, including nurses, learn and practice in accordance with MI in collaborative communication.

As the practice and guiding philosophy of MI evolved and expanded, psychologists William R. Miller and Stephen Rollnick (2013) found it helpful to provide three separate definitions of MI. The first definition concentrates on what the focus should be for a layperson learning and practicing MI, which is "a conversation about change" (p. 12). The focus at this level is on a collaborative conversation. The second definition is viewed from the lens of a practitioner and emphasizes the why and how of learning and applying MI in clinical practice. The last definition involves the technical aspects of how MI works.

Learning MI can help nurses activate and support behavior change effectively and efficiently, although developing this skill will take time and attention. Today's nurses are asked to do more at greater speed and with less (Aiken et al., 2012; Institute of Medicine, 2010), which can lead to poor health-care outcomes and increased resistance to new models of care. Nurses may mistakenly think of MI as an additional skill set to acquire rather than an evolution and improvement upon their current therapeutic communication skills. Dedicating time to learning something new may lead nurses to feel that they do not have the luxury of internalizing MI, although MI can help them practice more efficiently and effectively. Clearly, if a nurse only has a brief window of time to engage effectively with and activate patient behavior change, it behooves that nurse to be proficient in his or her communication and relationship-building skills.

A word of caution is necessary here: one cannot simply read a research article or a chapter in a book to become proficient in MI. Becoming effective with the collaborative, goal-oriented style of communication that is the very foundation and spirit of MI takes time, practice, mentoring, and patience with oneself. MI workshops and conferences are an effective way to learn specific techniques employed in the practice, although evidence shows that online workshops are also effective. Even the most seasoned MI clinicians experience days when they do not feel they are fully engaged in a collaborative MI-based conversation with their patients. Even with the best of intentions, nurses' busy lives realistically influence their ability to honor the spirit of MI in compassionate collaboration with their patients, practice acceptance of their patients as they are, and successfully evoke behavioral activation in the direction of healthy lifestyle changes. Miller and Rollnick (2013) emphasize the lifelong learning and mastery of MI: "In a very real sense, practicing MI over time teaches one this underlying spirit" (p. 23). As the use of MI was disseminated, Miller and Rollnick (2009) found it critical to identify to learners what is and is not MI-adherent practice to maintain fidelity to the model.

As a means of understanding specific nursing uses of MI and potential nursing contributions to the field of MI, this chapter will identify applications of MI from the perspective of multiple disciplines and explore recent research into the role of the nurse in MI practice. Historical perspectives influencing the drive toward collaborative communication, with the goal of behavior activation, will be presented. Extant evidence will be reviewed to assist students in identifying how to understand when MI is working well and what potential pitfalls to prepare for in practicing MI. Nurses are fully capable of adapting effective multidisciplinary tools and navigating obstacles with the goal of supporting patients' health behavior activation. An overview of the methods of evaluating one's MI practice to ensure treatment fidelity will be presented. Table 6-1 presents a brief overview of MI strategies, and the Case Illustration featured on page 97 at the end of the chapter provides an example of an MI interaction between patient and nurse.

HUMAN BEHAVIOR CHANGE AND MOTIVATION THEORIES

Miller & Rollnick (2013) recognized that the role of internally activated motivation has been observed for centuries, as per their inclusion of a quote by French mathematician and philosopher Blaise Pascal (1623–1662) at the beginning of a chapter, "People are generally better persuaded by the reasons which they themselves e discovered than by those which have come into the minds by others" (p. 25). A present-day example is when drivers typically obey traffic laws when a police officer or police car is visible (external motivation), but when no police officer is around, some disobey speed limits. The question that emerges is, Is learning how to help patients increase internal motivation for change possible? A more effective behavior change intervention could potentially help patients

Table 6-1 Overview of MI Strategies

Strategy	Description
Readiness Ruler	"On a scale of 0 to 10, how important is it to you to (behavior change)? And why are you at ____ and not at (lower number)?" (*This elicits change talk.*) "On a scale of 0 to 10, how confident are you that you could (behavior change)? And why are you at ___ and not at (lower number)? (*Answer indicates ability to make change.*)
Open Questions, Affirming, Reflecting, Summarizing (OARS)	Develop a patient-centered style of asking open-ended questions, affirming, and summarizing what is heard; facilitates the building of empathy and rapport
Reflective listening	Types: Simple Reflection: echo back what was said Complex Reflection: getting the "gist" of what was said; identifying the emotion, (Patient) "The doctor told me I have diabetes. I just don't know what I am going to do!" (Nurse) "Learning you have diabetes is really overwhelming you right now." Double-Sided Reflection: present both sides, "On the one hand, you want to quit smoking and, on the other hand, you feel like smoking relaxes you and you like to smoke." Amplified Reflection: Amplifies resistance that is heard, "If you quit drinking, you would lose all of your friends." Reframing: placing a different meaning on patient's statements, decrease resistance: (Patient) "My girlfriend is saying she will leave me if I don't stop drinking." (Nurse) "It feels to you that she is overreacting, but she might be really worried about you."
Recognizing Change Talk and Recognizing Sustain Talk	Change talk consists of statements that indicate the patient is considering making changes: "I could probably stop smoking inside my house and my car." Statements indicating resistance to change: "You all are overreacting. I don't drink that much."
Strengthening Change Talk	Supporting and goal setting without pressure: "If you were to decide to stop drinking, how would you go about it?"
Rolling with Resistance or Sustain Talk	Sustain talk consists of any client statements that support the status quo. Resistance examples: arguing, interrupting, discounting, or ignoring the nurse. Rolling with resistance: (Nurse) "I just realized that I probably have been pretty bossy about this with you and I don't want to do that. Can I get a do-over? I really want you to be healthy and not so short of breath all the time."
Developing a Change Plan	Desire, ability, reason, need, commitment (DARN-C) statements: "I really want to quit smoking (D)," "I can get my car detailed so it smells nice and I won't want to smoke in it (A)," "I'll be able to breathe easier when I quit smoking (R)," "If I am going to be able to keep up with my kids, I need to quit (N)," "We washed the walls in the house so it doesn't smell like smoke and that really helps me not smoke (C)."
Supporting Change	Anticipating challenges: "What might get in your way or trip you up?" "What could you do about that so that it doesn't trip you up?"

discover their own, internally driven need to make behavior changes.

Several mental health experts have heavily influenced how we approach behavior activation today. Sigmund Freud's early 20th-century theory of the human personality proposed that critical conscious and unconscious early childhood experiences shape our adult behavior. He developed psychoanalysis to treat and resolve mental and behavioral issues. In reaction to the field of psychoanalysis, B. F. Skinner focused on observable behavior and placed no importance on a person's inner psychological motivations. He developed a system of consequences (positive reinforcement, negative reinforcement, punishment, extinction) to facilitate behavior change. Carl Rogers placed heavy emphasis on the clinician, using a person-centered approach to psychotherapy to support patients as they continually improved their mental and physical functionality to reach one's full potential. Rogers's early work in the 1930s with child psychology transitioned into teaching mental health care and counseling for adults. Many experts in the field of psychology supported exploration into the internal and external motivations of individuals.

As the concept of motivation emerged among mental health treatment clinicians, the effect of clinician attitudes, beliefs, and behaviors became evident. In an early study of addiction treatment professionals, Leake and King (1977) randomized counselors into intervention and treatment groups. In this study, a randomized group of patients was assigned to a randomized group of counselors, with one group of counselors told that the patients they would see had a high alcohol recovery potential and expressed a belief in the patient's ability to achieve recovery. Unsurprisingly, this group of patients was more likely to demonstrate active progress toward recovery than the cohort of patients assigned to the cohort of counselors who provided treatment as usual. Clinicians believing in the possibility of patient recovery is very much aligned with MI core values.

In the field of addiction treatment, William Miller published an article in 1983 about the concepts foundational to MI that led to more than 30 years of ongoing collaboration with Stephen Rollnick to disseminate the core concepts and technical approaches of MI. Miller and Rollnick (2013) state, "[M]ore than 25,000 articles citing MI and 200 randomized clinical trials of MI have appeared in print, most of them published since the second edition" (p. vii) of the edition that was published in 2002.

Transtheoretical Model and MI

The transtheoretical model (TTM) of change (Velasquez, Maurer, Crouch, & DiClementi, 2001), sometimes called the stages of change (SOCs), is often associated with MI. These two models are separate but complementary concepts of facilitating behavior change. Briefly, SOC directs the clinician to assess each person's readiness to engage in behavior change. Movement through these stages is nonlinear and fluid, with the individual moving in and out of not being ready to change (precontemplation stage), getting ready to change (contemplation stage), being ready to change (preparation stage), making specific behavior changes (action stage), and sustaining change (maintenance stage) or returning to prior behaviors (relapse/recycle stage). MI is commonly used along with SOCs to help patients resolve inner ambivalence and make concrete plans to go from not thinking about changing to activating and sustaining behavior change. MI can help clinicians understand where to target interventions so clients can benefit the most from each encounter.

SUMMARY OF THE EVIDENCE FROM MULTIDISCIPLINARY STUDIES

Substantial health-care expenditures, time, energy, and attention are devoted to the treatment of chronic health-care conditions resulting from unhealthy behaviors. Other health-care expenses are related to illness or injury resulting from unsafe or risk-taking behaviors. Multidisciplinary research literature abounds on the use, efficacy, and clinical implications of MI in these situations. Thus, MI is used in patient care by virtually every health-care profession, including nursing.

Using MI to Encourage Health Behavior Change

Copeland, McNamara, Kelson, and Simpson (2015) completed a systematic review of 37 studies about health behavior change (excluding addictions). The authors also examined the studies with a focus on what elements of MI were effective. Overall, mechanisms such as "spirit of MI" and motivation were indicated as potentially beneficial to facilitating behavior change, and difficulties generalizing study qualities led to difficulties applying study results.

Christie and Channon (2014) performed a clinical review of the literature of nine studies about the use of MI with pediatric and adult patients who have diabetes and obesity. They found that a surprisingly small number of studies have been published about pediatric obesity and the use of MI to facilitate behavior change, and the few studies that have been published show mixed results of efficacy. MI did appear to lead to improvements in weight and metabolic control in adults with diabetes as well as children, despite the scarcity of pediatric studies. This review noted a lack of clarity about which MI skills were used, making it difficult to replicate and generalize the results.

Using MI to Treat Addiction

MI was first developed to treat addictions and substance use disorders more effectively. D'Amico et al. (2015) studied the use of MI in a group format with adolescents who used alcohol and marijuana. They found that talk of change among group members was associated with decreased alcohol use intentions, decreased alcohol use, and decreased heavy drinking 3 months after the group met. They also found that talk of sustaining use among group members was associated with less motivation to change, increased intentions to use marijuana, and increased positive expectancies of marijuana and alcohol. Even short sessions of MI can be effective, as found by Lindson-Hawley, Thompson, and Begh (2015) in treating adults who use tobacco. Novel uses of MI are readily found in the literature, such as the study by Mason et al. (2015) about text messaging using MI. These authors found that 72 adolescents used fewer cigarettes per day and voiced more intention not to smoke, and noted increased peer social support for behavior change from MI text messages sent to their phones. Accordingly, the possibilities of using MI in a variety of treatment settings become apparent with cohorts of patients of a variety of demographic backgrounds, as well as the possibilities of use among and within various disciplines.

PATIENT, INTERVENTION, CONTROL, OBSERVATION, AND TIME (PICOT) STATEMENT

As MI is increasingly used by multiple disciplines, the question becomes, Should nurses learn MI, and how can they best do so efficiently and effectively? U.S. nurses have regular contact with patients in virtually every treatment setting, so, MI could be an important therapeutic communication style and skill set for nurses to acquire to facilitate and support patient health behavior change. Nurses are ideally placed to activate patient behavior change by taking advantage of teachable moments through both brief and expanded patient interactions and developing novel nursing interventions. Activating and sustaining healthy behavior changes will improve the patient's overall quality of life, reduce patient morbidity and mortality, and decrease health-care costs.

Consider the following PICOT question: For nurses caring for patients who would benefit from health behavior change, does becoming proficient in MI result in positive patient health outcomes?

P: Nurses caring for patients who would benefit from health behavioral change
I: MI education and training for nurses
C: MI-naïve nurses
O: MI-competent nurses
T: Long-term and ongoing

Summary of the Evidence from Nursing Studies

Evidence on the use of MI to produce effective patient outcomes is generally but not universally positive. Some variation exists, possibly related to lack of fidelity of training to the MI core competencies, lack of support and mentoring of novice MI practitioners, inability of study design to reflect value added, and other factors. MI is commonly combined with other types of interventions such as cognitive behavior therapy (CBT), and study design may not adequately capture the nuances of each intervention. Variation of effectiveness may also be related to client differences based on age, gender, race, ethnicity, self-efficacy, and familial and community support. Diagnostic implications (e.g., severity, chronicity, patient resources) may also affect applications of MI interventions.

An exploration of nursing use of MI reveals a high degree of interest and abundant research activity. A wide variety of MI-oriented nursing actions are being studied in a range of clinical and academic settings. Research presented here demonstrates that MI research outcomes and efficacy are mixed, similar to the outcomes seen in non-nursing disciplines. Table 6-2 provides a variety of empirically tested tools that are commonly used in MI research and found in the literature.

Using MI to Encourage Health Behavior Change

In a systematic review of the literature conducted by nurses, Thompson et al. (2011) found 13 resources on the use of MI to improve cardiovascular health. The meta-analyses, systematic review, literature reviews, and primary studies included examined outcomes related to health behavior changes (e.g., obesity, smoking, diabetes, hypertension, physical activity, alcohol use). While the authors expected to find more studies about using MI

Table 6-2 Empirically Validated MI Evaluation Tools

MISC	Motivational Interviewing Skill Code, introduced by Miller and Mount as the first system for coding client and interviewer utterances within motivational interviewing (Miller & Rollnick, 2013, p. 410).
MITI	Motivational Interviewing Treatment Integrity coding system, simplified from the MISC and focusing on interviewer responses, to document fidelity to MI delivery (Miller & Rollnick, 2013, p. 410).
MI-SCOPE	MI Sequential Code for Observing Process Exchange (free download at https://casaa.unm.edu/download/scope.pdf).
BECCI	Behavior Change Counseling Index (https://doi.org/10.1016/j.pec.2004.01.003).
commMIt	Motivational interviewing training (comMIt).
MIACF	Motivational interviewing adherence and competency feedback form.

to improve cardiovascular outcomes, they posit that the use of MI is superior to treatment alone. Whether any of the resources studied nursing use of MI interventions for improving cardiovascular disease is unclear.

Al-Ganmi, Perry, Gholizadeh, and Alotaibi (2016) studied the use of MI-based interventions for supporting medication adherence among patients with cardiac disease. In the review of the literature, these nurse researchers found 14 studies meeting inclusion criteria. That is, the study should be a randomized control trial (RCT) or controlled clinical trial examining medication adherence and consist of both male and female patients with cardiac disease, with an intervention that could be performed by nurses; subjects were followed for at least 6 months, and medications were self-administered. Although results generally show promise that MI helps improve medication adherence in this population, significant heterogeneity was found in the results of each study, which restricts applicability of study interventions.

The use of MI by a variety of clinicians, including nurses, in a range of medical settings was the focus of a systematic review and meta-analysis by Lundahl et al. (2013). The authors included 48 studies with 9,618 participants and considered the use of MI for many health and health-related conditions, including HIV viral load, body mass index (BMI), dental outcomes, alcohol and tobacco use, sedentary lifestyle change, self-monitoring, and confidence in behavior change. An overall positive effect was found for the use of MI with these conditions. A positive effect was not found for using MI with eating disorders, self-care behaviors, or improvements in heart rate. In addition, brief MI interventions were found to be effective. The methods and type of clinician MI training were not clearly described.

In another literature review by Spoelstra, Schueller, Hilton, and Ridenour (2014), four articles with nurses as subjects were reviewed on the use of MI and CBT to improve medication adherence. These studies consisted of one RCT, four cohort studies, and one case study. The authors found support for the use of MI and CBT in five of the six studies. Discussion of how clinicians were trained to deliver MI or CBT was not included.

MI is also used by nurses in other treatment areas to help patients of all ages. Purath, Keck, and Fitzgerald (2014) conducted a systematic review of the literature about the use of MI to assist older adults with chronic health problems to change their behavior. The authors used the Preferred Reporting Items for Systematic Reviews and Meta-Analyses (PRISMA) guidelines to select eight articles for review. Articles were selected if MI was used as at least part of the study interventions, the study subject was a minimum of 60 years old, randomization was used in the study, pilot studies included a comparison group, the articles were published in English, and the study was completed in a primary-care setting. Although the authors found promise in the use of MI to facilitate behavior change in this cohort of patients, they reported that they considered MI to be a very fluid intervention, which is beneficial in that it allows for modifications to circumstances, but it does not lend itself well to clear descriptions of methods used or training fidelity to MI principles.

Using MI to Treat Addiction

Much of the early work in developing MI occurred in addictions treatment, and with many nurses specializing in addiction care, this is a natural area in which to expand nurse use of MI. O'May et al. (2016) studied two cohorts of bachelor's degree students (nurses and occupational therapists) to discover if they could be taught how to take advantage of teachable moments to deliver brief alcohol use interventions. After training, students agreed that they could serve in this role in practice. However, less than half of the group felt that they had the knowledge to provide patients with brief alcohol interventions. Although not identified by the authors, this may reflect a lack of adequate confidence to counsel others about social behaviors that students engage in during their academic pursuits.

Smoking is commonly addressed with MI interventions. Two studies were found addressing the nursing use of MI to help patients stop smoking. Bredie, Fouwels, Wollersheim, and Schippers (2011) conducted an RCT with high-risk cardiovascular patients and found at 3 months' follow-up that 26% of patients in the MI intervention group stopped smoking and another 31% decreased the amount they smoked. This compared favorably to the control group in which only 7% had quit at 3 months and 15% had decreased smoking. How the nurses were trained to deliver MI was not clearly identified. Osterlund Efraimsson, Fossu, Ehrenberg, Larson, and Klang (2012) conducted a prospective observational study of two videotaped MI intervention sessions delivered by nurses for 13 patients who smoke. At the conclusion of the study, the nurses tended to use (non-MI-adherent) direction-style interventions more than an MI-adherent style of evocation, collaboration, autonomy-support, and empathy. Nursing fidelity to delivering MI-adherent interventions was not objectively examined after training.

Nurses are not immune to benefitting from health behavior change and can also be subjects of studies. Mujika et al. (2014) studied 30 nurses who were randomized, with 15 placed in a control group and five into a group receiving an MI-based intervention. After four sessions, one nurse in each group had quit smoking; at the second time measurement (3 months post intervention), a total of six nurses from the intervention group had quit, but no one else from the control group had quit. This is important because nurses who smoke are less likely to offer smoking-cessation interventions (Essenmacher, Karvonen-Gutierrez, Lynch-Sauer, & Duffy, 2009).

Nurses are using MI more and more often to facilitate and support healthy patient behaviors. Robbins, Pfieffer, Maier, LaDrig, and Ber-Smith (2012) studied nurses working with middle school girls to increase their activity levels. The two school nurses received a two-day training (although only one nurse delivered the interventions) conducted by members of the Motivational Interviewing Network of Trainers (MINT), all of whom must adhere to standardized measures for trainings. Almost 92% (34 of 37) of the middle school girls completed all three intervention sessions. The secondary data analysis design study focused more on the process of training the school nurses than on the outcomes of behavior change. The authors noted that the school nurse's proficiency and fidelity to the core values and techniques of MI improved over time, although only about one-quarter of the nurse's reflections were complex (demonstrating proficiency with MI). No data were provided about the middle school girls' activity level, so whether the intervention was effective remains unknown. The authors observed that cost analyses should be performed in future studies.

Some nurses have provided sustained focus on the nursing use of MI to promote health behavior change. Brobeck, Bergh, Odencrants, and Hildingh (2011) conducted a descriptive design, qualitative method study by interviewing 20 primary-care nurses who learned and use MI. The nurses had an average of 26 years of experience, worked with patients to help them change lifestyle behaviors, and had been practicing MI for 3 to 10 years. The description of training the nurses in MI was not delineated, and discussion of the nurses' fidelity to the MI core values was likewise absent. Content analysis of the nurses' interviews reveals that the nurses felt MI is a valuable tool, although the demands of learning and practicing it must be considered. No outcomes about patient behavior change or cost analysis of MI practice were provided. These same authors (Brobeck, Odencrants, Bergh, & Hildingh , 2014) provided further examination of the nursing use of MI from the patient's perspective. Sixteen patients were interviewed by nurses who used MI to work with them to facilitate lifestyle changes. Transcripts of the interviews revealed themes categorized as the presumption of mutual interaction, creating a sense of well-being, and contributing to change. The authors noted the importance of meaningful discussion that supported that patient's self-determination and how without this support, "it would have been easy to delay the lifestyle change" (p. 5). Again, what the MI training consisted of for the nurses is unclear, and no patient outcomes or cost analyses were provided because neither were the focus of the study.

Ostlund, Wadensten, Haggstrom, Lindqvist, and Kristofferzon (2016) studied nurses trained in MI to determine if MI influenced their communication and their patients' responses. In a quantitative descriptive and predictive design study, 23 primary-care nurses provided 50 audiotapes of their interactions with 50 patients. The authors hypothesized that if the nurses' communication supported change talk, neutral talk, and sustain talk, then the patients would subsequently verbalize either change, neutral, or sustain talk accordingly. Two empirically validated MI measures were used to evaluate the audiotapes: Motivational Interviewing Skill Code (MISC) and Sequential Code for Observing Process Exchange (MI-SCOPE). The results reflected that, although the nursing communication supporting change predicted change talk in patients, the nurses mostly used neutral talk with patients. The authors posit that this may reflect the need for more MI training and support from managers for the nurses to learn MI. No cost-benefit analysis was completed with the study.

Noordman et al. (2012) conducted an observational study of primary-care nurses' use of MI in working with patients to make lifestyle changes regarding alcohol use, smoking, and physical exercise. Patient-care interactions were taped for 13 nurses as they engaged with 117 adult patients. The videos and transcripts were evaluated using the empirically validated Behaviour Change Counseling Index (BECCI), a common tool that rates clinician behaviors and techniques according to fidelity to MI core values and techniques. The depiction of the MI training that the nurse received is limited, described only as between a single half-day to six half-day trainings. Results demonstrate that the nurses did a good job of asking open-ended questions but regularly failed to follow up with empathic statements. Because the nurses were the focus of the study, no patient outcomes or cost analyses were provided.

Noordman, de Vet, van der Weijden, and van Dulmen (2013) also studied nurses' use of MI with the thought in mind of the patient's readiness for lifestyle change. The effect of readiness for change is often discussed in MI literature because the founders of MI emphasize the possibility of increasing an individual's readiness to activate behavior change (SOCs) as an area ripe for interventions facilitating change. In this study, 19 Dutch nurses were videotaped interacting with 103 patients to increase behavior changes regarding smoking, alcohol use, dietary habits, and physical activity. The authors found that the nurses tended to assess intuitively and be flexible with their MI strategies and interventions with patients depending on what SOC each nurse thought the patient was in during the interview. The implication is that nurses should be taught to assess and adapt MI strategies according to the patient's SOCs. Because the focus was on analyzing the nurses' application of MI depending on the patient's SOCs, the authors did not provide a clear description of the training and fidelity measures used to teach the nurses to use MI accurately. No cost analyses were performed.

Using MI to Increase Medication Adherence

By promoting education and treatment adherence, nurses have the potential to make a significant difference in the quality of patients' lives, improve treatment outcomes, and reduce health-care costs significantly. McKenzie and Chang (2015) conducted a pre- and posttest study with a convenience sample of 14 patients living with bipolar disorder to determine if an MI-based intervention by a psychiatric–mental health nurse practitioner (PMHNP) would improve medication adherence in this group. Study participants received a 45- to 60-minute MI intervention in which PMHNPs reviewed patient medications with the patient, assessed medication-taking patterns, measured effectiveness of the medications, evaluated patient-perceived importance of taking the medication, gauged patient confidence levels, and determined readiness to change. Participants were provided a journal to note any concerns about their medications, mood swings, and missing doses between pre- and posttesting. Participants were contacted twice over the next three weeks by phone, and nurses used an MI-based script to assess adherence. Five empirically validated measures were used to assess outcomes in the study. Medication adherence increased from 67.8% to 94.3% among the participants. Although positive outcomes were demonstrated in this study, limitations of the study, such as small sample size, convenience sampling, data captured by self-report, and lack of long-term follow-up, affect generalizability. Description of how the PMHNPs learned MI was not included, and their fidelity to the MI model was also not reported. Medication adherence has the potential to decrease health-care costs, but no cost-benefit analysis was performed as part of this study.

Hyrkas and Wiggins (2014) examined the outcomes of using MI to improve medication adherence and decrease readmission rates. These authors conducted a nonrandomized, nonconcurrent study on a convenience sample of 303 patients treated in an inpatient medical-surgical hospital. The control group included 98 patients who received treatment as usual, 137 patients who received patient-centered education ("teach-back") and medication tools (e.g., pill boxes), and 68 patients who received MI interventions. Patients were excluded if they were being started on new medication, enrolled in other studies, or had a mental health or substance abuse diagnosis. Twenty-two nurses were provided with an initial 16 hours of MI training by certified trainers, an additional 16 hours of intensive MI training, and four hours of coaching support in subsequent months. A specific MI algorithm for medication adherence was developed for the nurses to use to practice MI and to guide interactions with patients. Measurement instruments included discharge and post discharge surveys, self-reported medication screening scale, the Kim Alliance Scale (KAS), and the Patient Experience Scale (PES). Data were collected at discharge, 48 to 72 hours post discharge, and 30 days after discharge. Although patients in the MI group reported lower confidence with adhering to medications as ordered, they had fewer readmissions to the hospital. The authors noted that considerable time and resources are required to teach and train nurses to do MI; however, cost savings with fewer readmissions may mitigate or negate these expenses.

Using MI to Improve Metabolic Disorders

Nurses can have a substantial impact on improving quality of life and overall health and on decreasing health-care costs by providing effective interventions for persons with metabolic disorders, diabetes, and obesity. Several nurse-involved MI metabolic disorder intervention studies are found in the literature. Nurses have ideal opportunities to intervene and prevent childhood obesity.

Wong and Cheng (2013) studied the potential positive effects of using MI to improve health outcomes for 185 grade school children with obesity. This pre-post quasi-experimental design with repeated measures organized children into an MI-intervention group (n = 70), an MI-intervention plus telephone counseling for their parents' group (n = 66), and a control group who received no intervention. Both MI intervention groups of children showed significant improvements in obesity-related measurements and weight management–related behaviors. The control group saw deterioration in all the same measures. Of note, the children seemed to be willing to engage in behavior change, but whether the behavior change was sustained over time is unknown. Also unclear is how many registered nurses were trained to deliver the MI interventions, how the nurse(s) were trained, and whether fidelity to MI core principles was maintained during the interventions. No cost-benefit analyses were done with this study.

Lin et al. (2016) studied a cohort of older women with metabolic disorders to determine the effects of an MI-based lifestyle modification program. This RCT separated 115 middle- to older-age women into one of three groups: an experimental group who received an individualized MI-based program via telephone calls, a brief group who received a single lifestyle session with a brochure, and a usual care group. The experimental group participants realized significant improvements in their physical activity, a reduction in the percentage diagnosed with metabolic disorders, and a reduction in the number of metabolic risks. The brief group saw some improvements in the number of metabolic risks after the 12-week study. How the nurses were trained in MI and whether fidelity to the MI model was maintained is unclear, and no cost-benefit analysis was offered in the article.

El-Mallakh, Chlebowy, Wall, Myers, and Cloud (2012) were interested in how to train nurses in MI and maintain fidelity to the MI model. In this pilot intervention study, one Bachelor of Science Nurse (BSN) prepared nurse delivered MI-based self-care interventions to 26 patients diagnosed with type 2 diabetes (T2D). The authors randomly selected about one-quarter (n = 18) of 72 audiotaped intervention sessions and used an empirically validated scale, the Motivational Interviewing Treatment Integrity (MITI) scale, to assess the sessions for adherence to the MI model. The sessions covered topics such as physical activity, glucose monitoring, and diabetes medication adherence. The MI training that the nurse received was well described, including that the nurse was MI-naïve prior to the study and subsequently participated in four 3-hour training sessions, receiving standardized training materials in didactic and practicum experiences with early sessions focusing on MI philosophy and foundations, coaching and role-playing support, several telephone coaching sessions, and six simulated MI encounters. Because the purpose of this study was to determine the best method of teaching MI to nurses, no patient outcomes were provided, and the authors noted that the use of a single interventionist and a small sample size were major limitations to the study. No cost-benefit analysis was provided with this study.

Chen, Creedy, Lin, and Wollin (2012) also studied MI nursing intervention outcomes in people with diabetes. In this RCT with 3-month follow-up, 250 participants with T2D were randomly divided into an MI intervention group (n = 125) or a treatment-as-usual (TAU) group (n = 125). Several empirically validated measures were used to determine outcomes related to blood sugar monitoring, diet, exercise, psychological well-being, social relationships, confidence level, depression, anxiety, and environmental factors such as food availability. These measures included the Diabetes Self-Management Instrument (DSMI), the Diabetes Self-Efficacy Scale (C-DMSES), the World Health Organization Quality of Life brief scale, and the Depression Anxiety Stress Scale (DASS-21). The authors state that the nurse researcher who conducted the interviews for the intervention group was trained in MI, but no details of the training and no details of measurement to fidelity to the MI model are provided. Results showed an improvement in diabetes self-care, increased self-efficacy, improved quality of life, and improved blood sugar levels in the intervention groups versus the TAU group. The intervention group saw no improvement in depression, anxiety, or stress outcomes. No cost-benefit analyses were provided.

Lindhart et al. (2014) studied the effectiveness of MI training on 11 health-care providers, including nurses, who provide interventions for obese pregnant women. The providers attended a 3-day MI training (training methods were not defined) then were provided audiotapes of sessions they had with their patients. The sessions were evaluated using the empirically validated MITI, which identifies statements adherent to MI. Results showed that the providers generally (although not universally) changed their interventions to MI-adherent interventions. The authors posit that resistance to training all providers may be the result of time constraints, but that resistance would likely be tempered with demonstrated improved communication between provider and patients.

Not all nursing studies show clear benefit of MI interventions. Jansink et al. (2013a) used a cluster RCT to compare nurses trained in MI to nurses with no training in MI to help treat patients with diabetes. Sixty-five nurses from 58 randomly selected general practices participated in this study and were initially divided into intervention (n = 30) or TAU (n = 35) groups. Ultimately, the intervention group consisted of 15 nurses, and the TAU group consisted of 20 nurses. The intervention nurses received 4 half-day training sessions outside their clinical practice time, monthly follow-up calls were recommended, and the nurses received three quarterly coaching calls from trainers within the year following the initial training. An additional training session was added at 4 months after the initial training. The nurses' fidelity to MI was measured using BECCI. The intervention nurses were to submit five video recordings of consultations they delivered to patients with diabetes during the first 4 months after training and then again at about 1 year after the training. Audio recordings were accepted if no video capabilities were possible. Only 65% of the intervention nurses submitted recordings at the two required follow-up intervals. Significant difficulties in rating the audio recordings arose, so they were eventually disregarded. A total of 75 video recordings were examined from the intervention group versus 100 video recordings received from the TAU group. Of note, the intervention group of nurses had fewer years of practice experience (mean = 4.4 versus 9.7) than the control group. Small but significant changes were identified in the intervention group regarding the nurses inviting the patient to talk about behavior change and assessing the patient's confidence level for making lifestyle changes. No cost-benefit analyses were performed with this study.

Jansink and colleagues (2013b) also presented patient outcomes related to their study in another article. The authors examined patient outcomes related to blood sugar readings, physical activity, diet, patient's readiness to change her or his behavior, and quality of life. They determined no discernible difference in outcomes in the nursing intervention versus the TAU groups. The authors note the difficulty in comparing the quality of their MI trainings and support for nurses because they found no comparable studies. They posit that the difficulties may lie in the complexity of care for patients with diabetes.

Using MI to Treat Other Conditions

Other nursing applications of MI are more novel. Ream, Gargaro, Barsevick, and Richardson (2015) recruited 44 patients with cancer to study nursing-delivered interventions to support patient self-management of cancer-related symptoms, including chemotherapy fatigue, distress, anxiety, and depression. In a mixed-methods exploratory study, patients were randomized between an intervention group (n = 23) and a control group (n = 21). Patients in the intervention group received supportive telephone interventions. Results indicate that patients found the format of the intervention delivery to be feasible and acceptable and noted improvements in decreased fatigue intensity, distress, and anxiety, while improving self-care efficacy. The cancer nurse delivering the intervention had experience in working with cancer patients and completed a 10-week module to learn MI via computer-based distance learning and three practicum days at the college completing interviews and skills assessments. Fidelity to MI in this study is described as randomly reviewing 20% of the calls using a checklist (otherwise undefined). No cost-benefit analysis was provided.

Other novel uses of MI include counseling to decrease the risk of HIV transmission. Chen et al. (2016) studied the use of MI to reduce high-risk sexual behaviors among Chinese men who have sex with men. The authors randomized 80 men into an MI counseling intervention group versus a TAU group. The intervention group received a series of three MI counseling sessions with an emphasis on activating behavior change to use condoms consistently during sex with other men. Main goals and MI skills to be used were identified for each of the three sessions. Mixed logistic regressions indicate that participants in the intervention group were 5.7 times more likely to use condoms consistently compared to all study participants at baseline. Results of this study showed that this type of counseling was feasible, and condom use for anal sex increased over time, although condom use during oral sex remained the same. The MI training that the intervention nurses received was not fully described, and no cost-benefit analysis was provided.

Nurses are also exploring the use of MI to improve the treatment of pain. Mertens, Forsberg, Verbunt, Smeets, and Goossens (2016) sought to validate the fidelity of nurses delivering MI pretreatment interventions for patients receiving pain rehabilitation. In this two-armed RCT, two of four registered nurses (RNs) received 2 half-day MI trainings plus 3 half-day follow-up sessions and chronic pain rehabilitation instruction. The other two nurses delivered usual care for pain. The evidence-based MITI was used to evaluate 64 (20% of total) audiotaped patient-care sessions from all four provided over two rounds of interventions (n = 37 intervention tapes; n = 27 control tapes). The authors posit that, despite room for improvement in the quality of MI delivery and mixed inter-rater reliabilities of the MI fidelity scores, discerning the differences between the RN MI interventions and the usual-care RN interventions was possible. This study provided no cost-benefit analysis.

Nursing students are sometimes the recipients of MI interventions. McSharry and Timmins (2016) conducted an effectiveness study with 110 first-year undergraduate nursing students to determine if their health and well-being could be supported and improved during their coursework. An intervention promoting healthy lifestyle choices was designed and provided through a new course titled Teaching on Health and Well-Being. The students were randomized to either an intervention group (n = 55) or a control group (n = 55), and health behaviors were compared pre- and posttest. Statistically significant increases in psychological well-being were seen in the intervention group, with a corresponding decrease in well-being in the control group, and the intervention group increased physical activity, although this was not sustained over time. No cost-benefit analysis was provided with the study.

STRENGTHS AND LIMITATIONS OF EVIDENCE

From August 2015 to September 2016, a search was conducted of evidence-based databases including PubMed, Cumulative Index to Nursing and Allied Health Literature (CINAHL), the Motivational Interviewing (MINT) library web page, Proquest Nursing and Allied Health Source, and the Veterans Health Administration (VHA) National Desktop Library for publications about MI and its use by and with nurses. Only articles that described the nursing use of MI, MI studies conducted by nurses, and studies with nurses or student nurses as subjects of MI were selected. A total of 28 articles were found that met these criteria (Table 6-3).

Of the 28 articles, five consisted of reviews of the literature, systematic reviews of the literature, or meta-analyses. Eleven studies consisted of prospective observational designs, pilot studies, study protocol design, feasibility studies, intervention studies, or evaluation studies. Two studies were experimental and quasi-experimental, and one was a secondary analysis. Also included were six RCTs, one two-arm RCT, and one cluster RCT. Three studies were descriptive designs with qualitative methods.

Half of the articles were conducted with adult patients as participants. Eleven studies used nurses or nursing students as study subjects, another two studies examined the use of MI with older adults, and one study examined adolescent girls in an exercise program.

Nineteen of the studies provided no discussion or description of how the nurses who delivered MI interventions were educated or trained in MI principles. Another eight studies offered minimal discussion of the MI education and training of nurses intervening during the study. One study had adequately detailed discussion of MI training that the intervention nurses were engaged in prior to the onset of the study.

Providing a discussion of the costs and benefits of using MI was challenging. Twenty-seven of the articles contained no cost-benefit analysis. One study mentioned that health-care costs would be less if the MI intervention succeeded in lowering readmission rates.

Despite obvious limitations to the evidence, nurses are clearly interested in the potential benefits of using MI in their practice. As demonstrated in several of the articles, MI is useful for activating behavior change in a variety of clinical settings and for a variety of patient needs. These articles include the study by Thompson et al. (2011), who found the use of MI did result in some improvements to patients' cardiovascular health. In addition, Lundahl et al. (2013) found that HIV patients improved their self-care when nurses employed MI-based interventions. The study by Spoelstra et al. (2014) demonstrated improved medication adherence with the nursing use of MI strategies. Improvements were seen in geriatric patients' diet, weight, and physical activity levels with the nursing use of MI (Pruath & Fitzgerald, 2014). A novel use of MI has been demonstrated as effective in reducing stigma of mental health issues (Brobeck et al., 2011). Hyrkas and Wiggins (2014) demonstrated a positive effect of decreasing readmissions among patients with chronic disorders. Another unique use of the potential usefulness of MI is found in McSharry and Timmins's (2016) study of improving the well-being of nursing students.

RISKS, COSTS, AND BENEFITS OF APPLYING THE EVIDENCE

As noted above, a significant limitation to having all nurses educated and trained in using MI is that very few studies address the costs and benefits of adopting a more MI-adherent practice. Institutions require evidence of the cost and benefits for both the institution and its patients before planning to institute an MI program. Should MI be widely disseminated if it is costly and difficult to learn?

In a prospective single-blind RCT, Riegel, Creber, Hill, and Hoke (2016) offer a glimpse of potential cost savings and benefits that nurses can provide using MI with a convenience sample of patients who have heart failure (HF). The study aimed to determine if the rate of hospital readmission could be decreased for the patient's HF or other comorbid conditions. One hundred hospitalized patients with HF were recruited and randomly assigned on a 2:1 ratio to either an intervention (n = 70) or control (n = 30) group. Intervention group patients received a home visit by a nurse plus three to four follow-up telephone calls in which the patients received an MI-tailored intervention for HF (MITI-HF). Control group patients received education about self-care only. All patients completed the Self Care of HF Index, a questionnaire about improvements in self-care, and had their medical records reviewed for subsequent hospitalizations. Results showed fewer hospitalizations due to comorbid issues such as diabetes in the intervention group (with an overall 48% lower chance of having a non-HF-related readmission), although no difference was seen in the length of stay for patients who were hospitalized. The authors provide no specific dollar amount of cost savings, but hospital admission is universally accepted as expensive; therefore, any decrease in readmissions will result in general cost savings. Other than

Table 6-3 Summary of Nursing and MI Evidence

Citation	Source/Subjects Review of the Literature (ROL)	Discussion/Methods/Results
Thompson, D. R., Chair, S. Y., Chan, S. W., Astin, R., Davidson, P. M., & Ski, C. F. (2011). Motivational interviewing: A useful approach to improving cardiovascular health? *Journal of Clinical Nursing, 20*, 1236–1244.	ROL: 4 meta-analyses, 1 systematic review, 3 literature reviews, 5 primary studies.	8 sources were secondary analyses from National Heart, Lungs, & Blood Institute. MI found to be effective but not a panacea; patients had greater continuity of care; nurses had more opportunities to become proficient in MI.
Al-Ganmi, A. H., Perry, L., Gholizadeh, L., & Alotaibi, A. M. (2016). Cardiovascular medication adherence among patients with cardiac disease: A systematic review. *Journal of Advance Nursing*, 72(12), 3001–3014. doi: 10.1111/jan.13062	ROL: 14 met inclusion criteria (multifaceted education, received behavioral and educational counseling including MI completed by nurses).	Heterogeneity of samples prevents meta-analysis. MI-based nursing education via phone or text is a promising method to increase cardiac medication compliance.
Lundahl, B., Moleni, T., Burke, B. L., Buttons, R., Tollefson, D., Butler, C., & Rollnick, S. (2013). Motivational interviewing in medical care settings: A systematic review and meta-analysis of randomized controlled trials. *Patient Education and Counseling, 93*(2), 157–168.	Systematic ROL and meta-analysis of RCTs; 48 studies.	Modest promise held for increased behavior change for: improved HIV viral load, dental outcomes, body weight, alcohol and tobacco use, sedentary lifestyle, self-monitoring, confidence in change, and approach to treatment. Not very effective with eating disorders, self-care, or some medical outcomes.
Spoelstra, S. L., Schueller, M., Hilton, M., & Ridenour, K. (2014). Interventions combining motivational interviewing and cognitive behavior therapy to promote medication adherence: A literature review. *Journal of Clinical Nursing, 24*, 1163–1173.	Integrative literature review: 1 RCT, 4 cohort studies. 1 case study. Medication adherence.	Used self-report, pharmacy records, electronic pill bottles. Used Whittmore and Knafl method (2-point scale: high/low rigor; data relevance). Using combination of MI and CBT is effective for increasing medication adherence.
Purath, J., Keck, A., & Fitzgerald, C. E. (2014). Motivational interviewing for older adults in primary care: A systematic review. *Geriatric Nursing, 35*(3), 219–224.	Systematic ROL: 8 studies. PICOT focused ROL. PRISMA used for evaluation.	May be effective for improving geriatric diet, physical activity, weight control. Attrition bias; lack of blinding; difficult to tell if there is fidelity to MI model.
O'May, F., Gill, J., McWhirter, E., Kantartzis, S., Reese, C., & Murray, K. (2016). A teachable moment for the teachable moment? A prospective study to evaluate delivery of a workshop designed to increase knowledge and skills in relation to alcohol brief interventions (ABIs) amongst final year nursing and occupational therapy undergraduates. *Nursing Education in Practice, 6*(20), 45–53.	Developing study protocol; nursing and occupational therapy students.	Students deliver alcohol brief interventions (ABIs). Each profession agreed they should do it but less than half agreed they had appropriate knowledge to deliver effective ABIs.

(*continued*)

Table 6-3 Summary of Nursing and MI Evidence—cont'd

Citation	Source/Subjects Review of the Literature (ROL)	Discussion/Methods/Results
Bredie, S. J. H., Fouwels, A. J., Wollersheim, H., & Schippers, G. M. (2011). Effectiveness of nurse based motivational interviewing for smoking cessation in high risk cardiovascular outpatients: A randomized trial. *European Journal of Cardiovascular Nursing, 10*, 174–179.	Feasibility study. Intervention group = 46 (12 quit smoking). Control = 42 (3 quit smoking).	Developing a nurse-based MI (NBMI); also used Lifestyle Inventory with feedback. Quitters remained abstinent at 3 months. Participants who did not consent and participate had heavier use of tobacco. Did not record those who may have cut down. Time invested = 3.8 hours per patient, considered good investment.
Osterlund Efraimsson, E., Fossum, B., Ehrenberg, A., Larsson, K., & Klang, B. (2012). Use of motivational interviewing in smoking cessation at nurse-led chronic obstructive pulmonary disease clinics. *Journal of Advanced Nursing, 68*(4), 767–782.	Prospective observational study. Videotaped consultations. 13 patients who smoke.	Evaluated using MITI. Nurses received 4 days of training in MI. 5 parameters: evocation, collaboration, autonomy/support, empathy, direction. Direction scored highest; gave information; made closed information statements. Conclusion: nurses did not use MI.
Mujika, A., Forbes, A., Canga, N., de Irata, J., Serrano, I., Gasco, P., & Edwards, M. (2014). Motivational interviewing as a smoking cessation strategy with nurses: An exploratory randomized controlled trial. *International Journal of Nursing Studies, 51*, 1074–1082.	Exploratory trial stage parallel experimental design. 30 nurses who smoke (*n* = 15, MI intervention; *n* = 15 in usual care).	Data show highly addicted were less likely to quit. At 3 months, 6 nurses in intervention group remained quit (biologically validated).
Robbins L. B., Pfeiffer, K. A., Maier, K. S., LaDrig, S. M., & Berg-Smith, S. M. (2012). Treatment fidelity of motivational interviewing delivered by a school nurse to increase girls' physical activity. *The Journal of School Nursing, 28*(1), 70–78.	Secondary analysis 2 group pre-intervention post-intervention test quasi-experimental design. Delivered by one school nurse.	Nurse received 2-day MI training by MINT member; used an intervention manual. Program: Girls on the Move (after school activity club). 32 sixth- and seventh-grade girls; racially diverse. Focus of study on nurse competency (not on girls' outcomes). Reached beginning proficiency and proceeded to beyond competent; however, only 25% to 30% of reflections were complex. Conclusion: it takes more than 2 days of training for sustained competency.
Brobeck, E., Bergh, H., Odencrants, S., & Hildingh, C. (2011). Primary healthcare nurses' experience with motivational interviewing in health promotion. *Journal of Clinical Nursing, 20*, 3322–3330.	Descriptive design, qualitative methods. *N* = 20 RNs (not patient outcome focused).	Content analysis of interviews; health promotion practices for patients. Results: MI promotes caring relationship; valuable tool; must make more effort to practice MI skills; nurses state they can apply MI skills to other areas of care; nurses felt greater empathy toward patients.
Brobeck, E., Odencrants, S., Bergh, H., & Hildingh, C. (2014). Patients' experience of lifestyle discussions based on motivational interviewing: A qualitative study. *BMC Nursing, 13*(13). Retrieved from http://www.biomedcentral.com/1472-6955/13/13	Descriptive study, qualitative interviews. Convenience sample of 16 patient encounters with RNs.	Selection bias: all patients ready to change. Unclear what MI training was provided for nurses. Patients report often feeling shame about discussing lifestyles, but with MI, they felt liberated and able to speak freely; created a sense of well-being; contributed to behavior change; without support of RN it is easy to delay change; MI considered acceptable interaction.

Table 6-3 Summary of Nursing and MI Evidence—cont'd

Citation	Source/Subjects Review of the Literature (ROL)	Discussion/Methods/Results
Ostlund, A. S., Wadensten, B., Haggstrom, E., Lindqvist, H., & Kristofferzon, M. L. (2016). Primary care nurses' communication and its influence on patient talk during motivational interviewing. *Journal of Advanced Nursing*, 72(11), 2844–2856. doi: 10.1111/jan.13052	Descriptive predictive design. 50 audio-recordings between 23 primary-care nurses.	MI SCOPE used to evaluate recordings for fidelity. Nurses most often used neutral talk; did not use many open questions; did not use complex reflections, did not use change talk. Rigor of study discussed in-depth. 5 hypotheses about behavior change; 4 fully met.
Noordman, J., van der Lee, I., Nielen, M., Vlek, H., van der Weijden, T., & van Dulmen, S. (2012). Do trained practice nurses apply motivational interviewing techniques in primary care consultations? *Journal of Clinical Medical Research*, 4(6), 393–401.	Observational study of real-life encounters. 13 nurses; 117 patient encounters.	Used BECCI to evaluate fidelity to MI model. Scored highest in Domain 1: agenda setting and permission seeking. Scored lowest in asking open ended questions, discussing how to change and why change; failed to use empathetic statements. Very little description of MI training for nurses.
Noordman, J., van de Vet, E., van der Weijden, T., & van Dulmen, S. (2013). Motivational interviewing within the different stages of change: An analysis of practice nurse-patient consultations aimed at promoting a healthier lifestyle. *Social Science & Medicine*, *87*, 60–67.	Observational study of real-life encounters. 19 nurses; 103 patient encounters.	Used BECCI to evaluate fidelity to MI model. RNs flex MI strategies depending on stage of change that the patient is in; intuitively assess stage of change and tailor communication accordingly. Very little description of MI training for nurses.
McKenzie, K., & Chang, Y. (2015). The effect of nurse-led motivational interviewing on medication adherence in patients with bipolar disorder. *Perspectives in Psychiatric Care*, *51*, 36–44.	Pilot study, pre-intervention post-intervention test. 3-week intervention. 14 PMHNPs completed with goal of increasing medication adherence and decreasing admissions among patients with bipolar disorder.	Small group, homogenous, no control group, lack of follow-up. Used MI manual; face-to-face intervention plus 2 follow-up calls. Nonadherence decreased from mean of 4.3 (±2.6) to mean of 2.2 (±1.6); overall improvement from mean of 67.8% to mean of 94.3% adherent. Used Medication Adherence Rating Scale (MARS); Timeline Follow Back (TLFB); MI Rulers (ICR); Self-Efficacy and Appropriate Medication Use Scale (SEAMS); and patient satisfaction surveys.
Hyrkas, K., & Wiggins, M. (2014). A comparison of usual care, a patient-centered education intervention and motivational interviewing to improve medication adherence and readmissions of adults in an acute-care setting. *Journal of Nursing Management, 22*, 350–361.	Nonrandomized intervention study; prospective, longitudinal design with nonconcurrent convenience sample. 22 RNs; 303 patients.	Aim: increase medication adherence and decrease readmissions. 3 groups: n = 98 in usual care, *n* = 137 in teach back and medication tools, *n* = 68 in MI intervention T1 = upon discharge T2 = 48 to 72 hours later T3 = 30 days after discharge Results: MI was a significant predictor of fewer admissions and increased sense of importance and confidence about taking medications. No description of RN MI training.

(*continued*)

Table 6-3 Summary of Nursing and MI Evidence—cont'd

Citation	Source/Subjects Review of the Literature (ROL)	Discussion/Methods/Results
Wong, E. M. Y., & Chengh, M. M. H. (2013). Effects of motivational interviewing to promote weight loss in obese children. *Journal of Clinical Nursing, 22,* 2519–2530.	Pre-intervention post-intervention quasi-experimental design with repeated measures.	3 groups: *n* = 70 in MI group; *n* = 66 in MI plus counseling group plus telephone follow-up group; *n* = 49 in control group. Both MI and MI+ group and follow-up showed significant improvement in weight-related behavior changes and obesity anthropometric measures. No description of RN MI training.
Lin, C. H., Chiang, S. L., Heitkemper, M. M., Hung, Y. J., Lee, M. S., Tzeng, W. C., & Chiang, L. C. (2016). Effects of telephone-based motivational interviewing in lifestyle modification program on reducing metabolic risks in middle-aged and older women with metabolic syndrome: A randomized control trial. *International Journal of Nursing Studies, 60,* 12–23.	RCT with 3 parallel intervention groups. *N* = 115 older females with obesity.	Group 1: *n* = 38 (MI + lifestyle training for 12 weeks) Group 2: *n* = 38 (brief intervention) Group 3: *n* = 39 (usual care) Evaluated patient data with NCEP-ATPIII guidelines. Results: increased activity levels, although not to statistical significance (but clinically meaningful improvements); improved HDL; improved weight loss, decreased metabolic risks and less metabolic diagnoses. No description of RN MI training.
El-Mallakh, P., Chlebowy, D. O., Wall, M. P., Myers, J. A., & Cloud, R. N. (2012). Promoting nurse interventionist fidelity to motivational interviewing in diabetes self-care intervention. *Research in Nursing & Health, 35,* 289–300.	Pilot intervention study using one BSN-prepared RN. 72 audio-recordings with 28 patients.	Used MITI to evaluate audiotapes. 45-minute sessions. Results: training facilitates satisfactory MI progress toward proficiency. Provides detailed description of RN MI training.
Chen, S. M., Creedy, D., Lin, H-S., & Wollin, J. (2012). Effects of motivational interviewing on self-management, psychological and glycemic outcomes in type 2 diabetes: A randomized controlled trial. *International Journal of Nursing Studies, 49,* 637–644.	RCT pre-intervention post-intervention test. Intervention + 3-month follow-up group *n* = 104. Control group *n* = 110.	Aim: increase self-management, and psychological and glycemic outcomes. Nurse researcher with nursing background and extensively trained in MI; no description of RN MI training; no discussion of use of MI fidelity measures. Results: improved self-care, self-efficacy, QOL, HgbA1C but no improvement of depression, anxiety, or stress.
Lindhardt, C. L., Rubak, S., Mogensen, O., Hansen, H. P., Lamont, R. F., & Jorgensen, J. S. (2014). Training in motivational interviewing in obstetrics: A quantitative analytical tool. *Acta Obstetric Gynecology Scandinavia, 93,* 698–704.	Intervention study; pre-intervention post-intervention test. *N* = 11 OB, midwives, RNs with no prior MI experience.	3-day training in MI (very general description of details of training). MITI used to evaluate for fidelity of MI in recordings made by clinicians. Results: small but significant improvement but not universal; MI was more difficult to learn than anticipated; may note resistance from administration due to time and funding needed to train.
Jansink, R., Braspenning, J., Laurant, M., Keizer, E., Elwyn, G., van der Weijden, T., & Grol, R. (2013). Minimal improvement of nurses' motivational interviewing skills in routine diabetes care one year after training: A cluster randomized trial. *BMC Family Practice, 14,* 44.	Cluster RCT. Usual care group *n* = 35. MI treatment group *n* = 30. Focus on nursing outcomes.	Rural and urban setting diabetes care. Baseline and 14-month measures; used BECCI to evaluate recordings for MI fidelity. At baseline: 18 intervention nurses provided 90 recordings; 15 control nurses provided 75 recordings. At 14 months: 15 intervention nurses provided 75 recordings; 20 control nurses provided 100 recordings.

Table 6-3 Summary of Nursing and MI Evidence—cont'd

Citation	Source/Subjects Review of the Literature (ROL)	Discussion/Methods/Results
		Results: at 14 months, intervention group nurses improved 2 out of 24 MI skills; some general MI skills improved but minimal. Conclusion: Retention is minimal; may be due to complex care patients. Nurses received 16 hours of training spread out over 6 months; poorly described.
Jansink, R., Braspenning, J., Keizer, E., van der Weijden, T., Elwyn, G., & Grol, R. (2013). No identifiable HgbA1C or lifestyle change after a comprehensive diabetes programme including motivational interviewing: A cluster randomized trial. *Scandinavian Journal of Primary Health Care, 31*, 119–127.	Cluster RCT. Intervention group, *n* = 134 patients. Control group, *n* = 202 patients. Focus on patient outcomes.	Patients answered questionnaires, and medical records were reviewed. Results: no change in HgbA1C, diet (fat, fruit, vegetable intake), physical activity, or any metabolic measure; question usefulness of MI. Nurses had received 16 hours of training spread out over 6 months; poorly described; question effectiveness of delivery of training.
Ream, E., Gargaro, G., Barsevick, A., & Richardson, A. (2015). Management of cancer-related fatigue during chemotherapy through telephone motivational interviewing: Modeling and randomized exploratory trial. *Patient Education and Counseling, 98*(2), 199–206.	Mixed methods exploratory study. Guided adaptation of intervention: beating fatigue in cancer patients. 8 patients; 12 clinicians.	2 phases over 12 months. Focus groups: discuss the experience of fatigue, experience of usual care, intervention actions that decrease fatigue, and perceptions of phone-delivered treatment. MITI used to evaluate MI fidelity. Results: treatment group showed improvements in all except depression; control group showed increased depression and increased fatigue; beating fatigue intervention was deemed acceptable and feasible.
Chen, J., Li, X., Xiong, Y., Fennie, X. P., Wang, H., & Williams, A. B. (2016). Reducing the risk of HIV transmission among men who have sex with men: A feasibility study of the motivational interviewing counseling method. *Nursing Health Science, 18*(3), 400–407. doi: 10.1111/nhs.12287	RCT of 80 men who have sex with men (MSM). Intervention group, *n* = 40. Control group, usual treatment, *n* = 40.	Used MITI to evaluate audio recordings; all participants provided with condoms and lubricant. Results: recordings were MI adherent; increased condom use with anal but not oral sex; 5.7% more likely to use condoms (P = 0.006; 95% CI). No description of RN MI training.
Mertens, V. C., Forsberg, L., Verbunt, J. A., Smeets, R. E. J. M., Goossens, M. E. J. B. (2016). Treatment fidelity of a nurse-led motivational interviewing-based pre-treatment in pain rehabilitation. *Journal of Behavioral Health Services & Research, 43*(3), 459–473.	2-arm RCT. 2 RNs trained in pain control measures only (usual care). 2 RNs with history of MI experience and received 2 half-day training sessions in MI and pain control.	Used MITI to evaluate MI fidelity for 64 sessions (*n* = 37 MI/pain; *n* = 27 usual care). Results: proficiency exceeded only in 1 score (reflection to questions) and 1 measure (empathy); found MI fidelity was good but mixed inter-rater reliability; confirms need for rigor in studies. Limited description of RN MI training.
McSharry, P., & Timmins, F. (2016). An evaluation of the effectiveness of a dedicated health and well-being course on nursing students' health. *Nursing Education Today, 16*(44), 26–32.	Evaluation study of new educational module for undergraduate nursing students. *n* = 110.	Aim: improve physical health and well-being in undergraduate nursing students. *n* = 55 in treatment group *n* = 55 in control group Results: improved psychological well-being and physical activity, although not sustained over time. No description of MI training; no description of MI fidelity evaluation.

stating that the two RNs who provided the interventions were given a one-day training plus practice, no description of the specifics of MI training is provided.

Jassal, Riekert, Borelli, Rand, and Eakin (2016) completed post hoc analyses on an RCT for the use of MI with mostly African American, low-income individuals who provide care for 330 Head Start students. The primary aim of the study was to determine if cost savings related to reducing children's exposure to secondhand smoke (SHS) would be demonstrated at 3, 6, and 12 months. Significant cost savings in reduced emergency department visits were seen at the 12-month interval only, which did not overcome the additional costs of implementing MI to Head Start caregivers. The authors posit that this may be a very good long-term cost-savings strategy. Cost savings may not have been realized in the earlier intervals because caregivers may not have changed their behaviors immediately and/or the children had not yet had the time to benefit physically from less SHS exposure.

Patients with alcohol-use disorders being treated in the emergency department or trauma unit may also benefit from MI intervention. Shepard et al. (2016) studied the effect of including an MI intervention with an individual's significant other (SOMI) compared to providing MI to the individual only (IMI). In the full study, 406 patients (171 received interventions) were randomized, with the data evaluated using the Treatment Cost Assessment Tool. Costs of the intervention included employment of the staff who delivered the treatment as well as screening, recruitment, and baseline delivery of MI to the patient and significant other (SO). Client-based costs were assessed, including client travel time and the costs of treatment. The quality-adjusted life-year was also assessed. Encouraging results were realized, including a decreased rate of emergency department and trauma unit readmission. The authors report, "From baseline to 12-month follow-up, the percentage of hazardous drinking declined by 22.9% in SOMI and by 13.5% in IMI" (p. 835). In addition, a cost savings of $4.73 for every $1.00 spent providing SOMI was seen. No clear description of how staff members were trained to deliver SOMI and IMI was given, or what type of clinician delivered the intervention.

Hall, Staiger, Simpson, Best, and Lubman (2015) completed a systematic review of the literature to determine if training in MI helps clinicians achieve sustained practice changes in delivering substance use disorder (SUD) treatment, and, if they do, whether this had an impact on client outcomes. The PRISMA statement was used to evaluate the literature. Criterion for meeting sustained practice was determined as 75% of clinicians achieving beginning MI proficiency. Twenty studies were identified, but only two met the criterion. With such a limited sample, drawing conclusions about cost-benefit analyses was not possible. This speaks to the paucity of evidence about evaluating MI as a viable treatment option.

A possible path forward to studying the benefits of MI can be found in a study protocol for an RCT presented in the manuscript by Mertens, Goossens, Verbunt, Koke, and Smeets (2013). The aim was to provide a protocol for a study of 160 patients with chronic pain, one arm (n = 80) of which received a two-session MI intervention (MIP) to prepare and help motivate them to receive pain rehabilitation. The authors provide an in-depth description of their main research questions (i.e., effectiveness versus usual care, cost effectiveness and cost utility, feasibility of MIP regarding fidelity to MI model, and descriptions of patient and nurse experiences with MIP) as well as the methods and design of this parallel single-blind RCT. A description of the results of the patient experience is found in another article by these authors.

Potential risk associated with the use of MI is quite limited. Financial waste may be attributed to poorly executed programs that do not improve outcomes, such as treatment adherence and decreased readmission rates. Poorly delivered MI may increase treatment resistance. Training time can take staff members out of busy clinical areas, which in turn may decrease patient access to care. Any MI program must be well developed and executed.

Key Stakeholders

The buy-in from key stakeholders is critical to the success of implementing any training program. If frontline clinicians are to use MI to activate health behavior changes successfully, interested stakeholders must be provided with information about the use, cost effectiveness, methodology of implementation, and expected outcomes of MI. That becomes challenging when only limited numbers exist of well-implemented and measured rigorous studies of the nursing use of MI. Prior to approaching administrative stakeholders, it is vital to have a plan that addresses how clinicians (or students) will be taught, how fidelity to the model will be measured, how outcomes will be tracked, and how the outcomes will contribute to cost savings and/or satisfaction scores. Initial interest can originate from any level of clinical and nonclinical staff members, but buy-in from participants and supervisors is a first critical step in a successful program. For examples describing the effective study of the nursing use of MI, see the studies completed by Hyrkas and Wiggins (2014) and El-Mallakh et al. (2012).

Nursing Training and Fidelity to MI Core Values

Many factors affect the process of becoming proficient as a practitioner of MI. These factors can be discipline specific, clinician specific (e.g., years of academic preparation, years on the job, previous exposure to MI), patient specific (e.g., age, gender, race/ethnicity, diagnosis, resources, challenges), clinical setting–specific (e.g., primary care, mental health, pediatrics, geriatrics), and/or related to training and validating methodologies. The quality and fidelity of training is critical; as Miller and Rollnick (2013) observed, "It is unsurprising that MI would be ineffective when delivered with low fidelity" (p. 382). Studies that have been conducted in an assortment of countries and cultures show a variety of levels of MI skill acquisition.

Noordman and colleagues (2012, 2014) studied the training efforts necessary to assist nurses in gaining proficiency in using MI. In the 2012 study, the researchers conducted an observational study using 13 practice nurses from general practitioners' offices who interacted with 117 adult patients. The nurse's prior training with MI is described as between 1 half-day training and 6 half-day trainings. Whether the nurses had previous MI training is unclear. Video recordings were made of the nurse–patient encounters, and fidelity to MI was measured with BECCI. Results showed that the nurses exhibited some MI-adherent skills by asking open-ended questions but failed to meet significance in follow-up empathy statements.

Noordman, van der Weijden, and van Dulman (2014) found similar results in their study. This study examined pre- and posttest data from 17 Dutch nurses and 325 patients using videotaped interview sessions. MI fidelity was measured with the BECCI and the Maastrichtse Anamnese en Advies Scorelijst (MASS-Global). Improvements were found, including more attention to requests for help, better physical examinations, more understandable information provided to patients, and more attention paid to agenda-setting and permission seeking in communications with patients.

The authors note that, although this study did not universally increase all MI skills, it did show significant improvement in the nurses' communication skills. It may be more challenging to teach and train nurses working in busy practice settings than it is to prepare student nurses academically by teaching MI methods and techniques. Similar results were discovered by Bohman, Forsberg, Ghaden, and Rasmussen (2013), who found that 3½ days of training and systematic feedback on the use of MI did not result in the 36 nurses reaching a beginning level of proficiency with MI. The authors conclude that a one-time training with feedback may not be enough training for nurses to acquire MI skills. The case can also be made that certain areas of nursing practice are inherently more directive in style and might require a different way to employ MI skills.

A potentially effective model for teaching MI is found in Mallisham and Sherrod (2016), who designed, delivered, and evaluated an educational MI program conducted at least in part by psychiatric nurse practitioners for psychiatric nurses. The authors draw a distinction between patient-centered care and MI, which they describe as a more guided and directive approach than patient-centered care. Bachelor and associate degree nurses received an 8-hour MI training, role play, or observation during patient encounters, and 1:1 coaching and feedback. Participants were tested before and after part one of the training session, which focused on teaching MI core values through video examples, role play, and discussion of observation sheets. At the end of education and training sessions, performance was assessed with the MI training (comMIt) tool and the MI adherence and competency feedback (MIACF) form. Results from McNemar test and mean scores show statistically significant increases in MI knowledge and the use of knowledge into practice.

Cook at al. (2016) provided an excellent summary and evaluation of 10 years of interprofessional MI training. This manuscript reports on various disciplines, noting that nurses made up 20% of participants. They note that one discipline (mental health) accounted for most of the trainees in the early years, but by 2015 most training sessions included clinicians from five to nine separate disciplines. The authors provide an important discussion about the "trainability" of staff members who work in various clinical settings. For example, the training commitment (time, effort, funding, etc.) for some clinicians may exceed the resources they have available to receive training in one treatment modality, and some professions may simply require more directive and educationally directive interventions by staff members (e.g., pediatrics and adolescent care). Notably, many staff members are entering MI trainings with previous exposure and training in MI (in 2006, 0% of clinicians had previous MI exposure, but by 2013, 79% had some MI exposure), which may or may not affect study results.

The current study followed results from 394 participants in a variety of training settings, lengths, and delivery methods conducted from 2006 to 2015. The participants were given validated questionnaires to fill out after each session. The primary outcome measure of this study was the knowledge, attitudes, and beliefs (KAB) survey. Outcomes differed across disciplines, with higher outcomes noted in clinicians in direct practice versus nondirect health-care professionals. No consistent effect was noted with factors such as prior training, demographic variables, and training process differences, although years of clinical experiences predicted MI-consistent attitudes.

Some surprising results of this study include that the nurses in the study scored higher on the attitude scale of the KAB but lower on the behavior subscale, which has several possible implications. Nurses are theoretically aligned with MI core values (also known as the spirit of MI), but they may need more opportunities to practice specific MI techniques. In other words, they may know and accept MI in philosophy, but they may not practice it as much as they could and may benefit from having increased opportunities to engage with supervision or coaching.

This study recognizes some limitations, including having low internal validity due to participants not being part of a formal study and results being self-report measures. However, high external validity was achieved due to the large sample size.

Miller and Rollnick (2013) provide some recommendations for outcomes research that apply to improving the efficacy and outcomes of MI training. Although "there is no minimum or sufficient 'dose' of training to guarantee competence in MI" (p. 384), determining and documenting thresholds for competence and ongoing quality assurance in MI is vital. In addition, if a desired outcome exists, both provider and patient contributing factors must be included. Flexibility in the practice of MI is critical because human behavior change circumstances rarely fall within the confines of "one size fits all" and can lead to necessary innovation.

AREAS FOR FUTURE STUDY, IMPLEMENTATION, NURSING THEORY

Nurses are taught to be excellent, selfless teachers. However, the provision of external information alone does not activate or sustain behavior change. Particularly difficult is to resist, in the words of Miller and Rollnick (2013), "the righting reflex" (p. 6) of the well-intended use of a directive, information-laden style of communication to activate behavior change.

Miller and Moyers (2014) acknowledge that how MI results in good outcomes is not fully understood. They caution that "treatment outcomes are not likely to be improved greatly by searching for better specific content to prescribe in therapists' manuals" (p. 407). The relationship aspect of MI is emphasized, although they acknowledge that the context of an interpersonal relationship is inseparable from the technique. As previously noted, practitioner characteristics and patient characteristics indeed influence the dynamic. Practitioner characteristics include having an expectation (hope) of positive outcomes, the ability to form a relationship with the patient, good interpersonal skills (empathy), and clear fidelity to MI core values. Patient characteristics include initial optimism toward positive treatment outcomes, motivation to consider and make efforts to change, and confidence in their own ability to make changes occur. Miller and Moyer (2014) note that resistance to change is fairly normal and yet is "highly responsive to therapist style" (p. 406). The authors advocate for developing tools that can capture the elusive relational aspects of MI. The most useful MI intervention that nurses can readily learn and apply likely centers on learning reflective listening skills beyond the level typically taught in nursing schools due to time constraints. Providing an in-depth description of the various strategies and techniques that are taught for use in MI-adherent interventions is beyond the scope of this chapter; however, Table 6-1 provided a brief overview of MI strategies.

Many areas are ripe for future study of the application of MI in nursing practice, including topics related to nursing academic preparation, job-based teaching and training, the clinical setting of the practicing nurse, and nurse and patient demographics. Even as this chapter sought to answer questions about the nursing use of MI, a multitude of questions remain. Is teaching MI in academic settings prior to entering clinical practice more effective because practicing nurses are commonly overloaded with clinical responsibilities and have little time for additional learning? Will information-overloaded students retain MI skills once they enter clinical practice? Does the teaching and learning of MI differ among academic preparation (ADN, BSN, MSN, PhD/DNP)? Are factors such as gender, age, years of nursing experience, and other differences influencing the teaching and learning of MI?

Understand that implementation of any new approach is a process and not an event. A single MI training session for nurses provides an opportunity to explore and adopt new strategies, but it does not necessarily (or likely) install or sustain a new way of practice. Hall et al. (2015) identify the importance of establishing benchmarks and standardized methods of monitoring MI training. Without some sort of standardized yet flexible expectations, MI-based treatment outcomes are uncertain.

Nurses recognize the value of identifying nursing-specific models and theory supporting behavior change activation. Rosswurm and Larrabee (1999) discuss facilitating change in practitioner skills to effect patient behavioral change. These authors propose a six-step model of practitioner change in translating evidence into practice: (1) assess need for change in practice,

(2) link problem to interventions and outcomes, (3) synthesize best evidence, (4) design practice change, (5) implement and evaluate practice change, and (6) integrate and maintain change in practice. This model is useful when considering the implementation and study of MI nursing training and outcomes research.

An important nursing theory about behavior change is described by Ryan (2009), who proposes the Integrated Theory of Health Behavior Change (ITHBC). In this theory, behavior change activation "can be enhanced by fostering knowledge and beliefs, increasing self-regulation skills and abilities" (p. 161). The reader is tasked with developing a better understanding of human behavior change and appreciating what the nurse's role is in activating and sustaining health behavior change.

IMPLICATIONS FOR PRACTICE

Because the nursing experience itself widely varies, it would be naïve to think that MI will be learned and practiced the same way by every nurse. A quick search of nursing specialties shows that more than 100 separate areas of nursing practice exist, in both traditional and nontraditional settings. Some specialties, such as those focused on children and adolescents, might require MI techniques to be adapted with a more directive approach. The American Nurses Credentialing Center does not list any certification specific to MI, and how much, if any, content is dedicated to nurses being proficient in knowing about, understanding, or using MI is unclear.

Nurses are often charged with caring for patients who develop chronic health issues that worsen over time. Helping patients recognize and change health behaviors that cause or contribute to chronic health problems is imperative, as it saves time we would have to spend in the future. This requires that nurses develop more nuanced listening skills than what they likely possess, which may be a source of resistance. Today's nurses are inundated with necessary and required patient-care tasks and excessive documentation requirements—and they have only a short time in which to do it all. It is common for nurses to try to "fix" things and inadvertently contribute to more deeply entrenched unhealthy behaviors (e.g., "it's my only vice I have left"). The lack of patient activation to engage in collaborative nursing care perpetuates the cycle of chronic health-care problems that actually *adds* more time and effort.

When nurses are taught essential MI skills, especially listening skills, they learn to listen to patients for the purpose of understanding rather than for the purpose of responding with short-term, doomed to fail educational "fixes" that patients are not yet ready to hear. MI can help nurses move from thinking, "What's the *matter with* this patient? Doesn't she (or he) see what this is doing to their health?" to instead thinking, "What is it that *matters to* (motivates) this patient?" Getting at underlying motivation, i.e., see grandchildren graduate, being physically capable of continuing cherished hobbies, remaining independent in one's own home, etc., is much more likely to activate sustained behavior change. It is also a way of getting in tune with how patient's feel, as sometimes when they are discouraged and ready to give up on healthy behaviors, it is necessary to *lend them your hope* that they can achieve and sustain healthy goals.

A prime example of internal motivation is seen in present-day circumstances. The coronavirus epidemic may, unfortunately, provide some internal motivation for quitting smoking. Emerging evidence suggests that outcomes to this devastating illness may be complicated by a person's smoking status (Vardavas & Nikitara, 2020). Worries about coronavirus may motivate patients to make health behavior changes. Nurses need to be prepared with accurate information *and* the ability to listen for the purpose of understanding what this threat may mean for the individual. This will lead to support for quitting smoking even as the person's motivation waxes and wanes after the initial motivation.

NATIONAL GUIDELINES

A search of the use of MI in the Healthy People 2020 resources reveals that at least two initiatives use MI (https://www.healthypeople.gov/). One is the Healthy People 2020 at Work in the Community: Human Rights and Health available at: https://www.healthypeople.gov/2020/healthy-people-in-action/story/healthy-people-2020-work-community-human-rights-and-health. Because persons with mental illnesses use tobacco at higher rates, peer support specialists are a critical source of treatment support. This project identifies the usefulness of preparing, at least in part with MI core values, peer support persons to care for individuals who are trying to quit tobacco use.

Another initiative is the Colorado Heart Healthy Solutions (CHHS) Program, which helps reduce risk factors for cardiovascular disease. Information about this program can be found at https://www.healthypeople.gov/2020/healthy-people-in-action/story/colorado-heart-healthy-solutions-program-reduces-risk-factors. In this program, CHHS collaborates with community agencies and clinics, providing a network of skilled health-care workers who use MI skills to activate patient behavior change to reduce risks for health disease.

USEFUL RESOURCES

Specific MI learning opportunities (i.e., online, face-to-face, etc.) can be found in the MI internet link found in Table 6-4, which lists useful resources. A wealth of links to opportunities exist online using any search engine with the term *motivational interviewing* and the name of the state in which you wish to obtain training. Most academic settings that offer degrees and certification in health-care disciplines have dedicated MI courses that can be accessed by readers seeking to learn MI in academic settings as an elective course, which may or may not apply to degree completion credits. Nurses interested in learning more about MI would be well advised to engage in further reading. A list of recommended reading is available in Table 6-5.

Table 6-4 Useful MI Resources

Source	Link	Description
Motivational Interviewing (MINT)	http://www.motivationalinterviewing.org/	List of links to training; archive of articles; YouTube videos, presentation slides, and more.
Robert Wood Johnson Behavior Change Consortium	http://www.rwjf.org/en/library/grants/2000/11/promoting-health-through-the-behavior-change-consortium.html	Facilitate successful behavior change programs into practice; funding opportunities.
National Council for Behavioral Health	http://www.thenationalcouncil.org/	Represents the care of patients living with mental illnesses and addictions; improve access to care; trainings in mental health first aid.

Table 6-5 Recommended Reading

Citation	Description
Miller, W. R., & Rollnick, S, R. (2013). *Motivational interviewing: Helping people change* (3rd ed.). New York, NY: Guilford Press.	An update and restructuring around a four-process model of MI (engaging, focusing, evoking, and planning). The comprehensive primer of MI by original authors.
Dart, M. A. (2011). *Motivational interviewing in nursing practice: Empowering the patient.* Sudbury, MA: Jones and Bartlett.	Nursing text; guide for nurses to learn MI; focuses on patient with medical diagnoses, provides case exemplars with suggested MI-based language.
Miller, W. R,. & Rollnick, S. (2009). Ten things that motivational interviewing is not. *Behavioral and Cognitive Psychotherapy*, *37*, 129–140.	MI has been confused with other ideas, approaches, and theories over the course of its rapid dissemination. This article clearly defines what MI is and is not.
Miller, W. R., & Moyers, T. B. (2014). The forest and the trees: Relational and specific factors in addiction treatment. *Addiction, 110*, 401–413.	Emphasizes the importance of common aspects that are often dismissed, such as relational factors (i.e., empathy) because these factors can vary widely across providers and it is not clear how common they actually are.
Zuckoff, A. (2012). Why won't my patients do what's good for them? Motivational interviewing and treatment adherence. *Surgery for Obesity and Related Diseases*, *8*, 514–521.	Focuses the reader on: "A conceptual account of patient motivation for health change, highlighting the centrality of resolution of patient ambivalence through targeted conversation, is illustrated by thought exercises for the reader and supplemented by references to empirical data" (p. 514).
Mallisham, S. L., & Sherrod, B. (2016). The spirit and intent of motivational interviewing. *Perspectives in Psychiatric Care.* doi:10.1111/ppc.12161	Nurses can improve patient-centered communication skills that lead to improved treatment adherence.
Moyers, T. B. (2014). The relationship in motivational interviewing. *Psychotherapy*, *51*(3), 358–363.	Clarifies the significance of the relationship in MI with an important distinction: "MI is primarily concerned with helping clients to make a *decision* to change" (p. 358).
Isenhart, C., Dieperink, E., Thuras, P., Fuller, B., Stull, L., Koets, N., & Lenox, R. (2014). Training and maintaining motivational interviewing skills in a clinical trial. *Journal of Substance Use*, *19*(1–2), 164–170.	Describes eight steps to learning MI, with an emphasis on the first two steps (learning fundamental information about MI and practicing new skills with feedback to hone fidelity to the model).

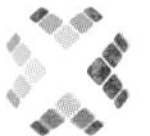

Case Illustration

Interactions between nurses and patients can take many directions, depending on the context and purpose of the visit. MI can help nurses interact effectively with patients to activate behavior change. Dialogue can be brief or extensive.

Mr. Smith, 68 years old, has smoked Pall Mall cigarettes for 53 years and smokes 18 to 20 cigarettes per day (cpd). Until 6 months ago, he smoked 30 to 40 cpd, but he decreased his tobacco use on his own. He is seen in primary care for shortness of breath and harsh, productive cough. He is angry about the referral to tobacco cessation services. He states, "I like smoking; it's my right to smoke; I will quit when the heavens open up and the angels begin to sing!"

RN Angela is Mr. Smith's nurse and has been trained in MI.

Interaction	**Interpretation**	**Comments**
RN: "I hear what you are saying: quitting smoking is not something that is on your radar and if you quit, it will be because you decided to, not something you were pressured to do."	Complex reflection: Validates Mr. Smith's autonomy and demonstrates an understanding of his irritation with being pressured to engage in treatment.	Uses the strategy, *rolling with resistance.* Mr. Smith appears to be in the precontemplation stage of change.
Mr. Smith: "That's right! I was doing it on my own and don't need your help."	Validates that he was correctly understood by RN.	
RN: "After all, if you want to quit, you'll continue to cut down or stop on your own."	Complex reflection: validates autonomy.	
Mr. Smith: "I can do this on my own."	Expressing need for autonomy.	
RN: "You are able to quit on your own without anyone helping you."	Amplified reflection: amplifies resistance that is heard.	Creates an opportunity for the patient to clarify and/or correct interpretation.
Mr. Smith: "Well, I don't know about that. I actually have tried to quit before and couldn't do it. These dang cigarettes!"	Less resistance verbalized, indicating that quitting was and remains *important* enough that he tried quitting in the past and is now less *confident* that he can be successful in quitting.	RN can focus on confidence-building strategies and not waste time trying to convince Mr. Smith that it is important to quit. More dialogue can be elicited via use of the Readiness Ruler.
RN: "So, on the one hand, it is important to you to quit and you've tried before, but on the other hand, you are frustrated that you were not able to quit when you tried on your own."	Double-sided reflection: presents an accurate picture of what is happening.	Validates RN is hearing and understanding Mr. Smith's past efforts and current frustration.
Mr. Smith: "Yeah, now you understand."	Building rapport.	
RN: "I wonder, if you decide to quit, how would you go about it?"	Strategy planning; respecting Mr. Smith's autonomy	
Mr. Smith: "Well, I guess I don't know. I mean, I quit drinking years ago, so maybe I could do some of the same things. Like, at first, not hanging around with my buddies who smoke."	Change talk: statements that indicate the patient is considering making changes.	Activating behavior change.
RN: "That was probably hard to do at first, but it sounds like you got the hang of it."	Reframing: placing a different meaning on patient's statements, decrease resistance.	Confidence building.

(*continued*)

Interaction	Interpretation	Comments
Mr. Smith: "Shoot, I can hang around folks who are having a drink or two without any problem at all nowadays."	Validating autonomy, building confidence.	
RN: "You really have some good ideas. Would it be okay with you if I brought up some other strategies that people who are quitting smoking sometimes find helpful. Like using a medication to quit or getting some counseling support?"	Asking permission to provide interventions validates Mr. Smith's autonomy.	
Mr. Smith: "Well, I'm not sure about some of that, but I'd like some ideas, as I am kinda stuck right now."	Open to strategy and goal planning; Mr. Smith has rapport and trust in RN.	Behavior activation and sustaining planning. Mr. Smith now appears to be in the preparation stage of change.

KEY POINTS

- This chapter provided an overview of the literature about the use of MI in a wide variety of nursing disciplines.
- Literature on nurses' use of MI provides mixed conclusions, likely because of the lack of fidelity in standardization and training.
- Other factors that influence the dissemination and implementation of MI to activate behavior change are clinician specific, patient specific, and setting specific.

Check Your Understanding

1. When used by practitioners, MI is defined as:
   A. A way to manipulate patients into doing what they should do for their health
   B. A person-centered counseling style for addressing the common problem of ambivalence about change
   C. A way to assess a patient's desire to activate behavior change
   D. All of the above
2. There are several ways to learn MI, including:
   A. Face-to-face training sessions
   B. Via coaching and mentoring
   C. Using roleplay
   D. All of the above in combination, as well as other methods
3. Motivational interviewing:
   A. Is very cost effective for nurses to use
   B. Is not cost effective for nurses to use
   C. Has not been well studied in regard to cost effectiveness for nursing use
   D. Is only cost effective when used in person
4. MI is effective in activating behavior change in people, including those living with:
   A. Cardiac diseases
   B. Diabetes
   C. Addictions
   D. Mental illnesses
   E. All of these, plus nursing students
5. MI and stages of change are:
   A. Conceptually the same thing
   B. Separate concepts
   C. Complimentary to each other
   D. Not to be used together in the same intervention
   E. B and C only
6. When considering implementing and/or studying an MI program, one should be mindful of clinician-specific factors such as:
   A. Area of clinical expertise
   B. Years of academic preparation
   C. Length of practice
   D. Previous exposure to MI
   E. All of the above

7. When considering implementing and/or studying an MI program, one should be mindful of patient-specific factors such as:
   A. Age and gender
   B. Race and ethnicity
   C. Diagnosis
   D. Availability of personal resources
   E. All of the above as well as challenges

8. When considering implementing and/or studying an MI program, one should be mindful of clinical setting–specific factors such as:
   A. Implications of practice in primary care
   B. Implications of practice in mental health settings
   C. Implications of practice with specific age cohorts
   D. All of the above, as well as implications of practice in inpatient and community settings

9. MI is best learned in:
   A. Academic settings as a student
   B. Clinical settings as a busy nurse
   C. Face-to-face trainings
   D. Other innovative settings and via the Web
   E. All of the above, although each presents different challenges

10. Elements that should be included in any MI training include:
    A. The spirit of MI
    B. MI strategies and techniques
    C. Coaching and follow-up
    D. Training fidelity measures
    E. All of the above

See "Reflections on Check Your Understanding" at the end of the book for answers.

REFERENCES

Aiken, L. H., Sermeus, W., Van den Heede, K., Sloane, D. M., Busse, R., McKee, M., . . . Kutney-Lee, A. (2012). Patient safety, satisfaction, and quality of hospital care: Cross sectional surveys of nurses and patient in 12 countries in Europe and the United States. *BMJ*, 344,e1717. doi: 10.1136/bmj.e1717

Al-Ganmi, A. H., Perry, L., Gholizadeh, L., & Alotaibi, A. M. (2016). Cardiovascular medication adherence among patients with cardiac disease: A systematic review. *Journal of Advanced Nursing*, 72(12), 3001–3014 doi: 10.1111/jan.13062

Bohman, B., Forsberg, L., Ghaden A., & Rasmussen F. (2013). An evaluation of training in motivational interviewing for nurses in child health services. *Behavioural and Cognitive Psychotherapy*, *41*(3), 329–343.

Bredie, S. J. H., Fouwels, A. J., Wollersheim, H., & Schippers, G. M. (2011). Effectiveness of nurse-based motivational interviewing for smoking cessation in high risk cardiovascular outpatients: A randomized trial. *European Journal of Cardiovascular Nursing*, *10*, 174–179.

Brobeck, E., Bergh, H., Odencrants, S., & Hildingh, C. (2011). Primary healthcare nurses' experience with motivational interviewing in health promotion. *Journal of Clinical Nursing*, *20*, 3322–3330.

Brobeck, E., Odencrants, S., Bergh, H.,& Hildingh, C. (2014). Patients' experience of lifestyle discussions based on motivational interviewing: A qualitative study. *BMC Nursing*, *13*(13). Retrieved from http://www.biomedcentral.com/1472-6955/13/13

Chen, S. M., Creedy, D., Lin, H-S., & Wollin, J. (2012). Effects of motivational interviewing on self-management, psychological and glycemic outcomes in type 2 diabetes: A randomized controlled trial. *International Journal of Nursing Studies*, *49*, 637–644.

Chen, J., Li, X., Xiong, Y., Fennie, X. P., Wang, H., & Williams, A. B. (2016). Reducing the risk of HIV transmission among men who have sex with men: A feasibility study of the motivational interviewing counseling method. *Nursing Health Science*, *18*(3), 400–407, doi: 10.1111/nhs.12287

Christie, D., & Channon, S. (2014). The potential for motivational interviewing to improve outcomes in the management of diabetes and obesity in paediatric and adult populations: A clinical review. *Diabetes, Obesity, and Metabolism*, *16*, 381–387.

Cook, P. F., Manzouri, S., Aagaard, L., O'Connell, L., Corwin, M., & Gance-Cleveland, B. (2016). Results from 10 years of interprofessional training on motivational interviewing. *Evaluation & the Health Professions*, *40*(2), 159–179. doi: 10.1177/0163278716656229

Copeland, L., McNamara, R., Kelson, M., & Simpson, S. (2015). Mechanisms of change within motivational interviewing in relationship to health behaviors outcomes: A systematic review. *Patient Education and Counseling*, *98*(4), 401–411.

D'Amico, E., Houck, J. M., Hunter, S. B., Miles, J. N. V., Osilla, K. C., & Ewing, B. A. (2015). Group motivational interviewing for adolescents: Change talk and alcohol and marijuana outcomes. *Journal of Consulting and Clinical Psychology*, *83*(1), 68–80.

Dart, M. A. (2011). *Motivational interviewing in nursing practice: Empowering the patient.* Sudbury, MA: Jones and Bartlett.

El-Mallakh, P., Chlebowy, D. O., Wall, M. P., Myers, J. A., & Cloud, R. N. (2012). Promoting Nurse interventionist fidelity to motivational interviewing in diabetes self-care intervention. *Research in Nursing & Health*, *35*, 289–300.

Essenmacher, C., Karvonen-Gutierrez, C., Lynch-Sauer, J., & Duffy, S. (2009). Staff's attitudes toward the delivery of tobacco cessation services in a primarily psychiatric Veteran Affairs Hospital. *Archives of Psychiatric Nursing*, *23*(3), 231–242.

Hall, K., Staiger, P. K., Simpson, A., Best, D., & Lubman, D. I. (2015). After 30 years of dissemination, have we achieved sustained practice change in motivational interviewing? *Addiction*, *111*, 1144–1150.

Hyrkas, K., & Wiggins, M. (2014). A comparison of usual care, a patient-centered education intervention and motivational interviewing to improve medication adherence and readmissions of adults in an acute-care setting. *Journal of Nursing Management*, *22*, 350–361.

Institute of Medicine. (2010).*The future of nursing: Leading change, advancing health.* Retrieved from http://books.nap.edu/openbook.php?record_id=12956&page=R1

Isenhart, C., Dieperink, E., Thuras, P., Fuller, B., Stull, L., Koets, N., & Lenox, R. (2014). Training and maintaining motivational interviewing skills in a clinical trial. *Journal of Substance Use*, *19*(1–2), 164–170.

Jansink, R., Braspenning, J., Keizer, E., van der Weijden, T., Elwyn, G., & Grol, R. (2013a). No identifiable Hb1Ac or lifestyle change after a comprehensive diabetes programme including motivational interviewing: A cluster randomised trial. *Scandinavian Journal of Primary Health Care*, *31*, 119–127.

Jansink, R., Braspenning, J., Laurant, M., Keizer, E., Elwyn, G., van der Weijden, T., & Grol, R. (2013b). Minimal improvement of nurses' motivational interviewing skills in routine diabetes care one year after training: A cluster randomized trial. *BMC Family Practice*, *14*, 44.

Jassal, M. S., Riekert, K. A., Borelli, B., Rand, C. S., & Eakin, M. N. (2016). Cost analysis of motivational interviewing and preschool education for secondhand smoke exposures. *Nicotine & Tobacco Research*, *18*(7), 1656–1664. doi: 10.1093/ntr/ntw001

Leake, G. J., & King, A. S. (1977). Effect of counselor expectations on alcoholic recovery. *Alcohol Health & Research World*, *1*(3), 16–22.

Lin, C. H., Chiang, S. L., Heitkemper, M. M., Hung, Y. J., Lee, M. S., Tzeng, W. C., & Chiang, L. C. (2016). Effects of telephone-based motivational interviewing in lifestyle modification program on reducing metabolic risks in middle-aged and older women with metabolic syndrome: A randomized control trial. *International Journal of Nursing Studies*, *60*, 12–23.

Lindhardt, C. L., Rubak, S., Mogensen, O., Hansen, H. P., Lamont, R. F., & Jorgensen, J. S. (2014).Training in motivational interviewing in obstetrics: A quantitative analytical tool. *Acta Obstetric Gynecology Scandinavia*, *93*, 698–704.

Lindson-Hawley, N., Thompson, T. P., & Begh, R. (2015). Motivational interviewing for Smoking cessation. Retrieved from http://www.thehealthwell.info/node/115326

Lundahl, B., Moleni, T., Burke, B. L., Buttons, R., Tollefson, D., Butler, C., & Rollnick, S. (2013). Motivational interviewing in medical care settings: A systematic review and meta-analysis of randomized controlled trials. *Patient Education and Counseling*, *93*(2), 157–168.

Mallisham, S. L., & Sherrod, B. (2016). The spirit and intent of motivational interviewing. *Perspectives in Psychiatric Care*, *53*(4), 226–233. doi: 10.1111/ppc.12161

Mason, M. J., Campbell, L., Way, T., Keyser-Marcus, L., Benotsch, E., Mennis, J., ... Stembridge, D. R. (2015). Development and outcomes of a text messaging tobacco cessation intervention with urban adolescents. *Substance Abuse*, *36*(4), 500–506.

McKenzie, K., & Chang, Y. (2015). The effect of nurse-led motivational interviewing on medication adherence in patients with bipolar disorder. *Perspectives in Psychiatric Care*, *51*, 36–44.

McSharry, P., & Timmins, F. (2016). An evaluation of the effectiveness of a dedicated health and well-being course on nursing students' health. *Nursing Education Today*, *16*(44), 26–32.

Mertens, V. C., Forsberg, L., Verbunt, J. A., Smeets, R. E. J. M., Goossens, M. E. J. B. (2016). Treatment fidelity of a nurse-led motivational interviewing-based pre-treatment in pain rehabilitation.*Journal of Behavioral Health Services & Research*, *43*(3), 459–473.

Mertens, V. C., Goossens, M. E. J. B., Verbunt, J. A., Koke, A. J., & Smeets, R. E. J. M. (2013). Effects of a nurse-led motivational interviewing of patients with chronic musculoskeletal pain in preparation of rehabilitation treatment (PREPARE) on societal participation, attendance level, and cost-effectiveness: Study protocol for a randomized control trial. *Trials*, *14*, 90. Retrieved from http://www.trialsjournal.com/content/14/1/90

Miller, W. R., & Moyers, T. B. (2014). The forest and the trees: Relational and specific factors in addiction treatment. *Addiction*, *110*, 401–413.

Miller, W. R., & Rollnick, S. R. (2009). Ten things that motivational interviewing is not. *Behavioural and Cognitive Psychotherapy*, *37*, 129–140. doi:10.1017/S1352465809005128

Miller, W. R., & Rollnick, S. R. (2013). *Motivational interviewing: Helping people change* (3rd ed.). New York, NY: Guilford Press.

Moyers, T. B. (2014). The relationship in motivational interviewing. *Psychotherapy*, *51*(3), 358–363.

Mujika, A., Forbes, A., Canga, N., de Irata, J., Serrano, I., Gasco, P., & Edwards, M. (2014). Motivational interviewing as a smoking cessation strategy with nurses: An exploratory randomized controlled trial. *International Journal of Nursing Studies*, *51*, 1074–1082.

Noordman, J., van der Lee, I., Nielen, M., Vlek, H., van der Weijden, T., & van Dulmen, S. (2012). Do trained practice nurses apply motivational interviewing techniques in primary care consultations? *Journal of Clinical Medical Research*, *4*(6), 393–401.

Noordman, J., de Vet, E., van der Weijden, T., & van Dulmen, S. (2013). Motivational interviewing within the different stages of change: An analysis of practice nurse-patient consultations aimed at promoting a healthier lifestyle. *Social Science & Medicine*, *87*, 60–67.

Noordman, J., van der Weijden, T., & van Dulmen, S. (2014). Effects of video-feedback on the communication, clinical competence and motivational interviewing skills of practice nurses: A pre-test posttest control group study. *Journal of Advanced Nursing*, *70*(10), 2272–2283.

O'May, F., Gill, J., McWhirter, E., Kantartzis, S., Reese, C., & Murray, K. (2016). A teachable moment for the teachable moment? A prospective study to evaluate delivery of a workshop designed to increase knowledge and skills in relation to alcohol brief interventions (ABIs) amongst final year nursing and occupational therapy undergraduates. *Nursing Education in Practice*, *6*(20), 45–53.

Osterlund Efraimsson, E., Fossum, B., Ehrenberg, A., Larsson, K., & Klang, B. (2012). Use of motivational interviewing in smoking cessation at nurse-led chronic obstructive pulmonary disease clinics. *Journal of Advanced Nursing*, *68*(4), 767–782.

Ostlund, A. S., Wadensten, B., Haggstrom, E., Lindqvist, H., & Kristofferzon, M. L. (2016). Primary care nurses' communication and its influence on patient talk during motivational interviewing. *Journal of Advanced Nursing*, *72*(11), 2844–2856. doi: 10.1111/jan.13052

Purath, J., Keck, A., & Fitzgerald, C. E. (2014). Motivational interviewing for older adults in primary care: A systematic review. *Geriatric Nursing*, *35*(3), 219–224.

Ream, E., Gargaro, G., Barsevick, A., & Richardson, A. (2015). Management of cancer-related fatigue during chemotherapy through telephone motivational interviewing: Modeling and randomized exploratory trial. *Patient Education and Counseling*, *98*(2), 199–206.

Resnicow, K., & McMaster, F. (2012). Motivational interviewing: Moving from why to how with autonomy support. *International Journal of Behavioral Nutrition and Physical Activity*, *9*(1), 9. Retrieved from http://www.ijbnpa.org/content/9/1/19

Riegel, B., Creber, R. M., Hill, J., & Hoke, L. (2016). Effectiveness of motivational interviewing in decreasing hospital readmission in adults with heart failure and multimorbidity. *Clinical Nursing Research*, *25*, 1–6. doi: 10.1177/1054773815623252

Robbins L. B., Pfeiffer, K. A., Maier, K. S., LaDrig, S. M., & Berg-Smith, S. M. (2012). Treatment fidelity of motivational interviewing delivered by a school nurse to increase girls' physical activity. *The Journal of School Nursing*, *28*(1), 70–78.

Rosswurm, M. A., & Larrabee, J. H. (1999). A model for change to evidence-based practice. *Image: Journal of Nursing Scholarship*, *31*(4), 317–348.

Ryan, P. (2009). Integrated theory of health behavior change: Background and intervention development. *Clinical Nurse Specialist*, *23*(3), 161–172. doi: 10.1097/NUR.0b013e3181a42373

Shepard, D. S., Lwin, A. K., Barnett, N. P., Mastroleo, N., Colby, S. M., Gwaltney, C., & Monti, P. M. (2016). Cost-effectiveness of motivational intervention with significant others for patients with alcohol misuse. *Addiction*, *111*, 832–839.

Spoelstra, S. L., Schueller, M., Hilton, M., & Ridenour, K. (2014). Interventions combining motivational interviewing and cognitive behavior therapy to promote medication adherence: A literature review. *Journal of Clinical Nursing*, *24*, 1163–1173.

Thompson, D. R., Chair, S. Y., Chan, S. W., Astin, R., Davidson, P. M., & Ski, C. F. (2011). Motivational interviewing: A useful approach to improving cardiovascular health? *Journal of Clinical Nursing*, *20*, 1236–1244.

Vardavas, C. I., & Nikitara, K. (2020). COVID-19 and smoking: A systematic review of the evidence, *Tobacco Induced Diseases*, *18*(March). doi: 10.18332/tid/119324

Velasquez, M., Maurer, G. G., Crouch, C., & DiClementi, C. C. (2001). *Group treatment for substance abuse: A stages of change therapy manual*. New York, NY: Guilford Press.

Wong, E. M. Y., & Cheng, M. M. H. (2013). Effects of motivational interviewing to promote weight loss in obese children. *Journal of Clinical Nursing*, *22*, 2519–2530.

Zuckoff, A. (2012). Why won't my patients do what's good for them? Motivational interviewing and treatment adherence. *Surgery for Obesity and Related Diseases*, *8*, 514–521.

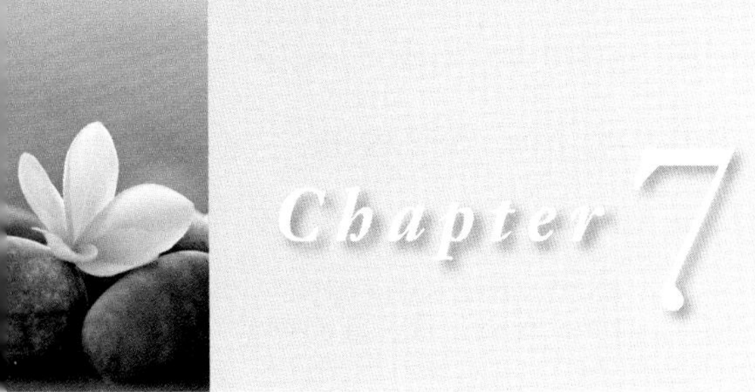

Health Screening and Counseling from Birth to Age 21

Margaret R. Colyar

LEARNING OBJECTIVES

After completing this chapter, the student will be able to:

1. Understand the components of health screening.
2. Determine age-related health screening tools.
3. Know the components of developmental screening.
4. Ascertain appropriate developmental screening tools by age group.
5. Identify key points for anticipatory guidance.
6. Ascertain appropriate health counseling for adolescents.

INTRODUCTION

Health screening of individuals from birth to age 21 years contributes to successful development and indicates when health-care professionals must intervene to correct deficits. Key components of health screening include immunizations, vital signs, blood components (lead and hematocrit), growth norms (height, weight, body mass index [BMI]), physical (fine motor, gross motor, dental, vision, hearing, body systems), developmental milestones, mental health, and nutrition. Healthy People 2020 has established objectives and health indicators for screening infants, children in early and middle childhood, and adolescents to increase the quality and years of a healthful life (Table 7-1).

This chapter will outline recommended immunizations for all age groups, then discuss general and specific growth and developmental screenings for infant, toddler, school-age, adolescent, and young adult groups. In addition, significant components of health counseling for adolescents will be outlined.

IMMUNIZATIONS

The Centers for Disease Control and Prevention (CDC) is dedicated to ensuring that everyone, everywhere shares in the benefits of immunization. Table 7-2 shows the current CDC recommendations for childhood immunization. Disease-specific information fact sheets on vaccinations for children can be found at https://www.cdc.gov/vaccines/schedules/hcp/imz/child-adolescent.html. Check the CDC for updates on immunization scheduling and when catch-up vaccines should be given.

Vaccination Research

Childhood and adult immunizations have been extensively researched. Current peer-reviewed studies agree that vaccines continue to be a safe and effective way to prevent serious disease. The American Academy of Pediatrics maintains a table of the latest evidence about vaccine safety so parents can review the data about common concerns. Key findings include the following:

Table 7-1 Healthy People 2020 Objectives and Goals

Objectives	Goals
Maternal/Infant/Child Health	**Improve health and well-being.**
Reduce rate of fetal and infant deaths. Reduce 1-year mortality rate for infants with Down syndrome. Reduce rate of child deaths. Reduce low birth weight and very low birth weight. Reduce preterm births. Increase early and adequate prenatal care. Increase abstinence from alcohol, cigarette, and illicit drugs among pregnant females. Increase the proportion of infants who are breastfed. Reduce the occurrence of fetal alcohol syndrome.	
Early and Middle Childhood	Document and track population-based measure of health and well-being for early and middle childhood populations over time in the United States.
Increase readiness for school in five domains of physical development; social-emotional development; and approaches to learning, language, and cognitive development. Reduce the proportion of children who have poor quality of sleep. Increase elementary, middle, and senior high school students that require school health education.	
Adolescent Health	Improve healthy development, health, safety, and well-being of adolescents and young adults.
Increase wellness checkups. Increase participation in extracurricular and/or out-of-school activities. Increase connection to parent or other positive adult caregiver. Increase transition to self-sufficiency. Increase education achievement.	
Mental Health and Mental Disorders	Improve mental health through prevention and by ensuring access to appropriate, quality mental health services.
Reduce suicide attempts by adolescents. Reduce the proportion of adolescents who engage in disordered eating behaviors. Reduce the proportion of persons who experience major depressive episodes. Increase the proportion of children with mental health problems who receive treatment. Increase the proportion of persons with co-occurring substance abuse and mental disorders who receive treatment for both disorders. Increase depression screening by primary-care providers.	

Source: https://www.healthypeople.gov/2020/topics-objectives

- "No significant correlation between exposure to antigens through vaccines and risk of developing a non-vaccine targeted infection" (Glanz et al., 2018)
- No evidence of a link between receipt of vaccines and development of autism spectrum disorders (Taylor, Swerdfeger, & Eslick, 2014)
- No evidence of safety concerns related to the Institute of Medicine's recommended child vaccination schedule (Hinshaw, 2013)

Prevenar 13 was first introduced for prevention of community-acquired pneumonia in infants and young

Table 7-2 Example Recommendations for Childhood Immunizations

Note: This table is provided as example of recommendations. Recommendations change as-needed. To review the most current immunization schedules, visit the CDC's website at http://www.cdc.gov/vaccines/schedules/index.html

Vaccine	Birth	2 Months	4 Months	6 Months	9 Months	12 Months	18 Months	4 TO 6 Years	11 TO 12 Years	16 Years
Hepatitis B, 3 doses	X	X		X	X	X				
Rotovirus, 3 doses by 6 months		X	X	X						
Diphtheria, tetanus, acellular pertussis		X	X	X		X	X		X	
Hemophilus (Hib)		X	X	X		X				
Prevnar 13 (PCV)		X	X	X						
Inactivated polio virus (IPV)		X	X	X	X	X		X		
MMR, 2 doses after 12 months old and after 4 years old						X		X		
Varicella, 2 doses after 12 months old and after 4 years old						X		X		
Hepatitis A, 2 doses 6 months apart						X	X			
Human papilloma virus (HPV), 2 doses 12 months apart									X X	
Meningicoccal									X	X
Pneumoccal 23								High risk only	High risk only	High risk only

Source: https://www.cdc.gov/vaccines/schedules/hcp/imz/child-adolescent.html

children in December 2009 in Europe and is approved for use in the United States (Atkinson, Wolfe, & Hamborsky, 2012). Randomized controlled studies have shown that Prevenar 13 coadministered with influenza vaccine has been effective and caused no ill effects (Frenck et al., 2012), and it has a significant impact on invasive pneumococcal disease and pneumococcal pneumonia throughout the world (Alderson, 2016).

Human papilloma virus (HPV) is very common and can cause cancers of the cervix, vagina, and vulva in women; cancers of the penis in men; and cancers of the anus and back of the throat, including the base of the tongue and tonsils (oropharynx), in both women and men. The Food and Drug Administration has approved a vaccine called Gardasil that prevents HPV. The CDC recommends that all children be vaccinated for HPV at age 11 or 12, although anyone can receive the vaccine up until age 26 (Centers for Disease Control and Prevention [CDC], 2019c).

PHYSICAL SCREENING

Health-care providers can compare the child's growth to growth charts developed for the United States by the CDC. The Center for Adoption Medicine has growth charts designed for children who were born in other nations, but many are limited to infant growth only.

Newborn through 12 Months

All infants should be screened for changes in length, weight, and head and chest circumference at each well-child visit. Newborns also need to be checked for gestational age and maturity. The Ballard scale is used to assess gestational age (Figure 7-1).

Neuromuscular Maturity

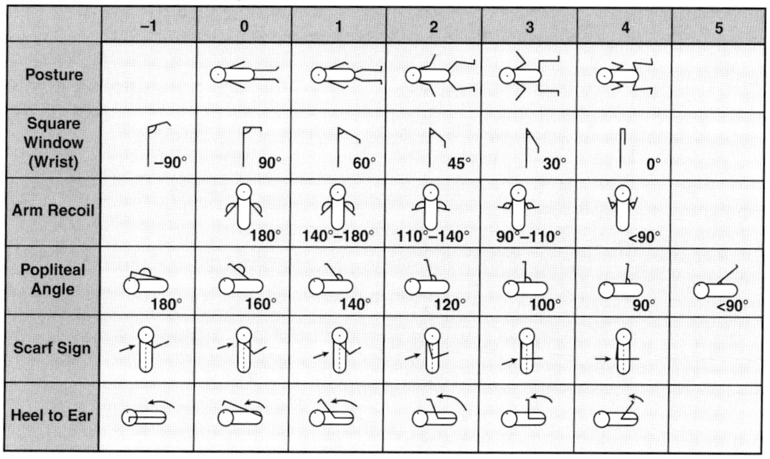

	−1	0	1	2	3	4	5
Posture							
Square Window (Wrist)	−90°	90°	60°	45°	30°	0°	
Arm Recoil		180°	140°–180°	110°–140°	90°–110°	<90°	
Popliteal Angle	180°	160°	140°	120°	100°	90°	<90°
Scarf Sign							
Heel to Ear							

Physical Maturity

Skin	Sticky; friable; transparent	Gelatinous; red; translucent	Smooth pink; visible veins	Superficial peeling or rash, few veins	Cracking; pale areas; rare veins	Parchment; deep cracking; no vessels	Leathery; cracked; wrinkled
Lanugo	None	Sparse	Abundant	Thinning	Bald areas	Mostly bald	
Plantar Surface	Heel-toe 40–50 mm:−1 <40 mm:−2	>50 mm no crease	Faint red marks	Anterior transverse crease only	Creases ant. 2/3	Creases over entire sole	
Breast	Imperceptible	Barely perceptible	Flat areola; no bud	Stippled areola; 1–2 mm bud	Raised areola; 3–4 mm bud	Full areola; 5–10 mm bud	
Eye/Ear	Lids fused; loosely:−1 tightly:−2	Lids open; pinna flat; stays folded	Slightly curved pinna; soft; slow recoil	Well-curved pinna; soft but ready recoil	Formed and firm; instant recoil	Thick cartilage; ear stiff	
Genitals (Male)	Scrotum flat, smooth	Scrotum empty; faint rugae	Testes in upper canal; rare rugae	Testes descending; few rugae	Testes down; good rugae	Testes pendulous; deep rugae	
Genitals (Female)	Clitoris prominent; labia flat	Prominent clitoris; small labia minora	Prominent clitoris; enlarging minora	Majora and minora equally prominent	Majora large; minora small	Majora cover clitoris and minora	

Maturity Rating

Score	Weeks
−10	20
−5	22
0	24
5	26
10	28
15	30
20	32
25	34
30	36
35	38
40	40
45	42
50	44

FIGURE 7–1 Ballard Scale: Neuromuscular Scale, External Physical Maturity Assessment Scale, and Maturity Score Sheet *Source:* Ballard, J. L., Khoury, L. C., Wedig, K., et al. (1991). New Ballard Score, expanded to include extremely premature infants. *Journal of Pediatrics*, *19*(3), 417–423.

Table 7-3 Apgar Scoring

Category	0	1	2
Breathing effort	Not breathing	Respirations slow (less than 30 breaths/min) or irregular	Infant cries well
Heart rate (by stethoscope)	None	Less than 100 beats/min	Greater than 100 beats/min
Muscle tone	Loose and floppy	Some muscle tone, weak flexion	Active motion, full flexion
Grimace response or reflex irritability (response to stimulation such as mild pinch)	No reaction	Grimacing	Grimacing and cough, sneeze, or vigorous cry
Skin color	Pale blue	Pink with blue extremities	Entire body is pink

Source: Medline Plus, U.S. National Library of Medicine, National Institutes of Health. Retrieved from http://www.nlm.nih.gov/medlineplus/ency/article/003402.htm

Apgar Score

The Apgar score of the child at 1 minute indicates the status in utero. The 5-minute Apgar score tells how the child reacts to extrauterine life. Apgar scoring gives parameters (appearance, pulse, grimace, activity, and respiratory effort) to assess successful transition to extrauterine life. Table 7-3 shows Apgar scoring. If the child has a poor score (<6) at 5 minutes, a 10-minute Apgar score should be completed: 0 to 3 is critical, 4 to 7 is worrisome, and 8 to 10 is excellent.

Disorder Screening

Box 7-1 shows various disorders for which newborns are screened prior to leaving the hospital. The list of these disorders varies from state to state.

BOX 7-1 Disorders for Which Newborns Are Screened Prior to Leaving the Hospital

- Phenylketonuria (PKU)
- Congenital hypothyroidism
- Galactosemia
- Sickle cell disease
- Biotinidase deficiency
- Congenital adrenal hyperplasia (CAH)
- Maple syrup urine disease (MSUD)
- Trosinemia
- Cystic fibrosis (CF)
- Medium-chain acyl-CoA dehydrogenase (MCAD) deficiency
- Severe combined immunodeficiency (SCID)
- Toxoplasmosis

Source: http://kidshealth.org/en/parents/newborn-screening-tests.html.

Hearing and Vision Screening

All newborns have a hearing screening before leaving the hospital. Vision for newborns and infants up to 3 months should be evaluated using black and white shapes (Figure 7-2). By age 3 months, the child starts developing tears; focuses on mouth, eyes, and simply colored shapes; can differentiate between red, green, and yellow; and has regular eye movements. Evaluate by checking for red reflex and corneal light reflex. As the child ages, other tests can be incorporated (Table 7-4).

Skin and Extremity Screening

Skin findings in newborns are shown in Table 7-5. Evaluate for birth trauma to the upper extremities (Table 7-6). Inspect for inequality in size and length of the legs, resistance to abduction, placement of medial thigh creases, and degree of flexion of the hips of the newborn to determine the presence of congenital hip dysplasia. Also Barlow and Ortolani maneuvers should be evaluated until the child is walking. Unstable hips present as the sound of clunks with hip manipulation.

Blood Disorder Screening

Anemia is a common problem in children who are African American, Native American, Alaska natives, infants living in poverty, immigrants from developing countries, preterm and low-birth-weight infants, and infants whose principal dietary intake is unfortified cow's milk.

Newborns should be screened for hemoglobinopathies (e.g., thalassemia and sickle cell disease) with hemoglobin electrophoresis. The U.S. Preventive Services Task Force recommends screening

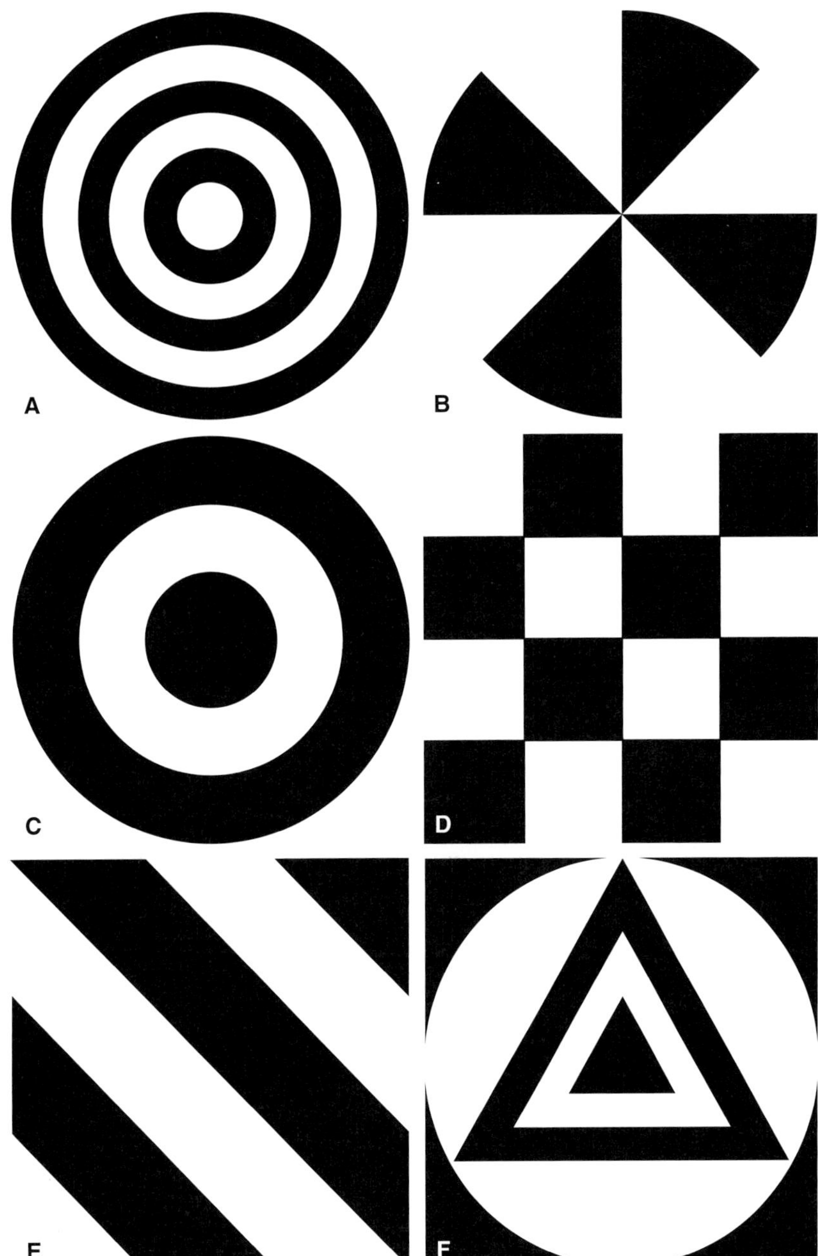

FIGURE 7–2 Newborns and Infants up to 3 Months Can Focus Well on Black and White Shapes

Table 7-4 Eye Examination Tests for Children

Age	Red Reflex	Corneal Light Reflex	Extraocular Movements	Cover/ Uncover	Visual Acuity
Newborn	X	X			
Infant, 2 to 9 months	X	X	Try		
Toddler, 1 to 3 years	X	X	X	Try	
Preschool child, 2 to 5 years	X	X	X	X	Picture

Table 7-5 Skin Findings in Newborns

Name of Skin Condition	Presentation	Location on Body
Café-au-lait spot	Pale tan macule	Entire body
Cavernous hemangiomas	Large, blood-filled, cystic papules	Scalp, face, and head
Erythema toxicum neonatorum	Pinpoint, re-based macules	Cheeks and trunk
Lanugo	Fine hair covering body	Entire body
Milia	White dots	Face and bridge of nose
Miliaria	Tiny, red, irritated lesions	Face and over any sweat gland
Mongolian spots	Hyperpigmented macules: gray, blue, or black	Lower back, buttocks, and shoulders; more common in African Americans, Asian Americans, and Hispanics
Port-wine stain (nervus flammeus)	Flat, red, purple, or jet black lesions	Face and scalp
Strawberry hemangioma	Soft, red, raised	Anywhere
Transient neonatal pustular melanosis	Brown or black spots	Anywhere; usually in African Americans
Vascular nevi Capillary hemangioma: stork bite or angel kiss	Pink, blanch easily	Eyelids, nose, nape of neck
Vernix caseosa	Cheesy white substance	Entire body

Source: Colyar, M. R. (2003). *Well-child assessment for primary care providers*. Philadelphia, PA: F.A. Davis.

Table 7-6 Birth Trauma of Upper Extremities: Three Common Types

Type	Presentation	Nerves Involved	Recovery
Erb's palsy	Cannot move the upper arm but still has palmar grasp	C5, C6	80%
Klumpke's paralysis	Hand and forearm are flaccid but upper arm moves; no palmar grasp	C7, C8, T1	<50%
Entire brachial plexus palsy	No movement in entire arm and hand	C5 to T1	Usually permanent

Source: Colyar, M. R. (2003). *Well-child assessment for primary care providers*. Philadelphia, PA: F.A. Davis.

hemoglobin or hematocrit between the ages of 6 and 12 months in high-risk infants. The American Academy of Pediatrics (AAP) recommends lead screening at ages 6, 9, or 12 months and prior to starting school. Normal hematocrit levels are found in Table 7-7.

Developmental Screening

AAP recommends that all children be screened for developmental delays and disabilities during regular well-child doctor visits at 9, 18, and 24 or 30 months. Research shows that early intervention treatment services can greatly improve a child's development and help children from birth through 3 years of age learn

Table 7-7 Hematocrit Normals as a Percentage of Packed Red Blood Cell Volume

Age	Range (%)
1 day	48–69
2 days	48–75
3 days	44–72
2 months	28–42
6 to 12 years	35–45
12 to 18 years	Boys: 37–39 Girls: 36–46

Source: Colyar, M. R. (2003). *Well-child assessment for primary care providers*. Philadelphia, PA: F.A. Davis.

important skills. Disorders such as attention deficit/hyperactivity disorder (ADHD) and autism can be detected early.

Infants

Developmental milestones for infants ages 2, 4, 6, and 9 months are shown in Tables 7-8 through 7-11.

Table 7-8 Developmental Milestones of 2-Month-Old Infants

Type of Skill	Red Flags
Gross Motor	
Head bobs + head lag + Moro reflex + asymmetrical tonic neck reflex Head or chest up when prone	Rolling over before age 3 months may indicate hypertonia
Fine Motor	
Grasp reflex is waning Hands unfisted about 50% of time May briefly hold object	Fisting after age 3 months is an early indicator of neuromotor dysfunction
Language	
Reciprocally coos Regards speaker	
Cognitive	
Piaget: Sensorimotor Tracking objects > 180 degrees	
Emotional	
Erikson: Trust versus mistrust May express interest, distress (hunger), or enjoyment (smiling)	Irritability
Social	
Reciprocal social smile Bonding by the parent Eyes follow moving person	Delay in social smile may be sign of visual or cognitive impairment or maternal depression

Source: Colyar, M. R. (2003). *Well-child assessment for primary care providers*. Philadelphia, PA: F.A. Davis.

Table 7-9 Developmental Milestones of 4-Month-Old Infants

Normal Infants	Red Flags
Gross Motor	
Moro reflex gone Asymmetrical tonic neck reflex gone Up on hands when prone, head erect Rolling front to back Head lag gone	Poor head control
Fine Motor	
Reaching for objects Holds objects	Persistent fisting
Language	
Laughs out loud Orients to voice Cry more distinctive to need Coos Listens to speaker	Absence of smile

(continued)

Table 7-9 Developmental Milestones of 4-Month-Old Infants—cont'd

Normal Infants	Red Flags
Cognitive	
Piaget: Sensorimotor Hand regard Regard objects when in hand Objects to mouth	Failure to reach for and grasp objects at age 4 to 5 months
Emotional	
Erikson: Trust versus mistrust Expresses anger, joy, pleasure, and displeasure	
Social	
Recognize the primary caregiver Attachment by the infant to the caregiver Smiles spontaneously	

Source: Colyar, M. R. (2003). *Well-child assessment for primary care providers*. Philadelphia, PA: F.A. Davis.

Table 7-10 Developmental Milestones of 6-Month-Old Infants

Normal Infants	Red Flags
Gross Motor	
No head lag present With sitting, the head is erect and spine is straight Sits with support, or propped on hands Rolls over in both directions Equilibrium response Bears weight while standing Stands with support	W-sitting Bunny hopping Poor head control
Fine Motor	
Grasping objects with both hands Transfers objects from hand to hand Rakes small objects Shakes, bangs, drops objects	Persistent fisting Hand dominance Failure to reach for objects
Language	
Babbling, using consonants Responds to name Using sound to get attention Responds to friendly versus angry tones Razzes (the raspberry sound)	Absence of babbling
Cognitive	
Object permanence developing, looks after dropped object	
Emotional	
Fear Emerging self-identity	
Social	
Stanger awareness Person preference Differential facial expressions	Absence of stranger awareness

Source: Colyar, M. R. (2003). *Well-child assessment for primary care providers*. Philadelphia, PA: F.A. Davis.

Table 7-11 Developmental Milestones of 9-Month-Old Infants

Normal Infants	Red Flags
Gross Motor	
Sits independently	Persistent standing on tiptoe
Crawling or creeping on hands and knees	Scissors motion on lower extremities
Sits with support, or propped on hands	Persistence of primitive reflexes
May pull to stand	
Weight bearing with standing	
Parachute response	
Fine Motor	
Maturing grasp: the inferior pincer grasp; may use fingertips	Persistence of primitive reflexes
Able to point at and pick up small object	
May be able to isolate the index finger and poke	
Feeds self with fingers	
Language	
Responds to own name	Inability to localize sound
May imitate sounds of others	
May say "mama" or "dada" but inappropriately	
Associating words with meanings	
May begin to integrate babble and intonation	
Looks where finger is pointing to rather than looking at the pointer	
Responds to "no"	
Cognitive	
Bangs objects on surface	
Learns object permanence	
Plays peekaboo	
Emotional	
Avoidance reaction	
Social	
Stanger awareness	Absence of stranger awareness
Separation anxiety	
Sense of self	

Source: Colyar, M. R. (2003). *Well-child assessment for primary care providers*. Philadelphia, PA: F.A. Davis.

Toddlers

Developmental milestones by age for toddlers are shown in Table 7-12.

Preschool Children

Developmental milestones for children ages 3 to 5 years are shown in Table 7-13.

Anticipatory Guidance Topics

Specific topics that should be discussed with new parents are presented in Box 7-2.

School-Age Screening

The CDC uses research data from the past two National Health and Nutrition Examination Surveys (NHANES I and II) to determine the reference for treating lead levels in children's blood. The reference value is checked every 4 years. Symptoms to screen for with children at risk for elevated lead levels are shown in Box 7-3. Current lead levels are shown in Table 7-14.

Children with early cavities are nearly three times more likely to develop cavities in their adult teeth. Risk factors are influenced by transmission of bacteria from mother to child, frequent sugar consumption, environment, and socioeconomic status. Normal dental development by age can be seen in Tables 7-15 and 7-16. AAP recommends the first dental screening at 3 years of age. The American Dental Association recommends that the first visit be at 1 year.

Table 7-12 Developmental Milestones by Age for Toddlers

Age, Months	Social	Fine Motor	Gross Motor	Language
12	Plays ball, imitates activities Drinks from a cup	Waves bye-bye Puts block in cup Fine pincer grasp	Stands, cruises, and takes a few steps	Says two or three words Says "mama" or "dada" Follows simple commands
15	Helps in house Removes garments Uses spoon or fork	Scribbles Dumps raisin-sized objects Builds tower of two cubes Messy self-feeding	Walks well Stoops and recovers Walks backward and sideways Climbs, bounces to music	Uses three to six words Naming Points
18	Little impulse control Temper tantrums start Feeds doll Undresses self Brushes teeth with help	Builds tower of four cubes Hand dominance Imitates vertical line Feeds self	Walks up steps holding on Runs Kicks ball forward	Uses 6 to 20 words Verbalizes wants Knows three body parts Receptive language developing Understands and follows commands Points to two pictures
24	Washes and dries hands Puts on clothing Protodeclarative behavior	Builds tower of six cubes Turns pages in book Imitates circle and horizontal line	Jumps up Throws ball overhand Walks up and down stairs with two feet per step	Combines words Names a picture Points to four pictures Knows six body parts Twenty-five percent to 50% of speech understandable

Source: Colyar, M. R. (2003). *Well-child assessment for primary care providers*. Philadelphia, PA: F.A. Davis.

Table 7-13 Developmental Milestones for Children Ages 3 to 5

Age	Cognitive	Social	Fine Motor	Gross Motor	Language
3	Preoperational. Use symbols to represent people, objects, and actions in the environment. Developing ability to represent the external world by means of arbitrary symbols that stand for objects. Tend to make inappropriate generalizations. Attribute feelings to inanimate objects; that is, clouds "cry". Prone to magical thinking. Believe thoughts are all-powerful;	Developing gender identity and self-esteem. Live in rich imaginary world.	Copy circle, draw a person with two to three parts, pick the larger line of two lines that are side by side.	Hop, broad jump, right a 3-wheeler, stand on one foot for 3 to 5 seconds, wash and dry hands, dress and undress with supervision.	Vocabulary 20 words. Two- to three-word sentences.

Table 7-13 Developmental Milestones for Children Ages 3 to 5—cont'd

Age	Cognitive	Social	Fine Motor	Gross Motor	Language
	for example, pet scratches them, they wish the cat dead, and the cat gets run over by a car, and the child believes his or her own thoughts caused the death of the pet. Unable to reason cause and effect of illness or injury logically.				
4	Same as 3-year-old.	Developing gender identity and self-esteem. Understands social rules but cannot always initiate self-control. Capable of feeling guilty about bad behavior.	Copy a cross.	Skip, walk on heels and toes, use alternating feet when descending stairs.	Vocabulary of 50 to 100 words. Well-formed sentences. Stuttering and baby talk occur frequently.
5	Same as 3- and 4-year-old.	Understands social rules but cannot always initiate self-control. Capable of feeling guilty about bad behavior.	Copy a square, draw a person with six parts.	Better coordination. Skip, walk on heels and toes, use alternation feet when descending stairs.	Vocabulary of 1,000 words Comprehension of speech 90% Can express feelings and thoughts Stuttering and baby talk occur frequently.

BOX 7-2 Anticipatory Guidance Topics

- Community interactions
- Family relationships
- Healthy habits
- Media exposure (TV, loud music)
- Motor vehicle safety
- Nutrition
- Oral health
- Prevention of illness
- School/vocational achievement
- Secondary smoke exposure
- Self-responsibility
- Sexuality
- Smoke detectors
- Social development
- Sun protection
- Violence prevention

BOX 7-3 Symptoms of Lead Poisoning

Abdominal discomfort
Anorexia
Blue line at gum margin
Constipation
Convulsions
Difficulty concentrating
Fatigue
Headache
Irritability
Lethargy
Metallic taste
Myalgia
Seizures
Tremor
Vomiting
Weight loss

Table 7-14 Indications Related to Lead Levels in the Blood

Blood Level (mcg/dL)	Indication/Action
< 9	No lead poisoning
10–14	Evaluate environment. Decrease exposure to lead. Follow up in 3 months.
15–19	Decrease lead exposure. Dietary interventions: • Increase iron • Increase calcium. • Eat regular meals (lead is absorbed more on empty stomach).
20–40	Decrease lead exposure. Continue dietary interventions.
20–41	Consider pharmacologic interventions.
>40	Chelation therapy within 48 hours.

Table 7-15 Temporary Teeth Eruption and Loss

	Eruption		Loss	
Tooth Name	**Upper**	**Lower**	**Upper**	**Lower**
	Months		Years	
Central incisor	6–8	5–7	6–7	5–6
Lateral incisor	8–11	7–10	8–9	7–8
Canine incisor	16–20	16–20	9–11	11–12
First molar	10–16	10–16	10–11	10–12
Second molar	20–30	20–30	10–12	11–13

Source: Colyar, M. R. (2003). *Well-child assessment for primary care providers*. Philadelphia, PA: F.A. Davis.

Table 7-16 Permanent Teeth Eruption and Loss

	Eruption	Loss
Tooth Name	**Upper (Years)**	**Lower (Years)**
Central incisor	7–8	6–7
Lateral incisor	8–9	7–8
Canine incisor	11–12	9–11
First premolar	10–11	6–7
Second premolar	10–12	11–13
First molar	6–7	6–7
Second molar	12–13	12–13
Third molar	17–25	17–25

Source: Colyar, M. R. (2003). *Well-child assessment for primary care providers*. Philadelphia, PA: F.A. Davis.

According to the CDC, 20% of children aged 5 to 11 years have at least one untreated decayed tooth. Children aged 5 to 19 years from low-income families are twice as likely (25%) to have cavities compared with children from higher-income households (11%) (CDC, 2019b). Left untreated, carious lesions can lead to expensive treatment, disruption of growth and development, pain, and life-threatening infections (American Dental Association [ADA], 2020).

Hearing Screening

Because hearing deficits cause developmental delays, infants should have hearing screening before leaving the hospital. Children in prekindergarten; kindergarten; and first, second, and third grades as well as all new students should have hearing screening via tympanometry or audiometry. The normal range of hearing is 10–20 decibels.

Vision Screening

Screening for impaired visual acuity could lead to interventions to improve vision, function, and quality of life. A visual acuity test (e.g., the Snellen eye chart) is the standard for screening for vision impairment in primary care, but its diagnostic accuracy is uncertain because no studies compare it against a clinically relevant reference standard (Chou, Dana, & Bougatsos, 2009).

Mathers, Keyes, and Wright (2010) reviewed multiple studies to determine the effectiveness of children's vision screening, when children should be screened, and which screening is most effective. Most studies suggested that children's vision screening was beneficial, although the components of the programs varied widely (e.g., tests used, screening personnel, and age at testing).

Vision characteristics by age are shown in Table 7-17, and eye examinations by age are shown in Table 7-18. Figure 7-3 shows the Snellen visual acuity charts that remain in use.

Table 7-17 Vision Characteristics by Age

Age in Years	Vision Characteristics
3	Visual acuity of 20/30
4	Color vision
5	Accommodates well Visual acuity of 20/30 Development of amblyopia is unlikely but it should be screened for
6	Visual acuity of 20/20

Table 7-18 Eye Examinations by Age

Age	Red Reflex	Corneal Light Reflex	Extraocular Movements	Cover/ Uncover Test	Visual Acuity Examination	Funduscopic Examination	Ishihara Color Test
Preschool	X	X	X	X	HTOV Illiterate E Picture LEA	X	Age 4
School age	X	X	X	X	Letter	X	Kindergarten
Adolescent	X	X	X	X	Letter	X	

X = examine

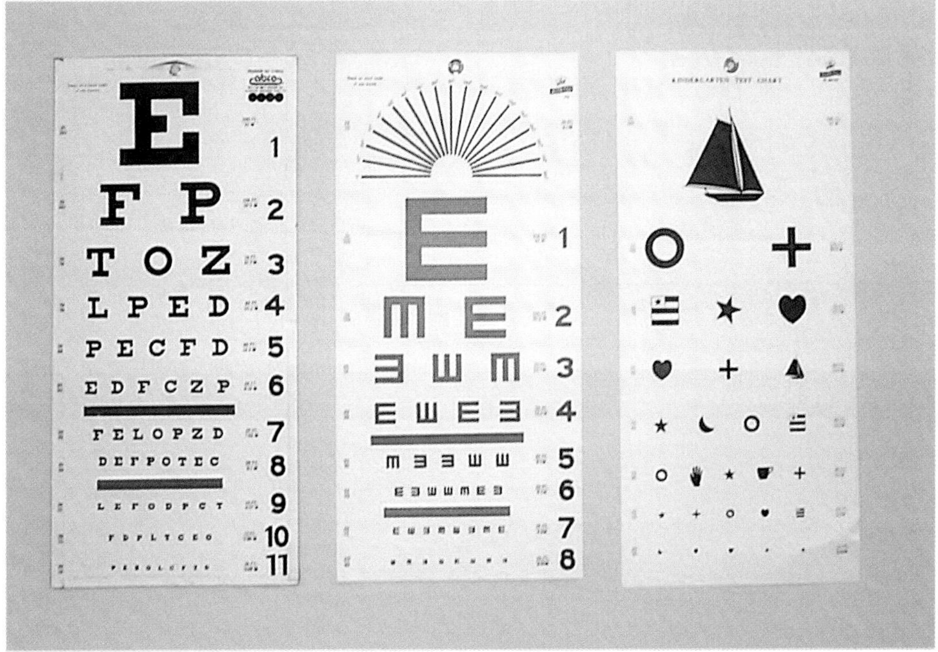

FIGURE 7–3 Eye Charts: Snellen, Illiterate E, and Pictorial Snellen

General Physical Assessment

A head-to-toe physical assessment should be done on all children to screen for physical problems. Auscultate the child's lungs for abnormal sounds and indications of acute respiratory effort (Table 7-19).

Cardiac screening

Evaluating the cardiovascular system involves classification of pulses (Table 7-20) and murmur detection (Tables 7-21 and 7-22).

Table 7-19 Abnormal Indications of Acute Respiratory Effort

Respiratory Problem	Description
Apnea	Periods of nonbreathing (periods > 15 seconds in newborns)
Drooling	Saliva flows outside the mouth
Dyspnea	Difficulty breathing
Grunting	Abnormal, short, deep, hoarse sounds in exhalation
Hyperpnea	Increased depth of breathing when required to meet demand
Hypopnea	Overly shallow breathing or an abnormally low respiratory rate
Intercostal retractions	Space between ribs pulls inward with inspiration
Muffled voice	Marbled quality of voice
Nasal flaring	Lateral margins or nares flares
Orthopnea	Must sit up to breathe
Stridor	High-pitched crowing sound with inspiration
Tachypnea	Faster breathing than normal for age
Tripoding	Sits in tripod position with chin forward
Wheezing	High-pitched musical sound caused by narrowed airways, heard on inspiration and expiration

Source: Colyar, M. R. (2011). *Assessment of the school-age child and adolescent*. Philadelphia, PA: F.A. Davis.

Table 7-20 Classification of Pulses

Numerical Classification	Description
0	Completely absent
1	Weak
2	Normal
3	Increased
4	Bounding

Source: Colyar, M. R. (2011). *Assessment of the school-age child and adolescent*. Philadelphia, PA: F.A. Davis.

Table 7-21 Types of Murmurs

Area	Type	Disorder
Systolic	Regurgitation, sounds like breath sound	Ventricular-septal defect
		Mitral insufficiency
		Tricuspid insufficiency
	Obstructive (organic), coarse and loud	Aortic and pulmonic stenosis

Table 7-21 Types of Murmurs—cont'd

Area	Type	Disorder
	Vibratory (innocent), musical, midpitch, and hum	Still's murmur
	Flow, sounds like vibratory murmur. In pulmonary area but has *fixed* split S2 and does *not* change with respiration.	Atrial septal defect
Diastolic	Regurgitation, all are organic	Aortic or pulmonic insufficiency
	Obstructive	Mitral or tricuspid stenosis
	Flow	Ventricular septal defect Atrial septal defect
	Continuous	Venus hum Patent ductus arteriosis

Source: Colyar, M. R. (2011). *Assessment of the school-age child and adolescent*. Philadelphia, PA: F.A. Davis.

Table 7-22 Innocent Murmurs by Age

Age Group	Murmur	Description
School age, 3 to 6 years old	Still's murmur	Low-pitched systolic ejection murmur. Musical or vibratory quality. Heard halfway between lower left sternal border and apex. Increases in intensity when supine; increases or disappears with change in position (turn to side) or valsalva. Louder with exercise and fever. Grade 1 to 3/6.
	Venus hum	Continuous blowing systolic and diastolic murmur. Heard right side of chest at level of clavicles. May be obliterated by turning head away from the side of the murmur or compressing internal jugular vein on side of murmur. Disappears in supine position.
	Carotid bruit	Harsh systolic ejection murmur. Heard best over right supraclavicular area and over carotids. Approaches aortic or pulmonic areas. Disappears in supine position. Increases with light pressure over carotid. Grade 1 to 3/6.
School age, 6 to 14 years old	Pulmonary murmur Ejection flow murmur	High-pitched, systolic ejection murmur. Heard best at upper left sternal border in supine position. Disappears when sitting and standing. Grade 1 to 3/6.
Any age	Hemic murmur	High-pitched systolic ejection murmur. Associated with anemia, fever, or increased cardiac output. Best heard over aortic and pulmonic areas. Disappears with stabilization of anemia, fever, or cardiac output. Common in pregnancy.

Source: Colyar, M. R. (2011). *Assessment of the school-age child and adolescent*. Philadelphia, PA: F.A. Davis.

Abdominal screening

Evaluating the abdomen should include common bulges (Table 7-23) and abnormal vascular sounds (Table 7-24).

Neurological screening

Assessment of cranial nerves (Table 7-25), lower and upper motor neuron lesions (Table 7-26), abnormal

Table 7-23 Common Abdominal Bulges in Children

Bulge	Description	Treatment
Umbilical hernia	Umbilicus protrudes, laxity around the umbilicus may be palpated.	None unless does not resolve by 5 years old.
Diastasis recti	Separation of the two rectus abdominis muscles from under breast to pubic area. When the child sits up, a ridge-like bulge appears.	Will disappear gradually.
Hernias		
Epigastric	Small, fatty nodule midline. Felt through linea alba from the xyphoid to the umbilicus. Caused by herniated fat.	Surgical correction may be needed if any of the hernias are painful.
Umbilical	Protrusion of the abdominal lining through the area around the belly button.	
Inguinal	Protrusion of the abdominal cavity contents through the inguinal canal.	
Femoral	Bulge in the upper part of the thigh, just below the groin, where the femoral artery and vein pass.	
Pyloric tumor	Olive-like muscle tumor in the right upper quadrant beneath the right rectus muscle.	Surgical correction.

Source: Colyar, M. R. (2011). *Assessment of the school-age child and adolescent*. Philadelphia, PA: F.A. Davis.

Table 7-24 Abnormal Vascular Sounds in the Abdominal Area

Sound	Problem
Harsh murmur, systolic or continuous	Aortic aneurysm
Soft, low-medium pitched murmur at midline and toward flank	Renal artery stenosis
Venous hum, periumbilical: medium pitch, continuous; heard with cirrhosis and portal hypertension	Partial obstruction, femoral arteries

Source: Colyar, M. R. (2011). *Assessment of the school-age child and adolescent*. Philadelphia, PA: F.A. Davis.

Table 7-25 Cranial Nerve Screening

Number And Name	Function(s)
I Olfactory	Sense of smell
II Optic	Sense of sight
III Oculomotor	Movement of the eyeball; constriction of pupil in bright light or for near vision
IV Trochlear	Movement of eyeball
V Trigeminal	Sensation in face, scalp, and teeth; contraction of chewing muscles
VI Abducens	Movement of eyeball
VII Facial	Sense of taste; contraction of facial muscles; secretion of saliva
VIII Acoustic (vestibulocochlear)	Sense of hearing; sense of equilibrium
IX Glossopharyngeal	Sense of taste; sensory for cardiac, respiratory, and blood pressure reflexes; sensory and motor to larynx (speaking); decreases heart rate; contraction of alimentary tube (peristalsis); increases digestive secretions
X Accessory	Contraction of neck and shoulder muscles; motor to larynx (speaking)
XI Hypoglossal	Movement of tongue

Source: Scanlon, V. C., and Sanders, T. (1995). *Essentials of anatomy and physiology* (2nd ed., p. 183). Philadelphia, PA: F.A. Davis.

movements (Table 7-27), and deep tendon reflexes (Table 7-28) should be included.

Musculoskeletal screening

The normal range of motion of all joints should be assessed (Table 7-29). Abnormalities that are prominent in children are genu varum/genu valgum (Figure 7-4A and B), Osgood-Schlatter (Figure 7-5A and B), intoeing/out-toeing (Figure 7-6A and B), and internal femoral torsion (Figure 7-7).

Table 7-26 Signs of Lower and Upper Motor Neuron Lesions

	Lower Motor Neuron Lesion	Upper Motor Neuron Lesion
Parameters	**Peripheral Nervous System**	**Central Nervous System**
Coordination	Weakness hinders movement	Impaired—cerebellum problems
Central Nervous System (CNS)	Impaired	Abnormalities—brain stem problems
Fasciculations	Presence—anterior horn cell problem	None
Intellect	Normal	Impaired—cortical problems
Power	Markedly reduced—neuromuscular junction problem	Slightly decreased
Reflexes	Difficult to elicit	Hyperactive—pyramidal problems
Sensation	Impaired	Intact
Tone	Reduced	Spastic—pyramidal problems

Source: Colyar, M. R. (2011). *Assessment of the school-age child and adolescent.* Philadelphia, PA: F.A. Davis.

Table 7-27 Abnormal Movements and Sensation—Choreiform Movements

Reflexes	Description
Involuntary posturing in unusual position	Dystonia
Quick nonrhythmic muscle contractions	Myoclonus
Repetitive movements without purpose or vocalizations	Tics
Writhing movements	Athetosis (seen with cerebral palsy)

Source: Colyar, M. R. (2011). *Assessment of the school-age child and adolescent.* Philadelphia, PA: F.A. Davis.

Table 7-28 Deep Tendon Reflex Response Scoring System

Score	Response	Indication
0	No response	Blocked somewhere in reflex arc
1+	Slight muscle contractions with little or no movement of the arm or leg	Normal, depending on other findings
2+	Visible muscle twitch and movement of arm or leg	Normal reflex
3+	Brisk, slightly exaggerated muscle twitch and movement of the arm or leg	Normal, depending on other findings
4+	Very exaggerated jerk of the muscle of arm or leg with repetitions (clonus)	Abnormal, lack of cortical inhibition

Source: Colyar, M. R. (2011). *Assessment of the school-age child and adolescent.* Philadelphia, PA: F.A. Davis.

Table 7-29 Normal Range of Motion of All Joints

Joint	Extension (Degrees)	Flexion (Degrees)	Right/Left (Degrees)
Temporomandibular Joints (TMJ)	3–6 cm		
Neck			
Forward	55	45	
Lateral bending			40
Rotation			70
Back	30	90	
Trunk			
Lateral bending			35
Rotation	30		
Hips			
Flexion with knee straight	0	90	
Flexion with knee flexed	0	120	
Supine			
Internal rotation	40		
External rotation	45		
Abduction	45		
Adduction	30		
Prone—hyperextension		15	
Prone—extension		0	
Knees	130	0	
Ankle			
Dorsiflexion		20	
Plantar flexion		45	
Eversion	20		
Inversion	30		
Shoulder			
Forward/back	50	180	
Internal rotation			90
External rotation			90
Abduction	180		
Adduction	50		
Elbow	0	180	
Pronation	90		
Supination	90		
Wrist	70	90	
Ulnar deviation	55		
Radial deviation	20		
Metacarpophalangeal Joint (MCP)	30	90	
Proximal Interphalangeal joints (PIP)	0	120	
Distal interphalangeal joints (DIP)	0–10	90	

Source: Colyar, M. R. (2011). *Assessment of the school-age child and adolescent.* Philadelphia, PA: F.A. Davis.

Skin screening

When a school nurse notices skin lesions, he or she should report the issue to the parents so they can seek treatment. The AAP reports that the gold standard for diagnosing head lice is finding a live louse on the head (Frankowski & Bocchini, 2010). The National Association of School Nurses (NASN) (2016) recommends management of head lice in the school setting and notes that the presence of lice should not disrupt the educational process. Children with nits should be allowed to stay in class to decrease absenteeism.

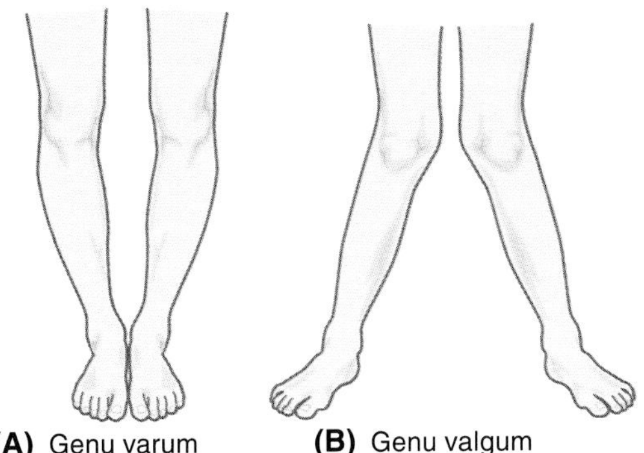

FIGURE 7–4 (A) Genu varum. (B) Genu valgum.

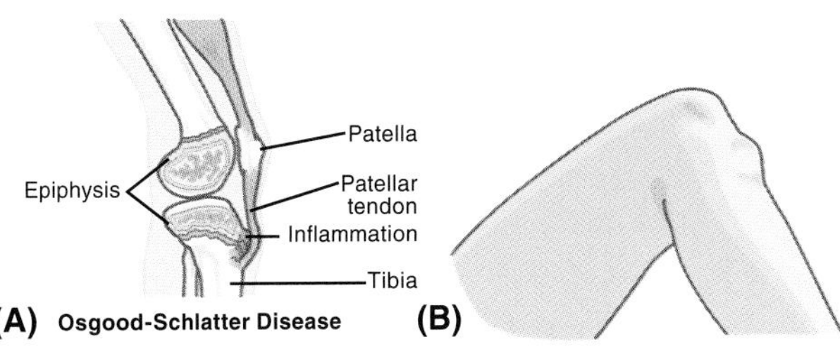

FIGURE 7–5 (A) Osgood-Schlatter. (B) Note the bony prominences below the patella.

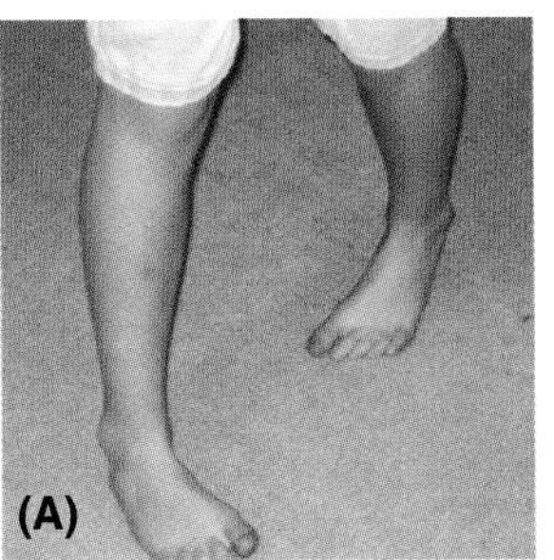

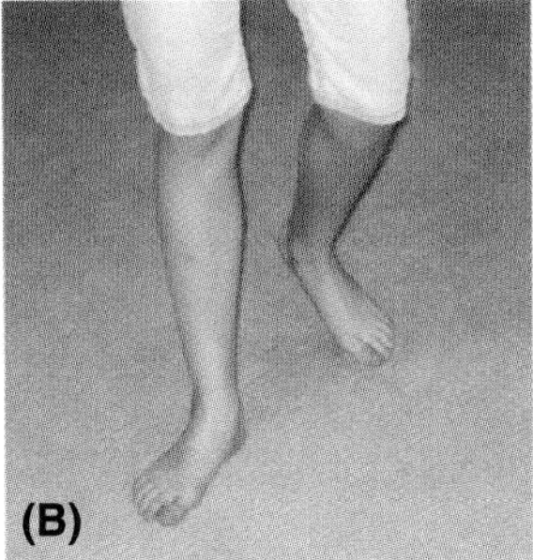

FIGURE 7–6 (A) Intoeing. (B) Out-toeing.

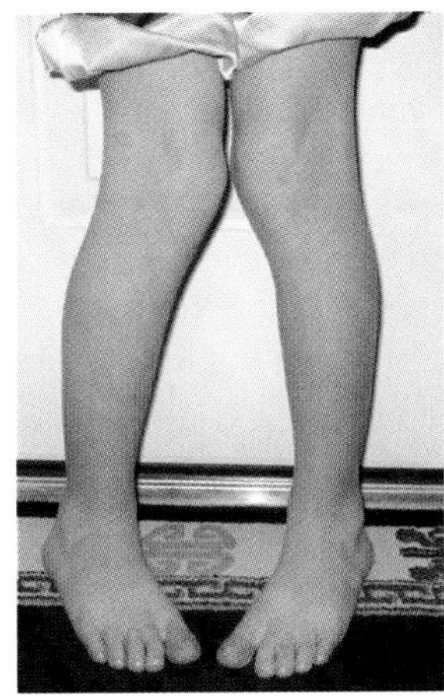

FIGURE 7–7 Internal Femoral Torsion

Table 7-30 Developmental Considerations

Age Group	Cognitive and Emotional Developmental Markers
Preschool	Attention gradually increases.
School age	Can sit and concentrate on their work for a period of time.
7 years	Thinking becomes more logical and systematic. Able to reason and understand.
12 to 15 years	Abstract thinking develops. Able to consider a hypothetical situation. Judgment begins to develop through experiences and education. Set of values is developed and is reflected in the child's thinking and actions.

Source: Colyar, M. R. (2011). *Assessment of the school-age child and adolescent*. Philadelphia, PA: F.A. Davis.

Mental Health

Mental health problems that may affect children include anxiety, depression, bipolar disorder, suicidal/homicidal thoughts, emotional distress, self-esteem issues, and acute psychosis. AAP provides a comprehensive list of mental health screening and assessment tools for primary care.

Cognitive and emotional development markers for preschool through adolescence are shown in Table 7-30. Behaviors that indicate the need for psychiatric referral are shown in Box 7-4. Information on abnormal thought content is given in Table 7-31, on thought process in Table 7-32, and on mood and affect in Table 7-33.

Nutritional Screening

In children, protein- and/or calorie-deficient diet results in underweight, wasting, lowered resistance to infection, stunted growth, and impaired cognitive development and learning. Signs of malnutrition are found in Table 7-34; grading of malnutrition is found in Table 7-35

Adolescent Screening

In addition to immunization surveillance and physical evaluation screening, specific screening of the adolescent includes secondary sexual characteristics, nutritional issues

BOX 7-4 School-Age Behavioral Checklist of Indications for Psychiatric Referral

Scoring: 0 = never; 1 = sometimes; 2 = often. Scoring is reversed for items followed by an asterisk. Scores between 15 and 22 indicate closer following; scores above 22 warrant psychiatric evaluation.

- Prefers to play alone
- Gets hurts in minor accidents
- Plays with fire
- Has difficulties with teachers
- Gets poor grades in school
- Is absent from school frequently
- Becomes angry easily
- Seems to be daydreaming
- Appears to be unhappy
- Acts younger than other children his or her age
- Does not listen to his or her parents
- Does not tell the truth
- Is unsure of him- or herself
- Has trouble sleeping
- Seems afraid of someone or something
- Is nervous and jumpy
- Has a nervous habit
- Does not show feelings
- Fights with other children
- Is understanding of other people's feeling
- Refuses to share
- Shows jealousy
- Takes things that are not his or hers
- Blames others for his or her troubles
- Prefers to play with children who are not his or her age
- Gets along well with grown-ups
- Teases others

Table 7-31 Adolescent Mental Status Evaluation—Thought Content Evaluation

Content	Description
Obsession	Persistent thoughts or impulses
Compulsion	Unwanted, repetitive acts
Delusion	False irrational beliefs
Hallucination	Sensory (visual, tactile, auditory, gustatory) perceptions are altered
Illusion	Misperception of existing stimulus
Phobia	Irrational fear of a situation or object
Hypochondriasis	Morbid worry about personal health without actual reason

Source: Colyar, M. R. (2011). *Assessment of the school-age child and adolescent*. Philadelphia, PA: F.A. Davis.

Table 7-32 Adolescent Mental Status Evaluation—Thought Process Evaluation

Process	Description
Blocking	Interruption of train of thought; inability to complete sentences
Confabulation	Fabrication to fill memory gaps
Neologism	Invented word with no real meaning
Circumstantiality	Excessive and unnecessary detail in speech pattern
Loosening associations	Shifts topics quickly even though unrelated
Flight of ideas	Continuous rapid skipping from topic to topic; speech is rapid
Word salad	Words, phrases, and sentences are mixed and are incoherent and illogical
Perseveration	Repetition of verbal or motor response
Echolalia	Mocking repetition of other people's words
Clanging	Choice of words is based on sounds, not meaning; use of rhyming

Source: Colyar, M. R. (2011). *Assessment of the school-age child and adolescent*. Philadelphia, PA: F.A. Davis.

Table 7-33 Mood and Affect

Types of Expression	Description
Flat	Blunted expression of feelings; voice is monotone
Depressed	Sad, gloomy, dejected
Ambivalent	Doesn't care about either side of an issue
Anxious	Apprehensive, worried, and uneasy
Fearful	Apprehensive, worried, and uneasy about an identified danger
Irritable	Impatient, annoyed, or easily provoked
Elated	Increased motor activity, overly confident and optimistic
Euphoric	Excessively cheerful or highly elated
Rage	Quickly shifting emotions
Inappropriate	Conflict between what the child does and what he or she is talking about (Example: laughs when talking about his broken leg)
Depersonalized	Estranged, perplexed, with loss of identity

Source: Colyar, M. R. (2011). *Assessment of the school-age child and adolescent*. Philadelphia, PA: F.A. Davis.

Table 7-34 Signs of Malnutrition

Body System	Normal Signs	Abnormal Signs	Deficiency or Excess
Weight	Weight in range for age group and gender.	Weight change in short time.	Fluid loss or gain.
Vital signs	Within normal limits for child's age.	Elevated blood pressure. Low blood pressure.	Fluid overload, high sodium intake, obesity. Dehydration.
Eyes	Corneas clear, shiny; membranes pink and moist, no sores at corners of eyelids.	Papilledema. Night blindness. Dryness, softening, pale or red conjunctivae, blepharitis. Foamy plaques of the cornea (Bitot's spots). Sunken eyeballs, dark circles, decreased tears.	Vitamin A excess. Vitamin A deficit. Dehydration.
Lips	Smooth.	Cheilosis (vertical cracks in lips), angular stomatitis (red cracks at sides of mouth).	B_2 (riboflavin), B_3 (niacin), B_6 (pyridoxine), iron.
Tongue	Red, not swollen or smooth, no lesions.	Glossitis, pale, papillary atrophy, papillary hypertrophy, magenta-colored or purplish tongue. Blunting of taste.	Zinc.
Gums	Reddish-pink, firm, no swelling or bleeding.	Swollen, ulcerated, or bleeding.	Vitamin C.
Nose	Sense of smell intact. Nasal mucosa pink, moist, and intact (without lesions).	Hyposmia (defect in sense of smell). Dry mucous membranes.	Zinc. Dehydration.
MS	Erect posture, no malformations, good muscle tone, can walk or run without pain.	Bending of ribs, epiphyseal swelling, bowlegs. Tenderness. Pain in calves, thighs; rickets; joint pain; muscle wasting.	Vitamin D deficiency, osteomalacia. Vitamin C deficiency.

(*continued*)

Table 7-34 Signs of Malnutrition—cont'd

Body System	Normal Signs	Abnormal Signs	Deficiency or Excess
Neuro	Deep tendon reflexes +2/4, senses intact, appropriate affect, no headache, awake, alert and orients x 3	Headaches. Drowsiness. Confusion, irritability. Disorientation. Peripheral neuropathy. Hyporeflexia. Tetany.	Vitamins A and D excess. Dehydration. Niacin, pyridoxine, Vitamin B_{12} deficits. Calcium, magnesium deficits.
Respiratory	Lungs clear, respirations normal.	Increased respiratory rate.	Iron deficiency anemia.
Cardiovascular	Regular rate and rhythm	Tachycardiac and systolic murmur.	Iron deficiency anemia.
Gastrointestinal	Abdomen soft, nontender, no organomegaly.	Hepatomegaly, ascites. Hyperactive bowel sounds.	Protein deficits, vitamin A excess. Hyperperistalsis with absorption problem.
Skin	Smooth, no rashes, bruises, or flaking	Poor skin turgor, edema, dry, flaking, scaling. Petechiae, ecchymoses. Dry bumpy skin. Cracks in skin, lesions on hands, legs, face, or neck. Hyperpigmentation of skin when exposed to sunlight. Nasolabial seborrhea. Acneiform forehead rash. Eczema. Xanthomas (excessive deposits of cholesterol). Purpura.	Vitamins A, B complex, linoleic acid. Vitamins. C and K. Vitamins A, linoleic acid. Niacin, tryptophan. Niacin. Riboflavin, B_6. B_6. Linoleic acid. Elevated cholesterol. Vitamin K excess.
Hair	Shiny, firm, does not fall out easily. Healthy scalp, even distribution of hair, no alopecia.	Dull, dry, sparse hair. Color changes, transverse pigmentation of hair shaft, hair easy to pluck, breaks easily, sparse hair distribution. Corkscrew hairs, unemerged hair coils.	Protein, zinc, linoleic acid. Copper, protein. Copper.
Nails	Smooth, pink	Brittle, ridged, or spoon-shaped nails, transverse ridges in nails. Splinter hemorrhages.	Iron. Vitamin C.

Source: Colyar, M. R. (2011). *Assessment of the school-age child and adolescent.* Philadelphia, PA: F.A. Davis.

Table 7-35 Assessment of Malnutrition

Grade of Malnutrition	Height/Weight as a Percentage of Standard
0	>90
1—Mild	81–90
2—Moderate	70–80
3—Severe	

Source: Colyar, M. R. (2011). *Assessment of the school-age child and adolescent.* Philadelphia, PA: F.A. Davis.

(eating disorders, obesity), depression, suicide, and risky behaviors (drugs, driving safety, gun safety, dating, and sexual coercion). The excellent book *The Teen Years Explained: A Guide to Healthy Development* (McNeely & Blanchard, 2010), from the Johns Hopkins Bloomberg School of Public Health, covers all aspects of adolescent development.

Physical Screening

Females are three to four times more prone to scoliosis problems that require treatment than are males. A joint position statement by the Scoliosis Research Society,

Pediatric Orthopaedic Society of North America, American Association of Osteopathic Colleges, and American Academy of Pediatrics recommends that screening be performed for females at ages 10 and 12 years of age. Males should be screened once at age 13 to 14 years (Hresko, Talwalkar, & Schwend, 2015). This is usually done during sports physicals. Table 7-36 outlines the steps and what to observe when doing postural screening.

Table 7-36 Procedure for Postural Screening

Steps	Observations
1. Ask the student to place his or her toes on a piece of tape that is on the floor. Instruct the student to stand erect with feet slightly apart, weight evenly distributed, hands hanging at sides, and looking forward.	Observe from the front, side, and back: • Is the head midline? • Are the shoulders at equal heights? • Is space between arms and body the same? • Are the hips (both sides of waist) at equal heights? • Are the knees at equal heights? • Is there exaggerated roundness of upper back? • Is there exaggerated arch in lower back? • Is one shoulder blade higher than the other? • Does the spine appear to curve?
2. While standing behind the student, have the student bend forward at the waist with arms hanging freely. Ensure that the student's feet are 2 to 3 inches apart and knees are straight. The student's back should be horizontal to the floor. (This is called the Adams Forward Bend Test.)	• Is one scapula higher than the other? • Is there a prominence or bulge on one side of the back? • Are the hip levels uneven? • Is there a curvature of the spine?* • [View from side] Are there spinal humps?
3. Have the student walk away from you a few steps and then turn and walk back.	• Is there asymmetry of movement on walking? • Do the knees come together and are the ankles abducted? (genu valgum—knock-kneed) • Do the knees abduct when the feet are together? (Genu varum—bow-legged)

* Some measure the curvature or degree of rotation using a scoliometer. It can be placed directly across the student's back where the irregularity is most prominent. The "0" should be directly over the top ridge of the spine. Do not press down on the device; any reading greater than 5 to 7 degrees should be rescreened or referred. A 5-degree angle of trunk rotation results in a referral rate of approximately 12%. Referral might also be made if there is asymmetry in two or more areas of visual assessment

Sources: (Ricci, Kyle, & Carman, 2017). Selekman, J., Shannon, R. A., & Yonkaitis, C. F. (2019). *School nursing: A comprehensive text* (3rd ed.). Philadelphia, PA: F.A. Davis.

Sexual maturity screening

Of the many ways to evaluate pubertal development (Shirtcliff, Dahl, & Pollak, 2009), the Tanner Scale is most often used for evaluating sexual maturity in adolescents (Figures 7-8 through 7-10). Characteristics of male and female maturity are found in Tables 7-37 and 7-38.

Body image screening

Severely distorted views of the body image can develop during adolescence. Box 7-5 outlines the screening procedure for eating disorders. Anorexia and bulimia are common during adolescence. Anorexia nervosa manifests as extreme weight loss and a fear of weight gain. Adolescents with anorexia show warning signs of dramatic weight loss and preoccupation with weight, food, calories, fat grams, and/or dieting. They usually diet excessively and exercise obsessively. Adolescents with bulimia nervosa eat large amounts of food and then vomit or take excessive amounts of laxatives to lose weight. Questions to ask regarding anorexia and bulimia are shown in Box 7-6.

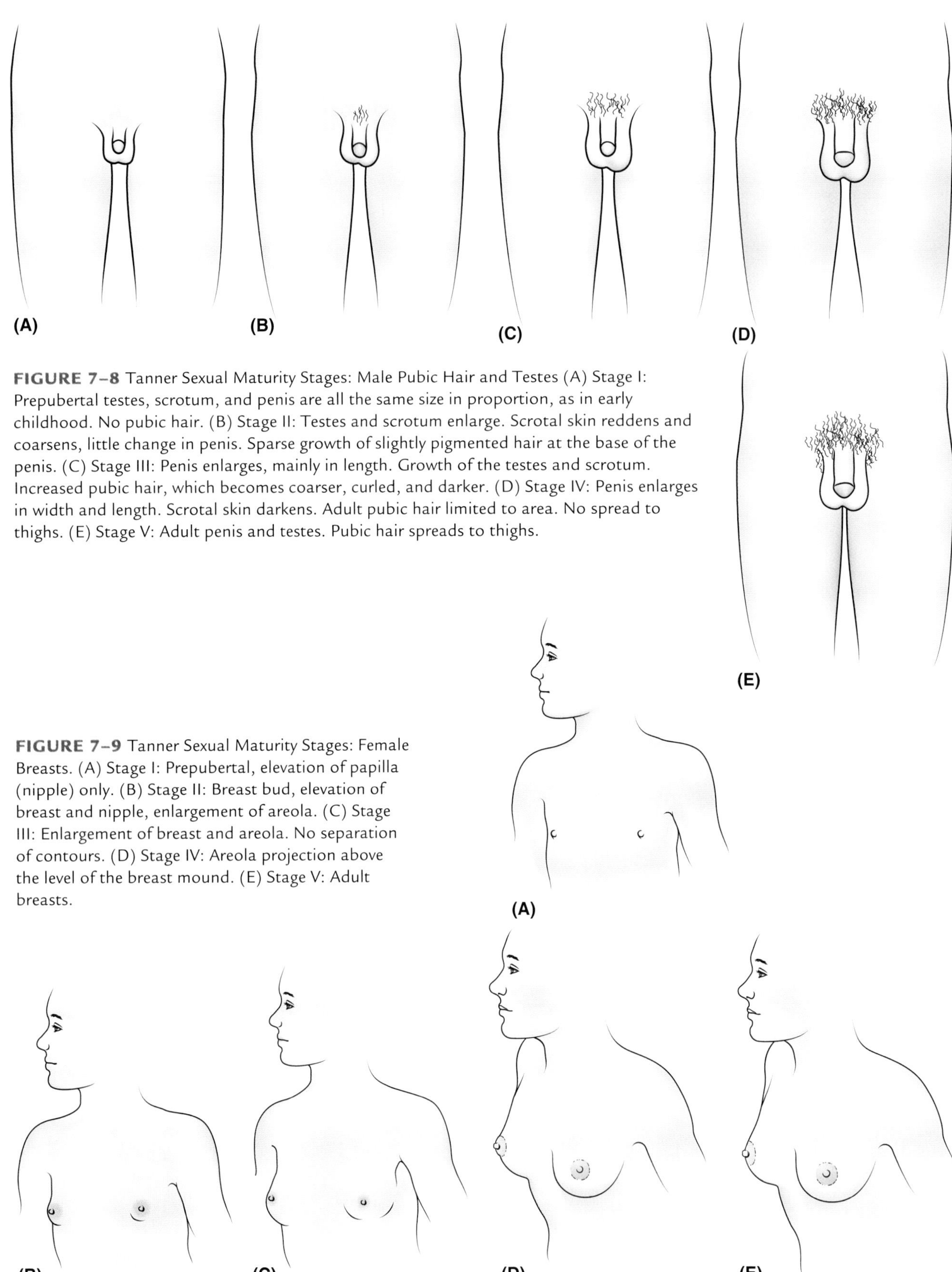

FIGURE 7–8 Tanner Sexual Maturity Stages: Male Pubic Hair and Testes (A) Stage I: Prepubertal testes, scrotum, and penis are all the same size in proportion, as in early childhood. No pubic hair. (B) Stage II: Testes and scrotum enlarge. Scrotal skin reddens and coarsens, little change in penis. Sparse growth of slightly pigmented hair at the base of the penis. (C) Stage III: Penis enlarges, mainly in length. Growth of the testes and scrotum. Increased pubic hair, which becomes coarser, curled, and darker. (D) Stage IV: Penis enlarges in width and length. Scrotal skin darkens. Adult pubic hair limited to area. No spread to thighs. (E) Stage V: Adult penis and testes. Pubic hair spreads to thighs.

FIGURE 7–9 Tanner Sexual Maturity Stages: Female Breasts. (A) Stage I: Prepubertal, elevation of papilla (nipple) only. (B) Stage II: Breast bud, elevation of breast and nipple, enlargement of areola. (C) Stage III: Enlargement of breast and areola. No separation of contours. (D) Stage IV: Areola projection above the level of the breast mound. (E) Stage V: Adult breasts.

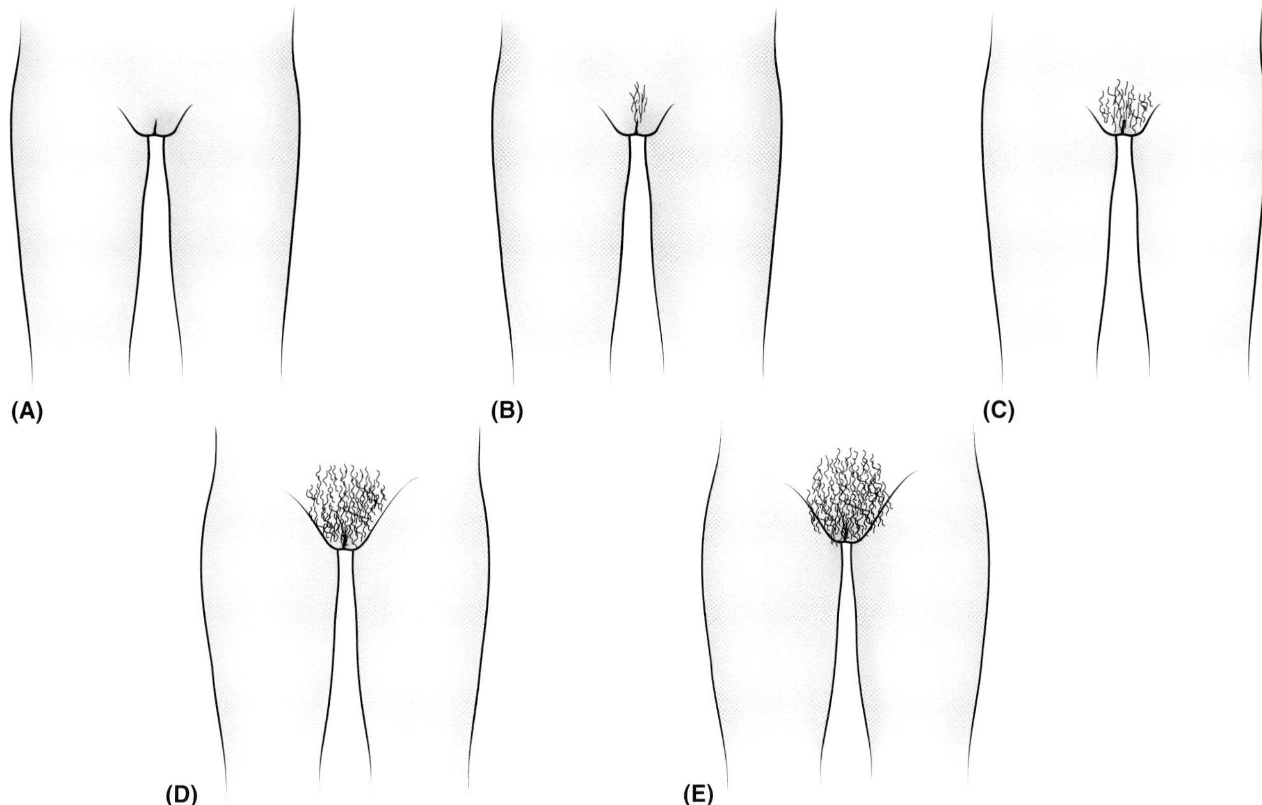

FIGURE 7–10 Tanner Sexual Maturity Stages: Female Pubic Hair. (A) Stage I: Prepubertal. No Pubic Hair. (B) Stage Ii: Sparse Growth of Slightly Pigmented, Downy Hair, Only Slightly Curled, Mainly Along Labia. (C) Stage Iii: Increased Hair Becoming Coarser, Curled, and Darker. (D) Stage IV: Adult Public Hair Limited to the Vulva, No Spread to Thighs. (E) Stage V: Adult Pubic Hair with Spread to Thighs.

Table 7-37 Characteristics Related to Male Sexual Maturity

Characteristic	Age of Onset
Growth of testes	11½–14½
Pubic and axillary hair	12–16
Growth of penis	12½–14½
Growth spurt	12½–16

Source: Colyar, M. R. (2011). *Assessment of the school-age child and adolescent*. Philadelphia, PA: F.A. Davis.

Table 7-38 Characteristics Related to Female Sexual Maturity

Characteristic	Age of Onset
Growth of breasts	11–13½
Pubic hair	11½–14
Axillary hair	2 years after pubic hair appears
Menarche	2 years after beginning breast development
Growth spurt	About 12; range is 11–13½

Source: Colyar, M. R. (2011). *Assessment of the school-age child and adolescent*. Philadelphia, PA: F.A. Davis.

Obesity is diagnosed when a child weighs more than 20 percent of the maximum recommended weight for his or her age. Children who are obese at the start of adolescence have a 1 in 4 likelihood of being obese as adults. Adolescents who are obese have a 28-to-1 likelihood of being obese as adults. Obesity rates have doubled since 1980 among children and have tripled for adolescents. Obesity in adolescents has increased from 5% to 18% in the last 20 years. Use the CDC growth charts to determine if an adolescent has a BMI equal to or greater than the 95th percentile. Issues that contribute to teen obesity are outlined in Box 7-7.

BOX 7-5 Eating Disorder Examination

QUESTIONS

1. Do you feel good about your body?
2. Do you feel you eat too much?
3. What do you do when you are over your goal weight? What do you do when you have eaten too much, or have eaten too many high-calorie foods?
4. Do you like to eat alone?
5. Do you need to take laxatives? If yes, how often?
6. Do you have a sore throat most of the time?
7. How often do you exercise?

PHYSICAL EXAMINATION MARKERS

- Height and weight
- Mouth and throat examination for palatal trauma (pharyngeal stimulation)
- Parotid gland examination (which is usually inflamed if there has been constant vomiting)
- Dental erosion due to tooth enamel being chemically "eaten" by hydrochloric acid from the stomach
- Metacarpal-phalangeal bruises/calluses due to constant abrasions (even scars) on the base of the index finger or the finger that is used to purge
- Vital signs, including bradycardia (a resting heart rate of 60 or less is often found in anorexics), bradypnea, hypotension, hypothermia, and poor capillary refill
- Hydration state
- Scaphoid abdomen or organomegaly
- Skin edema of extremities (indicates a loss of protein)

BOX 7-6 Questions to Ask Regarding Anorexia and Bulimia

1. Do you feel good about your body?
2. Do you feel you eat too much?
3. What do you do when you are over your goal weight? What do you do when you have eaten too much or have eaten too many high-calorie foods?
4. Do you like to eat alone?
5. Do you need to take laxatives? If yes, how often?
6. Do you have a sore throat most of the time?
7. How often do you exercise?
8. Examination of teens includes observation of the following:
   a. Height and weight
   b. Mouth and throat for palatal trauma (pharyngeal stimulation)
   c. Parotid gland, which is usually inflamed if there has been constant vomiting
   d. Dental erosion, such as enamel that is chemically "eaten" by hydrochloric acid from the stomach
   e. Metacarpal-phalangeal bruises/calluses, which result from constant abrasions, even scars on the base of the index finger or finger that purges
   f. Vital signs, bradycardia (a resting heart rate of 60 beats per minute or fewer is often found in anorexics), bradypnea, hypotension, hypothermia, and poor capillary refill
   g. Hydration state
   h. Scaphoid abdomen or organomegaly
   i. Skin edema of the extremities, which results from a loss of protein
9. Mental state, including apathy, psychomotor retardation, depression, anxiety, and obsessive-compulsive traits.

Source: Colyar, M. R. (2011). *Assessment of the school-age child and adolescent*. Philadelphia, PA: F.A. Davis.

BOX 7-7 Issues That Affect Obesity in Adolescents

- More high-fat, high-calorie foods and sugary drinks than nutritious, lower-calorie choices sold in schools.
- Low-income communities offer limited access to healthy food. Convenience stores are sometimes the only places to buy food.
- Sedentary lifestyle (sitting during school day, watching TV, or playing video games) and lack of exercise.
- School physical education programs have been slashed.
- Food product ads.
- Fast foods.
- Hormones, including contraceptives.
- Poor eating habits.
- Overeating or binging.
- Family history of obesity.
- Medical illnesses (endocrine, neurological problems).
- Medications (steroids, some psychiatric medications).
- Stressful life events or changes (separations, divorce, moves, death, abuse).
- Family and peer problems.
- Low self-esteem.
- Depression or other emotional problems.

Source: American Academy of Child and Adolescent Psychology. Guide/Obesity in children and teens (2016). Retrieved from https://www.aacap.org/AACAP/Families_and_Youth/Facts_for_Families/FFF-Guide/Obesity-In-Children-And-Teens-079.aspx

BOX 7-8 Stressors for Adolescents

- Breakup with boyfriend or girlfriend
- Increased arguments with parents
- Trouble with sibling(s)
- Increased arguments between parents
- Change in parents' financial status
- Serious illness or injury of family member
- Trouble with classmates
- Trouble with parents

Psychological and social contributors to the accumulation of problems and stressors:

- Loss experience such as a death or suicide of a friend or family member, broken romance, loss of a close friendship, or a family move
- Unmet personal or parental expectation such as failure to achieve a goal, poor grades, social rejection
- Unresolved conflict with family members, peers, teachers, coaches that results in anger, frustration, rejection
- Humiliating experience resulting in loss of self-esteem or rejection
- Unexpected events such as pregnancy or financial problems

Body dysmorphic disorder is an intense preoccupation with a perceived defect in one's appearance. Adolescents with this disorder have a perceived flaw that causes them significant distress and affects their ability to function in daily life. For example, they repeatedly check themselves in the mirror, groom, or seek reassurance, sometimes for many hours each day.

Muscle dysmorphia is a preoccupation with the idea that one's body is not sufficiently lean and muscular. Adolescents with muscle dysmorphia are excessively preoccupied with working out and weight lifting, often leading to steroid use. A growing body of evidence suggests that the prevalence of male body dissatisfaction and muscle dysmorphia is rising. Although there are no medications specifically to treat body dysmorphic disorder, medications used to treat other mental health conditions and cognitive behavior therapy can be effective (Mayo Clinic, 2020).

Mental status screening

Young people become stressed for many reasons, and stress and other negative emotions may develop into or exacerbate a mental health problem. Some of the main contributing factors to mental health disorders in teens are described in Box 7-8.

BOX 7-9 Clinical Manifestations of Depression in Children

Withdrawal from social activities
Sleep disturbance—too much or too little
Appetite disturbance—too much or too little
Multiple somatic complaints such as headaches and stomachaches
Decreased energy
Difficulty concentrating
Difficulty making decisions
Low self-esteem
Feelings of hopelessness

BOX 7-10 Personality Traits Seen with Depression in Adolescents

- Impulsive behaviors, obsessions, and unreal fears
- Aggressive and antisocial behavior
- Withdrawal and isolation, detachment
- Poor social skills resulting in feelings of humiliation, poor self-worth, blame, and feeling ugly
- Overachieving and extreme pressure to perform
- A depressed mood
- Loss of interest or pleasure
- Change in sleep, eating, energy, concentration, and self-image

Source: https://www.nimh.nih.gov/health/statistics/index.shtml

BOX 7-11 Risk Factors for Suicide

- History of previous suicide attempts
- Family history of suicide
- History of depression or other mental illness
- Alcohol or drug abuse
- Stressful life event or loss
- Easy access to lethal methods
- Exposure to the suicidal behavior of others
- Incarceration

Source: https://www.cdc.gov/violenceprevention/suicide/youth_suicide.html

Depression Screening

Box 7-9 and Box 7-10 review clinical and personality manifestations of children with depression. The actions in response to stress are also different for those who reported serious depression or a suicide attempt. Young people who are depressed are at much greater risk of attempting suicide than are youth who are not depressed. They report more anger; avoidance; passivity; and aggressive, antisocial behavior. Behaviors common among depressed adolescents include yelling, fighting, drinking, smoking, using drugs, sleep disturbances, and frequent crying.

Suicide and Risky Behavior Screening

Each year in the United States, thousands of teenagers commit suicide. Suicide is the third leading cause of death for 15- to 24-year-olds and the sixth leading cause of death for 5- to 14-year-olds. Cash and Bridge (2009) reviewed research on adolescent suicide and suicidal behavior by focusing on recent developments in our understanding of the epidemiology and established emerging risk factors (Box 7-11) of youth suicide and suicidal behavior. Personality traits that change dramatically over a 2-week period or longer, such as those listed in Table 7-39, can signify an elevated suicide risk. Other risky behaviors to screen for are drugs, driving safety, gun safety, dating, and sexual coercion.

Health Screening for Youth Ages 18–21 Years

Screening guidelines for youth ages 18 to 21 years are shown in Box 7-12.

KEY POINTS

- Health screening is an important component of wellness and healthy development from birth to age 21.

Table 7-39 Possible Warning Signs of Suicide

Warning Sign	Examples
Talking About Dying	Any mention of dying, disappearing, jumping, shooting oneself, or other types of self-harm.
Recent Loss	Death; divorce; separation; broken relationship; self-confidence; self-esteem; loss of interest in friends, hobbies, and activities previously enjoyed.
Change in Personality	Sad, withdrawn, irritable, anxious, tired, indecisive, apathetic.
Change in Behavior	Can't concentrate on school, work, routine tasks
Change in Sleep Patterns	Insomnia, often with early waking or oversleeping, nightmares.
Change in Eating Habits	Loss of appetite and weight, or overeating.
Fear of Losing Control	Acting erratically, harming self or others.
Low Self-Esteem	Feeling worthless, shame, overwhelming guilt, self-hatred, "everyone would be better off without me."
No Hope for the Future	Believing things will never get better, that nothing will ever change.

Source: American Psychological Association (2020). Teen suicide is preventable. http://www.apa.org/research/action/suicide.aspx

BOX 7-12 Screening Guidelines for Men and Women Ages 18 to 21

- Blood pressure screening: every 3 to 5 years.
- Cholesterol screening: Once after puberty.
- Diabetes screening: if blood pressure is elevated, family history of diabetes or if body mass index (BMI) is greater than 25.
- Dental exam: once or twice every year for an exam and cleaning.
- Eye exam: every year if diabetic.
- Immunizations: flu shot every year. After age 19, one tetanus-diphtheria and acellular pertussis (TdAP) vaccine as one of the tetanus-diphtheria vaccines. A tetanus-diphtheria (TD) booster every 10 years. Human papilloma virus (HPV) vaccine if not immunized prior.
- Chlamydia test: every year for sexually active women through age 24.
- HIV test: one time during adulthood.
- Depression: at each exam.
- Diet and exercise: at each exam.
- Alcohol and tobacco use: at each exam.
- Use of seat belts: at each exam.
- Use of smoke detectors: at each exam.
- Pelvic exam and pap smear (women only): screening for cervical cancer should begin at age 21, with a pelvic exam and Pap smear every 3 years.

Source: https://medlineplus.gov/ency/article/007462.htm

- Current research indicates that vaccines for children and adults are a safe, effective way to combat life-threatening communicable diseases.
- Infants and toddlers should be screened for developmental disabilities several times up until age 3.
- School-age children should receive physical, mental health, hearing, vision, and neurological screenings at each wellness visit.
- In addition to the screenings listed above, adolescents should be screened for risk-taking behaviors, depression, safe sex practices, nutrition, and suicidal ideation.

Check Your Understanding

1. Research on MMR vaccination shows:
   A. Multiple vaccines overwhelm and weaken the immune system.
   B. Children with inborn errors of metabolism experience adverse effects.
   C. There is an increased risk of pervasive disorders.
   D. There is no causal relationship between MMR and the number or amount of vaccinations.
2. Obesity is defined as:
   A. 20% above normal weight

B. Need to go on a diet
C. Doubled since 1980
D. BMI greater than or equal to 90th percentile

3. Screening of newborns includes all EXCEPT:
A. Vital signs
B. Skin lesions
C. Apgar
D. Visual acuity

4. Developmental screening includes all EXCEPT:
A. Language
B. Fine motor
C. Depression
D. Cognitive

5. Vision screening for school-age children includes:
A. Extraocular movements, cover/uncover
B. Black and white object recognition and corneal light reflex
C. Red reflex and corneal light reflex
D. Illiterate E and red reflex

6. Which of the following screenings should be done only once for men and women between the ages of 18 and 21?
A. Blood pressure
B. Depression
C. Dental
D. HIV

7. What musculoskeletal disorders should be checked for in infants?
A. Hip dysplasia
B. Intoeing
C. Genu valgum
D. Osgood-Schlatter

8. True or false: According to the National Association of School Nurses, children with head lice should be sent home from school.

9. Body dysmorphic disorder is seen in adolescents who:
A. Eat large amounts of food and vomit
B. Are obese
C. Are intensely occupied with a perceived body defect
D. Show a dramatic weight loss

10. The American Academy of Pediatrics recommends first dental screening:
A. At 3 years of age
B. At 1 year of age
C. When starting school
D. Two times per year

See "Reflections on Check Your Understanding" at the end of the book for answers.

REFERENCES

Alderson, M. R. (2016). Status of research and development of pediatric vaccines for Streptococcus pneumoniae. *Vaccine*, *34*(26), 2959-2961.

American Dental Association (2020). Statement on childhood caries. https://www.ada.org/en/about-the-ada/ada-positions-policies-and-statements/statement-on-early-childhood-caries

American Psychological Association (2020). Teen suicide is preventable. http://www.apa.org/research/action/suicide.aspx.

Atkinson, W., & Wolfe, S. and Hamborsky, J, eds. (2012). *Epidemiology and prevention of vaccine-preventable diseases. 12th edn. Washington DC: public health Foundation*.

Cash, S. J., & Bridge, J. A. (2009). Epidemiology of youth suicide and suicidal behavior. *Current Options in Pediatrics*, *21*(5), 613–619.

Centers for Disease Control and Prevention. (2019a). Childhood obesity facts. *Overweight & obesity*. Retrieved from https://www.cdc.gov/hpv/parents/vaccine.html

Centers for Disease Control and Prevention. (2019b). Children's oral health. *Oral health*. Retrieved from https://www.cdc.gov/hpv/parents/vaccine.html

Centers for Disease Control and Prevention. (2019c). Vaccinating boys and girls. *Human papillomavirus*. Retrieved from https://www.cdc.gov/oralhealth/basics/childrens-oral-health/index.html

Chou, R. Dana, T. & Bougatsos, C. (2009). Screening older adults for impaired visual acuity: A review of the evidence for the U.S. Preventive Services Task Force. *Annals of Internal Medicine*, *151*(1), 44–58, W11–W20.

Frankowski, B. L., & Bocchini, J. A., Jr. (2016). Clinical report: Head lice. Council on School Health and Committee on Infectious Diseases. National Association of School Nurses. Head lice management in the school setting—Position statement (revised).

Frankowski, B. L., Bocchini, J. A., & Council on School Health and Committee on Infectious Diseases. (2010). Head lice. *Pediatrics*, *126*(2), 392-403

Frenck, R. W., Gurtman, A., Rubino, J., Smith, W., van Cleeff, M., Jayawardene, D., & Schmöle-Thoma, B. (2012). Randomized, controlled trial of a 13-valent pneumococcal conjugate vaccine administered concomitantly with an influenza vaccine in healthy adults. *Clin. Vaccine Immunol.*, *19*(8), 1296-1303.

Glanz, J. M., Newcomer, S. R., Daley, M. F., DeStefano, F., Groom, H. C., Jackson, M. L., & Nordin, J. D. (2018).

Association between estimated cumulative vaccine antigen exposure through the first 23 months of life and non–vaccine-targeted infections from 24 through 47 months of age. *Jama*, *319*(9), 906-913.

Hinshaw, A., (2013). Institute of Medicine. The National Academy of Sciences.

Hresko, M. T., Talwalkar, V. T., & Schwend. R. M. (2015). Screening for the early detection for idiopathic scoliosis in adolescents. SRS/POSNA/AAOS/AAP position statement. *Pediatrics*, *126*, 2.

Mathers, M. I., Keyes, M., & Wright, M. (2010). A review of the evidence on the effectiveness of children's vision screening. *Child Care Health Development*, *36*(6), 756–780.

McNeely, C., & Blanchard, J. (2010). *The teen years explained: A guide to healthy adolescent development*. Baltimore, MD: Johns Hopkins Bloomberg School of Public Health.

Mayo Clinic (2020). Patient information https://www.mayoclinic.org/diseases-conditions/body-dysmorphic-disorder/diagnosis-treatment/drc-20353944

Shirtcliff, E. A., Dahl, R. E., & Pollak, S. D. (2009). Pubertal development: Correspondence between hormonal and physical development. *Child Development*, *80*(2), 327–337.

Taylor, L. E., Swerdfeger, A. L., & Eslick, G. D. (2014). Vaccines are not associated with autism: an evidence-based meta-analysis of case-control and cohort studies. *Vaccine*, 32(29), 3623–3629.

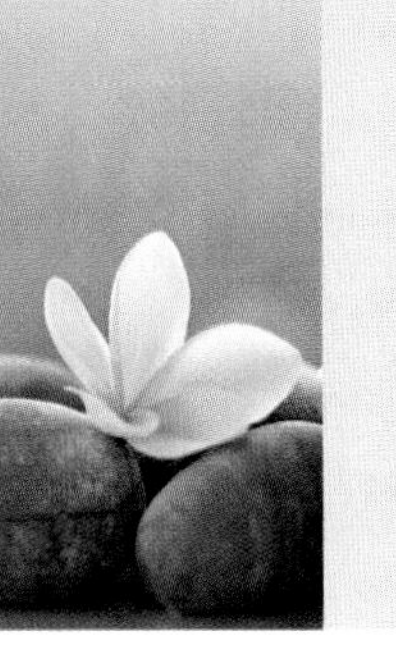

Chapter 8

Health Screening and Counseling: Adult and Older Adult

Vicky Stone-Gale and Diane John

LEARNING OBJECTIVES

After completing this chapter, the student will be able to:

1. Identify the evidence-based recommendations that address developmental issues for the adult and older adult.
2. Identify the recommended health-care screenings for the adult and older adult.
3. Review the risk factors for the adult and older adult.
4. Explain the prevention strategies that are appropriate for the adult and older adult.
5. Determine the health counseling needs for middle and older adults.

INTRODUCTION

Health screening of individuals from middle to older adulthood can promote prevention and thus help to avoid future medical issues, assist in the identification of risk factors that may lead to poor health, and detect disease early so progression can be delayed or halted. Evidence-based screening in the aging population, including recommended immunizations and screenings, can prevent acute and chronic illness. These screenings may include those for osteoporosis and breast and cervical cancer in women, abdominal aortic aneurysm in men, and lung cancer in those with a history of smoking. In addition, other age-related screenings may be performed based on memory deficits, physical changes, psychological problems, and functional issues.

This chapter will outline the developmental tasks, health determinants and prevention strategies, and health counseling for the middle and older adult populations. Screening tools for mental health, dementia and Alzheimer's, substance abuse, and falls will be provided. The elderly as a vulnerable population and screening for geriatric syndromes will be discussed.

DEVELOPMENTAL TASKS AND APPROACHES

The developmental tasks and approaches from middle to older adulthood result from changes in psychological, socioeconomic, and physical development. Developmental tasks and approaches are described using Erik Erikson's theory of psychosocial development and Robert Havighurst's developmental task theory. Erikson's theory holds that individuals travel through and ideally master specific developmental tasks in eight life stages. Havighurst's theory ascertains that individuals may achieve fulfillment in life when success is achieved as tasks are completed, or they may be unhappy and experience discontent if they fail.

Middle Adulthood

Middle adulthood is the age beyond young adulthood but before old age and ranges from age 40 to age 65, although some authors use a starting age of 45 years. Erikson defines this stage of life as the generativity versus stagnation stage (Table 8-1). Careers are established; relationships are stabilized; and children are raised and transitioning to adulthood, entering college, or starting careers. Many individuals in this stage become a meaningful part of society by getting involved in the community, achieving career success, and participating in organizations. However, if the person is unsuccessful or unproductive, stagnation can occur. Generativity crisis is a possibility at this stage of life. For example, divorce or job loss may lead to a change in finances or life circumstances, possibly creating the need to reenter the workforce and even causing the individual to rethink life choices (Schaie, 2016). The body starts to show signs of slowing down and aging during middle adulthood. Women transition into menopause, with accompanying physical changes, and the risk for medical problems such as cancer, hypertension, diabetes, and osteoporosis increases in both men and women. In this stage of life, individuals must accomplish specific developmental tasks. The middle age tasks according to Erikson are outlined in Table 8-2. Robert Havighurst describes similar middle age tasks in his developmental task theory.

Developing a Sense of Unity As a Couple

Unity with a partner is achieved when two individuals share a bond based on honesty and integrity, and join together with each other's needs in mind. In this life stage, with children leaving home and couples possibly facing an empty nest, conflicts can lead to disenchantment in the relationship, decreased intimacy, and even sexual dysfunction and affairs with other sexual partners. A relationship is in harmony when each person is creative in decision making, cognizant of the other partner's feelings and needs, and mindful of negative energy and feelings. Maintaining individual independence is important and healthy in a relationship and still enables the person to be giving, emotionally open, and willing to compromise when needed. Spending time alone and having an independent social life is healthy for a good relationship.

Table 8-1 Erikson's Generativity Versus Stagnation Stage

Signs of Generativity	Signs of Stagnation
Expresses confidence	Resentful
Productive in workforce	Life and work dissatisfaction
Tends to be their own person	Withdraws from others
Achieves set goals	Complains and blames others
Invests in next generation	Lack of physical care, obese
Takes charge and risks	Fatalistic attitude

Source: Adapted from Kropf, N., & Greene, R. R. (2017). Erikson's Eight Stages of Development.

Table 8-2 Middle-Age Developmental Tasks

Related to Family	Related to Self
• Developing a sense of unity as a couple • Helping children to transition to adulthood and leave the nest • Accepting grandparent role and keeping contact with children • Ensuring adequate living arrangements for elderly parents	• Adjusting to physical body changes • Ensuring financial and medical stability for retirement • Adjusting to career needs and achieving professional success • Creating a comfortable living environment • Maintaining a healthy lifestyle • Participating in community activities and civic duties

Helping Children Transition to Adulthood

Although many parents encourage their children to move out after graduating from high school or college, some feel ambivalence about children leaving home and have a hard time letting go. Adults who have recently become independent of their parents may have limited job stability and relationship experience. They may struggle with the challenges of finding appropriate adult roles and making positive life choices about work and relationships (Davis, Kim, & Fingerman, 2016). This can concern parents, who in turn struggle with their new role regarding their child or children. They want to instill their own values and may think back to their own transition period and try to identify with their children's struggles.

Accepting the Grandparent Role and Keeping Contact with Children

The role of grandparenting can be very satisfying and is classified as a highly generative activity. Grandchildren who engage in frequent interactions with their grandparents develop an emotionally close relationship (Baugh, Taylor, & Bates, 2016). Sometimes this closeness can be considered interference by the parents. Parents and grandparents may disagree on discipline, food choices, and social media interaction. Some grandparents take on the custodial grandparent role when parental absence requires them to provide full care. Although ideally a close relationship with their own children is expected in the middle-age years, when the parent-child relationship is jeopardized, the priority becomes the grandparent-grandchild relationship (Baugh, Taylor, & Bates, 2016). In this situation, grandparents may question their own child-rearing abilities when they see that their offspring lack the competency to raise their grandchildren. The grandparents may also face the emotional and behavioral issues that the children may experience because of parental loss (Table 8-3). Finally, they face the financial ramifications of raising children at a time in their lives when they might otherwise be saving their money for retirement.

Ensuring Adequate Living Arrangements for Elderly Parents

Taking care of elderly parents has grown to be a major concern for adult children. In 2011, roughly 62% of caregivers who responded to the National Study of Caregiving were described as female and one-third were either the daughter, daughter-in-law, or stepdaughter-in-law of the care recipient (Schulz & Eden, 2016). Not only is the middle-age adult responsible for his or her own children as they become independent, he or she may also be responsible for a parent who is becoming more dependent on care. This creates struggles that include time management between work, spouse, and parents; emotional conflict; and even financial burdens.

Serving as a caregiver can result in burnout, lost income, social isolation, depression, anxiety, and even marital distress. Not only does the caregiver experience many of these symptoms, elderly parents may also feel depressed and anxious about losing their independence and becoming a burden to their children. The caregiver's own children may experience conflict because the focus is not solely on them, even when they understand the need for their grandparents. If an elderly parent must move in with an adult child, financial concerns may arise as hired care is needed while the rest of the family works. Many times, adults caring for their aging parents retire early, quit their jobs, or limit their hours at work.

Adjusting to Physical and Physiological Body Changes

Entering middle age often requires the individual to understand that physical changes may be drastic but are a natural part of the aging process. Dissatisfaction with body image can affect well-being in the older adult. The 2016 qualitative study by Jankowski, Diedrichs,

Table 8-3 Custodial Grandparenting Problems and Outcomes

Child Emotional and Behavior Issues	Potential Outcomes
Anxiety	Social withdrawal, poor academic performance, isolation, lack of participation in school activities or sports, fear
Depression	Inadequate coping skills, fear, isolation, suicidal thoughts, guilt
Posttraumatic stress disorder	Social anxiety, psychosis, fear, anger, suicidal thoughts, social isolation
Anger outbursts	Fighting in school, stealing, acting out, jealous of peers' relationships with family

Source: Adapted from Grinwis, Smith & Dannison, 2004.

Williamson, Christopher, & Harcourt (2016) identified four major themes related to this dissatisfaction:

- Personal identity, capability, and social status are linked to appearance.
- Physical ability and health are more important than appearance.
- Appearance is linked to sociocultural norms and pressures.
- Culture and gender are related to differences in body image, with women often reporting more investment in appearance than men do.

Ensuring Financial and Medical Stability for Retirement

Retirement and enduring financial security are major priorities for this age group. As people near retirement, financial concerns can include the ability to pay the mortgage, afford health care, meet their everyday household and food expenses, and pay for medications and other medical needs. Many do not want to rely on living with their children, prefer to live in their own home, and cannot afford an assisted living facility (Baker, Sudano, Albert, Borawski, & Dor, 2002).

Health-care coverage can become a financial burden on many individuals in middle age as premiums increase and medication prices rise, which may lead to household debt and even bankruptcy (Dickman, Himmelstein, & Woolhandler, 2017; Baker, Sudano, Albert, Borawski, & Dor, 2001). As individuals begin to retire, health-care costs become their sole responsibility because these are no longer covered by employers. Some employer health plans continue to pay all or part of cost of insurance post retirement. Other retirement plans may include subsidies for health insurance. However, these options are not the norm. For most retirees, Medicare becomes their primary insurance. Medicare coverage differs from state to state. Most plans do not totally cover health care costs, and a supplementary policy, or a Medigap policy is necessary. Limited affordability may lead to lack of coverage and access to care concerns. Retirement and health care are top priorities that need to be considered in the early years of middle age so income adjustments can be made and retirement plans can be optimized for future needs.

Adjusting to Career Needs and Achieving Professional Success

By middle age, an individual's career has often been established. Some begin to question or regret their career decision and may wish they had achieved more success. Both men and women may also worry about how to balance family and career. Some middle-age adults may fear being replaced at work by a younger, less expensive employee. Health problems may also jeopardize the ability to retain a job. Middle-age individuals may have greater difficulty finding new employment because of these issues.

Creating a Comfortable Living Environment

As children leave home and middle-age adults become empty nesters, some begin to think about selling their homes or even moving to a different area. Today's older population, in comparison with earlier generations, carry more debt and use credit to maintain the lifestyle they are accustomed to living (Lewin-Epstein & Semyonov, 2016). Many individuals still carry a home mortgage beyond age 50. Mortgage debt is typically the largest household debt and may cause a middle-age individual to stay in the labor market rather than retiring (Lewin-Epstein & Semyonov, 2016). Paying down mortgage debt early in this phase of life can lead to a lessened financial burden and more comfortable retirement.

Maintaining a Healthy Lifestyle

Nurses must address both the physical and social components of health for adults in this age group. Behavior modification to decrease illness risk is key to maintaining a healthy lifestyle. The most common risks in this category include smoking, excessive alcohol consumption, decreased physical activity, lack of seat-belt use, and diets that are high in fat and low in fiber. The social support that individuals receive can have a significant impact on their well-being, whether at home or within the workplace, whereas lack of social support can impair the health of individuals who may have difficulty coping effectively, lack resources, and live in a stressful environment. Socioeconomic status, supportive social relationships, and cultural understanding about illness and health all influence a person's well-being.

Participating in Community Activities and Civic Duties

Family demands lessen as children leave home, and many adults strive to fill the void with social activities, travel, or activism. Retirees are more likely to volunteer than employed individuals. Women tend to do so to define their new identity in this stage of life, while men tend to volunteer with organizations of which they are already members. Women look at volunteering to cultivate social networks and enhance personal growth (Southby & South, 2016).

Success in this stage of development for some derives from making social and political contributions. In retirement, job satisfaction no longer provides meaning, and the middle-age adult may instead turn to social or leisure activities. The benefits derived from becoming a leader in the community; volunteering for fundraisers; working on committees; participating in civic organizations; and running for public office on the local, state, and national levels strengthen ties to the community and increase personal satisfaction, a key component of well-being. Retired individuals who had very social occupations are more likely to continue social activities when their work life ends by shifting their attention to civic activities (Pozzi, Marta, Marzana, Gozzoli, & Ruggieri, 2014). Social integration would be expected when a person shows active involvement in an organization versus only supporting that organization financially (Pozzi et al., 2014).

Older Adulthood

Older adulthood, age 65 years to death, is Erikson's eighth stage of psychosocial development, which he called ego integrity versus despair. By 2030, more than 20% of the population will be older than age 65. Never in our nation's history have so many people lived this long while remaining healthy and productive (American Psychological Association [APA], 2018). According to APA (2018), older adults who rate their health as good report more satisfaction with life than do those who rate their health as poor.

At this stage of development, older adults might begin to take stock of their lives and to reflect on their successes and get a sense of accomplishment and fulfillment, or they may replay their failures and become angry and bitter. Some fear death; others prepare to die peacefully. Ideally, older adults will not feel they wasted their lives, missed important opportunities, or chose the wrong path. Changes that begin in older adulthood are related to memory, physical changes, psychological problems, and functional issues.

Cognitive Changes

Many older adults worry about developing dementia or Alzheimer's disease, yet mild cognitive involvement (MCI) affects only about 15% to 20% of people age 65 years and older (Alzheimer's Association, 2020). These individuals with MCI have a higher risk (32%) of developing Alzheimer's in 5 years than individuals without MCI (Alzheimer's Association, 2020). Memory loss is common as we age, but not everyone that develops memory loss has dementia or Alzheimer's disease. Part of the aging process involves subtle cognitive changes in conceptual reasoning, processing speed, attention span, memory (the most common cognitive complaint), and verbal fluency (Harada, Natelson Love, & Triebel, 2013). Individuals with certain medical conditions or who take certain prescription medications can experience dementia-like symptoms such as depression, thyroid problems, alcohol abuse, and even vitamin deficiencies (Alzheimer's Association, 2020).

Dementia and Alzheimer's disease are often confused with one another, but they are separate illnesses. Dementia is a brain disorder that affects the individual's performance of daily activities and communication, and is characterized by loss of cognitive functioning such as reasoning, thinking, and remembering. This can range from mild to severe and can be caused by many reasons, depending on brain changes (National Institute on Aging [NIA], 2017b).

Alzheimer's disease is a specific form of dementia that is irreversible and affects parts of the brain that control thought, memory, and language (NIA, 2017b). The disease has three stages: (1) preclinical stage that begins a decade before symptoms are evident, (2) middle stage with mild cognitive impairment, and (3) final stage with the inability to communicate and dependence on others (NIA, 2017b). As more neurons die, additional areas of the brain become affected until there is widespread damage. No single test can prove an individual has Alzheimer's disease, and no cure is currently available (NIA, 2017b).

Older adults may not lose the ability to work or function socially, although it may take longer to process new information and retrieve old information, and they may need statements repeated. They may be slower at problem solving yet remain creative. Cognitive decline may be reduced in the setting of good health and education, yet faster cognitive decline can be apparent if the person has poor health, limited education, and blood pressure concerns (Harada et al., 2013).

Older Age Developmental Tasks

As with other stages of life, the transition into old age is characterized by adjustments to developmental tasks (Havighurst, 1972; Hutteman, Hennecke, Orth, Reitz, & Specht, 2014). Establishing an affiliation with others in the same age group, adopting and adapting to social roles, and establishing satisfactory living arrangements may have a positive impact on the individual's ability to complete developmental tasks. Conversely, when physical health declines, income is reduced, or a significant other is lost, these circumstances may limit the individual's ability to complete these tasks successfully. Havighurst identifies six tasks in his developmental task theory (Table 8-4).

Physical Changes

The physical changes that begin in middle age continue into older adulthood, including decreased bone mass, gray hair and hair loss, and skin changes. Sensory changes, especially hearing and vision, may affect the

Table 8-4 Later Maturity Stage Development Tasks

Devlopmental Tasks Adjusting To . . .	Situations
Decreased physical strength and health	• Acute and chronic diseases • Not being in perfect health • Dependency on others
Retirement and reduced income	• Managing money with reduced income • Starting new projects to stay fulfilled
Death of a spouse	• Caregiver to spouse • Death of spouse • Adjusting to loneliness • Moving to a different place
Establishing an affiliation with one's age group	• Identifying new developmental tasks • Leading a purposeful life
Adopting and adapting to social roles	• Contribute to the younger population and sharing knowledge • Doing civil duties and getting on committees
Establishing satisfactory living arrangements	• Living in a new location • Selling their home • Living with children

Source: Havighurst, 1972; Hutteman, Hennecke, Orth, Reitz & Specht, 2014.

individual's lifestyle and limit social activities, thus leading to social isolation.

Hearing difficulties occur in more than 48% of men and 37% of women in their older years (APA, 2018). Presbycusis can affect both ears, causing a decline in hearing high-pitched sounds and difficulty hearing conversations. Ear structures change, causing a decline in function, and tinnitus can develop as a side effect to diuretics; certain antibiotics, including vancomycin and erythromycin; and some cancer medications.

As eye structures change with aging, visual acuity declines and presbyopia becomes a common problem, leading to the need for bifocals, progressive lenses, or contacts. Reading can become more difficult, necessitating larger print and bright light. Floaters become more prominent, dry eyes can occur, and peripheral vision is reduced, making it more difficult and dangerous for the aging individual to drive. Cataracts, glaucoma, retinopathy, and macular degeneration can lead to visual loss and even blindness in older adults.

Taste and smell also begin to diminish as we age, and food preferences may change as the taste buds shrink and decrease in number. After age 70, the number of nerve endings decreases and mucous production slows, leading to a loss of smell, which may lessen interest in eating. This loss of smell also makes it more difficult to detect smoke, fumes, and other odors that could signify danger.

Pain, touch, and vibration sensations can be diminished due to a decrease in blood flow to the nerve endings, compromising the ability to differentiate hot and cold. Burns and frostbite are risks, as is peripheral neuropathy, a risk compounded in those with diabetes.

The older adult can experience neurological changes from brain atrophy; the gastrointestinal system slows, sometimes making constipation a chronic issue; and muscles weaken, causing lack of strength (APA, 2018). Activities of daily living become a struggle, with 53% of women and 40% of men over age 85 years needing assistance in this area (APA, 2018). Many individuals older than age 65 live productive, happy lives despite physical changes and resulting limitations that may occur (APA, 2018).

Decreased Physical Strength and Health

Daily exercise not only benefits a healthy older adult but also helps the frail elderly to become more strong and fit, reducing the risk for illness (APA, 2018). Acute and chronic disease can alter retirement plans of traveling and spending time with family as well as create the risk of becoming dependent on others. Being diagnosed with an illness can also be emotionally devastating, sometimes leading to mental health issues such as depression and anxiety. Depression is prevalent in 48% of the elderly diagnosed with a chronic medical problem such as hypertension (79%), diabetes (70%), and respiratory disease (80%), with no correlation with sociodemographic variables (Ghanmi et al., 2017).

Retirement and Reduced Income

During retirement, keeping busy and getting involved in new projects helps to fill the void of not working. Living on a reduced income can be difficult for the older person who was accustomed to higher earnings. For those without a sufficient retirement fund, a fixed income can be especially worrisome if a large mortgage or outstanding debt must be paid. Single women in lower socioeconomic groups who have not worked full-time are particularly affected by reduced finances during the retirement years (Nilsson, 2017).

Death of a Spouse

Losing a spouse can be devastating, and the subsequent loneliness and sadness can lead to depression (Fried et al., 2015). Mourning can continue for months and even years, with each person coping with loss in his or her own way. Bereavement can trigger depressive symptoms such as appetite and weight loss. Caregivers and clinicians should be aware of the symptoms, especially in individuals who have a history of depression. Widowhood mortality may be directly related to the wear and tear from taking care of the ill spouse. Health behavior changes may occur, including poor health choices such as drinking and smoking (Sullivan & Fenelon, 2014). Social activities change with the loss of a spouse. Finding a support system of caring friends and family members is critical for an individual struggling with the loss of his or her spouse.

Establishing an Affiliation with Peers

After working for many years and reaching retirement age, some older adults prefer to continue doing meaningful work. Others simply seek ways to stay socially and mentally engaged. Some must rely on public transportation to get around, and these transportation systems must focus on understanding the health changes and needs of older individuals. Many adults in this age group choose to work part-time to stay busy and socialize. Community involvement and volunteering help older adults maintain a sense of self and share experience and knowledge with younger generations. Teaching a class, lecturing on a specific topic, joining an organization where expertise can be shared, and joining organizational boards can all be fulfilling for a retiree.

Establishing Satisfactory Living Arrangements

With the income decrease that may accompany retirement, many older adults are unable to sustain their living arrangements. Baby boomers tend to work longer rather than avoid retiring to prevent a decline in their standard of living (Auerbach, Kotlikoff, Koehler, & Yu, 2017). Even if their home is paid off, the taxes and insurance may not be affordable. Because memories with children and grandchildren have been made in the family home, the prospect of selling it can be difficult for older adults and their adult children. Living in a retirement home may be necessary if the individual cannot live alone and has no family, and a nursing home may be needed if the older adult has a chronic illness. With loss of independence, a concomitant loss of self can occur. Low-income elderly adults may not own a home and must instead rent or live with their extended family. This group is often unable to retire due to financial constraints.

HEALTH DETERMINANTS AND PREVENTION STRATEGIES IN MIDDLE-AGE AND OLDER ADULTS

Healthy People 2030 is framed around determinants, equity, and disparities, which rely on data, evidence, and prevention (Office of Disease Prevention and Health Promotion [ODPHP] & American Public Health Association, 2017). The Healthy People 2030 plan of action is to identify regions and groups with poor health or who are at risk for poor health in the future and improve health and well-being for individuals of all ages.

To plan effective health services, understanding how current health needs are influenced by social, behavioral, developmental, and environmental risk factors is important. The World Health Organization [WHO] (2017) defines a risk factor as "an attribute, characteristic or exposure of an individual that increases the likelihood of developing a disease or injury." Significant concerns exist among primary-care doctors in the United States and nine foreign countries about how their practices can manage complex patient needs. Coordinating care and communicating with specialists, social service providers, home-care providers, and hospitals also pose challenges (Osborn et al., 2015).

Health Determinants

What factors make some people healthy and others unhealthy? How can we begin to understand the range of personal, social, economic, and environmental factors that influence health status, known as determinants of health? Health determinants fall under several broad categories: policy making, social factors, health services, individual behavior, biology, and genetics (ODPHP, 2014b).

Access to Health Care

Access to quality, comprehensive health-care services assists in preventing and managing disease as well as reducing unnecessary disability and premature death (ODPHP, 2014a). Some of the barriers to accessing quality and comprehensive health care include the high cost of care, lack of adequate insurance coverage, lack of available services, and lack of culturally competent care. Demographics pose additional challenges to accessing health care depending on one's age, race, ethnicity, socioeconomic status, sex, disability status, sexual orientation, gender identity, and residential location.

As individuals born between 1945 and 1964 age, they need providers who are knowledgeable and skilled in geriatric services. More education and resources are needed in geriatric training for health-care workers to provide care specific to this population.

Individuals living in rural areas have fewer services available. Individuals with disabilities are also at risk of experiencing problems accessing health-care services. Disability is increasing among middle-age adults and among older adults. Adults who are black and of lower socioeconomic status are also disproportionately affected (Miller, Kirk, Kaiser, & Glos, 2014).

Health-Care Costs

Based on a survey of a sample of the civilian noninstitutionalized population, the percentage of people in the United States who were uninsured declined in 2015 (9.1%), which was lower than the 2014 estimate (11.5%) and lower each year since 1997 (Ward, Clarke, Nugent, & Schiller, 2016). However, adults age 45 to 64 years accounted for the majority of individuals (6.6%) who did not receive medical care or who delayed seeking medical care because of cost (9.1%) (Centers for Disease Control and Prevention [CDC], 2017j). Individuals age 65 years and older fared somewhat better, with only 2.3% reporting that they did not receive medical care and 3.5% who delayed seeking medical care due to cost (CDC, 2017j). A similar trend is noted among middle-age adults with health insurance coverage. This group accounted for the highest percentage of individuals who did not receive and who delayed seeking medical care due to cost when compared to older adults age 65 years and older (CDC, 2017j).

Access to health care (did not receive or delayed seeking medical care due to cost) varies with gender, race, poverty status, family income, and current health status (Table 8-5). Females ranked higher in both categories when compared to males. White Americans face fewer barriers to care than do non-white Americans. Individuals near poverty status or with incomes less than $35,000 per year had the highest percentages in both categories of lack of access due to cost. People who live in the southern United States were more likely to have problems with access to health care due to cost, along with individuals considered to be in fair to poor health.

Prevention Strategies

Improving access to health care would include an increase in the number of insured adults. Policies are needed to increase access to health care and ensure that individuals have access to health-care workers who have the knowledge and skill to provide care for specific populations, such as older adults. The ACA was one such policy designed to provide access to health insurance coverage for Americans (U.S. Department of Health and Human Services [USDHHS], 2016a).

Preventive Screenings and Immunizations

Health-care providers can develop long-term, trusting relationships with patients that increase adherence to evidence-based preventive screenings and immunizations (see Boxes 8-1 and 8-2). Evidence-based screenings and immunizations prevent illness by (1) promoting healthy behaviors for those with and without risk factors; (2) providing protection to those who are at risk; and (3) identifying, treating, and managing people with risk factors before illness develops. The middle-age adult is at risk of the effects of poor diet, lack of exercise, and substance abuse that affect both present and future health. Preventive care is important for this population to delay or deter chronic diseases. Screenings for the older adult are multidimensional and include a multidisciplinary approach, with a focus on functional ability, physical health, cognition and mental health, and environmental and socioeconomic factors.

Chronic Conditions

Chronic conditions are among the most common, costly, and preventable of all health problems (CDC, 2017b). Eighty percent of adults over age 65 have at least one chronic condition and 65% have at least two (National Council on Aging, 2017). In fact, seven of the top 10 causes of death are the result of chronic diseases and their resulting complications. The CDC (2016b) reveals that one out of four adults in the United States has multiple chronic conditions, and this frequency increases to one out of three for adults 65 years and older. Common chronic conditions that most often manifest in middle age include diabetes, hypertension, heart disease, cancer, respiratory diseases, HIV, and kidney disease. Sleep health is also a concern for this population because more than one-third of adults are not getting enough sleep on a regular basis, resulting in chronic conditions. Sleep deprivation is linked not only to cardiovascular disease but also to diabetes, obesity, and arrhythmias (Tobaldini et al., 2017).

Older adults are also at a higher risk of chronic disease, with many individuals managing two or more

Table 8-5 Highest Percentage of Demographic Populations Who Did Not Receive Medical Care and Delayed Seeking Medical Care Due to Cost

Demographic Populations	Did Not Receive Medical Care Due to Cost	Delayed Seeking Medical Care Due to Cost
GENDER IDENTITY		
Females	4.8	6.9
Males	4.0	5.7
RACE		
American Indian or Alaskan Native and white (two or more races)	9.4	12.3
Native Hawaiian or other Pacific Islander	6.2	9.3
Black or African American	5.8	6.6
White	4.3	6.4
POVERTY STATUS		
Near poor	8.3	10.5
Not poor	2.7	4.7
ANNUAL FAMILY INCOME		
Less than $35,000	9.5	11.3
$35,000–$49,000	6.3	9.4
$50,000–$74,000	4.1	6.6
$75,000–$99,000	2.3	4.2
$100,000 or more	0.9	2.1
REGION		
South	5.2	6.7
West	4.4	6.3
Midwest	4.0	6.4
Northeast	3.3	5.2
CURRENT HEALTH STATUS		
Good	6.1	8.2
Fair or poor	13.1	15.9

Source: Adapted from CDC, Tables of Summary Health Statistics, 2017j.

chronic conditions (ODPHP, 2014d). Common chronic conditions among older adults include hypertension (58%); high cholesterol (47%); arthritis (31%); coronary artery disease (29%); diabetes (27%); mental health disorders, including depression, Alzheimer's disease, and dementia (25%); sensory impairment; and substance use and abuse disease (National Council on Aging, 2017). Obesity is also considered a chronic condition. All chronic conditions have an impact on the quality of life for older adults and are associated with increased mortality for this population.

Hypertension and Prevention Strategies

In 2014, the Joint National Committee (JNC) raised the guideline for initiating pharmacological treatment for blood pressure to 150/90 mm Hg or higher in adults ages 60 and older (Armstrong & Joint National Committee, 2014). Treatment in this age group is challenging, and the economic burden is rising as more than 80% of adults over 60 years old are considered hypertensive (Patel & Stewart, 2015). This reveals a critical need to reduce costs and improve patient outcomes. In patients older than age 60, isolated systolic hypertension is a

BOX 8-1 Recommended Screenings for Adults

Abdominal aortic screenings for men ages 65–75
Breast cancer screening for women ages 49–74
Cervical cancer screening for women ages 21–65
Hepatitis C vaccine for all adults born from 1945 to 1965
Osteoporosis screening for women ages 65 and older
Lung cancer screening for Adults ages 55–80 with a history of smoking

Source: Preventive Screenings for Adults. Adapted from Recommendations for Primary Care Practice, U.S. Preventive Services Task Force, May 2017. https://www.uspreventiveservicestaskforce.org/Page/Name/recommendations.

BOX 8-2 Recommended Immunizations for Adults

Influenza: annually
Td/Tdap: substitute Tdap or Td once, then Td booster every 10 years
Pneumococcal vaccination: 1 dose for those older than 65 years
Shingrix for those over age 50, or Zostavax if allergic to Shingrex and over age 60

Source: Adapted from Recommended Immunization Schedule for Adults Aged 19 Years or Older, by Vaccine and Age Group. United States, CDC, 2018. Retrieved from https://www.cdc.gov/vaccines/schedules/downloads/adult/adult-combined-schedule.pdf.

greater concern than diastolic hypertension due to cardiovascular risk. This age group benefits from even the slightest reduction in blood pressure (Patel & Stewart, 2015). Conservative treatment with nonpharmacological measures is a better option in the elderly because they are at higher risk for health issues when starting a new medication. Weight loss, regular exercise, diet control, sleep apnea treatment, and restricting dietary sodium are all effective conservative treatment options.

High Cholesterol and Prevention Strategies

High levels of low density lipoprotein (LDL) cholesterol have long been blamed for the development of heart disease in older adults. However, controversy now exists about the relationship between LDL cholesterol and heart disease. Researchers reviewed 19 studies and found that 80% of elderly patients who had lower LDL levels did not live as long as elderly patients who had higher LDL levels (Ravnskov et al., 2016). This will likely lead to reevaluation of guidelines for cardiovascular care, which have long called for statin use to control cholesterol (Ravnshov et al., 2016). It is well known that statins reduce the incidence of myocardial infarction and death in all age groups, yet many of the studies to support this have been done in older adults who are younger than age 74 (Felix-Redondo, Grau, & Fernandez Berges, 2013). With extension of life as a major goal for prevention, the most important outcome is mortality.

Arthritis and Prevention Strategies

Musculoskeletal conditions are among the most common problems affecting the elderly, and their prevalence increases with age. Arthritis is the most common cause of disability, and many patients report difficulty with everyday activities. Except for gout, most types of arthritis are more common in women than in men. Risk factors are listed in Box 8-3.

With advancing age comes increased bone frailty, decreased resilience of cartilage, reduced elasticity of ligaments, and decreased muscular strength, all significant factors in developing musculoskeletal conditions (Geno, Cepparo, Rosca, & Cotton, 2012). Chronic disease and being overweight or obese also increase this risk. Osteoarthritis (OA), one of the most common forms of arthritis, results from joint degeneration, which usually develops slowly and worsens over time. More than 30 million adults are affected (CDC, 2017g). The risk of developing OA increases with age, and until about age 55, the rate of developing osteoarthritis is similar in women and men. After age 55, many more women than men are affected by osteoarthritis. This may occur because women's broader hips increase stress on the

BOX 8-3 Arthritis Risk Factors

NONMODIFIABLE RISK FACTORS	MODIFIABLE RISK FACTORS
Age	Overweight and obesity
Gender	Joint injuries
Genetic	Infection
	Occupation

Source: Adapted from Centers for Disease Control and Prevention. (2017). Retrieved from https://www.cdc.gov/arthritis/basics/risk-factors.htm.

knees, one of the most common joints affected by OA (CDC, 2017g).

The CDC (2017b) has a goal to protect the health of 54.4 million men and women with arthritis so they can live to the fullest in minimal pain. The key focus areas on prevention and management include expanding the science base and collecting data, supporting state health departments, and reaching people through national programs. Examples of national programs funded by the CDC include the Y-USA and the National Recreation and Parks Association (NRPA). The Y-USA provides services and programs to improve healthy eating and active living to decrease modifiable risk associated with developing arthritis. The Y-USA also participates in a program to address health equity by bringing EnhanceFitness (an evidence-based group exercise program, targeting older adults to become more active) to low-income and underserved communities. NRPA supports local park agencies to deliver programs that focus on active living (walking and exercise programs) to encourage healthy lifestyles.

Chronic back conditions in the adult may result from a history of congenital anomalies, prior injury or illness, degeneration, or inflammatory processes. The results may be chronic pain, decreased mobility, and other comorbidities. Chronic back pain is a major public health concern and affects physical and mental health, limits functional status, and has a negative impact on an individual's quality of life (Lazkani et al., 2015). The prevalence of back pain increases as the population ages, and health-care visits for back disorders rise as the population ages up to 75 years (Watkins-Castillo & Anderson, 2014). Up to 31% of individuals with mobility issues note that their activities are limited by back pain. This rate increases for those ages 65 to 74 years.

Evidence supports the association between back pain and disability in adults ages 50 and older (Williams et al., 2015). In fact, many musculoskeletal conditions manifest during middle age and require medical intervention with health-care providers over many years. Preventive strategies vary in complexity, and many are specific to the chronic condition. A 2016 systematic review (Menichetti, Cipresso, Bussolin, & Graffigna, 2016) noted that different interventions appear to promote specific health outcomes such as physical health, cognitive functioning, or social health. No studies supported a holistic outcome comprising all three components.

Osteoporosis and Prevention Strategies

Osteoporosis is more common in women and affects one in four women ages 65 and older and about one in 17 men ages 65 and older (CDC, 2017h). Unfortunately, many people are unaware of osteoporosis until they sustain a fracture. Screening for osteoporosis and knowledge of risk can help prevent fractures and allow implementation of appropriate interventions to treat and manage the condition.

A risk assessment should be conducted for all women ages 65 years and older and all men ages 75 years and older with risk factors for osteoporosis (Box 8-4) (Jeremiah, Unwin, & Greenawald, 2015). The National Guideline Clearinghouse (NGC) (2015) recommends use of either the Fracture Risk Assessment Tool (FRAX), which is designed to assist clinicians in predicting the 10-year probability of fracture with or without the addition of femoral neck bone mineral density (BMD), or QFracture, which is designed to estimate an individual's 10-year risk of developing osteoporotic fractures of the hip, spine, and wrist without BMD measurement and is applicable to people ages 30 to 85 years.

Coronary Artery Disease and Prevention

Coronary artery disease (CAD) in the elderly has many potential risk factors, including chronic kidney disease (CKD). High phosphate levels, arterial stiffness, and vascular calcification contribute to the elevated risk of developing CAD among those with CKD (Gluba-Brzozka et al., 2015). In clients with CKD, the influenza vaccination could reduce the risk of recurrent cardiovascular events, potentially reducing hospital admissions (Chen et al., 2016).

Because of alcohol's association with hypertension, cardiac function and structure can be altered, leading

BOX 8-4 Risk Factors for Osteoporosis*

- Previous fragility fractures
- Alcohol intake of more than 14 units per week for women and more than 21 units per week for men
- Smoking history
- Lower level of sex hormones
- History of falls
- Current or frequent use of oral or systemic glucocorticoids
- Family history of hip fracture
- Other causes of secondary osteoporosis
- Low body mass index (BMI)
- Gender

* Women aged 65 years and over and men aged 75 years and over.

Source: Jeremiah, M. P., Unwin, B. K., & Greenawald, M. H. (2015). Diagnosis and management of osteoporosis. *American Family Physician, 92*(4), 261–268.

to alcoholic cardiomyopathy in patients who drink excessively (Goncalves et al., 2015). Alcohol is considered a "dose-dependent cardiac toxin" (Goncalves et al., 2015, p. 3). Although light to moderate drinking may have protective benefits, this is controversial. A positive correlation exists between high density lipoprotein (HDL) levels and alcohol consumption and a decrease in triglyceride/HDL ratio with alcohol consumption in both sexes (Goncalves et al., 2015). Alcohol leads to greater heart damage in women than in men, causing reduced systolic function and thus leading to alcoholic cardiomyopathy.

Obesity in the elderly has a distinct correlation with high mortality, especially among those with CAD (Sharma et al., 2016). An independent predictor of CAD in men with normal weight is the sagittal abdominal diameter, whereas in women waist-hip ratio and waist-hip-height ratio predict CAD risk (Carlsson et al., 2014).

A study by Chen et al. (2015) showed a significant correlation between CAD and parathyroid hormone and serum vitamin D levels in elderly Chinese women. Vitamin D levels <30 ng/ml may cause vascular endothelial damage in individuals with hypertension, potentially leading to CAD (Dhibar, Sharma, Bhadada, Sachdeva, & Sahu, 2016). During coronary angiography, the severity of CAD did not correlate with the severity of Vitamin D deficiency. Low testosterone levels in men are correlated with CAD, but the correlation between men and coronary artery calcifications (CACs) is unknown. Lai et al. (2015) studied the relationship of testosterone levels in men with CACs. Their findings showed low testosterone scores with high CAC scores, and vice versa. This determined that, even among men who have stable CAD, testosterone levels are independent predictors for severe CAC (Lai et al., 2015).

Limited prevention data exists for those ages 75 and older. Statin use may not be beneficial in this age group because of a high risk of side effects; the benefits of statins may not be evident for three to five years (Schwartz, 2015). Exercise in the elderly should be part of preventive therapy. Although comorbidities and the benefits of medications versus the risks need to be evaluated, it is important for patients to be involved in their care and to share decision making.

Diabetes and Prevention

Diabetes is a complex, chronic condition with multifactorial risks leading to poor glycemic control. The American Diabetes Association (ADA) (2018) reported that, among the 30.3 million adults with diabetes, approximately 7.2 million are undiagnosed. Adults 65 years of age and older account for 25.2% of those diagnosed and undiagnosed with diabetes. Unfortunately, diabetes was the seventh leading cause of death in 2015 (ADA, 2018). The total cost associated with diagnosed diabetes was $327 billion, with $237 billion related to direct medical costs and $90 billion associated with reduced productivity (ADA, 2018). American Indians, Alaska Natives, non-Hispanic blacks, Hispanics, and Asian Americans are disproportionately affected compared to their white counterparts.

According to the CDC (2017j), the risks associated with diabetes are based on the categories of diabetes (prediabetes, type 1 diabetes, type 2 diabetes, gestational diabetes). Prediabetes and type 2 diabetes are more common among adults who are middle-age and older, but type 1 diabetes can be diagnosed at any age. Risk factors associated with prediabetes and type 2 diabetes include:

- Being overweight or obese
- Being older than age 45
- A family history of type 2 diabetes
- A personal history of gestational diabetes
- Being African American, Hispanic/Latino American, American Indian, Alaska Native, Pacific Islander, or Asian American

Type 2 diabetes is also more prevalent among those who lead a sedentary lifestyle.

Type 1 diabetes is more likely to develop during childhood, adolescence, or young adulthood, but may develop at any age. Other risk factors for type 1 diabetes are a family history of type 1 diabetes and Caucasian ethnicity.

A national diabetes prevention program (DPP) is focused on implementing lifestyle changes that offer screening and referral and a list of lifestyle change programs accessible to everyone (CDC, National Diabetes Prevention Program, 2018). The goals of the national DPP are to:

- Deliver CDC-recognized lifestyle change programs.
- Ensure quality and adherence to proven standards.
- Train community organizations that can run a lifestyle program effectively.
- Increase referrals to and participation in lifestyle programs.
- Increase coverage by employer, private, and public insurers.

The goal of screening for diabetes is to identify people who have high blood sugar or diabetes so that they can be treated to avoid the comorbid medical and psychological conditions associated with uncontrolled diabetes. Diabetes is the number one cause of kidney failure, lower-limb amputations, and adult-onset blindness (CDC,

2017a). Treatment consists of controlling blood sugar levels through lifestyle modifications, including healthy eating and increased physical activity. Some people also take medications to help control their blood sugar levels.

ADA (2018) published guidelines indicating confirmation that the two-hour plasma glucose test is a more effective diagnostic tool for diabetes than fasting plasma and A1C cutoffs. However, the A1C test should be performed based on a method certified by the National Glycohemoglobin Standardization Program and the Diabetes Control and Complications Trial (DCCT) assay (ADA, 2018).

As the incidence and prevalence of diabetes grows and individuals who have this condition live longer, more adults over the age of 70 will be living with diabetes (Kaira & Sharma, 2018). The disease is also prevalent in long-term care facilities (Munshi et al., 2016). Although the diagnostic criteria for diabetes are similar among all populations, screening strategies for the elderly may vary.

Diabetes is more complex in this population because of the additional medical and psychosocial health issues. Because most of the common geriatric syndromes can be caused by diabetes, annual and opportunistic diabetes screening should be performed among the elderly (Kaira & Sharma, 2018). A comprehensive geriatric assessment includes a clinical analysis of the individual to determine how fit he or she is to manage self-care activities. This assessment includes an analysis of basic independent activities, advanced activities of daily living, functional status, comorbid conditions, and expected lifespan. This detailed assessment would help to identify and plan for supportive and therapeutic strategies. The main goal of providing diabetes care to the elderly is to achieve comfort, optimal quality of life, resolution of symptoms, and avoidance of acute complications (Kaira & Sharma, 2018).

Mental Health Problems and Prevention Strategies

Mental health is described as a state of well-being in which individuals realize their own abilities to cope with the normal stresses of life, work productively and fruitfully, and contribute to the community (Galderisi, Heinz, Kastrup, Beezhold, & Sartorius, 2015). Mental health is also described as essential to an individual's personal well-being, family and interpersonal relationships, and the ability to contribute to community and society (ODPHP, 2014c). Mental illness does not have a single cause but can be attributed to multiple factors, such as trauma, abuse, loneliness, alcohol abuse, chronic medical problems, and lack of social support.

Unfortunately, only an estimated 17% of adults are considered in a state of ideal mental health, which is especially concerning because of evidence that positive mental health is associated with improved health outcomes (CDC, 2017d). More than 64 million individuals seek medical treatment each year for mental illness (CDC, 2017d). Disorders of mental illness characterized by alterations in thinking, mood, and behavior exacerbate and are associated with increased morbidity and mortality. Stressors during the middle years increase the likelihood of developing mental health disorders; these stressors include marital relationships, health concerns, work-life balance, relationships with friends, and fear of aging (Suzuki, Takeda, Kishi, & Monma, 2017).

Adults in the middle years may care for others, including parents and grandchildren. An estimated 34.2 million adults provide unpaid caregiving services to someone age 50 or older. One in four caregivers provides care to an adult age 85 or older (Family Caregiver Alliance & National Center on Caregiving, 2016). These responsibilities make the middle-age adult prone to increased stress and depression. Risk for mental illness also increases with the potential for social isolation that occurs with aging. Depression is common and is often associated with chronic conditions. Mental illness in the older adult may be viewed as an inevitable result of aging and can cause difficulties in caregiving. Common mental disorders shown in Table 8-6 include depression, anxiety, bipolar disorder, schizophrenia, frequent mental distress, and Alzheimer's disease (CDC, 2013).

Historically, screening for mental illness has been emphasized; however, little has been done to protect the mental health of those not yet diagnosed. The prevention of mental illness should focus on emotional, psychological, and social well-being. Prevention strategies include (ODPHP, 2014c):

- Appropriate interventions in the early years (mental illness)
- Reducing substance use and substance abuse
- Violence prevention programs
- Preventive interventions for schizophrenia
- Improving family functioning
- School-based preventive interventions (improve academic outcomes)

Regular screenings for substance abuse and mental health disorders are recommended and should be performed in primary-care and other health-care settings on individuals of all ages. Many of these conditions are prevalent yet go undiagnosed and untreated. Screening tools for selected mental health disorders are shown in Table 8-7. Screening for dementia involves ruling out other conditions causing similar symptoms, such as vitamin B deficiencies, hydrocephalus, and depression (Box 8-5).

Table 8-6 Common Mental Disorders in the Middle-Age and Older Adult

Condition	Characteristic
Depression	• Approximately 6.7% of adults in the United States reported experiencing a major depressive episode. • Women (11.7%) reported experiencing greater percentages of lifetime major depression than did men (5.6%). • Among ethnic groups, whites (6.52%) reported increased percentage of lifetime depression when compared to blacks (4.57%) and Hispanics (5.1%).
Anxiety Disorders	• The estimated lifetime prevalence of any anxiety disorder is 15%, and the 12-month prevalence is more than 10%. • Women experience an increased frequency in anxiety disorders when compared to men. • The most common anxiety disorders include panic disorder, generalized anxiety disorder, post-traumatic stress disorder, phobias, and separation anxiety disorders.
Bipolar Disorder	• The results of the National Comorbidity study revealed that a lifetime prevalence of nearly 4% for bipolar disorder existed for the study participants. • Bipolar disorder is more common in women than men, with a ratio of 3:2, a median age of onset at 25 years, with men having an earlier age of onset than women. • Bipolar disorder accounts for the largest expense in behavioral health.
Schizophrenia	• The National Alliance on Mental Health reports an estimated 1.1% of adults in the United States live with schizophrenia (2017). • Among persons diagnosed with schizophrenia, by age 30, 9 out of 10 men, but only 2 out of 10 women, will manifest the illness. • There is a high rate of suicide for persons with schizophrenia, and approximately one-third of those diagnosed will attempt suicide.
Frequent Mental Distress	• Frequent mental distress is determined based on responses to a quality-of-life question ("Now thinking about your mental health, which includes stress, depression, and problems with emotions, for how many days during the past 30 days was your mental health not good?") and a report of 14 or more days of poor mental health. • Two time periods (1993–2001 and 2003–2006) revealed that 9.4% of U.S. adults experienced frequent mental distress. • Location may also have an impact on the degree of frequent mental distress with a higher prevalence in the Appalachian and the Mississippi valley regions of the United States.
Alzheimer's Disease/Dementia	• Alzheimer's disease, the most common type of dementia, has been identified as a disease with high mortality rates and is considered one of the leading causes of death in the United States; it is the fifth leading cause among persons age 65 years and older • An estimated 5.3 million Americans have Alzheimer's disease, and that number is projected to double due to the aging population by 2050. • It is estimated that the number of people living with dementia will double every 20 years, to number 65.7 million in 2030 and 115.4 million in 2050.

Sources: Centers for Disease Control and Prevention (2013). Burden of Mental Illness. U.S. Department of Health and Human Services. Retrieved from https://www.cdc.gov/mentalhealth/basics/burden.htm; Prince, M., Bryce, R., Albanese, E., Wimo, A., Ribeiro, W., & Ferri, C. P. (2013). The global prevalence of dementia: A systematic review and meta-analysis. *Alzheimer's & Dementia: The Journal of the Alzheimer's Association*, *9*(1), 63–75.

Sensory Impairments and Prevention Strategies

Sensory impairments include visual loss, hearing loss, and loss of balance. One in six older adults reports vision loss, and one in four reports hearing loss (CDC, 2015e). Sensory impairments increase with age, with reports of a 200% increase in vision and hearing impairment and a 40% increase in loss of sensation in the feet among those older than age 80 compared to their 70-year-old counterparts (CDC, 2015e). In addition, individuals with vision loss often report hearing loss, and some individuals with vision impairment, hearing impairment, or both report problems with balance.

Table 8-7 Mental Health Disorder Screening Tools

Disorder	Tools
Anxiety Disorders	General Anxiety Disorder (GAD7): seven-question screening tool PC-PTSD: Posttraumatic Stress Disorder: four-item screening tool
Depression	PHQ-9: Patient Health Questionnaire (most common)
Drugs And Alcohol	Alcohol Use Disorders Identification Test (AUDIT): 10-item questionnaire CAGE: five-question tool to determine need for further assessment AUDIT-C: three-question screening for hazardous or harmful drinking Drug Abuse Screen Test (DAST-10): 10-item, yes/no, 8-minute self-report screening
Bipolar Disorder	Mood Disorder Questionnaire: 13 questions, 5-minute self-report
Suicide	Columbia-Suicide Severity Rating Scale (C-SSRS): six questions Suicide Assessment Five-Step Evaluation and Triage (SAFE-T)
Trauma	LEC Event Checklist: 17-item self-report measure PCL-C: shorter version of PTSD checklist

Source: Substance Abuse and Mental Health Services Administration (SAMHS). (2015). U.S. Department of Health and Human Services. Retrieved from https://www.samhsa.gov/prescription-drug-misuse-abuse/specific-populations; Siu A.L., & The US Preventive Services Task Force (USPSTF) (2016). Screening for Depression in Adults. US Preventive Services Task Force Recommendation Statement. JAMA, 315(4), 380–387. doi:10.1001/jama.2015.18392.

BOX 8-5 Dementia and Alzheimer's Disease Screenings

Detailed medical history
Physical and neurological exam
MRI or CT scan to rule out other conditions causing symptoms
Mood assessment
Mini Mental Status Exam
Mini-cog
Cantab Mobile
Cognivue
Cognition and Automated Neuropsychological Assessment Metrics (ANAM) devices
EEGs

Laboratory tests

- Blood glucose test
- Thyroid function
- Hormone tests
- Cerebrospinal fluid analysis
- Drug and alcohol toxicity screen
- Urinalysis

Genetic testing (although not recommended)

Individuals with sensory impairments are more likely to report depression, falls, and cognitive impairment. Adults are at risk of sensory impairment because of physiological changes and environmental factors. Many individuals first notice a change in vision during middle age. Older adults with vision loss are more likely to experience comorbid conditions when compared to those without vision loss, which may lead to the inability to perform some tasks and to participate in social settings (Crews, Chou, Zhang, Zack, & Saaddine, 2014). Hearing loss in this population may be work-related. Occupational hearing loss is one of the most common work-related illnesses in the United States, and each year about 22 million workers are exposed to hazardous noise levels at work. Some workers are exposed to ototoxic chemicals that result in hearing loss.

Routine vision screenings are recommended for adults, especially those with chronic illnesses like diabetes. Wearing protective eyewear with sun exposure prevents some age-related vision conditions. Wearing protective gear when performing tasks that may result in eye injury is another preventive strategy.

Hearing loss prevention involves reducing noise exposure and limiting exposure to ototoxic agents that can affect hearing. The National Institute for Occupational Safety and Health (NIOSH) recommends that workers who are exposed to noise at a certain level or higher wear hearing protectors (CDC, 2016e). Some noise exposures may require workers to wear earplugs and earmuffs simultaneously. Several screening tests for hearing loss in older adults are performed in primary care (U.S. Preventive Services Task Force, 2017). Recent evidence with 125 subjects (mean age 72.4 years) demonstrated a 91% sensitivity with the finger rub test, in which the practitioner stands 70 cm behind the patient and rubs his or her fingers together sharply to create a sound (Strawbridge & Wallhagen, 2017).

Substance Use/Abuse and Prevention Strategies

Although substance use is highest among people in their late teens and twenties, a disturbing trend for middle-age adults reveals a twofold increase in illicit drug use, including nonmedical use of prescription drugs. Drug use has increased among those in their fifties and early sixties (National Institute on Drug Abuse [NIDA], 2015a). This increase is partly attributed to baby boomers whose rates of illicit drug use are much higher than previous generations (NIDA, 2015a). A similar trend is seen among older adults, with increased use of alcohol with prescription drugs posing a significant health risk (SAMHSA-HRSA, 2015).

The National Center on Addiction and Substance Abuse (2017) reported that one in four Americans who first smoked, consumed alcohol, or used other substances before age 18 develops a substance abuse problem as an adult. Young adults may turn to substance use because of the stress associated with child rearing, balancing a career with a family, and managing a household. For the middle-age adult, risks for addiction and substance use may emerge with financial pressure, divorce, empty nest syndrome, personal and family illness, stress of caring for an aging parent, or the death of a parent or loved one. Older adults have additional challenges like retirement, sudden or chronic illness, and the loss of independent living.

Most deaths from drug abuse are from opioid use (CDC, 2017f). From 2000 to 2015, more than half a million people died from drug overdoses and 91 Americans die every day from opioid overdose. Opioid misuse hospital stays increased 64% from 2005 to 2014 (U.S. Department of Health and Human Services, 2016b). Prevention includes improvement in opioid prescribing to reduce exposure to opioids, prevent abuse, and stop addiction (CDC, 2017f). The CDC guideline for prescribing opioids for chronic pain addresses the following (CDC, 2017f):

- Determining when to initiate or continue opioids for chronic pain (excluding cancer treatment, palliative care, and end-of-life care)
- Managing opioid selection, dosage, duration, follow-up, and discontinuation
- Assessing risk and addressing harms of opioid use

Prevention begins with routine screening for substance use, substance abuse, and addiction (National Center on Addiction and Substance Abuse, 2017). Because not everyone sees a health-care provider regularly, methods should be available for screening in other settings. NIDA (2015) provides a list of evidence-based screening tools for alcohol and drug use to be self-administered or clinician-administered (Table 8-8).

NIDA (2015b) also developed a general screening tool: NIDA-Modified ASSIST (NM ASSIST), which guides clinicians through a series of questions to identify

Table 8-8 Evidence-Based Screening Tools for Adults

Screening Tool	Substance Type		How Tool Is Administered	
	Alcohol	Drugs	Self-Administered	Clinician Administered
Prescreening				
NIDA Drug Use Screening Tool: Quick Screen	X	X		X
Alcohol Use Disorders Identification Test -C (AUDIT-C)	X		X	X
Opioid Risk Tool		X	X	
Full Screening				
NIDA Drug Use Screening Tool	X	X		X
Alcohol Use Disorders Identification Test (AUDIT)	X			X
CAGE-AID	X	X		X
CAGE	X			X
CRAFFT	X	X	X	X

Source: National Institute on Drug Abuse (2015). Chart of evidence-based screening tools for adults and adolescents. Retrieved from https://www.drugabuse.gov/nidamed-medical-health-professionals/tool-resources-your-practice/screening-assessment-drug-testing-resources/chart-evidence-based-screening-tools-adults.

risky substance use (alcohol, tobacco, prescription drugs for nonmedical reasons, illegal drugs) in adult patients. The tool allows clinicians to (1) identify drug use early and prevent the escalation to addiction; (2) increase awareness of the interaction of substance use with a patient's medical care, including potentially fatal drug interactions; and (3) identify patients in need and refer them to specialty treatment.

Obesity and Prevention Strategies

In 2014, more than 1.9 billion adults age 18 years and older were overweight and 600 million were obese (WHO, 2016). This equates to 39% of the adult population as overweight and 13% of the world's adult population as obese. WHO (2016) defines overweight in adults as a body mass index (BMI) greater than or equal to 25, and obesity as a BMI greater than or equal to 30. Obesity in the United States has reached epidemic proportions, with a prevalence of 36% from 2011 to 2014 (Ogden, Carroll, Fryar, & Flegal, 2015). Obesity was higher among women (38.3%) than among men (34.3%). The prevalence of obesity was higher among non-Hispanic white, non-Hispanic black, and Hispanic adults when compared to non-Hispanic Asian adults. Reducing the number of overweight or obese individuals is a public health concern because these conditions result in increased morbidity and mortality, with health consequences that include an increase in cardiovascular diseases, diabetes, musculoskeletal disorders, and some cancers.

Factors contributing to overweight and obesity include an increased intake of energy-dense foods high in fat and a decrease in physical activity (WHO, 2016). Among adults age 18 years and older, only 20.9% met the 2008 federal physical activities guidelines (CDC, 2016). Thirty-one percent were 18–24 years of age. Grade 1 obesity (BMI 30.0–34.9) increased from 17.9% to 20.6% between 1999–2002 and 2011–2014. Grade 2 obesity (BMI 35.0–39.9) rose from 7.6% to 8.8%, and grade 3 obesity (BMI 40 or higher) increased from 4.9% to 6.9% (Ogden et al., 2015).

A single solution to prevent obesity does not exist because it is a complex issue that requires a multifaceted approach (CDC, 2015b). Prevention strategies require approaches targeting individuals, families, and communities that address the issue of obesity and overweight with younger populations. Wing et al. (2016) conducted a randomized clinical trial examining the effectiveness of interventions to prevent and to reduce weight gain in young adults. The results revealed that participants who adopted interventions such as small changes lost an average of 1.2 pounds over a 2- to 3-year period, and participants who adopted large changes showed more profound results, with a weight loss of 5.2 pounds during the same time frame (Table 8-9). The intervention groups also attended 10 sessions for the first 4 months and were instructed to weigh and track their weight daily. Only 18% of the intervention group became obese compared to 17% in the control group receiving only information about preventing weight gain.

Because childhood obesity is associated with adult obesity, prevention strategies should include families and communities. Primary-care providers can play an effective role in preventing and treating obesity. In fact, the Institute of Medicine, in its 2012 report *Accelerating Progress in Obesity Prevention*, recommended expanding the role of health-care providers, insurers, and employers in obesity prevention and identified four strategies to

Table 8-9 Small Changes Versus Large Changes

Small Changes	Large Changes
Reduce daily caloric intake by 100 calories	Reduce daily caloric intake by 500 to 1,000 calories
Select lower-calorie drinks	Gradually increase moderate-intensity physical activity to 250 minutes a week
Reduce portion sizes	Frequent self-weighing
Gradually increase moderate-intensity physical activity to 250 minutes a week	
Use stairs, park further away from stores when shopping	
Pedometers used to monitor accumulation of 2,000 steps per day above regular activity	

Source: Wing, R. R., Tate, D. F., Espeland, M. A., Lewis, C. E., LaRose, J. G., Gorin, A. A., ... & Garcia, K. R. (2016). Innovative self-regulation strategies to reduce weight gain in young adults: The study of novel approaches to weight gain prevention (SNAP) randomized clinical trial. *JAMA Internal Medicine*, *176*(6), 755–762.

Table 8-10 Institute of Medicine (IOM) Strategies to Achieve the Goal of Preventing and Treating Obesity

STRATEGY 1	Provide standardized care and advocate for healthy community environments.
STRATEGY 2	Ensure coverage of, access to, and incentives for routine obesity prevention, screening, diagnosis, and treatment.
STRATEGY 3	Encourage active living and healthy eating at work.
STRATEGY 4	Encourage healthy weight gain during pregnancy and breastfeeding and promote breastfeeding-friendly environments.

Source: Committee on Accelerating Progress in Obesity Prevention; Food and Nutrition Board; Institute of Medicine (2012). Accelerating progress in obesity prevention: Solving the weight of the nation. D. Glickman D Editor, L. Parker L, LJ. Sim, et al. (Eds.) Washington, DC: National Academies Press. Retrieved from https://www.ncbi.nlm.nih.gov/books/NBK201138/

achieve this goal (Committee on Accelerating Progress in Obesity Prevention, 2012) (Table 8-10).

The prevalence of obesity among middle adults (39.5%) was higher compared to younger adults (30.3%) or older adults (35.4%) (Ogden, Carroll, Fryer & Flegal, 2015). For adults ages 40–59 years, the prevalence of obesity among women was higher than it was for men; for older adults, the gender differences were not significant. The Canadian Task Force on Preventive Health Care and the Agency for Healthcare Research and Quality (AHRQ) recommend measuring height, weight, and BMI, as appropriate, at primary-care visits (NGC, 2015). Health-care providers are strongly recommended to measure BMI during primary-care visits. In the prevention of weight gain, practitioners must use judgment to determine whether individuals with or at risk for comorbidities would benefit from being offered or referred to interventions for weight-gain prevention. On the other hand, for adults who express a concern or who are motivated to make lifestyle changes, practitioners should consider offering prevention interventions and consider individual values and preferences.

Weight screening has many advantages and benefits. Screening may help guide clinical practice to improve patients' health. In addition, in adults who are obese with obesity-related disease, a moderate weight loss of 5% to 10% of total body weight has been shown to improve management of the disease, a decrease in related symptoms, and a reduction in drug therapy. For adults who are obese and who do not have obesity-related disease, starting a regular exercise program can decrease the risk of developing obesity-related conditions. In adults who are overweight and otherwise healthy, adopting a healthy lifestyle may prevent obesity.

Injury and Violence Prevention

Injury and violence affect everyone, regardless of age, ethnicity, race, or socioeconomic status. Unfortunately, unintentional injury and violence significantly increase morbidity and mortality for all ages. Unintentional injuries are ranked as the leading causes of death for adults ages 35–44 years, the third leading cause of death for adults ages 45–64 years, and the seventh leading cause of death for adults ages 65 years or older (CDC, 2015). Injury prevention and control may be placed in the following categories: home and recreational safety, motor vehicle safety, prescription drug overdose, traumatic brain injury, and violence (Table 8-11).

Unintentional Poisoning and Prevention Strategies

Deaths from drug overdose have increased for the past two decades, and drug overdose is the leading cause of injury and death for adults in the United States (CDC, 2015d). These deaths may be listed as unintentional poisoning. Consider the safety tips shown in Table 8-12 to prevent unintentional poisoning.

Falls and Prevention Strategies

Adults ages 65 years and older are at a greater risk of falling when compared to other populations; however, fewer than half of these adults share a fall event with a health-care worker or a family member. Unfortunately, one out of five falls results in serious musculoskeletal or head injury. In addition, falls cause increased morbidity and health complications, leading to economic strain for individuals, families, and the health-care system. Unintentional fall-related deaths increased consistently from 2005 to 2014 among adults ages 65 years or older (CDC, 2017c). Most falls result from a combination of factors (Box 8-6).

Falls are preventable; screenings and interventions are available for individuals, families, communities, and health-care workers. The Stopping Elderly Accidents, Deaths, and Injuries Initiative (STEADI) provides information to assist in reducing the falls for this at-risk population. The STEADI toolkit is available at CDC .gov and includes material for health-care providers

Table 8-11 Unintentional Injury Deaths in Adults

Adults Ages 35–64 Years	Adults Ages 65 Years and Older
Poisoning	Fall
Motor vehicle/traffic	Motor vehicle/traffic
Suicide, firearm	Suicide, firearm
Suicide, suffocation	Unspecified
Homicide, firearm	Suffocation
	Poisoning
Fall	Adverse effects
Drowning	Fire/burn
Homicide, cut/pierce	Suicide, poisoning
Unspecified	Suicide, suffocation

Source: Centers for Disease Control and Prevention. (2015). Ten leading causes of death by age group, U.S. (2015). Retrieved from https://www.cdc.gov/injury/wisqars/pdf/leading_causes_of_death_by_age_group_2015-a.pdf.

Table 8-12 Prevention of Unintentional Poisoning

Drugs and Medicine	Household Chemicals and Carbon Monoxide
Only take prescription medications that are prescribed by a health-care professional.	Always read the label before using a product that may be poisonous.
Misusing or abusing prescription or over-the-counter medications is not a "safe" alternative to illicit substance abuse.	Keep chemical products in their original bottles or containers. Do not use food containers such as cups, bottles, or jars to store chemical products such as cleaning solutions or beauty products.
Never take larger or more frequent doses of medications, particularly prescription pain medications, to try to get faster or more powerful effects.	Never mix household products together. For example, mixing bleach and ammonia can result in toxic gases.
Never share or sell your prescription drugs. Keep all prescription medicines (especially prescription painkillers, such as those containing methadone, hydrocodone, or oxycodone), over-the-counter medicines (including pain or fever relievers and cough and cold medicines), vitamins, and herbals in a safe place that can be reached only by people who take or give them.	Wear protective clothing (Glasses, gloves, long sleeves, long pants, socks, shoes) if you spray pesticides or other chemicals.
Follow directions on the label. Read all warning labels. Some medicines cannot be taken safely when you take other medicines or drink alcohol.	Turn on the fan and open windows when using chemical products such as household cleaners.
Dispose of unused, unneeded, or expired prescription drugs.	
Turn on a light when giving or taking medicines at night.	
Keep medicines in the original bottles or containers.	
Monitor the use of medicines taken by individuals with cognitive impairment and visual impairment.	

Source: Centers for Disease Control and Prevention (2015). Tips to prevent poisoning. Retrieved from https://www.cdc.gov/homeandrecreationalsafety/poisoning/index.html

BOX 8-6 Conditions Leading to Falls

Lower-body weakness
Vitamin D deficiency
Use of medicines, such as tranquilizers, sedatives, or antidepressants. Even some over-the-counter medicines can affect balance and how steady people are on their feet.
Vision problems
Foot pain or poor footwear
Home hazards such as broken or uneven steps/throw rugs or clutter

Source: Centers for Disease Control and Prevention. (2017). Important facts about falls: Older adult falls. U.S. Department of Health and Human Services. Retrieved from https://www.cdc.gov/homeandrecreationalsafety/falls/adultfalls.html.

and materials for patients and their families (CDC, 2016). The Center for Clinical Practice at the National Institute for Health and Care Excellence (NICE) (2013) developed guidelines for health-care clinicians to consider in preventing falls in older adults who dwell in the community and preventing falls in older people during a hospital stay. The U.S. Preventive Services Task Force (2012) recommends exercise or physical therapy and vitamin D supplementation to prevent falls in community-dwelling adults ages 65 years or older who are at increased risk for falls.

The Centers for Medicare and Medicaid Services developed a quality reporting system called Physician Quality Reporting System (PQRS), and fall risks are one of the categories that has been identified as a gap in care. Screening tools are available to assess the patient at risk for and prevention of falls (Table 8-13).

Table 8-13 Screening Tools for Fall Risk

Screening Tools	Description
Hendrich II Fall Risk Model	Gives risk points for each of the following factors to determine overall level of risk for falls: • Confusion, disorientation • Depression • Altered elimination • Male sex • Vertigo or dizziness • Administration of, changes to, or discontinuation of antiepileptic drugs • Administration of benzodiazepines • Poor performance in Get Up and Go test
Morse Fall Scale	Determines risk of falls based on: • History • Other diagnosis • Mental status • Gait • IV • Use of ambulatory aid
Falls Efficacy Scale	Measures the fear of falling with a 10-item rating scale; assesses an individual's confidence in not falling during activities of daily living (ADLs)
Activities-specific Balance Confidence (ABC) Scale	Measures no confidence to complete confidence • 16-item scale rated 0% to 100%
Berg Balance Scale (BBS)	Assesses static balance and fall risk • 14-item measure
Timed Get Up and Go	Assesses mobility, balance, walking ability, and fall risk
Dynamic Gait Index	Measures ability to modify balance while walking in the presence of external demands
6-Minute Walk Test	Assesses distance walked over 6 minutes performed at fastest possible speed

Motor Vehicle Accidents and Prevention Strategies

The risk of being injured or killed in a motor vehicle accident increases with age. Involvement in crash fatalities begins increasing among drivers ages 70–74 years, with the highest incidence among drivers ages 85 years and older (CDC, 2017e). This trend is attributed to an increase in susceptibility to injury and an increase in medical complications (Insurance Institute for Highway Safety [IIHS], 2015). Age-related factors include visual impairment, a decline in cognitive functioning, and physical changes that may affect the driving ability of some older adults (CDC, 2017e). When considering all age groups, males have a substantially higher death rate when compared to females (IIHS, 2015).

Adults may prevent motor vehicle injuries by adhering to specific safety laws such as wearing seat belts, wearing helmets while on motorcycles and motorized vehicles, and limiting distractions while driving. Adults should also avoid driving while under the influence of substances and medications that may alter cognition and consciousness. In addition to the recommended safety interventions, older adults can prevent and reduce the number of traffic related injuries with a few simple tips (Box 8-7) (CDC, 2017e).

BOX 8-7 Prevention Tips for the Older Adult Driver

- Exercise regularly to increase strength and flexibility.
- Review of both prescription and over-the-counter medications by a health-care professional to reduce unwanted side effects and interactions.
- Get routine eye exams at least once a year. Wear glasses and corrective lenses as required.
- Drive during daylight and in good weather.
- Find the safest route with well-lit streets, intersections with left turn arrows, and easy parking. Plan the route before driving.
- Leave a large following distance between vehicles
- Avoid distractions while driving, such as listening to a loud radio, cell phone use (using a cell phone while driving may be illegal in some states), texting (texting and driving may be illegal in some states), and eating.
- Consider potential alternatives to driving, such as riding with a friend or using public transit.

Source: Centers for Disease Control and Prevention. (2017). Older adult drivers: Motor vehicle safety. Retrieved from https://www.cdc.gov/motorvehiclesafety/older_adult_drivers/index.html.

Geriatric Syndromes

By 2029, a projected 20% of the U.S. population will be 65 and older, and by 2056, the population 65 and over will become larger than the population ages 18 and younger (Colby & Ortman, 2014). This demographic change will have a significant impact on the health-care system because the workforce to care for the aging population will likely be insufficient (Bragg & Hansen, 2015).

The older adult is at higher risk for certain conditions based on his or her multifaceted health issues (U.S. Preventive Services Task Force, 2014b). Geriatric syndromes or those common health conditions among the older adult include (Smith & Shah, 2018):

- Delirium
- Falls
- Frailty
- Functional decline
- Incontinence
- Dizziness

Long-term services help individuals affected by geriatric syndromes manage activities of daily living and both chronic and acute health-care needs. Among surveyed older adults who used long-term care services, an estimated 63.7% utilized adult day services in 2014, 82.6% received home health services from an outside agency in 2013, 94.4% received hospice care in 2013, 84.95% were nursing home residents in 2014, and 92.95 % were residential care community residents in 2014 (CDC, 2016).

Geriatric Failure to Thrive and Prevention Strategies

Caring for the frail older adult poses a challenge for caregivers and health-care providers. The frail elder is often dehydrated, malnourished, or bedridden, and may be depressed. The complexity of clinical issues comprising loss of vitality, an apparent lack of will or desire to live, and a struggle to thrive in their current environment is referred to as geriatric failure to thrive (FTT) (Agarwal & Bruera, 2016). Failure to thrive describes a pathway that may lead to death, and therefore the goal to management is to identify contributing factors to modify or to reverse the situation (Agarwal & Bruera, 2016).

U.S. Preventive Services Task Force (2014a) reported about an approach (screening) to identify high-risk individuals with common risk factors for one or more geriatric syndromes. The screenings include home inspections, exercise and rehabilitation programs, multifactorial risk assessment and management, comprehensive geriatric

BOX 8-8 Signs of Elder Abuse

1. Bed sores
2. Violent or agitated behavior
3. Confusion or depression
4. Insomnia
5. Weight loss from inadequate food intake
6. Rocking motion, which could signify trauma
7. Unkempt appearance: dirty clothes, unwashed hair, body odor
8. Bruises, scars, welts, lacerations, broken eyeglasses, or other abuse marks
9. Not talking and appearing withdrawn
10. No longer participates in once-enjoyable activities

Source: National Institute on Aging. (2016). Elder abuse. Retrieved from https://www.nia.nih.gov/health/publication/elder-abuse.

Table 8-14 Elder Abuse Victims and Perpetrators

Victim Characteristics	Perpetrator Characteristics
Physically frail	Long history of conflict with victim
Functional impairment and poor physical health	Lived with victim in past
Women > men	Caregiver strain
Depression or other mental health issues	Mental illness history
Lack of support systems	Lack of support systems
Low Income or poverty	Family members (adult children or spouse)
Socially isolated	Socially isolated
Dementia, Alzheimer's disease	Home-care aides

Source: National Center on Elder Abuse. (2018). Statistics/data. Retrieved from https://ncea.acl.gov/whatwedo/research/statistics.html

assessment, and medication management programs. The intermediate outcome is a reduction in geriatric syndromes, and the health outcomes include a reduction in falls and improvement in functional limitations. Other outcomes include a reduction in fear of falling and improvement in balance, gait, and measures of mobility.

Elder Abuse

Elder abuse can take place in any environment—the individual's home, a skilled nursing facility, or even a hospital setting. Abuse may be physical but can also be emotional and verbal, and it can include abandonment, neglect, financial abuse, and sexual abuse, with the latter category disproportionately affecting female victims. Primary-care providers should ask patients directly whether they feel they are being mistreated and be suspicious if the caregiver refuses to have the patient be assessed alone. The patient may not understand that degrading verbal comments and yelling could be emotional abuse. Also important are questioning patients regarding inappropriate touching and asking who takes care of their finances and has access to their accounts. Box 8-8 lists signs of abuse; Table 8-14 gives victim and perpetrator characteristics.

KEY POINTS

- Health screenings assist in identifying risk factors, conditions, and diseases early when they are easier to treat and may decrease the burden of disease for the client.
- Age-related screenings may be performed based on memory deficits, physical changes, psychological problems, and functional issues.
- Developmental tasks are tasks that arise throughout the life span at certain periods and are the result of psychological, socioeconomic, and physical development.
- Erikson's theory of psychosocial development and Havighurst's developmental tasks theory assert that unsuccessful achievement of one task leads to the inability to perform another task later in life.
- Determinants of health include a range of factors that influence the health of individuals, communities, and populations. These factors are behavioral, biological, socioeconomic, and environmental.
- Prevention strategies such has screenings, immunizations, and counseling decrease the burden of disease for individuals, communities, and populations and lead to improved health-care outcomes.
- A variety of evidence-based screening tools exist for the middle-age and older adult that address age-related developmental, psychological, and physical issues.
- Screening for the elderly must include the associated geriatric syndromes that exist with this population.

Check Your Understanding

1. What are some of the barriers to accessing quality health care in the older adult?
   A. Receiving culturally competent care
   B. Socioeconomic status
   C. Lack of adequate insurance coverage
   D. Gender identity
2. What struggles are NOT seen in adult children faced with taking care of the dependent parent?
   A. Marital distress
   B. Time management
   C. Financial incentives
   D. Social isolation
3. The largest debt incurred by older adults includes:
   A. Medications
   B. Mortgage
   C. Helping children
   D. Credit card
4. What are some prevention strategies used to reduce motor vehicle injuries?
   A. Wearing seat belts
   B. Limit alcohol to one drink
   C. Take medications 2 hours before driving
   D. Use headphones with cell phone use
5. What are some factors affecting the need to individualize screening for older populations?
   A. Geriatric syndromes
   B. Client request
   C. Family request
   D. Aptitude test
6. Which population is at increased risk for mistreatment and abuse?
   A. Older adult
   B. Young adult
   C. Middle adult
   D. Adolescent
7. When should screenings be implemented?
   A. According to established guidelines and provider discretion
   B. Frequently and at least every 3 months
   C. Every 5 years for the middle adult and more frequently for the older adult
   D. Annually for the older adult and more frequently for the middle adult
8. Healthy People 2030 is focused on:
   A. Determinants, equity, and disparities
   B. Evidence to support each screening test
   C. Details for managing each client
   D. Resources, cost, and finances
9. Geriatric syndromes are:
   A. Often seen in the older adult
   B. Seen during the middle adult years
   C. Seen early with the young adult and progress over time
   D. Often manifest as conditions that are not avoidable
10. The ideal screening tool for mental health disorders should be:
   A. Based on the best evidence
   B. Brief and detailed
   C. Comprehensive and economical
   D. User friendly and paper-and-pencil

See "Reflections on Check Your Understanding" at the end of the book for answers.

REFERENCES

American Diabetes Association. (2018). Standards of medical care in diabetes—2018. *Diabetes Care, 41*(Supplement 1), S38–S50.

American Psychological Association. (2018). Older adults health and age-related changes. Retrieved from http://www.apa.org/pi/aging/resources/guides/older.aspx

Agarwal, K., & Bruera, E. (2016). Failure to thrive in elderly adults: Evaluation. Retrieved from UptoDate.com

Alzheimers' Association 2016. Dementia. Retrieved from https://www.alz.org/alzheimer_s_dementia

Auerbach, A. J., Kotlikoff, L. J., Koehler, D., & Yu, M. (2017). Is Uncle Sam inducing the elderly to retire? *Tax Policy and the Economy, 31*(1), 1 –42. Retrieved from https://www.journals.uchicago.edu/doi/abs/10.1086/691082

Baker, D. W., Sudano, J. J., Albert, J. M., Borawski, E. A., & Dor, A. (2001). Lack of health insurance and decline in overall health in late middle age. *The New England Journal of Medicine, 345*, 1106–1112. doi:10.1056/NEJMsa002887

Baker, D. W., Sudano, J. J., Albert, J. M., Borawski, E. A., & Dor, A. (2002). Loss of health insurance and the risk for a decline in self-reported health and physical functioning. *Medical Care, 40*(11), 1126–1131.

Baugh, E. J., Taylor, A. C., & Bates, J. S. (2016). Grandparents raising grandchildren. *Encyclopedia of Family Studies*, 1–9.

Bragg, E. J., & Hansen, J. C. (2015). Ensuring care for aging baby boomers: Solutions at hand. *Generations, 39*(2), 91–98.

Carlsson, A. C., Riserus, U., Arnlov, J. Borne, Y., Leander, K., Gigante, B., Hellenius, M. L., . . . de Faire, U. (2014). Prediction of cardiovascular disease by abdominal obesity measures is dependent on body weight and sex: Results from two community-based cohort studies. *Nutrition,*

Metabolism and Cardiovascular Disease, 24(8), 891–899. doi:10.1016/j.numecd.2014.02.001

Center for Clinical Practice at the National Institute for Health and Care Excellence (NICE). (2013). Falls in older people: assessing risk and prevention Retrieved from https://www.nice.org.uk/guidance/cg161

Centers for Disease Control and Prevention. (2013). Burden of mental illness. U.S. Department of Health and Human Services. Retrieved from https://www.cdc.gov/mentalhealth/basics/burden.htm

Centers for Disease Control and Prevention. (2015a). Strategies to prevent obesity. Overweight & Obesity. Division of Nutrition, Physical Activity, and Obesity. National Center for Chronic Disease Prevention and Health Promotion. Retrieved from https://www.cdc.gov/obesity/strategies/index.html

Centers for Disease Control and Prevention. (2015b). Ten leading causes of death by age group, U.S.: 2015. U.S. Department of Health and Human Services. Retrieved from https://www.cdc.gov/injury/wisqars/pdf/leading_causes_of_death_by_age_group_2015-a.pdf

Centers for Disease Control and Prevention. (2015c). Tips to prevent poisoning. Health & Recreational Safety. U.S. Department of Health and Human services. Retrieved from https://www.cdc.gov/homeandrecreationalsafety/poisoning/index.html

Centers for Disease Control and Prevention. (2015d, 2010). Vision, hearing, balance, and sensory impairment in Americans aged 70 years and over: United States, 1999–2006. U.S. Department of Health and Human Services. Retrieved from https://www.cdc.gov/nchs/products/databriefs/db31.htm

Centers for Disease Control and Prevention. (2016a). About CDC's STEADI (Stopping Elderly Accidents, Deaths, & Injuries) tool kit STEADI: Older adult fall prevention. U.S. Department of Health and Human Services. Retrieved from https://www.cdc.gov/steadi/about.html

Centers for Disease Control and Prevention. (2016b). All chronic surveillance systems: Chronic disease prevention and health promotion. U.S. Department of Health and Human Services. Retrieved from https://www.cdc.gov/chronicdisease/stats/index.htm

Centers for Disease Control and Prevention. (2016c). Leisure time physical activity. National Center for Health Statistics. U.S. Department of Health and Human Services. https://www.cdc.gov/nchs/data/nhis/earlyrelease/earlyrelease201605_07.pdf

Centers for Disease Control and Prevention. (2016d). Long-term care providers. Vital and Health Statistics Series 3, Number 38. U.S. Department of Health and Human Services. Centers for Disease Control and Prevention. National Center for Health Statistics. Retrieved from https://www.cdc.gov/nchs/data/series/sr_03/sr03_038.pdf

Centers for Disease Control and Prevention. (2016e). Noise and hearing loss prevention. The National Institute for Occupational Safety and Health (NIOSH). U.S. Department of Health and Human Services. Retrieved from https://www.cdc.gov/niosh/topics/noise/reducenoiseexposure/adminppe.html

Centers for Disease Control and Prevention. (2017a). Arthritis risk factors. Retrieved from https://www.cdc.gov/arthritis/basics/risk-factors.htm

Centers for Disease Control and Prevention. (2017b). Chronic disease overview. U.S. Department of Health and Human Services. Retrieved from https://www.cdc.gov/chronicdisease/overview/index.htm

Centers for Disease Control and Prevention. (2017c). Important facts about falls: Older adult falls. Home & Recreational Safety. U.S. Department of Health and Human Services. Retrieved from https://www.cdc.gov/homeandrecreationalsafety/falls/adultfalls.html

Centers for Disease Control and Prevention. (2017d). *Mental health*. Retrieved from https://www.cdc.gov/mentalhealth/learn/index.htm

Centers for Disease Control and Prevention. (2017e). Older adult drivers: Motor vehicle safety. U.S. Department of Health and Human Services. Retrieved from https://www.cdc.gov/motorvehiclesafety/older_adult_drivers/index.html

Centers for Disease Control and Prevention. (2017f). Opioid overdose. U.S. Department of Health and Human Services. Retrieved from https://www.cdc.gov/drugoverdose/index.html

Centers for Disease Control and Prevention. (2017g). Osteoarthritis fact sheet. U.S. Department of Health and Human Services. Retrieved from https://www.cdc.gov/arthritis/basics/osteoarthritis.htm

Centers for Disease Control and Prevention. (2017h). Osteoporosis. U.S. Department of Health and Human Services. Retrieved from https://www.cdc.gov/features/osteoporosis/index.html

Centers for Disease Control and Prevention. (2017i). Recommended immunization schedule for adults aged 19 years or older, by vaccine and age group: United States. U.S. Department of Health and Human Services. Retrieved from https://www.cdc.gov/vaccines/schedules/hcp/imz/adult.html

Centers for Disease Control and Prevention. (2017j). Tables of summary health statistics, Centers for Disease Control and Prevention. (2017j). Who's at risk? U.S. Department of Health and Human Services. Retrieved from https://www.cdc.gov/diabetes/basics/risk-factors.html

Centers for Disease Control and Prevention. (2018a). National Diabetes Prevention Program. U.S. Department of Health and Human Services. Retrieved from https://www.cdc.gov/diabetes/prevention/index.html

Centers for Disease Control and Prevention. (2018b). Recommended immunization schedule for adults aged 19 years or older, by vaccine and age group: United States. Retrieved from https://www.cdc.gov/vaccines/schedules/downloads/adult/adult-combined-schedule.pdf

Chen, C.-I., Kao, P.-F., Wu, M.-Y., Fang, Y.-A., Miser, J. S., Liu, J.-C, . . . Sung, L.-C. (2016). Influenza vaccination is associated with lower risk of acute coronary syndrome in elderly patients with chronic kidney disease. *Medicine*, *95*(5), e2588. Retrieved from http://doi.org/10.1097/MD.0000000000002588

Chen, W. R., Chen, Y. D., Shi, Y., Yin, D. W., Wang, H., & Sha, Y. (2015). Vitamin D, parathyroid hormone and risk factors for coronary artery disease in an elderly Chinese population. *Journal of Cardiovascular Medicine*, *(16)*6, 59–68. doi:10.2459/JCM.0000000000000094

Colby, S. L., & Ortman, J. M. (2014). The baby boom cohort in the United States: 2012 to 2060. *Population Estimates and Projections*, 1–16. U.S. Census. Retrieved from https://census.gov/content/dam/Census/library/publications/2014/demo/p25-1141.pdf

Committee on Accelerating Progress in Obesity Prevention; Food and Nutrition Board; Institute ... Washington (DC): National Academies Press (US); 2012 May.

Crews, J. E., Chou, C. F., Zhang, X., Zack, M. M., & Saaddine, J. B. (2014). Health-related quality of life among people aged ≥ 65 years with self-reported visual impairment: findings from the 2006–2010 Behavioral Risk Factor Surveillance System. *Ophthalmic Epidemiology*, *21*(5), 287–296.

Davis, E. M., Kim, K., & Fingerman, K. L. (2016). Is an empty nest best? Coresidence with adult children and parental marital quality before and after the Great Recession. *Journals of Gerontology Series B: Psychological Sciences and Social Sciences*, gbw022.

Dhibar, D. P., Sharma, Y. P., Bhadada, S. K., Sachdeva, N. & Sahu, K. K. (2016). Association of vitamin D deficiency with coronary artery disease. *Journal of Clinical & Diagnostic Reasoning*, *10*(9), doi:10.7860/JCDR/2016/22718.8526

Dickman, S. L., Himmelstein, D. U., & Woolhandler, S. (2017). Inequality and the health-care system in the USA. *The Lancet*, *389*(10077), 1431–1441.

Erik Erikson's Psycho-Social Stages of Development. Retrieved from http://socialscientist.us/nphs/psychIB/psychpdfs/Erikson.pdf

Family Caregiver Alliance & National Center on Caregiving. (0000). Retrieved from https://www.caregiver.org/caregiver-statistics-demographics

Felix-Redondo, F. J., Grau, M., & Fernandez Berges, D. (2013). Cholesterol and cardiovascular disease in the elderly: Facts and gaps. *Aging and Disease*, *4*(3), 154–169. Retrieved from https://www.ncbi.nlm.nih.gov/pmc/articles/PMC3660125/pdf/ad-4-6-154.pdf

Fried, E. I., Bockting, C., Arjadi, R., Borsboom, D., Amshoff, M., Cramer, A. O. J., . . . Stroebe, M. (2015). From loss to loneliness: The relationship between bereavement and depressive symptoms. *Journal of Abnormal Psychology*, *124*(2), 256–265. Retrieved from http://dx.doi.org/10.1037/abn0000028

Galderisi, S., Heinz, A., Kastrup, M., Beezhold, J., & Sartorius, N. (2015). Toward a new definition of mental health. *World Psychiatry*, *14*(2), 231–233.

Gell, N. M., Rosenberg, D. E., Demiris, G., LaCroix, A. Z., & Patel, K. V. (2013). Patterns of technology use among older adults with and without disabilities. *The Gerontologist*, *55*(3), 412–421.

Geno, R., Cepparo, Rosca, C, & Cotton A. (2012). Musculoskeletal disorders in the elderly. *Journal of Clinical Imaging Science*, *2*(39). doi:10.4103/2156-7514.99151

Ghanmi, L., Sghaier, S., Toumi, R., Zitoun, K., Zouari, L., & Maalej, M. (2017). Depression in the elderly with chronic medical illness. *European Psychiatry*, *41*, S651, Retrieved from https://doi.org/10.1016/j.eurpsy.2017.01.1086

Gluba-Brzozka, A., Michalska-Kasiczak, M., Franczyk-Skora, B., Nocum, M., Banach, M., & Rysz, J. (2015). Markers of increased cardiovascular risk in elderly patients with chronic kidney disease: A preliminary study. *Atherosclerosis*, *241* (1), e184., Retrieved from doi:https://doi.org/10.1016/j.atherosclerosis.2015.04.913

Goncalves, A., Jhund, P. S., Clagett, B., Shah, A. M., Konety, S., Butler, K., . . . Solomon, S. D., (2015). Relationship between alcohol consumption and cardiac structure and function in the elderly: The atherosclerosis risk in communities study. *Circulation: Cardiac Imaging*, *8*. Retrieved from https://doi.org/10.1161/CIRCIMAGING.114.002846

Grinwis, B., Smith, A. B., & Dannison, L. L. (2004). Custodial grandparent families: Steps for developing responsive health care systems. *Michigan Family Review*, *9*(1), 37–44.

Harada, C. N., Natelson Love, M. C., & Triebel, K. (2013). Normal cognitive aging. *Clinics in Geriatric Medicine*, *29*(4), 737–752. http://doi.org/10.1016/j.cger.2013.07.002

Havighurst, R. J. (1972). *Developmental tasks and education* (3rd ed.). New York, NY: David McKay.

Healthy People 2030. Development: An informational webinar. (2017). Retrieved from https://www.apha.org/~/media/files/pdf/webinars/2017/healthy_people_2030.ashx http://www.tandfonline.com/doi/abs/10.1080/21551197.2011.623931

Hutteman, R., Hennecke, M., Orth, U., Reitz, A. K., & Specht, J. (2014). Developmental tasks as a framework to study personality development in adulthood and old age. *European Journal of Personality*, *28*(3), 267–278.

Insurance Institute for Highway Safety. (2015). Fatality facts 2015, older people. Arlington, VA: IIHS. Retrieved from http://www.iihs.org/iihs/topics/t/older-drivers/fatalityfacts/older-people/2015

Jankowski, G. S., Diedrichs, P. C., Williamson, H., Christopher, G., & Harcourt, D. (2016). Looking age-appropriate while growing old gracefully: A qualitative study of ageing and body image among older adults. *Journal of Health Psychology*, *21*(4), 550–561.

Jeremiah, M. P., Unwin, B. K., & Greenawald, M. H. (2015). Diagnosis and management of osteoporosis. *American Family Physician*, *92*(4), 261–268.

Kaira, S., & Sharma, S. K. (2018). Diabetes in the elderly. *Diabetes Therapy*, 1–8.

Kropf, N. P., & Greene, R. R. (2017). Erikson's eight stages of development: 5. *Human Behavior Theory: A Diversity Framework*, 75.

Lai, J., Ge, Y., Shao., Y., Xuan, T., Xia, S., & Li, M. (2015). Low serum testosterone level was associated with extensive coronary artery calcification in elderly male patients with stable coronary artery disease. *Coronary Artery Disease*, *26*(5), 437–441. doi:10.1097/MCA.0000000000000260

Lazkani, A., Delespierre, T., Bauduceau, B., Pasquier, F., Bertin, P., Berrut, G., . . . Becquemont, L. (2015). Healthcare costs associated with elderly chronic pain patients in primary care. *European Journal of Clinical Pharmacology*, *71*(8), 939–947. doi:http://dx.doi.org.frontier.idm.oclc.org/10.1007/s00228-015-1871-6

Lewin-Epstein, N., & Semyonov, M. (2016). Household debt in midlife and old age: A multinational study. *International Journal of Comparative Sociology*, *57*(3), 151–172.

Menichetti, J., Cipresso, P., Bussolin, D., & Graffigna, G. (2016). Engaging older people in healthy and active lifestyles: A systematic review. *Ageing & Society*, *36*(10), 2036–2060.

Miller, N. A., Kirk, A., Kaiser, M. J., & Glos, L. (2014). Disparities in access to health care among middle-aged and older adults with disabilities. *Journal of Aging & Social Policy*, *26*(4), 324–346.

Munshi, M. N., Florez, H., Huang, E. S., Kalyani, R. R., Mupanomunda, M., Pandya, N., . . . Haas, L. B. (2016).

Management of diabetes in long-term care and skilled nursing facilities: A position statement of the American Diabetes Association. *Diabetes Care, 39*(2), 308–318.

National Center on Addiction and Substance Abuse (2015) Guide for Policymakers: Prevention, Early Intervention and Treatment of Risky Substance Use and Addiction retrieved from https://www.centeronaddiction.org/addiction-research/reports/guide-policymakers-prevention-early-intervention-and-treatment-risky

National Council on Aging. (2017). Retrieved from https://www.ncoa.org/resources/10-common-chronic-conditions-adults-65/

National Center on Elder Abuse (2018). Statistics/data. Retrieved from https://ncea.acl.gov/whatwedo/research/statistics.html.

National Guideline Clearinghouse. (2015, February 17). Guideline summary: Recommendations for prevention of weight gain and use of behavioural and pharmacological interventions to manage overweight and obesity in adults in primary care. Retrieved from https://www.guideline.gov

National Institute on Aging. (2016). Elder abuse. Retrieved from https://www.nia.nih.gov/health/publication/elder-abuse

National Institute on Aging. (2017a). Health & aging. Retrieved from https://www.nia.nih.gov/health/publication/elder-abuse

National Institute on Aging. (2017b). What is Alzheimer's disease? Retrieved from https://www.nia.nih.gov/health/what-alzheimers-disease

National Institute on Drug Abuse. (2015a). Nationwide trends. Retrieved from https://www.drugabuse.gov/publications/drugfacts/nationwide-trends

National Institute on Drug Abuse. (2015b). NIDA-Modified ASSIST (NM ASSIST). Retrieved from https://www.drugabuse.gov/nmassist/

National Institute on Drug Abuse. (2018). Chart of evidence-based screening tools for adults and adolescents. Retrieved from https://www.drugabuse.gov/nidamed-medical-health-professionals/tool-resources-your-practice/screening-assessment-drug-testing-resources/chart-evidence-based-screening-tools-adults

Nilsson, K. (2017). The ability and desire to extend working life. *In Healthy Workplaces for Women and Men of All Ages* (8), 31–49. Retrieved from http://lup.lub.lu.se/record/f9f246ac-6dcf-4afb-b057-3c63cb89d125

Office of Disease Prevention and Health Promotion. (2014a) Access to health services. Retrieved from https://www.healthypeople.gov/2020/topics-objectives/topic/Access-to-Health-Services

Office of Disease Prevention and Health Promotion. (2014b). Determinants of health. Retrieved form https://www.healthypeople.gov/2020/about/foundation-health-measures/determinants-of-health

Office of Disease Prevention and Health Promotion. (2014c). Mental health and mental disorders, 2017. Retrieved from https://www.healthypeople.gov/2020/topics-objectives/topic/mental-health-and-mental-disorders

Office of Disease Prevention and Health Promotion. (2014d). Older adults. Retrieved from https://www.healthypeople.gov/2020/topics-objectives/topic/older-adults

Office of Disease Prevention and Health Promotion & American Public Health Association (2017, June 22, 2017). Healthy People 2030: Development. Washington, DC: U.S. Department of Health and Human Services. Office of Assistant Secretary of Health. Retrieved from https://www.apha.org/~/media/files/pdf/webinars/2017/healthy_people_2030.ashx

Ogden, C. L., Carroll, M. D., Fryar, C. D., & Flegal, K. M. (2015, November). Prevalence of obesity among adults and youth: United States, 2011–2014. NCHS Data Brief. No. 219. Retrieved from https://www.cdc.gov/nchs/data/databriefs/db219.pdf

Osborn, R., Moulds, D., Schneider, E. C., Doty, M. M., Squires, D., & Sarnak, D. O. (2015). Primary care physicians in ten countries report challenges caring for patients with complex health needs. *Health Affairs, 34*(12). Retrieved from https://www.healthaffairs.org/doi/abs/10.1377/hlthaff.2015.1018

Patel, A., & Stewart, B. F. (2015). On hypertension in the elderly: An epidemiologic shift. *American College of Cardiology*. Retrieved from http://www.acc.org/latest-in-cardiology/articles/2015/02/19/14/55/on-hypertension-in-the-elderly

Pozzi, M., Marta, E., Marzana, D., Gozzoli, C., & Ruggieri, R. A. (2014). The effect of the psychological sense of community on the psychological well-being in older volunteers. *Europe's Journal of Psychology, 10*(4), 598–612.

Prince, M., Bryce, R., Albanese, E., Wimo, A., Ribeiro, W., & Ferri, C. P. (2013). The global prevalence of dementia: A systematic review and meta-analysis. *Alzheimer's & Dementia: The Journal of the Alzheimer's Association, 9*(1), 63–75.

Ravnskov, U., Diamond, D. M., Hama, R., Hamazaki, T., Hammarskjold, B., Hynes, N. . . . Sundberg, R. (2016). Lack of an association or an inverse association between low-density-lipoprotein cholesterol and mortality in the elderly: A systematic review. *BMJ Open, 6*,1–8. doi:10.1136/bmjopen-2015-01040

SAMHSA-HRSA. (2015). Center for integrated health solutions. Retrieved from https://www.integration.samhsa.gov/clinical-practice/screening-tools#anxiety

Schaie, K. W. (2016). Theoretical perspectives for the psychology of aging in a lifespan context. In *Handbook of the psychology of aging* (8th ed., pp. 3–13).

Schulz, R., & Eden, J. (2016). Older adults who need caregiving and the family caregivers who help them. Retrieved from https://www.ncbi.nlm.nih.gov/books/NBK396397/

Schwartz, J. B. (2015). Primary prevention: Do the very elderly require a different approach? *Trends in Cardiovascular Medicine, 25*, (3), 228–239. doi:https://doi.org/10.1016/j.tcm.2014.10.010

Sharma, S., Batsis J. A., Coutinho T., Somers V. K., Hodge D. O., Carter R. E., . . . Lopez-Jiminez, F. (2016). Normal-weight central obesity and mortality risk in older adults with coronary artery disease. *Mayo Clinic Proceedings, 91*(3), 343–351.

Siu A. L., & U.S. Preventive Services Task Force (USPSTF). (2016). Screening for depression in adults. U.S. Preventive Services Task Force Recommendation Statement. *JAMA, 315*(4), 380–387. doi:10.1001/jama.2015.18392

Smith, E. M., & Shah, A. A. (2018). Screening for geriatric syndromes: Falls, urinary/fecal incontinence, and osteoporosis. *Clinics in Geriatric Medicine, 34*(1), 55–67.

Southby, K., & South, K. (2016). Volunteering, inequalities, and barriers volunteering: A rapid evidence review.

Retrieved from http://eprints.leedsbeckett.ac.uk/3434/1/Barriers%20to%20volunteering%20-%20final%20 21st%20November%202016.pdf

Strawbridge, W. J., & Wallhagen, M. I. (2017). Simple tests compare well with a hand-held audiometer for hearing loss screening in primary care. *Journal of the American Geriatrics Society*, *65*(10), 2282–2284.

Sullivan, A. R., & Fenelon, A. (2014). Patterns of widowhood mortality. *The Journals of Gerontology: Series B*, *69B*(1), 53–62. Retrieved from https://doi.org/10.1093/geronb/gbt079

Suzuki, J., Takeda, F., Kishi, K., & Monma, T. (2017) The relationship between stressors and mental health among Japanese middle-aged women in urban areas. *Women & Health*. doi:10.1080/03630242.2017.1321606

Tobaldini, E., Constantino, G., Solbiati, M., Cogliati, C., Kara, T., Nobili, L., et al. (2017). Sleep, sleep deprivation, autonomic nervous system and cardiovascular diseases. *Neuroscience & Biobehavioral Reviews*, *74*(Part B), 321–329. Retrieved from https://www.sciencedirect.com/science/article/pii/S0149763416302184#!

U.S. Department of Health and Human Services. (2016a). Health workforce. Retrieved from https://bhw.hrsa.gov/grants/geriatrics

U.S. Department of Health and Human Services. (2016b). Opioid-related hospitalizations up 64 percent nationwide between 2005–2014: First state-by state analysis shows wide variations. In *Agency for HealthCare Research and Quality*. Retrieved from https://www.ahrq.gov/news/newsroom/press-releases/opioid-related-hospitalizations.html

U.S. Preventive Services Task Force. (2012). Falls prevention in older adults: Counseling and preventive medication. Retrieved from www.uspreventivesercicestaskforce.org

U.S. Preventive Services Task Force. (2014a, February). Analytic framework for older adults health topics. Retrieved from https://www.uspreventiveservicestaskforce.org/Page/Name/uspstf-analytic-framework-for-older-adults-health-topics

U.S. Preventive Services Task Force. (2014b). The guide to clinical preventive services. Retrieved from https://www.uspreventiveservicestaskforce.org/Announcements/News/Item/uspstf-releases-2014-guide-to-clinical-preventive-services

U.S. Preventive Services Task Force. (2017, May). *Preventive screenings for adults: Recommendations for primary care practice*. Retrieved from https://www.uspreventiveservicestaskforce.org/Page/Name/recommendations

Ward, B. W., Clarke, T. C., Nugent, C. N., & Schiller, J. S. (2016). Early researchers of selected estimate based on data from the 2015 National Health Interview Survey. Retrieved from https://www.cdc.gov/nchs/data/nhis/earlyrelease/earlyrelease201605.pdf

Watkins-Castillo, S. I., & Anderson, G. (2014). Impact on aging: The burden of musculoskeletal diseases in the United States. Retrieved from http://www.boneandjointburden.org/2014-report/iif0/impact-aging

Williams, J. S., Ng, N., Peltzer, K., Yawson, A., Biritwum, R., Maximova, T., . . . Chatterji, S. (2015). Risk factors and disability associated with low back pain in older adults in low- and middle-income countries: Results from the WHO study on global AGEing and adult health (SAGE). *PLoS One*, *10*(6), e0127880.

Wing, R. R., Tate, D. F., Espeland, M. A., Lewis, C. E., LaRose, J. G., et al. (2016). Innovative self-regulation strategies to reduce weight gain in young adults: The Study of Novel Approaches to Weight Gain Prevention (SNAP) randomized clinical trial. *JAMA Internal Medicine*. doi:10.1001/jamainternmed.2016.1236 [Epub ahead of print]. PMID: 27136493.

World Health Organization. (2016). Obesity to overweight. Retrieved from http://www.who.int/mediacentre/factsheets/fs311/en/

World Health Organization. (2017), Health promotion., Retrieved from http://www.who.int/topics/health_promotion/en/

Chapter 9

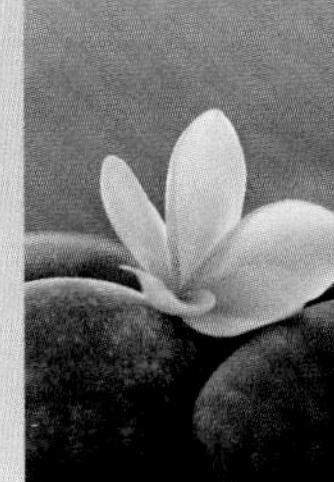

Family Health Promotion and Risk Reduction

Ruth Martin-Misener, Adele Vukic, and Christine Cassidy

LEARNING OBJECTIVES

After completing this chapter, the student will be able to:

1. Describe the complexity and shifting structure of the family unit.
2. Distinguish between families as the context of care and families as the unit of care.
3. Apply evidence to promote family health and reduce risk.
4. Integrate culturally competent care into assessments and interventions to promote the health of families.
5. Analyze the impact of interventions to promote family health and reduce risk.

INTRODUCTION

The potential for advanced practice nursing and clinical nurse leader roles to influence the health of families has never been greater. The two most common advanced practice nursing roles, the clinical nurse specialist and the nurse practitioner, are found in both Canada and the United States. Although differences exist in how the roles are funded, deployed, and regulated, overall, these roles share a fairly high degree of cross-country similarity. Graduate-level education is required for advanced practice nursing roles in both countries, and in many American states, the doctorate in nursing practice is now the entry to practice degree. Both Canada and the United States regulate and protect the nurse practitioner title and scope of practice; however, only the United States does this for clinical nurse specialists (Bryant-Lukosius et al., 2010). Title protection and separate regulation exists for nurse practitioners, and scope of practice is comparable across the two countries (Maier & Aiken, 2016).

A role introduced in the United States in 2003, clinical nurse leaders are generalist nurses with master's degrees who use evidence to improve the quality of clinical nursing care (Bender, 2014). According to the American Association of Colleges of Nursing (2007), clinical nurse leaders assume accountability for health-care outcomes for a specific patient group in a specific setting by assimilating and applying research-based information to plans of care by coordinating, delegating, and supervising the care provided by the health-care team. In Canada, the formal role of clinical nurse leader has not been defined or promoted, although some positions use the title. The Canadian Nurses Association (2009) recognizes the essential role of nurses in improving clinical outcomes and strongly endorses clinical leadership from all nursing roles.

In both countries, the number of APNs is increasing, particularly the nurse practitioner role (Canadian Institute for Health Information, 2016; Maier, Barnes, Aiken, & Busse, 2016), creating an unparalleled opportunity to promote family health and reduce inequities among populations experiencing unmet needs. APNs are well positioned to contribute to attainment of the United Nations General Assembly's (2015) sustainable development goals of good health and well-being, reduced inequalities, and increased partnerships to enable achievement of the goals. Working collaboratively across settings and sectors, APNs do this by improving access to health promotion and illness/injury preventive health services and treatment of illness and injury, thus creating the potential for a healthier life, especially for at-risk, hard-to-reach populations, and by developing intersectoral partnerships to achieve health, education, and economic goals (Bryant-Lukosius & Martin-Misener, 2016).

SOCIAL DETERMINANTS OF HEALTH

An individual's socioeconomic environment is an important social determinant of health. Families and other social support networks are at the core of this health determinant. Families exert a powerful influence on the health of family members and on the family unit as a whole through their customs, traditions, and beliefs. For example, the health of children is strongly influenced, sometimes for generations, by the social and economic background, health behaviors, and genetics of their parents and grandparents (Marmot et al., 2012). In turn, the health of one family member can affect the well-being of the family as a whole (Bevans & Sternberg, 2012; Pearson, 2015).

The science underpinning the social determinants of health calls attention to the inequities in health outcomes and the limitations of the health-care system. More and/or better health care will not improve health outcomes rooted in social inequities in income and education (Evans & Stoddart, 2016). And, powerful as they are, the social factors affecting health do not exist in isolation. The physical environment, genetic endowment, and human behavior or lifestyle also exert an influence on and interact with social factors (Evans & Stoddart, 2016). Understanding the complexity of these relationships is important to avoid blaming families for ill health among members. Families influence health, but they are not necessarily causative agents.

EVOLUTION OF FAMILY NURSING

In North America, working with families has been part of nursing since the early days of the profession, predating hospitals when home-based care was the norm (Wright & Leahey, 2009). It can also be seen in the work of pioneers of advanced practice nursing, such as Lillian Wald's work in the Henry Street Settlement in 1893 with immigrant families on the Lower East side of New York City, and Mary Breckenridge's service to underserved families in rural Kentucky from 1920 to 1950 through the Frontier Nursing Service (Keeling, 2015). In Canada, the legacy of outpost nurses working in remote northern communities began in 1893 with nurses arriving from England as part of the Grenfell Mission, led by British medical missionary Wilfred Grenfell (Kaasalainen et al., 2010).

The concept of family-centered care emerged following World War II; it grew out of greater public attention to psychological health and was facilitated by child health research (Jolley & Shields, 2009). Family-centered care and the related concept of patient-centered care have continued to evolve and are embraced by most health disciplines, including nursing, health organizations, and research institutes. Organizations such as the Institute for Patient and Family Centered Care (http://www.ipfcc.org/) and Accreditation Canada (https://accreditation.ca/client-and-family-centred-care) have been influential in pushing the philosophy of family-centered care forward in health service delivery systems. Although a definition has yet to be agreed on, commonly held principles of family-centered care include information sharing, respect, honoring differences, partnership and collaboration, negotiation, and care in the context of family and community (Kuo et al., 2012).

During the 1980s and 1990s, research and theory production that focused on the role of nurses in promoting family health accelerated; from this work emerged the field of family nursing and subsequently the concept of family systems nursing. This advanced practice of family nursing at its core is the focus of the family as a whole, or unit of care (Wright & Leahey, 1990). Several models have been developed to guide nurses and advanced practice nurses (APNs) in the practice of family systems nursing, such as the Calgary Family Assessment and Intervention Models (Wright & Leahey, 2013) and the Illness Beliefs Model (Wright & Bell, 2009). Over the years, more than 50 books and monographs and hundreds of articles have been published in this field (Bell, 2009). Supported by this robust base of scholarship, family nursing has been integrated in nursing practice and nursing education internationally (Denham, 2003; Leahey & Wright, 2016; Wright & Leahey, 2013). Family nursing is an important part of a growing interdisciplinary community of practice with a focus on improving family health (Bell, 2017).

While family nursing is concerned about individuals in the context of a family, the focus of family systems nursing is the whole family as the unit of care as well as individual family members (Kaakinen, Coehlo, Steele, & Robinson, 2018; Wright & Leahey, 2013). Interaction, reciprocity, and relationality are hallmarks of family systems nursing, and this level of therapeutic conversational practice generally occurs following education at the master's level (Wright & Leahey, 2013). Recent research has shown that, although family nurse practitioner programs in the United States include courses and clinical experiences that focus on the family as the context of care, similar opportunities do not exist for students to develop expertise in the therapeutic conversations that are the hallmark of family systems nursing (Nyirati, Denham, Raffle, & Ware, 2012). Although family nursing courses are not commonly included in Canadian nurse practitioner programs (Canadian Association of Schools of Nursing, 2012), the University of Montreal has incorporated a theoretical family nursing course along with a supervised practicum in its education programs for nurse practitioners and clinical nurse specialists (Duhamel, 2010). Perhaps not surprisingly, this university has been home to a family nursing unit since 1991, with established family nursing courses that include a supervised clinical practicum. This is far from common practice, however, and better integration of opportunities for advanced practice nursing students to develop clinical skills in therapeutic conversations with families are needed (Bell, 2016). This is particularly important insofar as training in family systems assessment and intervention is essential to being able to apply these skills in practice (Duhamel, Dupuis, Turcotte, Martinez, & Goudreau, 2015).

A key message that came out of work on social determinants and health inequities by the World Health Organization (WHO) was the need to "do something, do more, do better" (Marmot et al., 2012, p. 380). In writing this chapter, we offer a call to action for APNs and clinical nurse leaders who encounter families in their everyday work to exert the full potential of their advanced knowledge, skills, and capabilities to advocate for and improve the health of families. This means taking action every day in practice, one family at a time. It also means creating opportunities to develop, implement, and evaluate policies and programs that influence family health promotion within organizations, communities, and health and social systems. We believe that the well-worn saying "bloom where you are planted" holds true here. All APNs and clinical nurse leaders have an opportunity to promote family health through their own practice with individuals and families, as well as by building capacity in other nurses and health-care providers, and through policy development and implementation.

CHANGES IN FAMILY STRUCTURE AND DYNAMICS

North American families are changing. The dominant family structure of 50 years ago, a married man and woman living with biological and/or adopted children in the same residence, is less prevalent than ever before (Pew Research Center, 2015; Statistics Canada, 2012). Single parents and blended families are increasing as a consequence of climbing divorce rates, remarriage, and cohabitation/common-law arrangements. The extent of change varies among race and ethnic groups; for example, in the United States, more than 70% of Caucasian and Asian children, 55% of Hispanic children, and 31% of African American children live in households with two married parents (Pew Research Center, 2015). Reflecting shifting patterns in immigration and migration within and between countries, families are becoming more racially, ethnically, and culturally diverse.

Many immigrant and refugee families have unmet health needs and experience barriers in access to primary health care that are related to language, health literacy, and cultural differences (Kalich, Heinemann, & Ghahari, 2016; Woodgate et al., 2017). Some evidence shows that the stresses experienced by newly settled immigrant or refugee families may place their children at higher risk for maltreatment (LeBrun et al., 2016), and children with one or more parents with unauthorized immigration status face additional risks of poverty as well as reduced access to education and English language development (Capps, Fix, & Zong, 2016). The Truth and Reconciliation Commission (2015) report, in its call to action for culturally competent training for all health-care professionals, has stimulated awareness of the need for nurses to be inclusive of indigenous ways of knowing and being when working with families (p. 328).

Aided by reforms that legalized same-sex marriage, heteronormativity is slowly giving way to a broader perspective that recognizes and values created families, or families of choice (Gabrielson & Holson, 2014). Nevertheless, lesbian, gay, bisexual, trans, and queer/questioning (LGBTQ+) parents continue to face challenges with discrimination, stigmatization, and stereotyping in health and social systems that are heterocentric (Carabez, Pellegrini, Mankovitz, Eliason, & Scott, 2015; Goldberg, Ryan, & Sawchyn, 2009; Weber, 2009, 2010). Children of same-sex parents are at risk for internalizing stigma associated with homosexuality, with potential negative effects on physical and mental health (Trub, Quinlan, Starks, & Rosenthal, 2016).

This tapestry of family diversity, made even more intricate by the overlaps in the above characteristics, underscores the compelling simplicity and utility of Wright and Leahey's committed assertion that "the family is who they say they are" (Shajani & Snell, 2019 p. 55). Their more detailed definition is that a family is a unit with members who may or may not be biologically related, live together, or include children, and who are committed and attached to one another, functioning to safeguard, nurture, and socialize one another. Families do not exist in isolation. They are part of larger social, economic, and health systems that influence health and well-being. Around the globe, economic inequities continue to expand, with widening gaps between the rich and poor; populations are aging; technology is advancing; and people are living longer with chronic illnesses. In response, and driven by concerns about quality and costs, health-care systems are restructuring to shorten hospital stays and increase community and home-based services. Family nursing plays an important role in this paradigmatic shift in health-care systems.

We encourage readers to access the seminal texts of scholars who have written extensively on family systems nursing and the broader field of family nursing, for example, Denham (2003); Wright and Bell (2009); Wright and Leahey (2009, 2013); Gottlieb (2012); and Kaakinen,Coehlo, Steele & Robinson (2018). The remainder of this chapter provides a systematic review of family practice of APNs and clinical nurse leaders. Evidence tables present the findings from systematic reviews conducted to evaluate the impact of interventions using any type of family nursing intervention that promotes family health and/or reduces risk and findings from primary studies that focus on health promotion research with families of diverse cultures. These primary studies were grouped into four areas of focus relevant to the practice of APNs and clinical nurse leaders: (1) family health history, (2) family assessment, (3) family interventions/caring for families, and (4) family caregivers. For the remainder of this chapter, unless otherwise indicated specifically in the source, we use the term *family nursing* as an all-encompassing term that includes family systems nursing (Bell, 2013).

PATIENT, INTERVENTION, CONTROL, OBSERVATION, AND TIME (PICOT) STATEMENT

How and with what impact do APNs and clinical nurse leaders promote the health of families, particularly those of diverse cultures?

Methods

Our search strategy for relevant literature was developed in consultation with a library scientist. The strategy involved searching electronic databases and reference lists of seminal articles for appropriate studies. We searched PubMed (MEDLINE) and Cumulative Index to Nursing and Allied Health Literature (CINAHL) databases from January 1980 until January 2017. The search terms were then translated with the assistance of the library scientist and used in CINAHL for the same time period. A search of Google Scholar with no date restrictions was also conducted; only the first 100 hits (as sorted by relevance by Google) were screened. A separate targeted search on systematic reviews of family health promotion interventions using the PubMed Clinical Queries tool was conducted to identify outcomes of health promotion interventions. Only English language articles from Canada and the United States were included. The focus of the review was to identify the existing evidence of APNs working with families of diverse cultures. Studies were included if they focused on nursing and included family members in the study design.

FAMILY NURSING AND HEALTH IMPACT

More than 30 years of family nursing research has resulted in a considerable number of primary studies that have evaluated the effectiveness of various interventions designed to promote the health of families (Bell & Wright, 2015). Consequently, we elected to identify and summarize the published peer-reviewed systematic literature reviews that have been done in this area. Inclusive of all systematic literature review approaches, our search yielded nine papers, which are described in Table 9-1. Of these nine systematic reviews, two were narrative reviews (Chesla, 2010; Deek et al., 2016); one was an integrative review with thematic analysis (Östlund & Persson, 2014); and the remaining were traditional systematic reviews (Heo & Braun, 2014; Mattila, Leino, Paavilainen, & Astedt-Kurki, 2009; Van Sluijs, McMinn, & Griffin, 2007), three of which only reviewed randomized-controlled trials (RCTs) (Knowlden & Sharma, 2012; Marsh, Foley, Wilks, & Maddison, 2014; McBroom & Enriquez, 2009).

One review evaluated family systems nursing interventions (Östlund & Perrson, 2014). Using integrative review methods, the authors describe responses from families living with illness after having participated in family systems nursing interventions. Findings included improved understanding and capability, enhanced coping, improved mutual caring and caring more for each

Table 9-1 Systematic Reviews Highlighting the Family Health Promotion Interventions

Reference	Study Purpose	Study Design and Methods	Intervention(s)	Number of Articles Included in the Review	Impact of Family Health Interventions	Limitations
Chesla (2010)	To examine the evidence that family interventions improve health in persons with chronic illness and their family members, across the life span.	Narrative literature review of meta-analyses of RCTs.	Family psychosocial treatments of physical health conditions or chronic illnesses of a family member across the life span.	Not stated.	In adults, family-based interventions were significantly better than usual medical care for patient's physical and mental health, primarily depressive symptoms, and family member health or burden. Family-based multimodal interventions for childhood obesity demonstrated a moderate, significant, positive effect on child weight loss. Family intervention with childhood diabetes demonstrated a moderate, significant, positive effect on glucose control and a large, significant, positive effect on parents' diabetes knowledge. Multimodal interventions show greater promise in effecting change in complex conditions that require multiple lifestyle changes.	Search strategy was not provided. Risk of bias of primary studies was not assessed.

(*continued*)

Table 9-1 Systematic Reviews Highlighting the Family Health Promotion Interventions—cont'd

Reference	Study Purpose	Study Design and Methods	Intervention(s)	Number of Articles Included in the Review	Impact of Family Health Interventions	Limitations
Deek et al. (2015)	To identify elements of effective family-centered self-care interventions that are likely to improve outcomes of adults living with chronic conditions.	Narrative literature review of quantitative studies (RCTs and quasi-experimental designs).	Educational interventions on self-care that included sessions, handouts, or prescheduled visits provided to the patient and family caregivers.	10	Effective intervention elements: family-centered approach, active learning strategy, and transitional care with appropriate follow-up. Family involvement led to improved patient outcomes when the type of support (informational, instrumental, and emotional) was tailored to the patient's needs. Family-centered self-care interventions led to significant changes in readmission rates, medication adherence, and self-care behaviors.	Selection bias was avoided in only four studies. All but one study did not conceal allocation or blinding of participants. Detection bias was violated in all studies but one. The certainty of evidence was rated moderate. The limited number of studies conducted, heterogeneous populations, and the different clinical outcomes the interventions tested made it difficult to identify the effectiveness of family-centered interventions.

Table 9-1 Systematic Reviews Highlighting the Family Health Promotion Interventions—cont'd

Reference	Study Purpose	Study Design and Methods	Intervention(s)	Number of Articles Included in the Review	Impact of Family Health Interventions	Limitations
Heo and Braun (2013)	To investigate: (1) theoretical frameworks and strategies employed by interventions targeting Korean Americans, (2) cultural factors considered by these interventions, and (3) the extent of their success in engaging Korean participants and improving their health.	Systematic review of quantitative studies (RCTs, and quasi-experimental and observational designs).	Culturally tailored interventions of chronic disease targeting Korean Americans.	21 articles, with 16 unique interventions.	Intervention targets: cancer (n = 10), hypertension (n = 2), diabetes (n = 1), mental health (n = 1), tobacco cessation (n = 1), and general health (n = 1). Eleven interventions yielded significant effects among psychosocial variables, including health beliefs, self-efficacy, stage of readiness, satisfaction with interventions, and behavioral variables, including use of cancer screening, physiological outcomes (A1C, blood pressure), smoking quit rates. Each of these interventions provided social support via bilingual or ethnically matched lay health workers, nurses, nutritionists, peer group or family members during the intervention and/or the follow-up period.	The association between specific intervention components and intervention effectiveness could not be determined because the outcome variables in each study were not comparable. All confounding variables could not be identified. Operationalization of culturally sensitive strategies was not clearly described because many strategies were included in the intervention design or implementation processes. The studies did not consistently define the demographics of their populations.
Knowlden and Sharma (2012)	To systematically review and synthesize family and home-based interventions targeting treatment of childhood overweight and obesity.	Systematic review of RCTs.	Tertiary prevention interventions that targeted children in any weight category, which included at least one caregiver and a home-based component (clinical home visit or home-based activities).	10	The most common intervention delivery strategy was educational sessions that targeted parents. Targeting parents alone was found to be more effective than targeting both parents and children. All interventions included home-based activities to reinforce behavior modification. Home-based visits were found to be less effective than education sessions in changing adiposity measures.	The majority of studies did not include nontreatment control groups in their intervention designs, which makes it difficult to determine intervention effects across the primary studies. The review did not include gray/unpublished literature to address publication biases.

(continued)

Table 9-1 Systematic Reviews Highlighting the Family Health Promotion Interventions—cont'd

Reference	Study Purpose	Study Design and Methods	Intervention(s)	Number of Articles Included in the Review	Impact of Family Health Interventions	Limitations
Marsh et al. (2014)	(1) To examine the effectiveness of interventions with a family component that targeted reduction of sedentary time, including TV viewing, and video game and computer use, in children, with respect to decreasing sedentary time; (2) to investigate whether level of family involvement/ engagement affects this outcome.	Systematic review of RCTs.	Interventions with a family component that targeted reduction of sedentary time, including TV viewing, and video game and computer use, in children.	17	Level of parental involvement was found to be an important determinant of intervention success. Studies that included a parental component of medium to high intensity were consistently associated with statistically significant changes in sedentary behaviors. Participant age was found to be a determinant of intervention outcomes; all three studies conducted in preschool children demonstrated significant decreases in sedentary time. TV exposure was found to be related to changes in energy intake rather than physical activity.	The primary studies included in the review were assessed to be at low to moderate risk of bias. Due to heterogeneity, the quantitative synthesis of sedentary behavior outcomes was not feasible. Inadequate reporting made it difficult to establish risk of bias. Some included studies had small sample sizes and short follow-up periods, and not all measured change in sedentary time as their primary outcome. The definition of sedentary behavior varied across the studies.

Table 9-1 Systematic Reviews Highlighting the Family Health Promotion Interventions—cont'd

Reference	Study Purpose	Study Design and Methods	Intervention(s)	Number of Articles Included in the Review	Impact of Family Health Interventions	Limitations
Mattila et al. (2008)	To undertake a systematic review of nursing interventions studies on patients and family members published in international databases from 2001 to 2006. Research questions: • What are the main targets of these intervention studies? • What do these interventions involve? • What impacts do the interventions have?	Systematic literature review of quantitative (RCTs and observational), qualitative, and mixed methods study designs Analyzed by content analysis and the RE-AIM evaluation model, which includes five dimensions: reach, efficacy/effectiveness, adaptation, implementation, and maintenance.	Nursing interventions with adult (18 or over) patients and family members, or with family members only.	31	Interventions targeted patients with chronic diseases and individual family members. Interventions included elements of support, teaching, counseling, and education. *Support and teaching interventions:* Improved family member quality of life, decreased burden from patient's symptoms, and decreased family member burden. *Education and support interventions:* Helped family member to understand patient's behavior and to cope with everyday situations and problems. *Support and counselling interventions:* Reduced spouse's depressive symptoms. *Support and teaching interventions:* Improved family members' problem-solving skills, preparedness, vitality, mental health, involvement in patient care, social capacity, and reduced depressive symptoms. *Education and support intervention:* Reduced burden of care and improved self-efficacy and social support of family member. *Support intervention:* Improved relationship between patient and family member and patient's functional capacity.	The review focused on a cross-section of nursing interventions as opposed to selected patient groups and their family members, which may make the applicability of their results more difficult. The review did not search the Cochrane Database of Systematic Reviews, which may have included studies on intervention effectiveness.

(continued)

Table 9-1 Systematic Reviews Highlighting the Family Health Promotion Interventions—cont'd

Reference	Study Purpose	Study Design and Methods	Intervention(s)	Number of Articles Included in the Review	Impact of Family Health Interventions	Limitations
McBroom and Enriquez (2009)	To examine family-centered interventions that enhance the health outcomes of children with type 1 diabetes.	Systematic review of RCTs.	Family-centered interventions that aimed to enhance the health outcomes of children with type 1 diabetes including: • Behavioural Family Sytems Therapy (BFST) • Behavioural Family Sytems Therapy for Diabetes (BFST-D) • Family therapy (FT) • Multifamily group • Multisystemic therapy (MST) • Self-management training (SMT) • Teamwork (TW)	9	Family-centered interventions significantly improved A1Cs, enhanced family dynamics, and decreased family conflict. Intervention effectiveness appeared to increase when parent simulation was added as part of the intervention.	Very few studies reported information about race or ethnicity. The review did not include gray/unpublished literature to address publication biases.
Östlund and Persson (2014)	To describe responses from families living with illness after having participated in family systems nursing interventions.	Integrative review with thematic analysis of qualitative, quantitative (observational), and mixed methods study designs. Families' responses to family systems nursing interventions were categorized using the three domains of family functioning (Wright & Leahey, 2013): cognitive, affective and behavioral.	Interventions, based on family systems nursing theory, including an ill person or frail elderly and one or several family members.	17	Family response in the following domains: 1. Cognitive: Improved understanding, capability, and enhanced coping. 2. Affective: Caring more about each other and the family emotional well-being, and improved individual emotional well-being. 3. Behavioral: Caring more for each other and the family, improvement in interactions within and outside family, and healthier individual behavior.	The reported findings within and between the studies included families' responses on different levels of abstraction (i.e., close to raw data, researchers concluding the intervention to be a healing experience to families but not elaborating on this finding). The studies incorporated family systems nursing principles in a variety of ways, which may have affected their impact. The review did not include gray/unpublished literature to address publication biases.

Table 9-1 Systematic Reviews Highlighting the Family Health Promotion Interventions—cont'd

Reference	Study Purpose	Study Design and Methods	Intervention(s)	Number of Articles Included in the Review	Impact of Family Health Interventions	Limitations
van Sluijs, McMinn, & Griffin (2011)	To explore the effectiveness of interventions to promote physical activity (PA) in children and adolescents, developed in the family and community setting.	Mixed-methods strategy that involves a review of three systematic reviews and an updated systematic review of RCTs.	Interventions to promote PA in children and adolescents, developed in the family and community setting.	Three previous reviews, including 13 family-based and three community-based interventions. Six family-based and four community-based interventions were included in the updated review.	Significant positive effects on PA were observed for one community-based and three family-based studies. No distinctive characteristics of the effective interventions compared to ineffective interventions were identified.	Inadequate reporting made it difficult to determine randomization procedures and blinding at outcomes assessment. The brief intervention descriptions made it difficult to analyze potential effective components. There was a lack of precise and consistent PA outcome measures.

other and the family, improved interactions within and outside the family, and healthier individual behavior. The remaining eight reviews evaluated family-centered care (Deek et al., 2016; McBroom & Enriquez, 2009); family or family-based interventions (Chesla, 2010; Knowlden & Sharma, 2012), and interventions with a family component (Heo & Braun, 2014; Marsh et al., 2014; Mattila et al., 2009). These reviews evaluated nursing interventions that target the health of persons living with chronic illness and their families, self-care of patients and caregivers, childhood obesity, sedentary behaviors and physical activity in children, and the health of children with type 1 diabetes. Interventions included psychosocial, education, or mixed components. Culturally tailored interventions were evaluated in one review (Heo & Braun, 2014). The interventions had a positive impact on a variety of patient and family health outcomes, such as children's weight loss, parents' diabetes knowledge, medication adherence, self-care behaviors, quality of life, family member burden, problem-solving skills, and depressive symptoms as well as health system utilization outcomes such as readmission rates.

Assessing and Working with Families of Diverse Cultures

Underpinning the family nursing approach is the fundamental value of partnership between APNs or clinical nurse leaders and families, meaning that interventions are developed with, not for, families. Notwithstanding the importance of family nursing and its healing benefits, many generalists and APNs do not incorporate it into practice, often due to lack of time (Martinez, D'Artois, & Rennick, 2007; Wright & Leahey, 1999). Hence a number of practical strategies have been created to enable nurses to incorporate the therapeutic conversations that are a hallmark of family nursing into practice (Wright & Leahey, 1999, 2005).

Our intent in this section is not to review these seminal sources, many of which some readers of this chapter will have encountered in their undergraduate nursing education, but to present the evidence related to assessing and working with families of diverse cultures. Our search for published relevant primary research studies yielded papers in the following areas, all of which are germane to advanced practice nursing: family health history (n = 7), family assessment (n = 7), family interventions (n = 14), and family caregivers (n = 8).

Family Health History

Obtaining an accurate three-generational family history is an essential component of a comprehensive health assessment and serves as an inexpensive tool to promote health and prevent illness for the patient and family. The genetic predisposition of some families to specific diseases is well-established, and effective inquiry can identify potential health risks that may be preventable and/or treatable with good outcomes, especially with early detection. The explosion of genetic and genomic discoveries has heightened awareness of how knowledge of family history can benefit health. Despite this, many gaps preventing optimal use of family health history information persist, including lack of standardized documentation practices; uncoordinated health information systems, which prevent data sharing across settings; the inability to include influential nonbiological family members; linkage challenges within electronic medical records; and a lack of user-friendly information for families (Hickey, Katapodi, Coleman, Reuter-Rice, & Starkweather, 2017). APNs and clinical nurse leaders are well positioned to address these challenges and understand the importance of including biological, psychosocial, and environmental aspects when discussing family history with their clients. As Table 9-2 shows, families of diverse cultures may have their own definitions of family, and family members may differ in their knowledge of and ways of communicating about their family history. The need for APNs and clinical nurse leaders to examine their own biases and prejudices is advocated to provide culturally competent care (Hart & Mareno, 2014). It's important to be aware of and sensitive to ethnic and cultural specificities while avoiding stereotypes.

Family Assessment

Detailed approaches for family assessment are described in several well-known family nursing texts that are mindful of cultural differences (Denham, 2003; Gottlieb, 2012; Kaakinen, Coehlo, Steele, & Robinson , 2018 Wright & Leahey, 2013). Briefly summarized, family assessment involves consideration of a family's structure, function, development, and context. The assessment process does not merely consist of a series of questions but rather involves establishing a relationship of trust and mutuality with all family members (Wright & Leahey, 1999). The articles in our review illustrate how qualitative methods can be used to determine health needs and strategies for assessment of the family unit (Table 9-3). The articles reviewed report evidence of successful use of health assessment tools to assist APNs and clinical nurse leaders to view family health from contextual, structural, and functional perspectives. For example, the Family Assessment Device (FAD) is a self-report measure of perceived family functioning that measures structural, organizational, and transactional characteristics of the family

Table 9-2 Family Health History

Reference	Study Purpose	Study Design and Methods	Family of Interest	Intervention	Findings as They Relate to Advanced Practice Nursing
Corona, Rodríguez, Quillin, Gyure, & Bodurtha (2013)	To examine rates of family communication about family health history (FHH) of cancer, and predictors of community in a sample of English-speaking Latino young adults.	Descriptive.	224 Latino young adults, ages 18 to 25	Not applicable	Few study participants reported collecting information from their families to create an FHH (18%) or sharing information about hereditary cancer risk with family members (16%). More than half reported talking with their mothers about their FHH of cancer. Cancer worry, being female, and being older were associated with increased rates of collecting information from family members.
Hovick, Yamasaki, Burton-Chase, & Peterson (2015)	To examine family patterns of FHH communication, focusing on the perspectives of older African American adults.	Qualitative. 5 focus groups (*n* = 22) and 6 individual interviews.	African American	Not applicable	Four distinct patterns of FHH communication: 1. Noncommunication: Personal or family health was not a regular topic of discussion. 2. Open communication: Most participants strongly believed that health information could enable other family members to take better care of their health, especially health surveillance. 3. Selective communication: Some participants were selective about what and with whom they shared information (only communicated to certain people or about certain topics). 4. One-way communication: A smaller number of participants described communication with family members as one-way (communication not reciprocated by younger family members).

(*continued*)

Table 9-2 Family Health History—cont'd

Reference	Study Purpose	Study Design and Methods	Family of Interest	Intervention	Findings as They Relate to Advanced Practice Nursing
Maradiegue and Edwards (2006)	To discuss the importance of and the nursing practitioner's (NP) role in the assessment of ethnicity/family of origin in conducting a multigenerational family history in primary-care settings.	Literature review.	Not applicable	Not applicable	A multigenerational family is important for screening for a variety of disorders that are affected by genetic susceptibility, shared environments, and common behaviors. Patient's ethnicity/family of origin assessment is an integral part of the multigenerational family history, especially for the diagnosis of chronic diseases and the assessment of risk for genetic disorders. Challenges facing NPs and using a multigenerational family history: 1. Training clinicians on the correct assessment and utilization of a multigenerational family history. 2. Assessment of the subtleties of ethnicity and identifying family history. 3. Collection of the family history in a manner that is sensitive to the cultural beliefs of individuals. 4. Avoidance of stereotyping. Implications for practice: effectively conducting and evaluating the individual's and family's health risk with a multigenerational family history is important in the following stages of care: diagnosis, health promotion, disease prevention, and the determination for genetic counseling referral and predictive testing when appropriate.
Spruill, Coleman, Powell-Young, Williams, & Magwood (2014)	To describe the process, presentation, and adoption of a cultural symbol for inclusion of nonbiological family members in the FHH.	Descriptive analysis. Subsample of nurses who attended a genetic workshop at the National Black Nurses Association (NBNA) annual conference between 2008 and 2012.	Not applicable	Not applicable	All participants (n = 50) indicated challenges with the standard FHH in eliciting health information relating to important nonbiological family members. They identified collection of sensitive data in the FHH as the number one challenge. As such, a new symbol was developed that is sensitive to the dynamics of African American families and helps to guide risk-specific recommendations for disease management, prevention, and health promotion of common chronic disease.

Table 9-2 Family Health History—cont'd

Reference	Study Purpose	Study Design and Methods	Family of Interest	Intervention	Findings as They Relate to Advanced Practice Nursing
Thompson et al. (2015)	To examine African American women's definitions of family, family communication about health, and collection of FHH information.	Qualitative study. Individual interviews (*n* = 32).	African American	Not applicable	Participants defined family by biological relatedness, social ties, interactions, and proximity. Some use different definitions of family for different purposes (i.e., biomedical versus social). Health discussions took place between and within generations and were influenced by structural relationships (e.g., sister) and characteristics of family members (e.g., trustworthiness). Health discussion topics included disease prevention and wellness. There were generational differences in discussing and sharing health information. Older family members were less likely to discuss health information than were younger family members. Some participants felt the opposite. Denial is barrier to discussing health information. Family members did not want to talk or think about illness they had or could potentially contract. Participants described managing tensions between sharing health information and protecting privacy, particularly related to generational differences in sharing information. Few participants reported that anyone in their family kept formal FHH records.
Underwood and Kelber (2015)	To explore the collection, discussion, and use of FHH among a targeted group of men and women who reside in the midwestern United States.	Cross-sectional survey.	709 men and women participated, age of participants ranged from 18 to 88 years.	Not applicable	The clear majority (95%) of respondents believed that their FHH was important to their overall health. Only 60% had collected health information from their relatives to develop an FHH. Only 52% shared their FHH with their health-care providers. More targeted efforts by nurses and other health-care providers are needed to increase public awareness of the importance of discussing FHH and to promote the value and relevance of the FHH among clinicians in the practice setting.

Table 9-3 Family Assessment

Reference	Study Purpose	Study Design and Methods	Family of Interest	Intervention	Key Findings as they Relate to Advanced Practice Nursing
Buran, Sawin, Grayson, and Criss (2009)	To identify areas of need as perceived by parents of children with cerebral palsy (CP) in three domains. To evaluate internal reliability of the Family Needs Assessment Tool (FNAT)	Mixed methods: quantitative data and narrative data obtained from FNAT.	Parents of children with CP.	Family Needs Assessment Tool	Parents identified services (recreational/entertainment) as their greatest need, followed by information (plan for child's future, services available) and then obstacles to care (extensive travel). FNAT was found to be effective in identifying needs for families with a child who has CP. It may also be used to evaluate parents' perceptions of needs and provide clinicians with information for program planning and assessing needs central to providing quality care.
Denham (1999)	To identify ways economically disadvantaged families with young children defined family health within household contexts.	Qualitative interviews with family members (8 families, and 16 community informants; $n = 24$.	Economically disadvantaged families with young children from an Appalachian community in Ohio.	Not applicable	Three domains related to family health emerged from the data: (1) family environment (context of the family in the social and physical context), (2) family relationships (processes of communication, cooperation, and caregiving), and (3) family routines (daily structured health behaviors). The family environment, relationship process, and unique individual factors (i.e., health knowledge and beliefs) influenced health routines. Implications for family nursing practice: 1. Important to view family health from contextual, structural, and functional perspectives. 2. Family health is a complex construct that includes biophysical, relational, and contextual variables. 3. Family nurses should not use an "us versus them" stance or interfere with interventions intended to support family health. To promote family health, nurses need to foster a collaborative partnership between family and nurse, identify outcomes that the family views as meaningful, and develop a plan of care that families perceive to be achievable. Demonstrate mutual respect in client encounters and include a tolerance of difference and willingness to accept before expecting clients to change. Family nursing with diverse populations requires nurses to be culturally competent, overcome personal bias, and avoid stereotyping those who are different.

Table 9-3 Family Assessment—cont'd

Reference	Study Purpose	Study Design and Methods	Family of Interest	Intervention	Key Findings as they Relate to Advanced Practice Nursing
Eggenberger, Grassley, and Restrepo (2006)	To increase awareness of Mexican American cultural phenomena. To guide nurses in providing culturally competent nursing care that meets the needs of Mexican American women and their families.	Qualitative (no specific methodology). Interviews.	Mexican American family. Study participants: 6 women, ages 64 to 84.	Not applicable	The Mexican American women highlighted the importance of family, religion, and locus of control in the health beliefs, attitudes, and lifestyle practices in this culture. Nursing implications: 1. Listening to the voices of Mexican American women who can describe their history of social organization and environmental control can support culturally competent care. 2. Knowledge of this culturally relevant information and the significance of it in daily life is a starting point to delivering nursing care that is congruent with the Mexican American culture. It can also help to promote optimal health outcomes in Mexican American women and families. 3. Honor the significance of family values and roles in nursing care and consultation. 4. Using language and expressions familiar to the Mexican American family may improve family adherence to health teaching and treatment. 5. Screen for domestic violence because male dominance is found to be a common theme from the interviews. 6. Assess health locus of control (internal or external) to determine approach to health teaching.
Mansfield, Keitner, and Dealy (2015)	To describe family functions scores of a contemporary community sample, using FAD, and to compare this to a currently help-seeking sample.	Descriptive.	151 families from a community in southern New England. 46 families who completed FAD at their first family therapy appointment as part of their standard care at an outpatient family therapy clinic in an urban hospital.	Family Assessment Device (FAD) is a self-report measure of perceived family functioning. It assesses six dimensions of the McMaster Model of Family Functioning as well as a family's overall or general functioning.	FAD scores from the community families indicate satisfaction with family functioning. FAD scores from the help-seeking sample indicate dissatisfaction with family functioning. FAD continues to be a tool used to assess family functioning in clinical and research contexts.

(continued)

Table 9-3 Family Assessment —cont'd

Reference	Study Purpose	Study Design and Methods	Family of Interest	Intervention	Key Findings as they Relate to Advanced Practice Nursing
Marron and Maginnis (2009)	To identify any barriers that may exist when implementing family health assessments in practice.	Qualitative, hermeneutic approach. Focus groups.	Participants: 7 child health nurses.	Not applicable	Nurses identified several barriers to family assessment, including level of nurses' knowledge, skills and experience, and challenges related to time. Guidelines for conducting family assessment interviews are perceived as an enabler because they are relevant and contribute to improving practice. Nursing needs to be addressed: knowledge and skill development, and critical reflection about personal values and clinical practice.
McLeod, Tapp, Moules, and Campbell (2010)	To identify and interpret the family nursing practices that address family concerns and distress and that support meaningful involvement of family members in the care of their loved ones.	Qualitative, interpretive hermeneutics. Interviews with 30 nurses and 19 families. Participant observations in 3 adult cancer care settings: ambulatory care, palliative-care unit, and an in-patient unit.	Families with one person in an adult cancer care setting.	Not applicable	Two key interpretations of family nursing practices were: 1. Coming to know a family and being known by the family: nurses opened relational space for families to become involved in the care of their loved ones and gained an understanding of the family by reading nonverbal and paraverbal cues. 2. Attending to family concerns and distress: nurses guided families by being a bridge, helping families to conserve relationships, and negotiating competing family agendas.
Nichols and Tafuri (2013)	To determine how experts promote a systematic perspective when conducting a structural family assessment.	Qualitative, video recordings of 10 initial consultations conducted by three widely recognized structural family therapists.	Five two-parent families, two blended families, and three couples. Six families were Caucasian, three were Hispanic, and one was African American.	Not applicable	Twenty-five distinct techniques for promoting a systematic perspective when conducting a structural family assessment were found. Most commonly used techniques were (1) initiates an enactment (directs family members to talk with each other), (2) describes an organizational problem in the family, (3) describes a family member's role in an interactional problem, (4) describes a problematic interactional pattern involving the roles of two family members, (5) suggests how family members should behave differently to improve their actions, (6) praises family members for behaving productively in the sessions, and (7) asks about the emotion and feeling behind a family member's actions.

unit (Epstein, Baldwin, & Bishop, 1983). Despite the utility of assessment tools, nurses describe several barriers to conducting a family assessment, including their level of knowledge, skills, and experience as well as challenges related to time (Marron & Maginnis, 2009). Nonetheless, APNs and clinical nurse leaders can use such tools not only as a starting point for their family assessment but also to assist in developing a collaborative partnership with families to create meaningful plans of care.

Family Interventions

As with family assessment, family interventions are detailed in the texts noted above (Denham, 2003; Gottleib, 2012; Kaakinen , Coehlo, Steele and Robinson, 2018; Wright & Leahey, 2013) and others. Many family nursing interventions are rooted in therapeutic conversations and include specific strategies such as commending families on their strengths, normalizing responses, and facilitating exchanges among family members (Wright & Leahey, 2013). The goal of these conversations is to reduce family suffering and promote emotional, psychological, and spiritual healing (Wright & Leahey, 2005). Recent discoveries in neuroscience have shown that these conversations can alter the brain biologically, creating neural connections that change how illness is remembered and experienced, thereby enabling sustainable change (Wright, 2015).

Table 9-4 presents studies in which interventions were implemented with first-time mothers, military families, Asian Indian immigrants, single-parent families, and low-income first-time mothers. For example, the Nurse Family Partnership (NFP) and Family Check Up (FCU) are programs that target low-income first-time mothers and parenting support services, respectively (Jack et al., 2012, 2015; Miller, 2015; Stormshak et al., 2011). Some studies examine nurses caring for families of diverse cultures and highlight the importance of providing culturally competent care. Barriers to the implementation of this type of care in practice include learning about numerous cultures and cultural preferences, lack of time and training, language barriers, and challenges overcoming personal prejudices and biases (Hart & Mareno, 2014).

Family Caregivers

Caregivers are a critical component of the family unit. They provide care for family members at both ends of the life cycle and sometimes in between. Table 9-5 describes studies that include Mexican, Chinese, African American, and immigrant families and the impact of chronic illness on the health of caregivers. The caregivers in these studies are providing care for family members with Alzheimer's disease, cancer, stroke, and renal disease requiring dialysis. Families with caregivers require targeted nursing interventions to promote the health and well-being of the caregiving family member and the remainder of the family. Nursing interventions should focus on assessing the caregivers' perceived health status and partnering with the caregiver to develop health promotion strategies (Byers, Wicks, & Beard, 2011). Caregiver health promotion strategies may include developing problem-solving and coping skills that focus on time management, role overload, and emotion control and incorporating these skills into caregivers' daily care demands (Honea et al., 2008).

STRENGTHS AND LIMITATIONS OF THE BODY OF EVIDENCE

The preceding sections presented evidence on the outcomes of family nursing interventions and evidence related to assessing and working with families of diverse cultures in four areas germane to advanced practice nursing, including family health history, family assessment, family interventions, and family caregivers. The breadth and depth of family nursing interventions is revealed in the nine systematic reviews covered. The impacts of these interventions included multiple improvements in physiological (e.g., weight loss, glycemic control), behavioral (e.g., smoking rates, cancer screening), psychosocial (e.g., health beliefs, self-efficacy, family dynamics), and health system (e.g., readmission rates) outcomes. The primary studies that examined assessing and working with families of diverse cultures used qualitative and quantitative methods to describe and explore aspects of family health history, family assessment, family interventions, and family caregivers in a variety of cultures. The studies shed light on differences in the patterns of communicating family health histories and reinforce that, although some differences exist between groups of people of varying cultural backgrounds, differences likewise exist within families who share the same cultural background.

A common theme across studies is the importance of providing culturally competent care while also attending to and overcoming personal biases and stereotype avoidance. The primary studies address families with a broad range of ethnic and cultural backgrounds, families facing particular health and/or socioeconomic challenges, and families with same-sex parents. Some studies corroborated findings from family nursing theory and other research on the importance of relational aspects of promoting family health. Other studies describe the development of an intervention designed to reach out to a particular population with a family service. Included studies provide direction to improve nursing care and

Table 9-4 Family Nursing Interventions

Reference	Study Purpose	Study Design and Methods	Family of Interest	Intervention	Key Findings as They Relate to Advanced Practice Nursing
Agazio et al. (2013)	To describe the experience of military mothers and their children during wartime deployments, with clinical implications for NPs in military or community settings.	Qualitative, grounded theory. Interviews with 37 active duty and reserve component military women.	Military families.	Not applicable	NPs are ideally positioned to support military families before, during, and after deployment. Implications for NPs: • Before deployment: anticipatory guidance related to detachment from family (healthy coping versus symptoms of anxiety, depression, guilt); encourage healthy discussions between mother and child and mother and spouse. • Deployment: focus may shift to care of the children and their caregiver. • After deployment: before and at reintegration, NPs are in a key position to intervene early for post-traumatic stress and to support family readjustment.
Aston et al. (2015)	To explore the experiences of public health nurses (PHNs) and mothers who participated in either the targeted or universal home visiting program.	Feminist poststructuralism. Face-to-face interviews with 16 PHNs, 16 mothers, and 4 managers.	First-time mothers who had received a minimum of one home visit in either of the programs.	Postpartum home visits.	Importance of relationships: provided a foundation to facilitate meaningful learning and created a space to establish trust and support. The how-to of relationship development (the how-to was discussed by both PHNs and mothers): • Friendly and approachable. • Client led (tailor visit to needs of client as opposed to coming with set agenda). • Strength-based approach (focuses on mothers identifying and making decisions about the health of their families and themselves). • Respect: “She wasn’t invasive.”

Table 9-4 Family Nursing Interventions—cont'd

Reference	Study Purpose	Study Design and Methods	Family of Interest	Intervention	Key Findings as They Relate to Advanced Practice Nursing
De Gagne (2015)	To explore health-care experiences among Asian Indian immigrants living in the southeastern United States.	Concurrent triangulation mixed methods. Focus groups survey.	135 Asian Indian immigrants, ages from 40 to 64 years.	Not applicable	Barriers to health-care services: high costs, dissatisfaction with services, and inconvenience in accessing services. Participants identified needs in the health-care system, including self-management and community-based health programs, and culturally tailored health-care services. Important to understand immigrants' experiences of health-care utilization, perceptions of the health-care system, and the needs for health maintenance and promotion programs at the community level.
Ford-Gilboe (1997)	To examine the extent to which selected aspects of family health potential (strengths, motivation, and resources) predicted health work (health-related problem solving and goal attainment behaviors) in a sample of 138 female-headed single-parent Canadian families and two Canadian parent-families.	Cross-sectional. Survey instruments sent via the postal service. The mother and one child (ages 10 to 14) completed the mailed self-report instruments.	Single-parent families (headed by a mother) and two-parent families that consisted of male-female couples.	Not applicable	The independent variables (family cohesion, family pride, mother's nontraditional sex role orientation, general self-efficacy, internal health locus of control, network support, community support, and family income) predicted 22% to 27% of the variance in health work in the total sample and each family type, holding the mother's education level constant. Family cohesion was the most consistent predictor of health work (8% to 13% of the variance).

(continued)

Table 9-4 Family Nursing Interventions—cont'd

Reference	Study Purpose	Study Design and Methods	Family of Interest	Intervention	Key Findings as They Relate to Advanced Practice Nursing
Hart and Mareno (2014)	To discover and describe challenges and barriers perceived by nurses in providing culturally competent care in their day-to-day encounters with diverse populations.	Qualitative descriptive (part of a larger prospective, cross-sectional, descriptive survey design). Mailed a research packet containing a research survey to nurse participants.	Patient- and family-centered care.	Not applicable	Three themes emerged from the data: (1) great diversity (numerous cultures and different cultural preferences), (2) lack of resources (time, money, training) and language barriers, and (3) prejudices and biases (nurses should examine their own prejudices and biases to practice culturally competent care).
Jack et al. (2015)	To describe the complex process for moving the Nurse Family Partnership (NFP) from the research arena to full implementation in Canada.	Process evaluation component of larger-scale project that involved: (1) adapting the intervention, (2) piloting the intervention in small-scale feasibility and acceptability studies, and (3) conducting an RCT and process evaluation through a study called the British Columbia Healthy Connections Project (BCHCP).	Low-income first-time mothers.	NFP is a program of intensive prenatal and postnatal home visitation by registered nurses that targets low-income mothers and their first children. NFP's goals are to help parents improve: (1) prenatal health and pregnancy outcomes; (2) child health and development through more sensitive and competent care; and (3) parental life course by developing and fulfilling a vision for their future, planning future pregnancies, completing education plans, and finding work.	Adaptation of NFP home-visit materials is a continuous process. In Canada, it was most appropriate for public health agencies to implement NFP and for public health nurses to deliver the intervention. NFP was well-received by clients, their family members, and health-care providers.

Table 9-4 Family Nursing Interventions—cont'd

Reference	Study Purpose	Study Design and Methods	Family of Interest	Intervention	Key Findings as They Relate to Advanced Practice Nursing
Jack et al. (2012)	To determine whether the NFP can be implemented in Canada with fidelity to the U.S. model. To identify the adaptations required to increase the acceptability of the intervention for service providers and families.	Qualitative case study. Interviews with mothers. 7 focus groups with health care providers (HCPs). 80 documents were reviewed to identify implementation challenges.	108 low-income, first-time mothers in Hamilton, Ontario.	See Jack et al. (2015) study above.	The NFP intervention can be implemented in Canada with fidelity to 16 of the 18 model elements. The primary adaptation required was to reduce nurse caseloads from 25 to 20 active clients. HCPs expressed frustration about the limited eligibility criteria, especially with the provision of universal health services in Canada.
Miller (2015)	To project how NFP will affect the lives of pregnant women and the lives of their babies.	Synthesis of 39 evaluation reports of NFP (21 reports on 3 RCTs).	Low-income, first-time mothers.	See Jack et al. (2012, 2015) studies above.	By 2031, NFP program enrollments in 1996–2013 will prevent an estimated 500 infant deaths, 10,000 preterm births, 13,000 dangerous closely spaced second births, 4,700 abortions, 42,000 child maltreatment incidents, 36,000 intimate partner violence incidents, 90,000 violent crimes by youth, 594,000 property and public order crimes (e.g., vandalism, loitering) by youth, 36,000 youth arrests, and 41,000 person-years of youth substance abuse. They will reduce smoking during pregnancy, pregnancy complications, childhood injuries, and use of subsidized child care; improve language development; increase breastfeeding; and raise compliance with immunization schedules. Trial findings replicate across cultures.

(*continued*)

Table 9-4 Family Nursing Interventions—cont'd

Reference	Study Purpose	Study Design and Methods	Family of Interest	Intervention	Key Findings as They Relate to Advanced Practice Nursing
Niska, 1999	To assess the similarity of nursing interventions to previously used ways of enhancing family processes of nurturing, support, and socialization. To inquire whether young parents would be receptive to nurses intervening in their families.	Ethnography. Researcher lived within the research area with an elderly Mexican American couple who were not study participants for 5 weeks. Parents rated 20 ways of offering nursing interventions according to dimensions of similarity and acceptability and then offered explanatory comments.	23 Mexican American families.	Nursing interventions were assessed as they relate to the family processes of nurturing, socialization, and support.	A. Family Nurturing Sixty-one percent to 70% reported that the three nursing techniques for enhancing family nurturing were similar to the ways their own parents helped nurture their family. Reasons for the unacceptability of the way of enhancing family nurturing: 1. Family members perceived the nurse as an outsider with unfamiliar ideas. 2. Family members relied on keeping tight family boundaries intact. 3. Family members preferred habitual ways of behaving rather than receiving new information. B. Family Socialization The three ways of enhancing family socialization were perceived to be similar to existing ways of socialization (43% to 78% of families). Reasons for the unacceptability of the way of enhancing family socialization: 1. Family members expected nurses to work in a restricted role of caring for the sick rather than in expanded or advanced practice roles. 2. Family members relied on keeping tight family boundaries intact. 3. Family members preferred habitual ways of behaving rather than receiving new information.

Table 9-4 Family Nursing Interventions—cont'd

Reference	Study Purpose	Study Design and Methods	Family of Interest	Intervention	Key Findings as They Relate to Advanced Practice Nursing
					C. Family Support Families identified similarities in informational support, but only 35% to 78% would want a nurse to intervene in their families. Reasons for the unacceptability of the way of offering emotional support: 1. Family members admitted a sense of family vulnerability. 2. Family members relied on keeping tight family boundaries intact. 3. Family members preferred habitual ways of behaving rather than receiving new information. Reasons for the unacceptability of the way of offering informational support: Same three reasons as emotional support and family members expected nurses to work in restricted roles of caring for the sick rather than advanced practice roles. D. Nursing Implications 1. Nurses can help families link with the community. 2. Nurses can use media to publicize family health promotion resources in the community, register families for community programs, and collaborate with families to create protective networks for children. 3. Nurses need to obtain permission to inquire and continue the topic if they become involved within the family boundaries. They need to be sensitive to potential vulnerability of the family members. 4. Nurses need to be aware of how families receive intergenerational advice. 5. Nurses can educate families about expanding nursing roles and help family members become familiar with the advanced skills and knowledge that nurses share with families.

(continued)

Table 9-4 Family Nursing Interventions—cont'd

Reference	Study Purpose	Study Design and Methods	Family of Interest	Intervention	Key Findings as They Relate to Advanced Practice Nursing
Park and Chesla (2010)	To describe the strengths and challenges in Asian American family management of mental illness in a member from the perspective of health providers.	Interpretive phenomenology. 20 mental health care providers who treated mentally ill Asian American patients and their families.	Asian American families.	Not applicable.	Strengths in working with families: (1) persistent and loyal engagement in care of the mentally ill member, (2) able to create a space for the ill member in everyday productive life. Challenges in working with families: (1) difficulties in transitioning the patient into and out of professional care, (2) family involvement that was so intense that it potentially inhibited patient improvement, (3) family care practices that highlighted the patient's needs but demonstrated little regard for the well-being of people outside the family, and (4) family difficulties in revising expectations for the ill member.
Robinson (1998)	To explore both the process and outcome of nursing interventions offered with a nursing practice to families experiencing difficulties with chronic illness.	Grounded theory. Data collection: transcriptions of research conversations, videotapes of therapeutic sessions, outcome studies completed after therapeutic work was finished, and field notes.	14 families experiencing difficulties with chronic illness.	Not applicable	Four-stage theory of the women's evolving relationships with the family member experiencing chronic illness: 1. Women, families, and chronic illness (overwhelming illness burden for these women that led to difficult life balance). 2. Women falling down and falling apart (after an illness-related loss). 3. Nurses helping them to help themselves (help to enable healing, move beyond and overcome problem). 4. Taking charge of one's life (address each woman's new, evolving relationship with self).

Table 9-4 Family Nursing Interventions—cont'd

Reference	Study Purpose	Study Design and Methods	Family of Interest	Intervention	Key Findings as They Relate to Advanced Practice Nursing
Robinson and Wright (1995)	To identify and describe family nursing interventions that families describe as making a difference that matters in living with a chronic condition.	Qualitative (from previous grounded theory study). Data collection: transcriptions of research conversations, videotapes of therapeutic sessions, outcome studies completed after therapeutic work was finished, and field notes.	Families experiencing emotional and/or physical suffering who visited the family nursing unit.	Not applicable	Two stages of the therapeutic change process and the associated nursing interventions: 1. Creating the circumstances for change *Interventions:* a. Bringing the family together. b. Establishing a therapeutic relationship between nurse and family (draw forth comfort, demonstrate trustworthiness). 2. Moving beyond and overcoming problems *Interventions:* a. Invite meaningful conversation. b. Notice and distinguish family and individual strengths and resources. c. Explore concerns with careful attention. d. Put illness and illness problems in their place (help describe a new family story that highlights the family's influence on both illness and illness problems).
Stormshak et al. (2011)	To examine the impact of FCU and linked intervention services on reducing health risk behaviors and promoting social adaptation among middle school youth.	Quasi-experimental.	593 middle school adolescents and their families.	FCU intervention: a brief three-session intervention based on motivational interviewing. FCU was offered to all families who were randomly assigned to the intervention group.	Families who engaged in the intervention had youth who reported lower rates of antisocial behavior and substance use over time than did a matched control sample. A family-centered approach to supporting youth in the public school setting reduced the growth of antisocial behavior, alcohol use, tobacco use, and marijuana use throughout the middle school years.

(*continued*)

Table 9-4 Family Nursing Interventions—cont'd

Reference	Study Purpose	Study Design and Methods	Family of Interest	Intervention	Key Findings as They Relate to Advanced Practice Nursing
Weber (2009)	A review of the current literature to determine the fundamental issues facing alternate families that include sexual minority parents and their children. To explore the unique nursing needs of families with LGBTQ+ parents in the field. These families are critically examined for direct relevance to psychiatric nursing practice.	Literature review.	Families in which parents are lesbian, gay, bisexual, or transgender.	Not applicable	Clinical issues in providing nursing care to children and adolescents: • Nurses need to understand the needs of the child but also understand those needs within the context of the family unit. • Parents may choose not to disclose their sexual orientation to HCPs (may worry about latent homophobia, bias, and possibility of flawed care; may not honor their confidentiality). • Nurses are challenged to create an environment in which the family feels confident, relaxed, and comfortable enough to disclose and discuss their sexual orientation and family constellation. To establish a supportive health-care environment, clinicians should: • Examine their own attitudes toward gay and lesbian parenting. • Create an office environment to set the tone of a supportive, safe environment for children of diverse families and their parents (gender-neutral language, posters of a wide range of family types and compositions). • Make resources available from the clinical environment (books about gay and lesbian parenting, community and national resources). Nursing implications: • Nurses can challenge and help change social attitudes and public policy that can be harmful to their clients who are gay, lesbian parents, or their children. • Nurses can become familiar with local and national programs that are receptive to, welcoming, and supportive of alternative families. • Nurses can provide guidance to gay and lesbian parents regarding child care and counsel regarding school environments. • Nurses can embrace professional responsibility to care for and support all families to achieve health and social adjustment.

Table 9-5 Family Caregivers

Reference	Study Purpose	Study Design and Methods	Family of Interest	Intervention	Key Findings as They Relate to Advanced Practice Nursing
Byers et al. (2011)	To provide an overview of depressive symptoms and health promotion behaviors of African American women who are family caregivers of hemodialysis patients.	Descriptive cross-sectional.	75 African American women caring for a relative receiving chronic hemodialysis therapy.	Not applicable	Caregiver scores reflected no depressive symptoms, but one-third of participants indicated mild to severe levels of distress. Nursing interventions should focus on: (1) health promotion strategies to help caregivers maintain or achieve optimal health; (2) assessing caregivers' perceptions of their health status; and (3) developing interventions to help the caregiver decrease depressive symptoms and anxiety levels, and improve health promotion strategies.
Gonzalez, Polansky, Lippa, Walker, and Feng (2011)	To examine the characteristics, perceived burden, activities, and challenges of high-risk information caregivers of persons diagnosed with Alzheimer's disease.	Descriptive cross-sectional. High-risk family caregivers with poor health and one medical condition were compared with low-risk family caregivers.	Family caregivers of persons diagnosed with Alzheimer's disease.	Not applicable	Caregivers with low income, depressive symptoms, and high care demands are more likely to be in the high-risk group. Age was not a risk factor for poor health in this population. Nurses should screen family caregivers for depression and monitor those with high care demands.
Honea et al., 2008	To review critically and synthesize the evidence regarding assessment tools and interventions aimed at reducing caregiver strain and burden in the oncology population.	Literature review.	Caregivers of oncology patients.	Types of interventions: 1. Psychoeducational 2. Supportive psychotherapy 3. Cognitive behavioral 4. Massage 5. Healing touch 6. Respite or adult day care 7. Multicomp-onent interventions to improve recipient competence	No intervention can be recommended for nursing practice as an evidence-based strategy to reduce strain and burden in caregivers of patients with cancer. Intervention likely to be effective: psychoeducational, supportive psychotherapy. These interventions may lead to a decreased level of anxiety, greater knowledge, self-efficacy, and confidence in performing caregiving roles. Nurses can further assist caregivers by: • Encouraging them to challenge negative thoughts and engage in positive activities. • Developing problem-solving abilities that focus on time management, role overload, and emotional control. • Incorporating problem-solving and coping skills into day-to-day care demands.

(continued)

Table 9-5 Family Caregivers—cont'd

Reference	Study Purpose	Study Design and Methods	Family of Interest	Intervention	Key Findings as They Relate to Advanced Practice Nursing
Rote, Angel, and Markides (2015)	To identify which types of impairment (functional, psychological, and cognitive) in the elderly individual are associated with family caregiver depressive symptoms.	Correlational.	626 caregiver/care recipient dyads (elderly Mexican American adults and their caregivers).	Not applicable	More severe mobility limitations, social disability, neuropsychiatric disturbances related to cognitive decline, and depressive symptoms in the elderly subject are positively associated with caregiver psychological distress. Perceived social stress partially accounts for these associations. Multicomponent interventions that focus on reducing subjective feeling of overload and burden, while taking into account physical and mental health care, and assessment of the needs of caregivers by gender and socioeconomic standing may reduce caregiver burden and psychological distress and improve health outcomes for Mexican American family caregivers.
Stewart et al. (2006)	To share relevant insights from individual and group interviews with immigrant women family caregivers, service providers, and policy influencers, and discuss these in relation to immigration, health, and social policy, and program trends in Canada.	Qualitative. Individual interviews with immigrant family caregivers (n = 29) and two group interviews with women family caregivers (n = 7) and two group interviews with service providers and policy makers (n = 15).	Immigrant women family caregivers.	Not applicable	Immigrant women experienced barriers to health and social services similar to Canadian-born family caregivers, particularly those who have low incomes, jobs with limited flexibility and heavy caregiving demands. Additional barriers for immigrant women family caregivers to access formal services include information, transportation, language, attitudinal, and network barriers. Participants recommended changes to policies and programs to address issues with information, transportation, language, attitudinal, and network barriers.

Table 9-5 Family Caregivers—cont'd

Reference	Study Purpose	Study Design and Methods	Family of Interest	Intervention	Key Findings as They Relate to Advanced Practice Nursing
Yeung et al. (2015)	To explore the experiences and needs of Chinese stroke survivors and family caregivers as they return to community living using the Timing It Right Framework as a conceptual guide.	Qualitative interviews.	Five Chinese Canadian stroke survivors and 13 Chinese Canadian caregivers.	Not applicable	Two main themes emerged from the data: 1. Participants' education and support needs change over time. 2. Chinese resources are needed in care settings (i.e., access to care in their preferred language, traditional Chinese medicine, and Chinese food during recovery and rehabilitation). Health-care professionals should provide timely and accessible education and be aware of the role of Chinese diet and traditional medicine in stroke survivors' rehabilitation.
Zhan (2004)	To examine the experiences of Chinese American caregivers who provide care for family members with Alzheimers' disease (AD) and associated disorders. To identify factors that hinder or facilitate Chinese American caregivers in obtaining an AD diagnosis and receiving services.	Qualitative Interviews.	Four Chinese American caregivers who provided care for family members with AD.	Not applicable	Findings highlight cultural knowledge and insights for nurses working with Chinese American patients and their families. Four main themes emerged from the data: 1. Initial awareness of the signs and behaviors of AD. 2. Descriptions of cultural views on AD (Chinese community stigmatized AD and dementia). 3. Perceived barriers (not knowing about AD at the early stage of the disease, strong stigma attached to AD, lack of family and community support, negative interactions with health-care and service providers, language difficulties and lack of culturally specific AD services) and facilitators (Medicaid program, Chinese home-care agencies, the Alzheimer's Association; and valuing care for older adults) for obtaining diagnosis. 4. Reflections on their caregiving experiences.

health outcomes while simultaneously identifying the challenges to providing culturally competent care.

Limitations of the body of evidence are attributable to the quality of the evidence and the search parameters. The majority of studies focus on female participants, leaving questions about the family health perspectives of men and children. Few studies outline best practices for nurses working with families of diverse cultures, particularly indigenous cultures, and families with same-sex parents. Many studies highlight the importance of nurses' roles but provide limited information on the "how" of role enactment.

Our search parameters limited studies to those from Canada and the United States and published in English. Studies conducted elsewhere or in other languages may have yielded additional important information. Our search parameters were restricted to nursing interventions; thus, studies conducted by or for other professions that have application to nursing practice were not included.

Important Client Differences to Consider in Applying the Evidence in Practice

The evidence clearly demonstrates that every family is different, and striving to be inclusive of the diversity of family compositions is essential. Nurses must skillfully engage with individuals and families to ask them about their perspectives and goals and avoid judgments and assumptions. It means rethinking and revising the messaging and language in organizational policies, procedures, and forms, as well as aspects of environments that can communicate exclusion, such as signage and reading materials in community clinics, health-care offices, waiting room areas, and hospitals. And it means being mindful of the hegemony of race, class, and gender and taking action to make changes that promote family health for all.

Areas Where Further Research Is Needed

Further research is needed in family nursing intervention studies providing outcomes. The evidence provides some examples of effective approaches to working with families; however, it is limited in scope, focusing primarily on chronic illness with little attention to other aspects of health and well-being such as mental health. More studies that focus on diverse family groups and tailored interventions are also needed.

The evidence recognizes the need for family assessments, yet research is limited on the context of these assessments and best approaches (Marron & Maginnis, 2009). Full caseloads and productivity expectations are realities of the workplace, and APNs and clinical nurse leaders are challenged to justify the length of time that they spend with patients (Martin-Misener et al., 2016). The healing power of conversations comes up against these practical considerations. Thus, more research is needed to develop and evaluate high-impact strategies and tools that meet the needs of diverse families and practice contexts and enable APNs and clinical nurse leaders to translate family nursing theory into clinical practice and health benefits for families (Duhamel et al., 2015). Using electronic medical records and other information technology to integrate family health assessments is an important component of this knowledge translation (Hickey et al., 2017). Related to this, research is needed to understand how advanced practice nursing and clinical nurse leader roles, and the roles of other health-care professionals, can be optimized in interventions to promote family health and reduce risk, especially for families who are disadvantaged. The potential of high-functioning collaborative interprofessional teams to address family health promotion is a promising innovation.

Advanced practice nursing is a growing field and graduate education programs are needed that prepare nurses with the knowledge and skills to work with increasingly diverse families in restructured health-care systems. Research to explore how graduate education should respond to these changes is likewise needed. Currently, in the United States and Canada, family nursing education for nurse practitioners is limited (Duhamel et al., 2015; Nyirati et al., 2012). Whether clinical nurse specialists or clinical nurse leaders receive more extensive training in family nursing is unknown.

Risk, Costs, and Benefits of Applying the Evidence

The risks and costs of not applying the evidence are substantial, especially because the evidence indicates that health outcomes are improved when nurses incorporate health-promoting family interventions in their practice. Chelsa (2010) concludes that family-based interventions are significantly better than usual medical care. Outcomes of programs such as the Nurse Family Partnership Program (Jack et al., 2015; Miller, 2015) identify reduced negative health outcomes and increased positive healthy lifestyles for all family members, suggesting that investing in family nursing could reduce the high cost of medical interventions. Similarly, the Family Check Up model (Stormshak et al., 2011) links intervention services to reduced health risk behaviors and positive healthy development among middle school children. With these interventions, the high cost for childcare services, the justice system, and education system to respond to youth who are in trouble could be decreased exponentially.

Feasibility and System Issues to Consider in Applying the Evidence

Barriers for nurses to provide health promotion interventions include lack of resources, time, training, experience, and language barriers (De Gagne, Oh, So, Haidermota, Lee, 2015; Hart & Mareno, 2014; Zhan, 2004). Systems issues include the lack of availability of graduate nursing education programs that incorporate family nursing theory and practice opportunities as well as cultural competence training. APNs and clinical nurse leaders can take the lead in advocating for organizations to focus on family health promotion and a shift in the reallocation of current resources to invest in system changes that respond to family health needs.

Key Stakeholders in Making Evidence-Based Practice Changes

The key stakeholders involved in making evidence-based practice changes are APNs, clinical nurse leaders, families, cultural leaders, academics, policy makers, researchers, and government health and social departments at all levels. The need for stakeholders to form partnerships to collaborate on evidence-based practice changes is relevant to implementing family interventions to increase public health awareness of the importance of family health histories (Underwood & Kelber, 2015), develop more culturally relevant services (De Gagne et al., 2015; Eggenberger, Grassley, & Restrepo, 2006), and relieve family caregiver stress and burnout (Byers et al., 2011).

Safe and Effective Care-Planning Implications

APNs and clinical nurse leaders play a key role in promoting the health of individuals and families in practice settings spanning the care continuum. The opportunities afforded for nurses to work with families can have an important impact on positive health outcomes. Nurses can strategically advance their practice to affect change with diverse families and relieve the burdens of family caregiver stress.

Interprofessional Health Education Implications

The potential for interprofessional practice teams to promote family health in diverse cultures is promising. APNs and clinical nurse leaders could initiate practices that promote interprofessional practice through advocacy with organizations and mentorship in the field. Interprofessional education experiences, including simulation, that incorporate family theory and promote relationship-based family care and enhanced communication between health-care providers can potentially optimize health outcomes of the family unit.

HEALTHY PEOPLE 2020 AND NATIONAL GUIDELINES RELATED TO CARE OF FAMILIES

The only Healthy People 2020 (U.S. Department of Health and Human Services [USDHHS], Office of Disease Prevention and Health Promotion, 2017) family health goal is to improve pregnancy planning and spacing and prevent unintended pregnancy. The National Guideline Clearinghouse (USDHHS, Agency for Healthcare Research and Quality, 2017) has a number of guidelines related to family caregiving, treatment of families during invasive procedures, and person- and family-centered caregiving. The following list is not a part of these guidelines. The list offers specific tools, strategies, and helpful information for APNs and clinical nurse leaders.

Assessment Tools

- http://extensionpublications.unl.edu/assets/pdf/g1881.pdf Strength-based inventory. Provides a tool to identify family strengths when working with families from a strength-based approach. Gottlieb, L. (2013). *Strength-based nursing care: Health and healing for person and family.* New York, NY: Springer Publishing Co.
- http://www.stress.org/holmes-rahe-stress-inventory/ Stress Inventory, Holmes and Rahe Stress Scale. Measures the stress according to Holmes and Rahe that apply to events in the past year. The inventory assists family members in determining their levels of stress in the past year. Family members can assist in problem solving, making healthy decisions and supporting one another in times of high stress.
- Ryan (2005). *Evaluating and treating families: The McMaster approach.* New York, NY: Routledge. This book contains a copy of the family assessment device (FAD) along with information on the properties and measure. FAD (Epstein, Baldwin, & Bishop, 1983) is a 60-item questionnaire based on the McMaster Model of Family Functioning. Each item is a statement about families. Participants rate the extent to which the statement describes their family. FAD includes a general functioning (GF) scale. Higher scores indicate poorer functioning, which helps APNs identify where to focus their interventions.

- Eggenberger, Grassely, & Restrepo (2006). Culturally competent nursing care for families: Listening to the voices of Mexican-American women. *Online Journal of Issues in Nursing.*11(3). doi:10.3912/OJIN.Vol11No03PPT01. This article provides an interview guideline for ascertaining a family's views of health beliefs.

Client Education Materials

- http://www.familypact.org/Resources/client-education-materials/published-client-education-materials/outreach-materials Family health providers have access to a wide range of easy-to-read, culturally appealing client education materials.
- http://nutritionandaging.org/tools-forms-templates/client-education-materials/ This Web site is culturally appropriate and provides brochures, facts and tip sheets, videos, and other resources that may be useful in helping older adults understand various topics related to healthy eating and healthy lifestyles. Spanish language versions are available for many of the educational tip sheets.
- http://healthfinder.gov Helpful information on most health topics from A to Z. Available only in English yet framed in an easy-to-read and easy-to-follow format.
- www.lalecheleague.org Available in several different languages and provides families with support and frequently asked questions for breastfeeding .
- https://medlineplus.gov/ Available in Spanish and offers a variety of health education material on health wellness and disorders, and medications in many formats, including videos, interactive games, and quizzes.

Web Sites

- http://www.cdc.gov/genomics/ Case studies for health professionals working with families doing family histories. The case studies focus on genetic issues and discuss developing genograms and the need to follow up with families. Provide examples to illustrate the importance of doing family trees and mapping out family health histories. The example provided is with breast and ovarian cancer related to the genetic factor, which reinforces the need for all female family members to have follow-up care. Also provide the general public with reliable information for understanding family health histories such as cardiac illnesses, diabetes, stroke in families, and the need for interventions.
- http://fcrc.albertahealthservices.ca/publications/cultural/Cultural-Competence-Check-Card-2012.pdf A basic communication tool to ensure cultural competence, with 10 guiding questions to establish a basis for family's understanding of illness.
- http://www.cno.org/Global/for/rnec/pdf/CompetencyFramework_en.pdf Nurse Practitioner Competency framework outlining the four categories of core competencies for advanced practice nursing inclusive of working with families and practicing cultural safety. The categories describing the core competencies are: 1. professional role, responsibility and accountability, 2. health assessment and diagnosis, 3. therapeutic management, and 4. health promotion, and prevention of illness and injury.
- https://www.cno.org/Global/docs/prac/41040_CulturallySens.pdf Includes case studies and guidelines for providing culturally competent care with families. The guidelines are framed within Leininger's transcultural theory, with emphasis on culture care preservation, culture care accommodation, and culture care repatterning.
- http://dspace.ucalgary.ca/handle/1880/44060 A repository of free publications from the Family Nursing Unit at the University of Calgary.
- htttp://www.mcgill.ca/nursing/about/model/Offers abstracts, publications and background on the McGill Model of family nursing.
- http://janicembell.com/bibliography-family-systems-nursing/ A list of family systems nursing publications, updated February 2020 from the Web site of Janice M. Bell, RN, PhD.

KEY POINTS

- The family as a whole, including its individual members, is the focus when family is viewed as the unit of care. Family as context and family as unit of care are equally important.
- The family unit is complex. Increasing numbers of families living alone, lone parent and blended families, LGBTQ+ families, and immigrant and refugee families are shifting the traditional family structure.
- Family nursing uses a reciprocal, relational, and interactional approach for health promotion and healing.
- Family history can influence family health for generations.
- Family assessment and interventions need to be tailored to cultural understandings.

- Family assessment tools exist to assist APNs and clinical nurse leaders in understanding the family's structure, function, development, and context.
- Family interventions have a positive impact on individual and family health, including physiological, behavioral, and psychological outcomes as well as health systems outcomes.
- More research is needed to design, implement, and evaluate high-impact strategies and tools for APNs and clinical nurse leaders to use for translating family nursing theory into clinical practice.

Check Your Understanding

1. Which of the following best facilitates the understanding of family in the context of advanced practice nursing?
   A. A family is who they say they are.
   B. A family consists of two or more people who live together.
   C. The nurse relies on the legal definition of family.
   D. A family consists of a bond between two or more people.
2. According to the evidence, barriers for advanced practice nurses to provide culturally competent family nursing interventions are:
   A. Lack of knowledge of different cultural values, beliefs, and traditions
   B. Potential to stereotype families of different cultures
   C. Lack of awareness of their own values and beliefs
   D. All of the above
3. Which of the following aspect(s) should APNs and clinical nurse leaders consider when conducting family health histories?
   A. Most families, from all cultural backgrounds, are open to communicating about their family health histories.
   B. Nurses should consider only the genetic component of family health histories.
   C. Denial is a barrier to discussing health information.
   D. None of the above
4. When APNs and clinical nurse leaders work with families, the need for family assessment is critical. Which of the following is relevant when doing a family assessment?
   A. Conduct a comprehensive assessment inclusive of structure, development, context, and function to develop appropriate health interventions at all times.
   B. The focus is on employing a reciprocal, interactive, and relational approach.
   C. The focus is on identifying the nurse's goals for the family.
   D. The focus is on employing assessment tools to determine family functioning at all times.
5. An APN is working closely with an 88-year-old woman with several comorbidities and her 90-year-old husband, who is also her primary caregiver. Which of the following nursing actions are relevant?
   A. Conduct a family assessment that focuses on the family unit's structure, function, development, and content.
   B. Partner with the husband to develop health promotion strategies that would benefit him.
   C. Focus on developing problem-solving and coping skills.
   D. All of the above.

See "Reflections on Check Your Understanding" at the end of the book for answers.

REFERENCES

Agazio, J., Hillier, S. L., Throop, M., Goodman, P., Padden, D., Greiner, S., & Turner, A. (2013). Mothers going to war: The role of nurse practitioners in the care of military mothers and families during deployment. *Journal of the American Association of Nurse Practitioners, 25*(5), 253–262. https://doi.org/10.1111/j.1745-7599.2012.00811.x

American Association of Colleges of Nursing. (2007). *White paper on the education and role of the clinical nurse leader.* Retrieved from http://www.aacn.nche.edu/publications/white-papers/ClinicalNurseLeader.pdf

Aston, M., Price, S., Etowa, J., Vukic, A., Young, L., Hart, C., . . . Randel, P. (2015). The power of relationships: Exploring how public health nurses support mothers and families during postpartum home visits. *Journal of Family Nursing, 21*(1), 11–34. https://doi.org/10.1177/1074840714561524

Bell, J. M. (2009). Family systems nursing: Re-examined. *Journal of Family Nursing, 15*(2), 123–129. https://doi.org/10.1177/1074840709335533

Bell, J. M. (2013). Family nursing is more than family centered care. *Journal of Family Nursing, 19*(4), 411–417. https://doi.org/10.1177/1074840713512750

Bell, J. M. (2016). The central importance of therapeutic conversations in family nursing: Can talking be healing? *Journal of Family Nursing, 22*(4), 439–449. https://doi.org/10.1177/1074840716680837

Bell, J. M. (2017). Social media and family nursing scholars: Catching up with 2007. *Journal of Family Nursing, 23*(1), 3–12. https://doi.org/10.1177/1074840717694524

Bell, J. M., & Wright, L. M. (2015). The Illness Beliefs Model: Advancing practice knowledge about illness beliefs, family healing, and family interventions. *Journal of Family Nursing, 21*(2), 179–185. https://doi.org/10.1177/1074840715586889

Bender, M. (2014). The current evidence base for the clinical nurse leader: A narrative review of the literature. *Journal of Professional Nursing: Official Journal of the American Association of Colleges of Nursing*, *30*(2), 110–123. https://doi.org/10.1016/j.profnurs.2013.08.006

Bevans, M., & Sternberg, E. M. (2012). Caregiving burden, stress, and health effects among family caregivers of adult cancer patients. *Journal of the American Medical Association*, *307*(4), 398–403.

Bryant-Lukosius, D., Carter, N., Kilpatrick, K., Martin-Misener, R., Donald, F., Kaasalainen, S., . . . & DiCenso, A. (2010). The clinical nurse specialist role in Canada. *Nursing Leadership*, *23*, 140–166.

Bryant-Lukosius, D., & Martin-Misener, M. (2016). *Advanced practice nursing: An essential component of country level human resources for health*. Policy Paper for the International Council of Nurses. Retrieved from http://www.icn.ch/what-we-do/hrh-policy-briefs/

Buran, C. F., Sawin, K., Grayson, P., & Criss, S. (2009). Family needs assessment in cerebral palsy clinic. *Journal for Specialists in Pediatric Nursing*, *14*(2), 86–93. https://doi.org/10.1111/j.1744-6155.2008.00176.x

Byers, D. J., Wicks, M. N., & Beard, T. H. (2011). Depressive symptoms and health promotion behaviors of African-American women who are family caregivers of hemodialysis recipients. *Nephrology Nursing Journal*, *38*(5), 425–431.

Canadian Association of Schools of Nursing. (2012). *Nurse practitioner education in Canada: National framework of guiding principles & essential components*. Retrieved from https://casn.ca/wp-content/uploads/2014/12/FINALNPFrameworkEN20130131.pdf

Canadian Institute for Health Information. (2016). *Regulated nurses 2015*. Retrieved from https://secure.cihi.ca/estore/productSeries.htm?pc=PCC449

Canadian Nurses Association. (2009). *Position statement: Nursing leadership*. Retrieved from https://www.cna-aiic.ca/~/media/cna/page-content/pdf-en/nursing-leadership_position-statement.pdf?la=en

Capps, R., Fix, M., & Zong, J. (2016). *A profile of U.S. children with unauthorized immigrant parents* (Fact Sheet). Washington, DC: Migration Policy Institute.

Carabez, R., Pellegrini, M., Mankovitz, A., Eliason, M., & Scott, M. (2015). Does your organization use gender inclusive forms? Nurses' confusion about trans* terminology. *Journal of Clinical Nursing*, *24*(21–22), 3306–3317. https://doi.org/10.1111/jocn.12942

Chesla, C. A. (2010). Do family interventions improve health? *Journal of Family Nursing*, *16*(4), 355–377. https://doi.org/10.1177/1074840710383145

Corona, R., Rodríguez, V., Quillin, J., Gyure, M., & Bodurtha, J. (2013). Talking (or not) about family health history in families of Latino young adults. *Health Education & Behavior: The Official Publication of the Society for Public Health Education*, *40*(5), 571–580. https://doi.org/10.1177/1090198112464495

Deek, H., Hamilton, S., Brown, N., Inglis, S. C., Digiacomo, M., & Newton, P. J. (2016). Family-centered approaches to healthcare interventions in chronic diseases in adults: A quantitative systematic review. *Journal of Advanced Nursing*, 72(5), 968–979. https://doi.org/10.1111/jan.12885

De Gagne, J. C., Oh, J., So, A., Haidermota, M., & Lee, S.-Y. (2015). A mixed methods study of health care experience among Asian Indians in the southeastern United States. *Journal of Transcultural Nursing*, 26(4), 354–364. https://doi.org/10.1177/1043659614526247

Denham, S. A. (1999). Part 3: Family health in an economically disadvantaged population. *Journal of Family Nursing*, *5*(2), 184–213. https://doi.org/10.1177/107484079900500205

Denham, S. A. (2003). *Family health: A framework for nursing*. Philadelphia, PA: F. A. Davis.

Duhamel, F. (2010). Implementing family nursing: How do we translate knowledge into clinical practice? Part II: The evolution of 20 years of teaching, research, and practice to a Center of Excellence in Family Nursing. *Journal of Family Nursing*, *16*(1), 8–25. https://doi.org/10.1177/1074840709360208

Duhamel, F., Dupuis, F., Turcotte, A., Martinez, A.M., & Goudreau, J. (2015). Integrating the Illness Beliefs Model in clinical practice: A Family Systems Nursing knowledge utilization model. *Journal of Family Nursing*, *21*(2), 322–348. https://doi.org/10.1177/1074840715579404

Eggenberger, S. K., Grassley, J., & Restrepo, E. (2006). Culturally competent nursing care for families: Listening to the voices of Mexican-American women. *Online Journal of Issues in Nursing*, *11*(3).

Epstein, N. B., Baldwin, L. M., & Bishop, D. S. (1983). The McMaster family assessment device. *Journal of Marital and Family Therapy*, *9*(2), 171–180. https://doi.org/10.1111/j.1752-0606.1983.tb01497.x

Evans, R.G., & Stoddart, G.L. (2016). Producing health, consuming health care. In M. L Barer, G. L. Stoddart, K. M. McGrail, & C. B. McLeod (Eds.), *An undisciplined economist: Robert G. Evans on health, economics, health care policy, and population health* (pp. 386–428), Montreal, Canada: Queens University Press.

Ford-Gilboe, M. (1997). Family strengths, motivation, and resources as predictors of health promotion behavior in single-parent and two-parent families. *Research in Nursing & Health*, *20*(3), 205–217.

Gabrielson, M.L. & Holson, E.C. (2014). Broadening definitions of family for older lesbians: Modifying the Lubben Social Network Scale. *Journal of Gerontological Social Work*, 57,198–217.

Goldberg, L., Ryan, A., & Sawchyn, J. (2009). Feminist and queer phenomenology: A framework for perinatal nursing practice, research, and education for advancing lesbian health. *Health Care for Women International*, *30*(6), 536–549.

Gonzalez, E. W., Polansky, M., Lippa, C. F., Walker, D., & Feng, D. (2011). Family caregivers at risk: Who are they?? *Issues in Mental Health Nursing*, *32*(8), 528–536. https://doi.org/10.3109/01612840.2011.573123

Gottlieb, L. (2012). *Strengths-based nursing care: Health and healing for person and family*. New York, NY: Springer.

Hart, P. L., & Mareno, N. (2014). Cultural challenges and barriers through the voices of nurses. *Journal of Clinical Nursing*, *23*(15/16), 2223–2233. https://doi.org/10.1111/jocn.12500

Heo, H. H., & Braun, K. L. (2014). Culturally tailored interventions of chronic disease targeting Korean Americans: A systematic review. *Ethnicity & Health*, *19*(1), 64–85. https://doi.org/10.1080/13557858.2013.857766

Hickey, K. T., Katapodi, M. C., Coleman, B., Reuter-Rice, K., & Starkweather, A. R. (2017). Improving utilization of the family history in the electronic health record. *Journal of Nursing Scholarship: An Official Publication of Sigma Theta Tau International Honor Society of Nursing*, *49*(1), 80–86. https://doi.org/10.1111/jnu.12259

Honea, N. J., Brintnall, R., Given, B., Sherwood, P., Colao, D. B., Somers, S. C., & Northouse L. L. (2008). Putting evidence into practice: Nursing assessment and interventions to reduce family caregiver strain and burden. *Clinical Journal of Oncology Nursing*, *12*(3), 507–516. https://doi.org/10.1188/08.CJON.507-516

Hovick, S. R., Yamasaki, J. S., Burton-Chase, A. M., & Peterson, S. K. (2015). Patterns of family health history communication among older African American adults. *Journal of Health Communication*, *20*(1), 80–87. https://doi.org/10.1080/10810730.2014.908984

Jack, S. M., Busser, D., Sheehan, D., Gonzalez, A., Zwygers, E. J., & Macmillan, H. L. (2012). Adaptation and implementation of the nurse-family partnership in Canada. *Canadian Journal of Public Health (Revue Canadienne De Santé Publique)*, *103*(7 Suppl 1), eS42–eS48.

Jack, S. M., Catherine, N., Gonzalez, A., MacMillan, H. L., Sheehan, D., Waddell, D., & British Columbia Healthy Connections Project Scientific Team. (2015). Adapting, piloting and evaluating complex public health interventions: Lessons learned from the Nurse-Family Partnership in Canadian public health settings. *Health Promotion and Chronic Disease Prevention in Canada: Research, Policy and Practice*, *35*(8–9), 151–159.

Jolley, J., & Shields, L. (2009). The evolution of family-centered care. *Journal of Pediatric Nursing*, *24*(2), 164–170. https://doi.org/10.1016/j.pedn.2008.03.010

Kaakinen, J. R., Coehlo, D. P., Steele, R., & Robinson, M. (Eds.). (2018). *Family health nursing: Theory, practice, and research* (6th ed.). Philadelphia, PA: F. A. Davis.

Kaasalainen, S., Martin-Misener, R., Kilpatrick, K., Harbman, P., Bryant-Lukosius, D., Donald, F., ... DiCenso, A. (2010). An historical overview of the development of advanced practice nursing roles in Canada. *Canadian Journal of Nursing Leadership*, *23*(SI), 35–60.

Kalich, A., Heinemann, L., & Ghahari, S. (2016). A scoping review of immigrant experience of health care access barriers in Canada. *Journal of Immigrant and Minority Health*, *18*(3), 697–709. https://doi.org/10.1007/s10903-015-0237-6

Keeling, A. W. (2015). Historical perspectives on an expanded role for nursing. *Online Journal of Issues in Nursing*, *20*(2), 2.

Knowlden, A. P., & Sharma, M. (2012). Systematic review of family and home-based interventions targeting paediatric overweight and obesity. *Obesity Reviews: An Official Journal of the International Association for the Study of Obesity*, *13*(6), 499–508. https://doi.org/10.1111/j.1467-789X.2011.00976.x

Kuo, D. Z., Houtrow, A. J., Arango, P., Kuhlthau, K. A., Simmons, J. M., & Neff, J. M. (2012). Family-centered care: Current applications and future directions in pediatric health care. *Maternal and Child Health Journal*, *16*(2), 297–305. https://doi.org/10.1007/s10995-011-0751-7

Leahey, M., & Wright, L. M. (2016). Application of the Calgary family assessment and intervention models: Reflections on the reciprocity between the personal and the professional. *Journal of Family Nursing*, *22*(4), 450–459.

LeBrun, A., Hassan, G., Boivin, M., Fraser, S.-L., Dufour, S., & Lavergne, C. (2016). Review of child maltreatment in immigrant and refugee families. *Canadian Journal of Public Health*, *106*(7 Suppl 2), eS45–eS56.

Maier, C. B., & Aiken, L. H. (2016). Expanding clinical roles for nurses to realign the global health workforce with population needs: A commentary. *Israel Journal of Health Policy Research*, *5*, 21. https://doi.org/10.1186/s13584-016-0079-2

Maier, C. B., Barnes, H., Aiken, L. H., & Busse, R. (2016, September). Descriptive, cross-country analysis of the nurse practitioner workforce in six countries: Size, growth, physician substitution potential. *British Medical Journal Open*, *6*(9), e011901.

Mansfield, A. K., Keitner, G. I., & Dealy, J. (2015). The family assessment device: An update. *Family Process*, *54*(1), 82–93. https://doi.org/10.1111/famp.12080

Maradiegue, A., & Edwards, Q. T. (2006). An overview of ethnicity and assessment of family history in primary care settings. *Journal of the American Academy of Nurse Practitioners*, *18*(10), 447–456. https://doi.org/10.1111/j.1745-7599.2006.00156.x

Marmot, M., Allen, J., Bell, R., Bloomer, E., Goldblatt, P., on behalf of the Consortium for the European Review of Social Determinants of Health and the Health Divide. (2012). WHO European review of social determinants of health and the health divide. *Lancet*, *380*, 1011–1129.

Marron, C. A., & Maginnis, C. (2009). Implementing family health assessment: Experiences of child health nurses. *Neonatal, Paediatric & Child Health Nursing*, *12*(1), 3–8.

Marsh, S., Foley, L. S., Wilks, D. C., & Maddison, R. (2014). Family-based interventions for reducing sedentary time in youth: A systematic review of randomized controlled trials. *Obesity Reviews*, *15*(2), 117–133. https://doi.org/10.1111/obr.12105

Martinez, A. M., D'Artois, D., & Rennick, J. E. (2007). Does the 15-minute (or less) family interview influence family nursing practice? *Journal of Family Nursing*, *13*(2), 157–178. https://doi.org/10.1177/1074840707300750

Martin-Misener, R., Kilpatrick, K., Donald, F., Bryant-Lukosius, D., Rayner, J., Valaitis, R., . . . Lamb, A. (2016). Nurse practitioner caseload in primary health care: Scoping review. *International Journal of Nursing Studies*, *62*, 170–182. https://doi.org/10.1016/j.ijnurstu.2016.07.019

Mattila, E., Leino, K., Paavilainen, E., & Astedt-Kurki, P. (2009). Nursing intervention studies on patients and family members: A systematic literature review. *Scandinavian Journal of Caring Sciences*, *23*(3), 611–622. https://doi.org/10.1111/j.1471-6712.2008.00652.x

McBroom L. A., & Enriquez M. (2009). Review of family-centered interventions to enhance the health outcomes of children with type 1 diabetes. *Diabetes Educator*, *35*(3), 428–438. https://doi.org/10.1177/0145721709332814

McLeod, D. L., Tapp, D. M., Moules, N. J., & Campbell, M. E. (2010). Knowing the family: Interpretations of family nursing in oncology and palliative care. *European Journal of Oncology Nursing: The Official Journal of European Oncology Nursing Society*, *14*(2), 93–100. https://doi.org/10.1016/j.ejon.2009.09.006

Miller, T. R. (2015). Projected outcomes of nurse-family partnership home visitation during 1996–2013: USA. *Prevention Science: The Official Journal of the Society for*

Prevention Research, *16*(6), 765–777. https://doi.org/10.1007/s11121-015-0572-9

Nichols, M., & Tafuri, S. (2013). Techniques of structural family assessment: A qualitative analysis of how experts promote a systemic perspective. *Family Process*, *52*(2), 207–215. https://doi.org/10.1111/famp.12025

Niska, K. J. (1999). Family nursing interventions: Mexican American early family formation . . . third part of a three-part study. *Nursing Science Quarterly*, *12*(4), 335–340.

Nyirati, C. M., Denham, S. A., Raffle, H., & Ware, L. (2012). Where is family in the family nurse practitioner program? Results of a U.S. family nurse practitioner program survey. *Journal of Family Nursing*, 18(3), 378–408.

Östlund, U., & Persson, C. (2014). Examining family responses to family systems nursing interventions: An integrative review. *Journal of Family Nursing*, *20*(3), 259–286.

Park, M., & Chesla, C. (2010). Understanding complexity of Asian American family care practices. *Archives of Psychiatric Nursing*, *24*(3), 189–201. https://doi.org/10.1016/j.apnu.2009.06.005

Pearson, C. (2015). *The impact of mental health problems on family members*. Ottawa, Canada: Statistics Canada. Retrieved from http://www.statcan.gc.ca/pub/82-624-x/2015001/article/14214-eng.htm

Pew Research Center. (2015). *Parenting in America: Outlook, worries, aspirations are strongly linked to financial situation*. Retrieved from http://www.pewsocialtrends.org/files/2015/12/2015-12-17_parenting-in-america_FINAL.pdf

Robinson, C. A. (1998). Women, families, chronic illness, and nursing interventions: From burden to balance. *Journal of Family Nursing*, *4*(3), 271–290. https://doi.org/10.1177/107484079800400304

Robinson, C. A., & Wright, L. M. (1995). Family nursing interventions: What families say makes a difference. *Journal of Family Nursing*, *1*(3), 327–345. https://doi.org/10.1177/107484079500100306

Rote, S., Angel, J. L., & Markides, K. (2015). Health of elderly Mexican American adults and family caregiver distress. *Research on Aging*, *37*(3), 306–331. https://doi.org/10.1177/0164027514531028

Shajani, Z.& Snell,D. (2019*). Wright & Leahy's nurses and families: A guide to family assessment and intervention* (7th ed). Philadelphia, P.A: F.A Davis

Spruill, I. J., Coleman, B. L., Powell-Young, Y. M., Williams, T. H., & Magwood, G. (2014). Non-biological (fictive kin and othermothers): Embracing the need for a culturally appropriate pedigree nomenclature in African-American families. *Journal of National Black Nurses' Association*, *25*(2), 23–30.

Statistics Canada. (2012). *Fifty years of families in Canada: 1961 to 2011*. Retrieved from https://www12.statcan.gc.ca/census-recensement/2011/as-sa/98-312-x/98-312-x2011003_1-eng.cfmfrom

Stewart, M. J., Neufeld, A., Harrison, M. J., Spitzer, D., Hughes, K., & Makwarimba, E. (2006). Immigrant women family caregivers in Canada: Implications for policies and programmes in health and social sectors. *Health & Social Care in the Community*, *14*(4), 329–340.

Stormshak, E. A., Connell, A. M., Véronneau, M.H., Myers, M. W., Dishion, T. J., Kavanagh, K., & Caruthers, A. S. (2011). An ecological approach to promoting early adolescent mental health and social adaptation: Family-centered intervention in public middle schools. *Child Development*, *82*(1), 209–225. https://doi.org/10.1111/j.1467-8624.2010.01551.x

Thompson, T., Seo, J., Griffith, J., Baxter, M., James, A., & Kaphingst, K. A. (2015). The context of collecting family health history: Examining definitions of family and family communication about health among African American women. *Journal of Health Communication*, *20*(4), 416–423. https://doi.org/10.1080/10810730.2014.977466

Trub, L., Quinlan, E., Starks, T. J., & Rosenthal, L. (2016). Discrimination, internalized homonegativity, and attitudes toward children of same-sex parents: Can secure attachment buffer against stigma internalization? *Family Process*. https://doi.org/10.1111/famp.12255

Truth and Reconciliation Commission of Canada. (2015). Truth and Reconciliation Commission of Canada: Calls to Action. Retrieved from http://www.trc.ca/websites/trcinstitution/File/2015/Findings/Calls_to_Action_English2.pdf

Underwood, S. M., & Kelber, S. (2015). Enhancing the collection, discussion and use of family health history by consumers, nurses and other health care providers: Because family health history matters. *Nursing Clinics of North America*, *50*(3), 509–529. https://doi.org/10.1016/j.cnur.2015.05.006

United Nations General Assembly. (2015). *Transforming our world: The 2030 agenda for sustainable development*. Retrieved from www.un.org/ga/search/view_doc.asp?symbol=A/70/L.1&Lang=E

U.S. Department of Health and Human Services, Agency for Healthcare Research and Quality (2017). *National guideline clearinghouse*. Retrieved from https://www.guideline.gov/search?q=Family

U.S. Department of Health and Human Services, Office of Disease Prevention and Health Promotion. (2017). *Healthy people 2020*. Retrieved from https://www.healthypeople.gov/2020/topics-objectives/topic/family-planning

Van Sluijs, E. M., McMinn, A. M., & Griffin, S. J. (2007). Effectiveness of interventions to promote physical activity in children and adolescents: Systematic review of controlled trials. *British Medical Journal*, *335*(7622), 703.

Weber, S. (2009). Policy aspects and nursing care of families with parents who are sexual minorities. *Journal of Family Nursing*, *15*(3), 384–399. https://doi.org/10.1177/1074840709339594

Weber, S. (2010). A stigma identification framework for family nurses working with parents who are lesbian, gay, bisexual, or transgendered and their families. *Journal of Family Nursing*, *16*(4), 378–393. https://doi.org/10.1177/1074840710384999

Woodgate, R. L., Busolo, D. S., Crockett, M., Dean, R. A., Amaladas, M. R., & Plourde, P. J. (2017). A qualitative study on African immigrant and refugee families' experiences of accessing primary health care services in Manitoba, Canada: It's not easy! *International Journal for Equity in Health*, *16*(1), 5. https://doi.org/10.1186/s12939-016-0510-x

Wright, L. M. (2015). Brain science and illness beliefs: An unexpected explanation of the healing power of therapeutic conversations and the family interventions that matter. *Journal of Family Nursing*, *21*(2), 186–205. https://doi.org/10.1177/1074840715575822

Wright, L. M., & Bell, J. M. (2009). *Beliefs and illness: A model for healing*. Calgary, Alberta, Canada: 4th Floor Press.

Wright, L. M., & Leahey, M. (1990). Trends in nursing of families. *Journal of Advanced Nursing*, *15*, 148–154.

Wright, L. M., & Leahey, M. (1999). Maximizing time, minimizing suffering: The 15-minute (or less) family interview. *Journal of Family Nursing*, *5*(3), 259–274. https://doi.org/10.1177/107484079900500302

Wright, L. M., & Leahey, M. (2005). The three most common errors in family nursing: How to avoid or sidestep. *Journal of Family Nursing*, *11*(2), 90–101. https://doi.org/10.1177/1074840704272569

Wright, L. M., & Leahey, M. (2009). *Nurses and families: A guide to family assessment and intervention* (5th ed.). Philadelphia, PA: F.A. Davis.

Wright, L.M., & Leahey, M. (2013). *Nurses and families: A guide to family assessment and intervention* (6th ed.). Philadelphia, PA: F.A. Davis.

Yeung, E. H. L., Szeto, A., Richardson, D., Lai, S., Lim, E., & Cameron, J. I. (2015). The experiences and needs of Chinese-Canadian stroke survivors and family caregivers as they re-integrate into the community. *Health & Social Care in the Community*, *23*(5), 523–531. https://doi.org/10.1111/hsc.12164

Zhan L. (2004). Caring for family members with Alzheimer's disease: Perspectives from Chinese American caregivers. *Journal of Gerontological Nursing*, 30(8), 19–29.

Mental Health Promotion

Joanne DeSanto Iennaco

LEARNING OBJECTIVES

After completing this chapter, the student will be able to:

1. Explain differences between mental health and mental illness in the contexts of both mental health promotion and mental illness prevention.
2. Identify common approaches to mental health promotion across the life span.
3. Discuss common contexts for mental health promotion needs assessments and activities, including the family, schools, workplace, and community.
4. Describe and evaluate evidence-based interventions to promote mental health and prevent mental illness.
5. Differentiate strategies used in translating evidence-based practices to actual communities and populations.

INTRODUCTION

Mental health promotion is an important focus for nursing intervention given the proportion of individuals who present with problems directly or indirectly related to their mental health. It is estimated that the worldwide burden of disease from mental and substance use disorders is higher than that of any other health problem, accounting for 22.9% of all years lived with disability in the global population. In addition, this burden increased by 37.6% from 1990 to 2010 (Whiteford et al., 2013). Global Health 2035 is an effort to promote health and prevent morbidity and mortality. It includes a focus on noncommunicable diseases, which in turn includes behavioral health risk factors (smoking, substance use, and physical activity) (Jamison et al., 2013).

Mental health refers to a state of mental or emotional wellness required for good physical health and overall well-being. Mental health is broader than the absence of a diagnosable mental illness or disorder, encompassing everything from how we cope with life's ups and downs to our ability to achieve goals and form healthy relationships with others. Mental health promotion, a tool used to prevent movement on a continuum from mental wellness to mental illness, focuses on encouraging health behaviors and lifestyles that lower or limit the risk of future mental health problems or illness. Strategies of mental health promotion include interventions focused on stress management; coping skills; relationship skills; and interpersonal, economic, and environmental supports.

Mental illness prevention is focused on common mental disorders such as depression, anxiety, and substance use disorders. Prevention may also include interventions focused on crisis and disaster management to limit the negative impact of trauma on individuals, families, and communities.

This chapter first describes areas of mental health promotion and identifies how each intersects with the systems or ecologic context. Then, common areas of mental illness prevention are briefly identified. Finally, an evidence-based patient, intervention, control, observation, and time (PICOT) question is identified for a mental health promotion activity: home visiting to improve attachment and mental health outcomes in early childhood. The evidence for the intervention is presented, evaluated, and discussed in terms of its applicability and readiness for implementation.

MODELS OF MENTAL HEALTH PROMOTION

Ecological models envision mental health with an interactive systems framework. This approach considers the holistic context of an individual and his or her interactions with and relationships to multiple levels or spheres, including the self, significant others, social supports, vocational and avocational activity, community, culture, economics, and the environment. Early systems theory, developed by von Bertalanffy (1975), provided a template for considering the varied and dynamic interactive effects of different levels of any system, positing that changes in any single level of the system have ripple effects on other aspects of the system. Each sphere involves an assortment of interactions that require good mental health for effective functioning as well as positive quality of life for both individuals and communities. The interdependence across levels of a system is important to consider, and the ideas of systems seeking balance or homeostasis and using feedback to evolve or maintain function continuously are important concepts of systems theory that can be applied to the understanding of mental health.

To define mental health promotion, we must define mental health. A healthy mental state requires that individuals have the capacity to negotiate social and environmental contexts. Many skills are prerequisite to this capability, including the development of initial attachments to and bonds with others, the ability to manage emotion and behavior, and competency in communication. These skills are the foundation for developing interpersonal relationships and concomitant healthy group and community support systems. They are used to cope with adversity and provide a sense of positive self-esteem, social inclusion, and mastery.

Individual-level competence is needed for social interaction, emotional control, and the ability to manage interpersonal relationships and behavior. Coping with the normal stress of life, working productively, and contributing to social and community groups are important outcomes of mental health. Examples of individual mental health promotion activities may include coping skills, stress management, communication skills, building healthy relationships, and involvement in support groups or activities. These groups may be specific to common challenges in life such as grief, relationship changes, or activities that promote social inclusion.

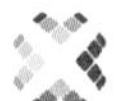

Case Illustration

Denise is a 15-year-old high school student who presents for care at the community health center urgent-care department; she has sustained a bloody nose after an argument with her boyfriend, Carl. Denise reports they had been arguing about his involvement with an older friend who dropped out of school and had been in trouble recently with the police. Denise and Carl have been together about 2 months and she describes the relationship as "up and down." She relates that he has a bad temper and gets into fights a lot at school. This is the first time that an argument became physical.

Denise lives with her two younger siblings and her parents in a three-family house, and her grandparents live downstairs. Her father was recently laid off. Denise reports that he has been out a lot lately looking for work, and her mother has been working more to make ends meet. She identifies that she has had a good relationship with both parents; however, recently neither parent has been around much, and she has often had to manage the household when her parents were at work or away from home.

Denise is referred to the school health clinic where she can see a counselor and the nurse practitioner to follow up on her injury. She is encouraged to use the counselor as a support to help her work out issues in her relationship with Carl. The provider gives Denise information about resources related to intimate partner violence in their area, including a support group for teen victims of abuse that focuses on improving coping, self-esteem, communication skills, and relationship skills.

Mental health promotion activities might include a focus on attachment; adaptation to developmental transitions; cognitive development; communication skills; interpersonal relationships; sense of self (self-esteem); emotion and mood regulation; regulation and control of behavior; sleep; nutrition; stress management and coping; activity, achievement, and meaning; spirituality; intimacy and healthy intimate relationships; parenting skills; anger management; assertiveness training; sexuality; diversity; environmental opportunities; and economic supports. These activities are necessary for good mental health, and some clearly overlap with physical health promotion. Areas of prevention focus on preventing negative outcomes and limiting disability associated with anxiety disorders, substance use and abuse, depression, suicide, and psychosis.

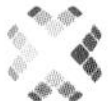

Case Illustration

Denise meets with the nurse practitioner, who asks about Denise's relationship with Carl and whether they are sexually active. She denies any plans to have sex with Carl, and reports that things had not gone very far with them beyond kissing. She reports he is interested in more, but she is not and does not want to take this step with him. She notes that she is a good student and plans to go to college and does not want to get involved with Carl in this way because she thinks it would interfere with her future plans. The nurse invites Denise to return to care if she is considering sexual activity with Carl and provides her with condoms for protection in case she gets involved in a situation where they are needed.

Levels of Prevention

It is important to consider the context of public health intervention through the lens of health promotion and the levels of disease prevention. One framework uses a matrix of interventions in public health (Gordon, 1983) that specifies the groups or populations that would benefit from each level of intervention. Integrated into this model is the public health model, which identifies three levels of prevention: primary, secondary, and tertiary. Health promotion is considered part of the first level, an aspect of primary prevention that occurs prior to disease development.

Other interventions at the primary prevention level include vaccines that prevent the development of a disease or disorder. In the primary prevention of psychiatric disorders, we are not able yet to prevent specific disorders or illnesses definitively through vaccines or other methods; however, consideration and attention to the mental health promotion activities described above may improve resilience, resistance, and individual outcomes should a psychiatric disorder occur.

Secondary prevention involves early identification and intervention to reduce morbidity from psychiatric disorders. Psychiatry has made progress in limiting morbidity using models to identify and intervene earlier in psychosis. For example, the Specialized Treatment Early in Psychosis (STEP) model, a collaboration between the Connecticut Department of Mental Health and Addiction Services and the Yale University Department of Psychiatry, centers on an interdisciplinary team to provide comprehensive care when initial symptoms of psychosis develop. They strive to prevent the disabling effects of further symptoms. Treatment starts with comprehensive assessment to understand the individual, followed by strategies including community coaching, individual and group therapy, medication management, and support for family and friends (Yale School of Medicine, 2020).

Substance use is another area with clear programs for early intervention. One of the most common implementation strategies in this realm is the Screening, Brief Intervention, and Referral to Treatment (SBIRT) model. Using this model, providers from any specialty learn to deliver a brief intervention that uses motivational interviewing and cognitive behavioral techniques to promote reduced risky substance-related behaviors (SAMHSA-HRSA Center for Integrated Health Solutions, 2020).

Tertiary prevention involves the limitation of disability and further morbidity associated with diseases or disorders, with interventions such as a visiting nurse, direct care, and assessment to identify further complications; treatment to improve the signs and symptoms of chronic conditions; and health teaching about diseases, treatments, and ways to reduce risk of complications. The levels of prevention are aligned with the absence or presence of disease as well as the severity of the illness associated with the condition. Many health conditions change in severity over time and exist on a continuum with improvements and exacerbations, without a clear starting point or consistent level of severity. This is also true for psychiatric disorders. Many psychiatric disorders do not start with a clear indicator but with a gradual series of changes that may culminate in crisis, after which a disorder is diagnosed.

Another approach to mental health promotion is to evaluate the focus or target of the intervention, which Gordon (1983) identified in a matrix of levels of intervention from universal strategies designed to have an impact on anyone in a population, to selective or targeted interventions that focus on particular groups at risk for a specific disorder, to indicated preventive interventions where persons with very high risk due to the presence of some symptom or condition are the focus of intervention or health promotion activity. Culture, environment, and access to economic opportunity are important predisposing factors that affect an individual's ability to function at her or his highest level of adaptation. Offering mental health promotion activities as a universal strategy ensures that individuals at greatest

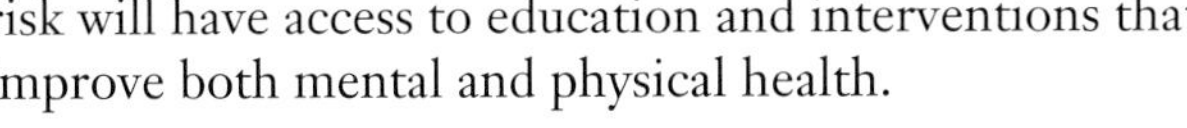

risk will have access to education and interventions that improve both mental and physical health.

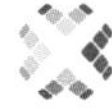

Case Illustration

Before leaving the appointment, the nurse also asks about Denise's follow-up with the counselor and a relationships skills support group. The support group would be considered a secondary level of intervention because Denise has already experienced some violence at the hands of her partner, and the group would be expected to help prevent further relationship problems. From the perspective of the matrix of interventions, this intervention is a selective or targeted one, offered to individuals at risk for further violence in relationships.

Levels of Care

Levels of care include health promotion activities purely for wellness, acute supportive activities aimed at reducing distress and treating acute issues, and intervention to manage diagnosable mental health conditions that require attention over time. Wellness or mental health promotion activities may focus on improving coping skills or developing support systems and include structuring activities that promote adaptation both developmentally and with expected life transitions. Acute supportive activities promote continued coping and resilience when traumatic events, losses, or stressors push individuals beyond their normal ability to manage feelings, maintain healthy relationships, or function in expected roles. Interventions for diagnosable conditions involve treatments that support continued function individually, in relationships, and within roles.

Along with consideration of actual areas of mental health promotion, nurses must recognize that mental illness comes with stigma and stereotypes that are embedded in our society. Activity to promote mental health is often marginalized and given lower priority than physical health promotion initiatives. However, reports by the Surgeon General and World Health Organization (WHO) clearly delineate the importance and integral nature of mental health to good health (U.S. Department of Health and Human Services, 1999; World Health Organization, 2005). For example, most individuals and health plans consider a yearly physical examination an important feature of health promotion and maintenance; however, there is no equivalent annual examination of mental health and well-being.

MENTAL HEALTH PROMOTION PRIORITIES

Priorities for mental health promotion are important across the life span; however, experiences in our most formative years have a serious impact on later life. Adverse and traumatic events in childhood are known to affect our ability to develop a healthy sense of self, regulate emotion and behavior, engage in healthy relationships, benefit from social supports, and manage the challenges we face in life. The Adverse Childhood Experiences (ACEs) study (SAMHSA, 2016) provides evidence that childhood trauma has a major impact on adult health and mental health. While 63% of individuals reported experiencing one or more types of childhood trauma, 20% experienced three or more types. These experiences account for 50% to 67% of serious drug problems. As the number of traumatic experiences increases, so does the risk of substance use, smoking, obesity, sexually transmitted diseases (STDs), depression, post-traumatic stress disorder (PTSD), and hallucinations, in addition to chronic diseases like chronic obstructive pulmonary disease (COPD) and ischemic heart disease (IHD) (Bright, Knapp, Hinojosa, Alford, & Bonner, 2016; Feliti et al., 1998; SAMHSA, 2016; Schilling, Aseltine, & Gore, 2007). Efforts to reduce these experiences could have a major impact on reducing health and mental health problems in later life.

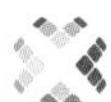

Case Illustration

Denise meets with the school counselor and reports that she is worried about Carl, who has been using more substances recently and often seems to be on edge. She reports that they got together after realizing that they both were having a bad time with their families and could relate to each other about this. She tells the counselor that she is worried that Carl is throwing away his future by becoming more involved with substance use and other drug-related activity and missing a lot of school. Denise explains that Carl lives with his mother and siblings and that his father, who is a cocaine addict, was recently incarcerated for beating his mother. The counselor encourages Denise to bring Carl to a future appointment so that she can engage him in services also.

Attachment and Promotion of Healthy Relationships

An important aspect of mental health is our ability to relate to others, convey our thoughts and feelings and feel understood, and provide reflection and empathy in response to others. This important area is often not addressed directly in health-promoting activities, even though effective communication is the cornerstone of all human experience.

Attachment may be the most important aspect of relationships because it forms a foundation for all such interactions across the life span. From our initial bonding with caregivers to relationships we form over time, we develop patterns of relating that contribute to our sense of security, competency, and self-esteem. Bowlby (1969) developed a theory of attachment focusing on relationship quality and access to attachment figures and their connection to a child's experience of competency, security, and feeling loved. Similar patterns of attachment can be seen in intimate relationships in adulthood, which also means that attachment has an impact on parenting.

Parenting

Relationships with caregivers are important, and interventions that support parenting may have a positive impact on the mental health of children later in life. Morgan, Brugha, Fryers, and Stewart-Brown (2012) found that caring, supportive relationships with parents were protective of children's adult mental health and that overcontrol in relationships increased the risk of poor mental health, regardless of socioeconomic status. When the impact of attachments and family relationships is considered in relation to adult development and resilience, it is striking that our culture has no universal commitment to a paradigm of preparation for parenting. However, several programs are available to provide education and support in developing parenting skills. Minding the Baby (Sadler et al., 2013) is a program that provides psychoeducation and support in promoting secure attachment, developing reflective parenting skills, and enhancing the self-efficacy of mothers in caring for their children. This program also promotes the physical health and development of the child and maternal health by providing home visits, with a nurse practitioner and a social worker, from pregnancy through early childhood.

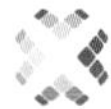

Case Illustration

Denise attends the relationship skills group and finds that it helps her share her views more assertively with Carl on the activities they engage in when they are together. In her follow-up appointment with the nurse practitioner, Denise discloses that at times they go further sexually than she plans to, and she reports that she is worried that she missed her period this month. A pregnancy test reveals that Denise is pregnant. The nurse refers Denise to a school-based parenting program and offers to meet with Denise and her boyfriend or parents if she would like to discuss her plans.

Interpersonal Relationships and Social Supports

People are innately social beings and an aspect of health relates to the ability to connect with and relate to others. Programs exist to encourage development of interpersonal and social skills in children. Many schools offer social learning programs to enhance the learning from the home environment, such as the "Stop and Think" Social Skills Program (Knoff & Batsche, 1995), Primary Mental Health Project (Cowen et al., 1963; Cowen, Zax, Izzo, & Trost, 1966), the EQUIP program (Gibbs, Potter, & Goldstein, 1995), the PREPARE curriculum (Goldstein, 1988), and the ACCEPTS program (Walker, 1983. In a meta-analysis of social and emotional learning programs in schools, Durlak, Weissberg, Dymnicki, Taylor, and Schellinger (2011) found an average effect size in the intervention groups of 0.22 and 0.24 for reducing conduct problems and emotional distress, respectively ($p \leq 0.05$ for both). These results generally agree with prior reviews on these outcomes.

Intimate relationships and sexuality are also of significant importance to mental health across the life span. Often, information that would serve to enhance intimate relationships and have an impact on levels of domestic and intimate partner violence is lacking or unavailable.

Sense of Self, Communication Skills, Emotions and Mood, and Behavioral Regulation

From early childhood through adulthood, we continually learn about ourselves and build self-esteem through experiences and interactions with others. Self-esteem is our assessment and acceptance of who we are by acknowledging our strengths and limitations. It involves believing in our own worth and not relying too heavily on the judgment of others. Having skill in the ability of relating to others is important. Knowledge of the various components of communication helps individuals ensure that the messages they intend to communicate are conveyed and received and that they allow for feedback if interpretation is not straightforward.

Within relationships, emotions may be triggered that complicate communication. Emotional regulation, which involves learning to recognize, identify, and manage emotions, is an important developmental milestone. Behavioral regulation allows us to manage the ups and downs of life as well as changes in rules and roles. Anger management and assertiveness education are helpful in reducing aggressive behavior and its impact on individuals, families, and groups. Emotional and social skill programs assist learners to develop these important interpersonal skills further.

Self-Efficacy and Resilience

Self-efficacy is the perception that one is competent and able to manage life. Bandura's concept of self-efficacy provides a framework focused on an individual's confidence in her or his ability to manage future situations (Bandura, 1998). Positive self-efficacy leads to resilience in coping with difficult life situations. Resilience refers to adapting well to adversity despite the traumatic events, pain, sadness, and distress we may experience. Characteristics of resilient individuals include optimism and the ability to balance negative and positive emotions. These concepts are important outcomes of mental health promotion activity. In their review, Mann, Hosman, Schaalma, and de Vries (2004) found lower self-esteem in childhood predicts later life depression, plays a role in anxiety and eating disorders, and increases risk for substance abuse (p. 361). On the other hand, they found positive self-efficacy and resilience are associated with avoidance of high-risk behaviors (p. 362).

Stress Management

Cannon (1914) first described "fight or flight" as the physiologic response to a challenging or dangerous situation that promotes secretion of catecholamines or a sympathetic adrenal medullary response. Modern threats, however, typically don't require the physical exertion for which this adrenaline response prepares us, which means this reaction most often occurs in response to social threats. Perceptions of stress are correlated with physiologic responses (Frankenhaeuser, 1988; Fujiwara et al., 2004 & Lundberg, Holmberg), such as adrenal dysregulation, which changes cortisol and catecholamine levels that are associated with chronic physical and mental disorders, including diabetes, depression, and heart disease.

Understanding the physiologic and psychologic responses to stressful situations is important because of the connections between stress and health. As with other conditions, predisposing, precipitating, and perpetuating factors affect our ability to adapt to or manage stressors. Stress management interventions can include mindfulness techniques, meditation, or relaxation training. A multitude of other topics might be included in the frame of mental health promotion, including attention to healthy levels of sleep, nutrition, activity, and exercise. Meeting higher-level needs related to sense of meaning and purpose as well as spirituality are also important to mental health.

Substance Use and Abuse

SBIRT is a program that offers mechanisms for early identification of harmful and hazardous substance use and intervention to reduce risky behavior that may ultimately result in substance abuse and its negative sequelae (Kaner et al., 2018). The focus of the program is first to assess for the presence and severity of harmful or hazardous use of alcohol or substances. Next steps involve increasing awareness of and motivation to change behavior and identifying steps that could be taken to reduce the risk of negative outcomes (SAMHSA, 2017). The integration of SBIRT into clinical settings provides greater access to early intervention that may help to prevent problems and reduce the impact of substance abuse.

Suicide

Suicide is one of the leading causes of death, and for each suicide death, 25 people make suicide attempts (Drapeau & McIntosh, 2016). Suicide is related to many other problems, including mental illness, trauma, violence, and substance abuse, so suicide prevention efforts must be comprehensive and coordinated to have an impact on the many risk factors. Prevention strategies developed nationally include many of the kinds of programs already described that promote mental health. In addition, public awareness is important so that individuals in every community are knowledgeable of the risks for suicide and can encourage individuals at risk to seek help. Health providers must be able to recognize suicide risk and identify accurately, intervene, and refer individuals to the appropriate care needed to prevent suicide attempts and death.

Tools exist for use in a variety of settings to screen for and assess the nature and need for referral of suicide-related behaviors, including the Columbia Suicide Severity Rating scale (Posner et al., 2011). In addition, tools for use in psychiatric or behavioral settings, such as the Collaborative Assessment and Management of Suicidality (CAMS) clinical framework and Suicide Status Form (SSF) (Jobes, 2009) can guide treatment. Treatment promotes social support, problem-solving skills, resilience, and intervention for commonly comorbid problems such as depression and anxiety.

Early Treatment of Psychosis

A variety of factors contribute to the risk of psychosis, including brain development, genetics, and substance use. In 2016, more than 1 million people in the United States were diagnosed with schizophrenia, and the prevalence of 0.3% is similar to that in other countries (Charlson et al., 2018). Despite the lower prevalence compared to other disorders, the burden of disease associated with schizophrenia is high, contributing 13.4 million years of life lived with disability (YLD) globally in 2016 (Charlson, et al., 2018).

Current thought suggests that if individuals with either prodromal or mild symptoms were identified early, the course of the illness trajectory could be changed beneficially with intervention (Srihari et al., 2014). Innovative programs such as the STEP program that provide specialized services to those in their first episode of illness have been successful in significantly reducing the number of inpatient hospitalizations as well as improving global functioning and vocational outcomes (Srihari et al., 2015).

Traumatic Events

Traumatic events such as natural disasters occur with some regularity. Approximately a third of individuals with severe exposure to trauma may develop PTSD or some other mental health problem (North & Pfefferbaum, 2013). Given that trauma is ubiquitous, disaster planning efforts must include ways to identify individuals most in need of mental health care and provide services to assist in prevention of further morbidity and treatment of needs. Several programs have been developed to prevent negative sequelae after disasters or traumatic events. These include psychological first aid, crisis counseling, and psychological debriefing. A review by North and Pfefferbaum (2013) concluded that insufficient evidence exists to establish whether these programs are beneficial in disaster settings. However, identification, triage, and intervention plans should be included in care planning efforts for individuals after a disaster or traumatic event (North & Pfefferbaum, 2013).

This chapter has reviewed a range of potential areas for mental health promotion and prevention of complications from mental disorders. Evidence-based practice should help guide the planning of mental health programs and interventions. An area of importance is in parent-child attachment and whether interventions that promote attachment and parenting skills have an impact on mental health outcomes in children.

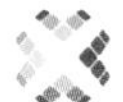

Case Illustration

Denise has decided to have the baby, and her parents are supportive of her decision. She will be able to live in her family home and raise the baby with the support of her parents and grandparents, who can provide some child care while Denise is at school. Denise enrolled in the school-based program for teen parents and is continuing her studies during her pregnancy. In her fifth month, she was referred to a home-based parenting support program for teen mothers. They provide regular home visits prenatally and into the second year of the baby's life. The focus of the program is helping Denise to have as healthy a pregnancy as possible and provide support for her coping and parenting skills. Denise and Carl broke up the month after Denise learned she was pregnant because Carl believed she should have an abortion. Denise did not agree, however, because it conflicted with her and her family's religious views.

PICOT QUESTION AND EVIDENCE: THE EFFECTS OF HOME-VISITING ATTACHMENT INTERVENTIONS ON PEDIATRIC MENTAL HEALTH

Given that attachment forms the basis for all future relationships, an important area for mental health promotion is parent-child attachment, bonding, and parenting skills. Families with limited resources to manage the multiple changes that occur with childbirth and child rearing are vulnerable. At even higher risk for adverse consequences are low-income, single-parent families. Programs that support this high-risk population could possibly improve outcomes for healthy births and child development, and promote healthy parent-child relationships to reduce children's risk of mental health disorders, including depression, anxiety, PTSD, and conduct and oppositional defiant disorders.

This is a difficult population to engage in interventions, and home-visiting programs have been found to be successful in reaching those most in need, improving mother-child attachment, and improving parenting skills (Kitzman, 2007). Interest in this question drove the evidence-based review PICOT question:

P: In single-parent, low-income households, does
I: home-visiting intervention from pregnancy through the first year of life,
C: compared to the usual prenatal and postnatal care,
O: improve attachment, bonding, physical health, and mental health outcomes
T: in early childhood (to age 5 years)?

Background

Low-income, single parents are a vulnerable population, subject to risks that have an impact on child outcomes. Interventions that enhance the quality of life and relationships for at-risk populations can improve outcomes for both the parent and child. The child outcomes are of particular interest given that negative outcomes could interfere with children's ability to learn and develop into healthy children, adolescents, and adults. Many programs have been identified and tested for impact on child health outcomes, including group interventions (Constantino et al., 2001; Heinrichs, Kliem, & Hahlweg, 2014; Niccols, 2008), video feedback interventions (Cassibba, Castoro, Constantino, Sette, & van Ijzendoorn, 2015; Kalinauskiene et al., 2009; Landry, Smith, & Swank, 2006; Negrao, Pereira, Soares, & Mesman, 2014; Velderman, Bakermans-Kranenburg, Juffer, & van Ijzendoorn, 2006), and center-based education programs for young children (Bradley, McKelvey, & Whiteside-Mansell, 2011). A difficulty with many of these programs is the inability of high-risk, low-income families to participate in center-based studies due to their lack of supports and resources. As a result, many programs have high attrition or do not include younger single mothers from low socioeconomic status contexts.

Home-based visiting programs have been successful in bringing resources and support into single-parent homes to improve parent and child outcomes (Akai, Guttenta, Baggett, Willard Noria, & Centers for the Prevention of Child Neglect, 2008; Cooper et al., 2009; Eckenrode et al., 2010; Fraser, Armstrong, Morris & Dadds, 2000; Heinicke et al., 1999; Kitzman et al., 1997; Kitzman et al., 2010; Olds, Henderson, Chamberlin, & Tatelbaum, 1986; Olds et al., 1997; Olds et al., 1998; Olds, 2002; Olds et al., 2002; Olds, Holmberg, et al., 2014; Olds, Kitzman, et al., 2014; Sadler et al., 2013; Van den Boom, 1995). These effects include reduced rates of substance abuse among mothers (Olds et al., 1997; Olds et al., 2010); lower rates of subsequent pregnancy (Landsverk et al., 2002; Olds, 2002); and improved occupational and financial outcomes for families (Olds, 2002), with reduced reliance on Aid to Families with Dependent Children (AFDC) (Olds et al., 2010).

Given the dual nature of the intervention (for both mother and child), it is important to understand the impact of the intervention on the child in the low-income, single-parent household. Prior reviews of cross-sectional and longitudinal studies have found an association between attachment and child mental health outcomes, including improved attachment security (Bakermans-Karnenburg, van Ijzendoorn, & Juffer, 2003; Brumariu & Kerns, 2010; Colonnesi et al., 2011; De Wolff & van Ijzendoorn, 1997; Fraley, 2002; Fukkink, 2008; Groh et al., 2014; Madigan, Atkinson, Laurin, & Benoit, 2013; Schneider, Atkinson, & Tardif, 2001). This observational data has evaluated outcomes in children from as early as 12 months to 19 years (Bakermans-Karnenburg et al., 2003; Brumariu & Kerns, 2010; Colonnesi et al., 2011; De Wolff & van Ijzendoorn, 1997; Fearon, Bakermans-Kranenburg, van Ijzendoorn, Lapsley, & Roisman, 2010; Groh et al., 2014). Prior studies have shown a particular increase in strength of this relationship at older ages (Brumariu &Kerns, 2010; Colonnesi et al., 2011; Schneider et al., 2001). These results provide some foundation for the idea that interventions that affect parenting, maternal sensitivity, and attachment security have the potential to improve childhood physical and mental health outcomes.

Evidence supports the impact of home-visiting interventions from prenatal to early childhood and that those impacts seem to be stronger as the child ages, so the PICOT question was revised to: In single-parent, low-income households does home-visiting intervention from pregnancy through the first year of life, compared to usual prenatal and postnatal care, improve mental health outcomes in childhood and adolescence?

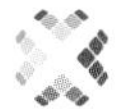

Case Illustration

Denise continues to have the nurse home visitors for a year after the birth of her child, a girl that she named Ariel. She has not been involved in a relationship since breaking up with Carl. The baby is healthy, and Denise has been able to continue with school, with the support of her parents and grandparents. Denise reports that she has learned a lot about how to care for her child from the home-visiting program and that she feels like she has her own coach to offer her tips and ideas about how to manage as a single mom and help her baby stay heathy and reach developmental milestones. Denise reports she is doing well in school and still hopes to attend college when she finishes high school.

Review of Evidence

To answer this PICOT question, a systematic evidence review was completed of randomized controlled trials providing home-visiting intervention to promote children's mental health. Databases, including Medline, Psych Info, and Cumulative Index to Nursing and Allied Health Literature (CINAHL) from 2000 to 2016, were searched. Search terms included: *pregnancy*, *prenatal care*, *parenting skills*, *parenting*, and combined with *attachment*, *bonding*, *parent-child relationships*; *mental health*; and limited to *parent* or *child*; *child development*, *low-income*; *home-visiting interventions*, and *randomized controlled trials* (RCTs).

A total of 14 reviews, systematic reviews, and meta-analyses were found that involved the variables of interest; 10 of these were excluded because they did not review RCTs, which left four reviews. Of these, one was a report of RCTs from an investigator that was included in the review of individual RCTs (Olds, 2002). Two were discussions of evidence and did not present methods or search criteria that would be expected in a systematic review (Kitzman, 2007; Olds, Sadler, & Kitzman, 2007), although they were specific to the PICOT question and provided information on studies implemented in the field from 1982 to the present and included discussion of RCTs on home-visiting programs from pregnancy to age 2. Both provided a narrative review of attachment and child mental health outcomes. The remaining review by Fukkink (2008) was of video feedback interventions, most of which were implemented after infancy and many in families referred due to clinical need; thus, this review did not meet the required focus on preventive intervention.

The search strategy identified a total of 36 individual studies. The results included 27 RCTs as well as quasi-experimental, longitudinal, cross-sectional, and case reports of home-visiting interventions and reports of associations between attachment and health outcomes in children. From the 27 RCTs, only 12 involved home-visit interventions from pregnancy to 2 years, and child mental health or cognitive development outcomes were reported in only 10 studies. Of the 10, only five represented unique studies with unique samples; the others were reports from extended follow-ups over time (up to age 20) of the original interventions implemented from pregnancy to age 2 years. Another four included interventions initiated close to birth, although only one included discussion of child mental health or cognitive development.

One RCT review involving home visiting specifically focused on videotaped parenting programs. Some studies also included cognitive development and child mental health as outcomes (Fukkink, 2008). Of the 29 studies reviewed by Fukkink (2008), 13 were RCTs, although most involved interventions initiated later in childhood rather than during pregnancy. Of the four RCTs reported whose interventions were initiated prior to the child reaching 6 months of age, only one study followed children more than 1 year, and the study duration fell short of 18 months for follow-up. Results from this review suggested that short but powerful interventions were more effective, which supports results of reviews on other outcomes (Bakermans-Kranenburg et al., 2003). Results on children's behavior had a small to moderate effect size of 0.33 ($p < 0.05$); however, effects for those during the prenatal to early childhood period were not broken out for analysis, so the impact of intervention during this period cannot be identified.

Kitzman (2007) offers a narrative discussion of home-visiting interventions for low-income families that raises many of the same concerns about evidence of effect identified by Olds (2007). These concerns include the lack of consistency of results, small effect sizes, and the difficulty in comparing programs implemented and outcomes tracked in disparate ways. Programs have had a beneficial impact on reducing pregnancy and improving maternal health and behavior during pregnancy, as well as improved maternal sensitivity and attachment outcomes. Mixed results have been found in reducing child abuse and neglect, injury and ingestions, and cognitive development. Results suggest that those who benefit most are adolescent, low-income, and socially disadvantaged mothers with their first child. It is difficult to determine the specific aspects of intervention that are most effective because of the heterogeneity of interventions and outcomes studied.

Olds, Sadler, & Kitzman (2007) published a review of intervention studies of home visiting from pregnancy to age 3, and the effects of this intervention on both child health and development. They report overall that nurse home visitors had the strongest evidence of improvement of prenatal and postnatal physical and mental health for both mother and child (Olds et al., 2007, p. 383). Reviewing interventions that had mixed results, Olds, Sadler, and Kitzman (2007) point out the difficulties in evaluating the results of studies that use varied models of intervention and suggest researchers ground interventions in theory and carefully ensure that the elements of the intervention are replicated in randomized controlled trials to determine the effect in varied populations. They identify the promise that program interventions by professional and nurse home visiting specifically seem to have on children's health and development. Olds, Sadler, and Kitzman (2007) identify several programs as having positive outcomes on child development and mental health:

- The Infant Health and Development Program (IHDP) intervened with 1 year of home visiting from birth followed by two years of group or center-based interventions. This intervention had a positive impact on academic achievement at age 3 and risky behaviors at age 18. However, this impact was evident only for the babies at the highest weight, and thus at the lowest risk.
- Healthy Family Alaska (HFAK) offered home visits by paraprofessionals for at-risk families and children. The intervention group, at 2 years old, scored higher on cognitive development, and these children were reported to have fewer behavior problems by their mother. Lower-risk families at baseline also had better outcomes with the intervention.
- Healthy Family San Diego (HFSD) used home visitors with higher levels of education than the HFAK and HSP programs and found that at 1 and 2 years, the children tested higher on mental functioning, but there was no significant difference at 3 years.
- Early Head Start (EHS) involved multiple modalities, including home visiting by paraprofessionals, center-based care, and parent education, although specific programs vary. Children in EHS had better cognitive and language development and better emotional engagement and attention, and parents reported less aggressive behavior than controls, although home-visit-only programs did not have significant effects for children at age 3.
- The New Zealand Early Start program, consisting of postnatal home visits by nurses and social workers, showed beneficial effects on parenting measures and use of health services, but child measures were not included.
- The UCLA Family Development project involves home visiting from pregnancy to age 2 by mental health professionals and a support group program for mothers of first children at risk. At age 12 months, intervention children were more likely to have secure attachment, more task endurance, greater sense of separate self, and less noncompliance than the control group, although there were no significant differences in development.
- The Nurse-Family Partnership (NFP), a series of interventions implemented in three different sites chosen for the ability to evaluate effectiveness of the intervention in a rural low-income population (Elmira, New York), in a low-income, minority urban population (Memphis, Tennessee), and with paraprofessional as well as nurse home visitors (Denver, Colorado).
    - In the Elmira, New York, trial, youth in the intervention group at age 12 years had fewer arrests and adjudications than the control group, with greater effects in those at highest risk, although there were no effects on behavior problems.
    - In the Memphis, Tennessee, trial, children had fewer injuries and ingestions at age 6, they had higher intellectual functioning and vocabulary with fewer behavior problems, and those in some higher-risk groups were less aggressive and had better academic achievement (math).
    - In the Denver, Colorado, arm, home visiting by paraprofessionals (versus nurses) was evaluated. Paraprofessionals did not produce the same outcomes as nurses, although parent sensitivity and home environments were improved. Nurse-visited children had fewer language delays, particularly in those with higher risk, who at ages 2 and 4 had better language and cognitive development, as well as behavioral adaptation versus a control group. This trial showed that paraprofessional visitors had approximately half the effect of nurse home visitors.
    - The economic costs of NFP were beneficial, with a $17,000 return on investment when the three trials were examined.
- The Early Intervention Program (EIP) served adolescent mothers and provided home visits from mid-pregnancy to approximately 1 year, supplemented with a group pregnancy intervention. Compared to public health nursing visits (two prenatal and one postnatal visit), results were promising, with beneficial effects on rate of hospitalization involving injuries versus the control group.
- The Baltimore program for drug-exposed infants found nurse-visited children had fewer parent reports of behavioral and emotional problems using the Child Behavior Checklist (CBCL) versus the control group.

Some programs reviewed by Olds, Sadler, and Kitzman (2007) had mixed or no significant difference from the control group:

- The Hawaii Healthy Start Program (HSP), which provided paraprofessional home visits for 3 to 5 years to vulnerable families identified during pregnancy, did not have effects on psychomotor development to age 3. Mixed results on other variables may have resulted from family dropouts and variability in the intervention across study sites.
- Parents as Teachers (PAT), involving home visiting during pregnancy or near birth up to 3 years, was able to improve school readiness in pilot studies in California trials, including one with teen mothers. Intervention children had more advanced cognitive development and better social development and self-help skills than those reported by mothers in the control group; however, there was no difference on the Bayley test scores, and some trials did not have effects on children.
- The PAT model augmented with the Born to Learn model had mixed effects, with only low socioeconomic status (SES) families exceeding the control group in cognitive development and adaptive behavior at 2 years, but not 3 years, although social skills were better at 3 years in the PAT children.
- The Comprehensive Child Development Program (CCDP) used paraprofessional home visitors and center-based education to age 5 years with no effect on child achievement or behavior.

Overall recommendations from the review by Olds, Sadler, and Kitzman (2007) are that programs of intervention have specific piloting and development prior to investment in larger RCTs, so that efficacy studies and then effectiveness trials can evaluate outcomes based on pilots that offer the most promising results. In addition, replication of interventions must be careful to follow the original models to build the foundation of evidence-based practice methods to benefit mothers and children at risk. The importance of carefully testing and following up for effects on child development and mental health are important prior to making investments in delivering these programs on a wide basis in communities at risk.

Results from Randomized Controlled Trials

Individual studies were evaluated that met inclusion criteria for this review. Eckenrode et al. (2010); Kitzman et al., (1997, 2010); Olds, Holmberg, et al. (2014); and Olds, Kitzman, et al. (2014) report on interventions of the NFP on child development and mental health outcomes at ages 2, 6, 9, 12, 15, 19, and 20 years for programs implemented in Elmira, New York; Memphis, Tennessee; and Denver, Colorado. All studies had relatively good follow-up with minimal attrition given the length of follow-up in some instances (from 2 years to 20 years later).

Olds (2002) reported on a series of RCTs implemented in Elmira, New York; Memphis, Tennessee; and Denver, Colorado, using NFP intervention that involved home visiting from pregnancy to 2 years after birth. Data from the Colorado study were not available in the 2002 report; however, results from the Elmira and Memphis sites were reported from a total of 1,535 families; cognitive development of the child at age 2 and 4 years and mental health outcomes at 15 years were evaluated. Results from the Elmira trial found significant benefit in the NFP intervention group for both cognitive development and mental health outcomes. Kitzman et al. (1997, 2010) reported on cognitive development and mental health outcomes of the NFP intervention in Memphis at age 2 years (Kitzman et al., 1997) and age 12 years (Kitzman et al., 2010). Eckenrode et al. (2010) reported on results from NFP in Elmira at age 19 in participants. Olds later reported on results from the NFP in youth at ages 6 and 9 (Olds, Holmberg, et al., 2014, Denver, Colorado) and age 20 years (Olds, Kitzman, et al., 2014, Memphis, Tennessee).

Kitzman et al. (1997) followed up on the Memphis sample, an urban African American population, at age 2 and found no overall differences between groups for cognitive development or behavior problems. However, in families where mothers were at greatest risk due to lower psychological resources, children's responsiveness to their mothers was greater and homes were found to be more conducive to child development in the intervention group using the HOME scale ($p = 0.003$).

In later follow-up, Kitzman et al. (2010) found that 12-year-old children showed significantly less substance use in the past 30 days (cigarettes, alcohol, and marijuana) (Odds Ratio (OR) = 0.31, $p = 0.04$), fewer days of use (OR = 0.18, $p = 0.02$), and fewer internalizing disorders (22.1% in the intervention group versus 30.9% in the control group, $p = 0.04$). While there were no significant differences with externalizing or behavioral problems in these groups, for the low-resource mothers, the children had higher academic achievement scores on both the Peabody Inventory Achievement test (88.78 versus 85.7, $p = 0.009$) and standardized testing (reading and math, 40.52 versus 34.85, $p = 0.02$).

In the Denver trial reported by Olds, Holmberg, et al. (2014), which compared paraprofessional intervention versus nurse intervention with follow-up at ages 6 and 9, there were no significant effects on emotional and behavior problems. However, nurse-visited children were less likely to have emotional problems at 6 years (Relative Risk (RR) = 0.45, p = 0.08), and less internalizing (RR = 0.44, p = 0.08) and fewer attention problems (RR = 0.34, p = 0.07) at 9 years. Children of mothers with few resources had significantly better language (averaged age 2, 4, and 6 years; d = 0.30, p = 0.01) and sustained attention (age 4, 6, and 9 years; d = 0.36, p = 0.006). There were no significant effects on externalizing, intellect, or academic achievement, although there were stronger effects of nurse intervention in adverse neighborhoods.

Eckenrode et al. (2010) and Olds, Kitzman, et al. (2014) evaluated outcomes at age 19 years in the Elmira, New York, study and at age 20 years in the Memphis, Tennessee, study. In the Elmira study, only girls in the intervention group were at decreased risk of criminal involvement (10% intervention group versus 30% in the control group) or arrest (4% intervention versus 20% in the control group), resulting in a relative risk of 0.33 (95% Confidence Interval (CI) 0.15–0.82) and 0.20 (95% CI of 0.05–0.85) for each outcome, respectively. There were no differences in educational achievement between groups. In the Memphis study, at age 20, there had been fewer deaths from preventable causes (including Sudden Infant Death Syndrome (SIDS), injury, and homicide), with no deaths in the intervention group versus 1.6% in the control group.

Heinicke et al. (1999, 2001) evaluated the PAT program for outcomes at ages 6 months and 1 year for attachment and cognitive development, as well as at 2 years for cognitive development and mental health. No effect was found for cognitive development in either follow-up study; however, there were changes to the scale used between follow-up assessments that may have affected analyses. At 12 and 24 months (Heinicke et al., 2001), there was a significant difference in both the child's sense of separate self and less child noncompliance in the intervention versus control group, with an increasing effect size over time. At 24 months, there was greater child positive affect (d = 0.74, p = 0.004), and significantly better child task involvement as well as less externalization for intervention versus control families (p < 0.0001).

The last study was based in South Africa and involved community health worker home visits to mothers in pregnancy and up to 6 months postpartum based on WHO program principles (Improving the Psychosocial Development of Children, and the Social Baby). This sample included both low-risk (home had electricity) and higher-risk (no electricity in home) mothers, all of whom were living in poverty and low-resource areas. There were no significant differences overall in cognitive development, although the Bayley Mental Development Index scores were higher in the intervention group than in the control group (mean = 85.2 and 83.1, respectively; d = 0.20, p = 0.09).

Discussion of the Evidence

The results of these RCTs suggest that these programs benefit child cognitive development as well as mental health, particularly those programs with nurse home visitors and higher-risk mothers. These results are less consistent than the beneficial effects found from home-visiting interventions on parenting, maternal attachment, and sensitivity outcomes, as well as pregnancy and birth outcomes that are more specific to the intervention and fall closer in time to the end of the intervention period.

Results in higher-risk families offer interesting information about the impact of these interventions on child development and mental health. For example, the intervention in South Africa involved an extremely vulnerable population due to differences in basic resources such as housing and electricity compared to U.S.-based interventions. The Murray, Cooper, Arteche, Stein and Tomlinson (2016) study found that the families most improved by the intervention were those in the less vulnerable group, which was defined by the presence of electricity in the home, which in turn would likely make this group analogous to the highest-risk groups in the United States.

Strengths and Limitations

Strengths of the evidence include a large number of studies that have had some outcome measures for child cognitive development and child mental health, although the results have been mixed. In addition, several of the studies offer repeated evaluation of the same model, such as NFP (Eckenrode et al., 2010; Kitzman et al., 1997; Kitzman et al., 2010; Olds et al., 2002, Olds, Holmberg, et al., 2014; Olds, Kitzman, et al., 2014) and PAT (Heinicke et al., 1997, 2001). The development and replication of these models offers information about both efficacy and effectiveness, particularly in the NFP studies, which provide replication of the model with some aspects that vary, including the population served (rural, urban, minority) and the provider of home visits (nurse, professional, paraprofessional).

Limitations do exist in the evidence; for example, that the intervention does not specifically focus on preventing problems with child cognitive development or mental health. Several differences can also be identified that may affect results. First, outcome measures are variable across even the same studies based on differences in how cognitive ability, development, and mental health are evaluated across age groups. Next, studies used paraprofessionals, mental health or child development professionals, community workers, and nurses to deliver the home-visiting intervention. It can be debated which individuals might be best suited to intervene with different populations, although it does appear that the most consistent evidence of beneficial impact comes from interventions with well-trained professionals in mental health or nursing.

Applying Evidence to Practice

It is important to consider both the costs and benefits to underserved populations who may benefit from the intervention. The programs that showed the most consistent results were also cost-effective, suggesting that implementing these interventions can result in government savings. The interventions seem most beneficial to at-risk families who have adolescent single mothers living in low-income areas with few psychological resources. Identification of these risk factors in young mothers and referral to programs that offer parenting skills and intervention as well as home-based programs are promising. However, additional evidence is needed to replicate the models that have had beneficial impact on child mental health and to discern more exactly how the intervention affects these outcomes. It is possible that other kinds of interventions more specifically focused on child mental health and cognitive development will offer equal or more benefit.

KEY POINTS

- Mental health and substance abuse result in higher systemic costs worldwide than any other chronic health issue.
- Mental health refers to a state of emotional well-being beyond the simple absence of mental illness.
- Mental health promotion focuses on encouraging behaviors and lifestyles that lower the risk of future mental illness.
- Mental health promotion includes interventions focused on stress management; coping skills; relationship skills; and interpersonal, economic and environmental supports.
- An interactive systems approach to mental health considers the holistic context of an individual and his or her relationships to multiple spheres, including the self, significant others, social supports, vocational and avocational activity, community, culture, economics, and environment.
- Adverse and traumatic events in childhood affect our ability to develop a healthy sense of self, regulate emotion and behavior, engage in healthy relationships, benefit from social supports, and manage life's challenges.
- Home-visit nurse interventions to low-income, single-parent households designed to have an impact on parenting, maternal sensitivity, and attachment can potentially improve childhood physical and mental health outcomes.

Check Your Understanding

1. A prevention strategy that is focused on early identification of depression by screening with a scale like the PHQ-9 in a primary-care setting is an example of which level of prevention?
   A. Health promotion
   B. Primary prevention
   C. Secondary prevention
   D. Tertiary prevention
2. Mental health promotion is a priority because:
   A. The burden of disease from mental illness has decreased since 1990.
   B. Mental and substance use disorders account for more than 20% of all years lived with disability.
   C. Depression is the leading cause of death in the United States.
   D. Schizophrenia is the most common mental disorder.
3. Which of the following is an example of a universal preventive intervention to promote mental health?
   A. Early intervention in youth showing signs of psychosis
   B. Group smoking cessation programs for smokers
   C. Vocational programs to promote individuals with mental illness to return to work
   D. Disaster preparedness planning and education campaigns
4. The ACEs study found that, as the number of traumatic experiences in childhood increases, the risk of all of the following also increase EXCEPT:
   A. Breast cancer
   B. COPD
   C. Depression and PTSD
   D. Obesity

5. All of the following are programs to promote social skills and social learning EXCEPT:
   A. Stop and Think
   B. EQUIP
   C. SBIRT
   D. ACCEPTS
6. Resilient individuals have characteristics that help them adapt to adversity, including which of the following?
   A. Behavioral regulation
   B. Pessimism
   C. Aggressive behavior
   D. Optimism
7. Cannon described the fight or flight response, which involves physiologic responses due to secretion of:
   A. Insulin and glucose
   B. Growth hormones and testosterone
   C. Catecholamines and cortisol
   D. IgG and IgM

See "Reflections on Check Your Understanding" at the end of the book for answers.

REFERENCES

Akai, C. E., Guttenta, C. L., Baggett, K. M., Willard Noria, C. C., & Centers for the Prevention of Child Neglect. (2008). Enhancing parenting practices of at-risk mothers. *Journal of Primary Prevention, 29*, 223–242.

Bakermans-Kranensburg, M. J., van Ijzendoorn, M. H., & Juffer, F. (2003). Less is more: Analyses of sensitivity and attachment interventions in early childhood. *Psychological Bulletin, 129*(2), 195–215.

Bandura, A. (1998). Health promotion from the perspective of social cognitive theory. *Psychology and Health, 13*, 623–649.

Bowlby, J. (1969). *Attachment*. New York, NY: Basic Books.

Bradley, R.H., McKelvey, L.M., & Whiteside-Mansell, L. (2011). Does the quality of stimulation and support in the home environment moderate the effect of early education programs? *Child Development, 82*(6), 2110–2122.

Bright, M. A., Knapp, C., Hinojosa, M. S., Alford, S. & Bonner, B.. (2016). The comorbidity of physical, mental, and developmental conditions associated with child adversity: A population based study. *Maternal and Child Health Journal, 20*, 843–853. doi:10.1007/s10995-015-1915-7

British Columbia Schizophrenia Society. (2003, May 15). Discover the facts: Educational kit for family and friends (Figure; J.A. Lieberman Relative prevalence of Schizophrenia) http://www.bcss.org/wp-content/uploads/relativeprevalence.jpg). Retrieved from http://www.bcss.org/resources/topics-by-audience/family-friends/2003/05/discover-the-facts/

Brumariu, L. E., & Kerns, K. A. (2010). Parent-child attachment and internalizing symptoms in childhood and adolescence: A review of empirical findings and future directions. *Development and Psychopathology, 22*, 171–203.

Cannon, W. B. (1914). The emergency function of the adrenal medulla in pain and the major emotions. *American Journal of Physiology, 33*, 356–372.

Cassibba, R., Castoro, G., Costantino, E., Sette, G., van Ijzendoorn, M. H. (2015). Enhancing maternal sensitivity and infant attachment security with video feedback: An exploratory study in Italy. *Infant Mental Health Journal, 35*(1), 53–61.

Charlson, F. J., Ferrari, A. J., Santomauro, D. F., Diminic, S., Stockings, E., Scott, J.G. . . . Whiteford, H. A. (2018). Global epidemiology and burden of schizophrenia: Findings from the Global Burden of Disease Study 2016. *Schizophrenia Bulletin*, https://doi.org/10.1093/schbul/sby058

Colonnesi, C., Draijer, E. M., Stams, G. J. J. M., Van der Bruggen, C. O., Bogels, S. M., & Noom, M. J. (2011). The relation between insecure attachment and child anxiety: A meta-analytic review, *Journal of Clinical Child & Adolescent Psychology, 40*(4), 630–645.

Constantino, J. N., Hashemi, N., Solis, E., Alon, T., Haley, S., McClure, S., . . . Carlson, V. K. (2001). Supplementation of urban home visitation with a series of group meetings for parents and infants: Results of a "real-world" randomized controlled trial. *Child Abuse & Neglect, 25*, 1571–1581.

Cooper, P. J., Tomlinson, M., Swartz, L., Landman, M., Molteno, C., Stein, A., . . . & Murray, L. (2009). Improving quality of mother-infant relationship and infant attachment in socioeconomically deprived community in South Africa: Randomized controlled trial. *British Medical Journal, 338:b974* doi:10.1136/bmj.b974.

Cowen, E. L., Izzo, L. D., Miles, H., Telschow, E. F., Trost, M. A., & Zax, M. (1963). A preventive mental health program in the school setting: Description and evaluation. Journal of Psychology: Interdisciplinary and Applied, *56*, 307–356.

Cowen, E. L., Zax, M., Izzo, L. D., & Trost, M. A. (1966). Prevention of emotional disorders in the school setting: A further investigation. *Journal of Consulting Psychology, 30*, 381–387.

De Wolff, M. S., van Ijzendoorn, M. H., (1997). Sensitivity and attachment: A meta-analysis on parental antecedents of infant attachment. *Child Development, 68*(4), 571–591.

Drapeau, C. W., & McIntosh, J. L. (for the American Association of Suicidology). (2016). U.S.A. suicide 2015: Official final data. Washington, DC: American Association of Suicidology. Retrieved from http://www.suicidology.org

Durlak, J. A., Weissberg, R. P., Dymnicki, A. B., Taylor, R. D., & Schellinger, K. B. (2011). The impact of enhancing students' social and emotional learning: A meta-analysis of school-based universal interventions. *Child Development, 82*, 405–432.

Eckenrode, J., Campa, M., Luckey, D. W., Henderson, C. R., Cole, R., Kitzman, H., . . . Olds, D. (2010). Long-term effects of prenatal and infancy nurse home visitation on the life course of youths: 19-year follow-up of a randomized trial. *Archives of pediatric and Adolescent Medicine, 164*(1), 9–15.

Fearon, R. P., Bakermans-Kranenburg, M.J., van Ijzendoorn, M. H., Lapsley, A. M., & Roisman, G. I. (2010). The significance of insecure attachment and disorganization in the development of children's externalizing behavior: A meta-analytic study. *Child Development, 81*(2), 435-456.

Felitti, V. J., Anda, R. F., Nordenberg, D., Williamson, D. F., Spitz, A. M., Edwards, V., . . . Marks, J. S. (1998). Relationship of childhood abuse and household dysfunction to many of the leading causes of death in adults: The Adverse Childhood Experiences (ACE) study. *American Journal of Preventive Medicine, 14*, 245–258.

Fraley, R. C. (2002). Attachment stability from infancy to adulthood: Meta-analysis and dynamic modeling of developmental mechanisms. *Personality and Social Psychology Review, 6*(2), 123–151.

Fraser, J. A., Armstrong, K. L., Morris, J. P., & Dadds, M. R. (2000). Home visiting intervention for vulnerable families with newborns: Follow-up results of a randomized controlled trial. *Child Abuse & Neglect, 24*(11), 1399–1429.

Fujiwara, K., Tsukishima, E., Kasai, S., Masuchi, A., Tsutsumi, A., Kawakami, N., . . . Kishi, R. (2004). Urinary catecholamines and salivary cortisol on workdays and days off in relation to job strain among female health care providers. *Scandinavian Journal of Work, Environment, & Health, 30*(2), 129–138.

Fukkink, R. G. (2008). Video feedback in widescreen: A meta-analysis of family programs. *Clinical Psychology Review, 28*, 904–916.

Gibbs, J. C., Potter, G. B., & Goldstein, A. P. (1995). *The EQUIP program: Teaching youth to think and act responsibly through a peer-helping approach.* Chicago, IL: Research Press.

Goldstein, A. P. (1988). The Prepare Curriculum: *Teaching prosocial competencies*. Champaign, IL: Research Press.

Gordon, R. S. (1983). An operational classification of disease prevention. *Public Health Reports, 98*(2), 107–109.

Groh, A. M., Fearon, R. P., Bakermans-Kranenburg, M. J., van Ijzendoorn, M. H., Steele, R. D., & Roisman, G. I. (2014). The significance of attachment security for children's social competence with peers: A meta-analytic study. *Attachment Human Development, 16*(2), 103–136.

Heinicke, C. M., Fineman, N. R., Ponce, B. A., & Guthrie, D. (2001). Relation-based intervention with at-risk mothers: Outcome in the second year of life. *Infant Mental Health Journal, 22*(4), 431–462.

Heinicke, C. M., Fineman, N. R., Ruth, G., Recchia, S. L., Guthrie, D., & Rodning, C. (1999). Relationship-based intervention with at-risk mothers: Outcome in the first year of life. *Infant Mental Health Journal, 20*(4), 349–374.

Heinrichs, N., Kliem, S., & Hahlweg, K. (2014). Four-year follow-up of a randomized controlled trial of Triple P group for parent and child outcomes. *Prevention Science, 15*, 233–245. doi:10.1007/s11121-012-0358-2

Jamison, D. T., Summers, L. H., Alleyne, G., Arrow, K. J., Berkley, S., Binagwaho, A., . . . Yamey, G.. (2013). Global health 2035: A world converging within a generation. *Lancet, 382*, 1898–1955.

Jobes, D. A. (2009). The CAMS approach to suicide risk: Philosophy and clinical procedures. *Suicidology, 14*, 3–7.

Kalinauskiene, L., Cekuoliene, D., Van IJzendoorn, M. H., Bakermans-Kranenburg, M. J., Juffer, F., & Kusakovskaja, I. (2009). Supporting insensitive mothers: The Vilnius randomized control trial of video-feedback intervention to promote maternal sensitivity and infant attachment security. *Child: Care, Health and Development, 35*(5), 613–623.

Kaner, E. F. S., Beyer, F. R., Muirhead, C., Campbell, F., Pienaar, E. D., Bertholet, N., . . . Burnand B. (2018). Effectiveness of brief alcohol interventions in primary care populations. *Cochrane Database of Systematic Reviews, 2*(CD004148). doi:10.1002/14651858.CD004148.pub4.

Kitzman, H., Olds, D., Henderson, C., Hanks, C., Cole, R., Tatelbaum, R., . . . Barnard, K.. (1997). Effect of prenatal and infancy home visitation by nurses on pregnancy outcomes, childhood injuries and repeated childbearing. *JAMA, 278*, 644–652.

Kitzman, H. J. (2007). Effective early childhood development programs for low-income families: Home visiting interventions during pregnancy and early childhood. *Encyclopedia on Early Childhood development*. Retrieved from http://www.child-encyclopedia.com/sites/default/files/textes-experts/en/794/effective-early-childhood-development-programs-for-low-income-families-home-visiting-interventions-during-pregnancy-and-early-childhood.pdf

Kitzman, H. J., Olds, D. L., Cole, R. E., Hanks, C. A., Anson, E. A., Arcoleo, K. J., . . . Homberg, J. R. (2010). Enduring effects of prenatal and infancy home visiting by nurses on children: Follow-up of a randomized trial among children at age 12 years. *Archives of Pediatric & Adolescent Medicine, 164*(5), 412–418.

Knoff, H. M., & Batsche, G. M. (1995). Project ACHIEVE: Analyzing a school reform process for at-risk and underachieving students. *School Psychology Review*, 24, 579–603.

Landry, S. H., Smith, K. E., & Swank, P. R. (2006). Responsive parenting: Establishing early foundations for social, communication, and independent problem-solving skills. *Developmental Psychology, 42*(4), 627–642.

Landsverk, J., Carrilio, T., Connelly, C. D., Ganger, W. C., Slymen, D. J., Newton, R. R., & Jones, C (2002). *Healthy families San Diego clinical trial technical report*. San Diego, CA: Child and Adolescent Services Research Center, San Diego Children's Hospital and Health Center.

Lundberg, U., Holmberg, L., & Frankenhaeuser, M. (1988). Urinary catecholamines: Comparison between HPLC with electrochemical detection and fluorophotmetric assay. *Pharmacology, Biochemistry and Behavior, 31*, 287–290.

Madigan, S., Atkinson, L., Laurin, K., & Benoit, D. (2013). Attachment and internalizing behavior in early childhood: A meta-analysis. *Developmental Psychology, 49*(4), 672–689.

Mann, M., Hosman, C. M. H., Schaalma, H. P., & de Vries, N. K. (2004). Self-esteem in a broad-spectrum approach for mental health promotion. *Health Education Research, 19*(4), 357–372.

Morgan, Z., Brugha, T., Fryers, T., & Stewart-Brown, S. (2012). The effects of parent-child relationships on later life mental health status in two national birth cohorts. *Social Psychiatry and Psychiatric Epidemiology.* doi 10.1007/s00127-012-0481-1

Murray, L. Cooper P., Arteche, A., Stein, A., & Tomlinson, M. (2016). Randomized controlled trial of a home-visiting intervention on infant cognitive development in peri-urban South Africa. *Developmental Medicine & Child Neurology, 58*, 270–276.

Negrao, M., Pereira, M., Soares, I., & Mesman, J. (2014). Enhancing positive parent-child interactions and family functioning in a poverty sample: A randomized control trial. *Attachment & Human Development, 16*(4), 315–328.

Niccols, A. (2008). 'Right from the Start': Randomized trial comparing an attachment group intervention to supportive home visiting. *Journal of Child Psychology and Psychiatry, 49*(7), 754–764.

North, C. S., & Pfefferbaum, B. (2013). Mental health response to community disasters: A systematic review. *JAMA, 310*(5), 507–518.

Olds, D. (2002). Prenatal and infancy home visiting by nurses: From randomized trials to community replication. *Prevention Science, 3*, 153–172.

Olds, D. L., Eckenrode, J., Henderson, C. R., Kitzman, H., Powers, J., Cole, R., . . . Luckey, D. (1997). Long-term effects of home visitation on maternal life course and child abuse and neglect: Fifteen-year follow-up of a randomized trial. *JAMA, 278*(8), 637–643.

Olds, D. L., Eckenrode, J., Henderson, C. R., Cole, R., Eckenrode, J., Kitzman, H., . . . Powers, J. (1998). Long-term effects of nurse home visitation on children's criminal and antisocial behavior: Fifteen-year follow-up of a randomized controlled trial. *JAMA, 280*(14) 1238–1244.

Olds, D. L., Henderson, C. R., Chamberlin, R., & Tatelbaum, R. (1986). Preventing child abuse and neglect: A randomized trial of nurse home visitation. *Pediatrics, 78*, 65–78.

Olds, D. L., Holmberg, J. R., Donelan-McCall, N., Luckey, D. W., Knudtson, M. D., & Robinson, J. (2014). Effects of home visits by paraprofessionals and by nurses on children: Follow-up of a randomized trial at ages 6 and 9 years. *JAMA Pediatrics, 168*(2), 114–121.

Olds, D. L., Kitzman, H. J., Cole, R. E., Hanks, C. A., Arcoleo, K. J., Anson, E.A., . . . Stevenson, A.J. (2010). Enduring effects of prenatal and infancy home visiting by nurses on maternal life course and government spending: Follow-up of a randomized trial among children at age 12 years. *Archives of Pediatrics and Adolescent Medicine, 164*, 419–424.

Olds, D. L., Kitzman, H., Knudtson, M. D., Anson, E., Smith, J. A., & Cole, R. (2014b). Effect of home visiting by nurses on maternal and child mortality: Results of a 2-decade follow-up of a randomized clinical trial. *JAMA Pediatrics, 168*(9), 800–806.

Olds, D., Robinson, J., O'Brien, R., Luckey, D., Pettitt, L., Henderson, C., . . . Talmi, A. (2002). Home visiting by paraprofessionals and by nurses: A randomized controlled trial. *Pediatrics, 110*, 486–496.

Olds, D., Sadler, L., & Kitzman, H. (2007). Programs for parents of infants and toddlers: Recent evidence from randomized trials. *Journal of Child Psychology and Psychiatry, 48*(3/4), 355–391.

Posner, K., Brown, G. K., Stanley, B., Brent, D. A., Yershova, K. V., Oquendo, M. A., . . . Mann J. J. (2011). The Columbia-Suicide Severity Rating Scale: Initial validity and internal consistency findings from three multisite studies with adolescents and adults. *American Journal of Psychiatry, 168*(12), 1266–1277.

Sadler, L. S., Slade, A., Close, N., Webb, D. L., Simpson, T., Fennie, K., & Mayes, L. C. (2013). Minding the Baby®: Improving early health and relationship outcomes in vulnerable young families in an interdisciplinary reflective parenting home visiting program. *Infant Mental Health Journal, 34*(5), 391–405.

SAMHSA. (2016). Center for the Application of Prevention Technologies. The role of adverse childhood experiences in substance abuse and related behavioral health problems. Retrieved from https://www.samhsa.gov/capt/sites/default/files/resources/aces-behavioral-health-problems.pdf

SAMHSA. (2017). About screening, brief intervention and referral to treatment. Retrieved from https://www.samhsa.gov/sbirt/about

SAMHSA-HRSA Center for Integrated Health Solutions. (2020). SBIRT: Screening, brief intervention, and referral to treatment. Retrieved from https://www.integration.samhsa.gov/clinical-practice/SBIRT

Schilling, E. A., Aseltine, R. H., & Gore, S. (2007). Adverse childhood experiences and mental health in young adults: A longitudinal survey. *BMC Public Health*, 7(30). doi:100.1186/1471-2458/7/30

Schneider, B. H., Atkinson, L., & Tardif, C. (2001). Child-parent attachment and children's peer relations: A quantitative review. *Developmental Psychology, 37*(1), 86–100.

Srihari, V. H., Tek, C., Kucukgoncu, S., Phutane, V. H., Breitborde, N. J. K., Pollard, J., . . . Woods, S. W. (2015). First-episode services for psychotic disorders in the U.S. public sector: A pragmatic randomized controlled trial. *Psychiatric Services, 66*(7), 705–712. doi:10.1176/appi.ps.201400236

Srihari, V. H., Tek, C., Pollard, J., Zimmet, S., Keat, J., Cahill, J. D., . . . Woods, S. W. (2014). Reducing the duration of untreated psychosis and its impact in the U.S.: The STEP-ED study. *BMC Psychiatry, 14*, 335. Retrieved from http://www.biomedcentral.com/1471-244X/14/335

U.S. Department of Health and Human Services. (1999). *Mental health: A report of the Surgeon General*. Rockville, MD: U.S. Department of Health and Human Services, Substance Abuse and Mental Health Services Administration, Center for Mental Health Services, National Institutes of Health, National Institute of Mental Health.

Van den Boom, D. C. (1995). Do first-year intervention effects endure? Follow-up during toddlerhood of a sample of Dutch irritable infants. *Child Development, 66*, 1798–1816.

Velderman, M. K., Bakermans-Kranenburg, M. J., Juffer, F, van Ijzendoorn, M. H. (2006). Effects of attachment-based interventions on maternal sensitivity and infant attachment: Differential susceptibility of highly reactive infants. *Journal of Family Psychology, 20*(2), 266–274.

von Bertalanffy, L. (1975). General systems theory. In B. D. Ruben & J. Y. Kim (Eds.), *General systems theory and human communication*. Rochelle Park, NJ: Hayden Book Co.

Walker, H. M. (1983). *The Walker social skills curriculum: The ACCEPTS Program*. Austin, TX: Pro-Ed.

Whiteford, H. A., Degenhardt, L., Rehm, J., Baxter, A. J., Ferrari, A. J., Erskine, H.E., . . .Vos, T. (2013). The global burden of mental and substance use disorders: findings from the global burden of disease study 2010. *The Lancet, 382*, 1575–1586. doi:10.1016/S0140-6736(13)61611-6

World Health Organization. (2005). *Promoting mental health: Concepts, emerging evidence, practice*. Report of the World Health Organization, Department of Mental Health and Substance Abuse in collaboration with the Victorian Health Promotion Foundation and the University of Melbourne,. Geneva, Switzerland: World Health Organization.

Yale School of Medicine. (2020). Specialized treatment early in psychosis (STEP). Retrieved from https://medicine.yale.edu/psychiatry/step/

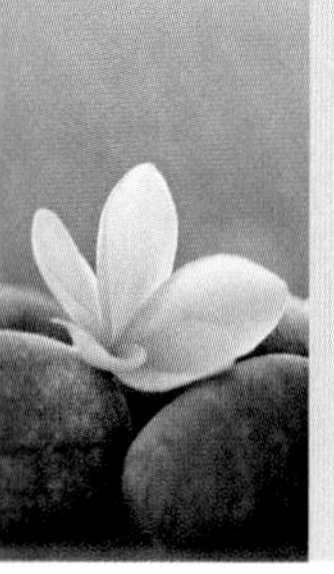

Chapter 11

Assessing Learning Needs and Health Literacy

Terri Ann Parnell

LEARNING OBJECTIVES

After completing this chapter, the student will be able to:

1. Develop a PICOT question for health literacy.
2. Discuss the implications of low health literacy for health promotion.
3. Discuss the value of health literacy, culture, and language assessment in all health promotion plans and activities.
4. Differentiate best practices to close the health literacy gap between nurses and clients.

INTRODUCTION

Health literacy is the currency for success in everything we do in health, wellness and prevention.

Dr. Richard H. Carmona, 17th surgeon general of the United States from 2002 to 2006

Most often defined as the ability of individuals to obtain, process, and understand their health information and make appropriate decisions, health literacy has a significant impact on overall health and well-being. Health literacy is a necessary skill across the life span for successfully functioning in daily life as well as in a health-care environment. It requires a constellation of abilities, including reading and comprehending written information, math skills to understand concepts such as risks and benefits of treatment options, and effective communication skills to obtain accurate information from and to educate patients (Ad Hoc Committee on Health Literacy, 1999; Baker, 2006). The link between low health literacy and poor outcomes has been clearly established (Berkman, Sheridan, Donahue, Halperin, & Crotty, 2011; Yin, Jay, Maness, Zabar, & Kalet, 2015), leading organizations such as the U.S. Department of Education; The Joint Commission; the Agency for Healthcare Research and Quality (AHRQ); the National Academies of Sciences, Engineering and Medicine (NASEM); the American Academy of Nursing; the American Medical Association; the World Health Organization (WHO); and others to consider health literacy a critical issue. Healthy People 2020 focuses specific objectives on improving health providers' communication skills (U.S. Department of Health and Human Services [USDHHS], 2010a). The Centers for Disease Control and Prevention (CDC) provides numerous planning and evaluation tools, guidelines, standards, and research summaries focusing on health literacy (CDC, 2016). The National Action Plan (2010) identified overarching goals and strategies that all sectors should pursue to create a health literate society. And in an effort to reduce disparities when obtaining quality health care, the National Prevention Strategy fosters the provision of person-centered information and services that are health literate, and culturally and linguistically appropriate (National Prevention Council, 2011).

National data has reported that only 12% of U.S. adults have proficient health literacy skills (U.S. Department of Education, 2006). In 2012, the Program for the International Assessment of Adult Competencies (PIAAC), a cyclical, large-scale study, assessed adults from 24 participating countries on literacy, numeracy, and problem-solving using technology. Although the PIAAC did not include a specific health literacy section, inadequate numeracy and literacy skills have a direct relationship on a person's health literacy skills. The results revealed that only 13% of U.S. adults scored in the highest literacy levels and 10% in the highest numeracy level. The 2012 and 2014 reports on literacy indicated no improvements in literacy rates from a decade prior (U.S Department of Education, 2012).

The concept of health literacy continues to evolve toward a collaborative partnership among the clinician providing care and education, the individual client, and the health-care system. There is a progressive consensus regarding the complex nature of health literacy as well as its dependency on both individual and system factors (Rudd, 2010). Brach, Dreyer, et al. (2012) defined the concept of a health literate health care organization and subsequently identified 10 attributes (Brach, Keller, et al., 2012) with suggested guidelines and strategies to assist organizations with making it easier for individuals to access, navigate, and use information and services to enhance their health.

The benefits of an emphasis on health literacy extend beyond each health-care encounter to the daily necessity of illness prevention and health promotion. Health promotion does not exist solely when nursing professionals are delivering care; it's also an essential part of the quality of life in every community. As such, health literacy has also been defined as "the personal, cognitive, and social skills, which determine the ability of individuals to gain access and understand, and use information to promote and maintain good health" (Nutbeam, 2000; WHO, 1998, p. 10).

Primary prevention strategies must provide access to health information that is easy to understand and meaningful to the end user. Encouraging the use of preventive strategies depends equally on the alignment of health-care systems and clinicians providing the appropriate services, the individual's understanding of the preventive care benefits, and the level of engagement and activation (National Prevention Council, 2011). Secondary prevention measures to treat or eliminate existing disease should also be addressed through a health literacy lens (Institute of Medicine [IOM], 2011b). Advanced practice clinicians and nursing leaders have a vital role in providing person-centered care that supports the vision of the National Prevention Strategy, to improve quality of life for all individuals and communities (National Prevention Council, 2011).

BRIEF HISTORY AND DEMOGRAPHIC TRANSFORMATION

The concept and practice of health literacy is a complex, dynamic, crosscutting priority that involves behavior change across the entire life span. Low health literacy skills are associated with less healthy choices, poorer health, more hospitalizations, and increased health-care costs (IOM, 2004). Low health literacy is also associated with poor management of chronic illness and has a negative impact on an individual's ability to optimize his or her health outcomes (Edwards, Wood, Davies, & Edwards, 2012).

While low health literacy can affect everyone, it is more prevalent among older adults, individuals with less education, and those who have limited English proficiency (IOM, 2004). When addressing health literacy, nurses must be cognizant of the impact that health-care professionals, health policies, and health-care systems have on an individual's health literacy skills.

In addition, older adults are the fastest-growing age group in North America, and for the first time ever the population of seniors will be greater than that of children younger than 18. In 2050, the number of Americans age 65 and older is projected to be 88.5 million, more than double its projected population of 40.2 million in 2010 (Ortman, Velkoff, & Hogan, 2014). This increase will necessitate a greater demand for preventive and health-care services.

The United States is becoming more diverse in terms of race, ethnicity, and language, and is experiencing a dramatic demographic shift. Minority groups are the fastest growing demographic, currently accounting for one-third of the U.S. population (Betancourt, Renfrew, Green, Lopez, & Wasserman, 2012). Diversity also occurs within various ethnic and racial groups with respect to immigrant status, primary language, socioeconomic status, education, and cultural norms. Respecting the health-care beliefs and practices of culturally and linguistically diverse patients can help enhance positive health outcomes (Parnell, 2015). Culture gives meaning to an individual's perception and definition of health and illness. It may influence interactions with his or her health-care provider and the health-care system. Cultural beliefs also determine how one describes illness and explains symptoms, as well as who we go to for care and how we feel about the care we receive (Karnick, 2016). The fluid nature of health literacy and culture means that health-care interactions are rich with differences that are continuously evolving.

In addition to respecting and understanding an individual's culture, nurses must be able to communicate effectively with each client in his or her preferred language. Preferred written and spoken language is defined as the self-selected language the client wishes to use to communicate with health-care providers (National Quality Forum, 2009). The number of limited English proficient (LEP) persons in the United States grew by 80% between 1990 and 2010. In 2010, Spanish-speaking LEP individuals made up 66% of the total U.S. LEP population (Pandya, Batalova, & McHugh, 2011). As reported by the 2003 International Adult Literacy and Skills Survey (IALSS), administered in English and French to Canada's adult population, the average scores on the health literacy scale were lower for immigrants and those who did not speak English or French well (Rootman & Gordon-El-Bihbety, 2008).

Health care, including the provision of health information, must be understandable to recipients regardless of their cultural and linguistic preferences. It is vital to understand how people obtain, interpret, and use health information so that advanced nurse practitioners can truly understand the potential impact of health literacy (IOM, 2004).

The rapid growth of an aging population, increased racial and ethnic diversity, and an increased LEP population present opportunities for nursing leaders to focus on the assessment of learning needs and providing all persons with the capacity to obtain, process, understand, and communicate about information needed to make informed health decisions (Berkman, Davis, & McCormack, 2010). Health literacy is essential to engaging individuals in their health care; therefore, all engagement strategies should also integrate efforts to improve health literacy (Coulter, 2012). Providing clients with culturally and linguistically appropriate information in alignment with their health literacy skills gives them the tools and knowledge they need to adopt healthy behaviors (National Prevention Council, 2011).

CURRENT SYSTEMIC APPROACHES FOR IMPROVING HEALTH LITERACY

Health literacy has evolved from the implication that the health consumer holds the sole responsibility for obtaining, processing, and understanding basic health information and services to an understanding of the relevant social, environmental, and systemic factors that necessitate a public health approach (Freedman et al., 2009). Low health literacy skills are linked to suboptimal health outcomes, including a decreased ability to understand medication labels and health messages, increased use of emergency services, more hospitalizations, and worse overall health status (Koh et al., 2012). While most people are affected by low health literacy skills at some point, these negative outcomes disproportionately affect minorities, LEP individuals, the elderly, and those of lower socioeconomic status (IOM, 2004; Koh et al., 2012).

Health literacy has continued to evolve as an area of research over the past several decades, and it is now more widely recognized as a dynamic systems issue (Rudd, 2010). Leaders from diverse expertise areas collaborated to increase the awareness and implications of low health literacy and participated in developing common health literacy goals and strategies. In 2010, several major initiatives were created to bring the health literacy agenda to a tipping point. The Affordable Care Act (ACA) addressed health literacy by incorporating health literacy training for professionals and by streamlining the enrollment processes for Medicaid, Children's Health Insurance Plans, and state-based insurance exchanges (Somers & Mahadevan, 2010). The ACA also created health-care delivery models that assist with chronic disease management and self-management, and address the need to communicate health information so that it is understandable, culturally appropriate, and patient-centered.

The National Action Plan to Improve Health Literacy presents a similar vision with unified health literacy goals and strategies to create a health literate society. The National Action Plan is based on two main principles: Everyone has the right to health information that helps them make informed decisions, and health services should be delivered in a way that is understandable and beneficial to health and quality of life (USDHHS, 2010b).

A new federal agency requirement was passed in 2010 called the Plain Writing Act, and it is designed to improve the effectiveness and accountability of all federal agencies to the public by promoting clear government communication that everyone can use and understand. Under this act, federal agencies are expected to develop procedures, staff training, and regular compliance reports that must be posted on their plain language Web pages. These plain writing strategies will assist all agencies in achieving their mission of improving service to the public.

In 2010, the Joint Commission (2010) published "Advancing Effective Communication, Cultural Competence and Patient and Family Centered Care: A Roadmap for Hospitals." This monograph provides hospitals with methods to ensure that all patients, regardless of preferred language, communication needs, mobility needs, cultural preferences, health literacy level, or sexual identity, receive the same safe, high-quality care. It provides recommendations along the continuum of care with suggested practice examples.

Also in 2010, Healthy People 2020 was released with revised goals and objectives for health promotion and disease prevention for the nation (USDHHS, 2010a). Healthy People 2020 includes objectives related to system-level changes such as health-care providers' use of the teach-back method, the level of shared decision making between patients and providers, and access to personalized e-health tools. The teach-back method helps the educator to ensure that what has been explained to the patient was delivered in a method that the patient understood. In this method, the patient explains the instructions back in her or his own words (Farris, 2015; Koh et al., 2012). Integrating health literacy strategies into all health-care policies and processes is a key component of helping all individuals live a healthy life. See Table 11-1 to review select health literacy guidelines, laws, standards and resources.

Table 11-1 Select Health Literacy Guidelines, Laws, Standards, and Resources

GUIDELINES	YEAR	DESCRIPTION
National Institutes of Health and National Cancer Institute, "Pink Book"	2004	Practical approach for planning and implementing health communication related to cancer
U.S. Government, Federal Plain Language Guideline (PLAIN)	2011	Works with federal agencies to make sure citizens receive clear communications from the government
National Institutes of Health, Clear Communication: An NIH Health Literacy Initiative	2017	Supports research efforts on health literacy concepts, theory, and interventions as these relate to USDHHS public health priorities
LAWS		
U.S. Government, The Plain Language Writing Act	2010	Signed by President Obama in 2010, it requires federal agencies to use clear communication that the public can understand and use
Patient Protection and Affordable Care Act	2010	Health literacy is directly and indirectly implied throughout many of the provisions
STANDARDS		
Joint Committee, National Health Education Standards	2007	Identifies what students should know and be able to do by grades 2, 5, 8, and 12 to promote personal, family, and community health
Department of Health and Human Services, Office of Minority Health, National Culturally and Linguistically Appropriate Services (CLAS)	2013	Helps organizations address cultural and language differences between providers and the people they serve
RESOURCES		
Department of Health and Human Services, National Action Plan to Improve Health Literacy	2010	Sets forth a vision and seven goals to improve health literacy and create a health literate society
National Academies of Sciences, Engineering and Medicine, Ten Attributes of a Health Literate Health Care Organization	June 2012	After obtaining feedback from *Attributes of a Health Literate Organization* Discussion Paper, January 2012, decreased attributes of a health literate organization to 10 and provided rationale and suggested strategies
National Academies of Sciences, Engineering and Medicine, Roundtable on Health Literacy	2015	Collaborates to inform, inspire, and activate a wide variety of stakeholders in the development, implementation, and sharing of evidence-based health literacy practices and policies
CDC, Clear Communication Index	2015	A research-based tool to help in the development and assessment of public communication materials
AHRQ, Patient Education Materials Assessment Tool	2017	A tool that helps evaluate and compare the understandability and actionability of patient education materials

THE ROLE OF NURSING CARE

IOM has defined health as "a state of well-being and the capability to function in the face of changing circumstances" (IOM, 2011a, p. 37). Health as a concept includes social, personal, and physical abilities and resources. Nurses are uniquely positioned to enable their clients to increase control over and improve their health. The proliferation of this strategy, called health promotion, can ultimately bridge the existing health literacy gap.

"Health literacy strategies need to be woven into prevention efforts at all levels. Building one's health literacy should be thought of as a lifelong process. Even simple, small initiatives and interventions can dramatically improve health literacy and outcomes and associated costs" (IOM, 2011b, p. 81). A health-care provider must always strive to provide clear, culturally, and linguistically appropriate health information and education. Fostering a nursing culture that uses a health literacy "universal precautions approach" is one that always assumes everyone may have difficulty understanding health information (AHRQ, 2017). Using plain language when communicating is one of the most important ways clinicians can reduce health disparities related to low health literacy (Sudore & Schillinger, 2009). Furthermore, eliminating obstacles to health promotion by changing the way health-care providers communicate health information at the individual, community, and systemic levels offers the best opportunity to achieve a health-literate society.

PICOT QUESTION AND EVIDENCE: PRINT MATERIALS AND SELF-MANAGEMENT PROGRAMS

According to the CDC, 60 percent of American adults have a chronic disease, and 40 percent have two or more chronic conditions (CDC, 2018). Chronic diseases are some of the most costly and preventable of all health conditions. Not only do chronic and mental health conditions account for an estimated 90 percent of health-care spending, they represent the leading causes of death and disability in the United States (CDC, 2018). In addition, patients now take on more responsibility with self-management of their chronic diseases. Person-centered patient education is essential when fostering the development of successful health behavior changes.

For clients managing chronic disease, a common aim of patient education is to improve overall adherence to medication and treatment regimens and ultimately enhance lifestyle behaviors. The economic implications of low health literacy are of major concern in the United States. Chronic medical conditions decrease overall quality of life, increase mortality, and are costly for the health-care system (Hossain, Ehtesham, Salzman, Jenson, & Calkins, 2013).

Heart failure affects nearly 6 million Americans, and total direct medical costs exceed $21 billion (McNaughton et al., 2015). This condition predominately affects individuals over the age of 65 and leads to more hospitalizations for older adults than any other health condition (Chen, Yehle, Plake, Murawski, & Mason, 2011). With the aging of the U.S. population and with increasing technological and pharmaceutical innovations in the treatment of disease, the prevalence of chronic diseases will continue to rise, making enhanced health literacy more important than ever.

Generic written patient education material as a method of teaching self-care and management is ineffective for many patients with chronic disease because the management strategies that must be explained are often complex. For example, heart failure self-management training must include information on recognizing changes in symptoms, weight monitoring, salt restriction, exercise, adherence to medications, and following an action plan when heart failure symptoms are exacerbated (Baker et al., 2011). The patient, intervention, control, observation, and time (PICOT) question below can assist in further exploration about the implications of low health literacy among patients managing a chronic disease such as heart failure:

P: For clients with congestive heart failure, does
I: print educational material,
C: compared to a self-management program,
O: improve program goals
T: over a year-long period?

A search of the literature focusing on heart failure, health literacy and self-management was performed and provided a variety of results. In a multi-method study completed between 2006 and 2010, "The Impact of Cultural Differences on Health Literacy and Chronic Disease Outcomes," the researchers assessed health literacy and chronic disease self-management among 296 patients from four different ethnic groups: Vietnamese, African American, white, and Latino (Shaw, Armin, Torres, Orzech, & Vivian, 2012). The researchers identified a range of chronic disease self-management abilities among the participants with limited education and/or low health literacy. With culturally diverse patients, nurses must assess and consider their patients' cultural understanding of health to anticipate more accurately their ability to understand, adhere to, and maintain self-management of chronic disease.

Several articles referred to the lack of research regarding the relationship between literacy or health literacy and adverse outcomes in heart failure (Peterson et al., 2011; Wu et al., 2013). Self-care requires integration and application of knowledge and skills. Heart failure is more common in people older than age 65 who have limitations in physical and/or cognitive function, so clinicians are uniquely challenged when determining the learning and educational needs of heart failure patients (Robinson et al., 2011). In one study, low health literacy was significantly associated with higher overall mortality (Peterson et al., 2011). Others suggested new ways to assess the health literacy of older adults as well as interventions to mitigate literacy-related disparities in outcomes.

Self-management of chronic disease can be complex and challenging for all but particularly for those with low health literacy. For example, patients with diabetes must take medication as directed and understand adverse side effects, manage dietary restrictions, and be aware of complications such as foot ulcers and vascular issues. For these patients, a clinician's communication style can either enhance and facilitate patient empowerment or become a barrier to education and information exchange (Edwards et al., 2012).

Nurses should strive to communicate with all patients in plain language and organize information delivery effectively. It is often best to start by answering patient questions, then presenting the definitive "need to know" information. Omit nonessential information to avoid overwhelming the patient with facts that are not currently relevant. Avoid medical jargon and acronyms, and be consistent with your word choices to help mitigate patient confusion. For example, when teaching a heart failure patient, stick to the term *sodium* when referring to a low-sodium diet rather than switching back and forth between *sodium* and *salt*. Rather than relying on conceptual words such as *often*, *normal*, or *frequently*, be specific when discussing time frames and other key information. Provide specific examples, such as, "Walk once in the morning and once in the evening."

Knowledge and understanding are essential elements for patient empowerment and successful self-management (Driscoll, Davidson, Clark, Huang, & Aho, 2009). In addition to verbal patient education as described above, easy-to-read print resources about symptoms, lifestyle behaviors, and medications can facilitate successful self-management. Written materials with a large font, pictures and illustrations to enhance the text, limited use of medical jargon, and a clear focus on several action steps provide meaningful and understandable information to clients and assist them in enhancing adherence to treatment regimens. Testing these materials with low literacy clients during development will help ensure that they meet all patient needs.

Family support can be helpful in self-management of chronic illness, especially for patients with low health literacy. However, clients may perceive family support in both positive and negative ways. Barriers to family support include the family members' coping abilities, emotional readiness to receive information, availability and involvement in the patient's life, and their own health literacy abilities. On the other hand, facilitators include a family member's capacity to communicate the information adequately and appropriately. Therefore, clinicians should be alert to family barriers to self-care in addition to available family support, even in families that seem to have good overall function (Rosland, Heisler, Choi, Silveira, & Piette, 2010; Short, McCormack, & Copley, 2014).

Teach-back is a strategy that can help ensure that your teaching is effective while remaining respectful to the patient and family. For example, you could ask a patient to role-play explaining his activities during recovery to a loved one, noting that you want to make sure that you were clear with your instructions. If the client was able to teach back the information as he explains to you what he would tell his wife, it's a good indicator that your teaching was effective.

Clinicians can enhance the goals of self-management education by reducing the cognitive burden of the client and bridging the health literacy gap that exists between patients and providers. Health is not merely the absence of disease or infirmity; it is a state of complete physical, mental, and social well-being (WHO, 2006). With this definition in mind, providers must truly integrate patients and their families as active participants in care to achieve optimal health outcomes (Smith, Fitzpatrick, & Hoyt-Hudson, 2011). While patients may not have all the resources, knowledge, or tools to promote their own health or prevent disease, they can turn the knowledge they have into belief, action, and ultimately behavior change (Smith et al., 2011). Meeting our patients where they are in terms of health literacy, providing information and services in an understandable and actionable way, and partnering with them to conquer health-related challenges helps to improve outcomes.

STRENGTHS AND LIMITATIONS OF THE BODY OF EVIDENCE

For the past several decades, health literacy research has provided a vast body of evidence that documents

BOX 11-1 Effects of Health Literacy

DIMINISHED HEALTH LITERACY	ADEQUATE HEALTH LITERACY
Lack of knowledge about disease management	Increased awareness
Inability to locate information on disease	Increased self-advocacy
Inability to understand medical information	Ability to understand health information and to access services
Feelings of shame and embarrassment	Better communication with providers
Decrease in self-management	Greater compliance and disease management
Decrease in health decision making	Improved health status
More likely to make medication errors	Less probability of hospitalization
Decrease in compliance	Reduced health disparities
Higher incidence of hospitalization	Reduced financial burden on family and system
Increased health-care burden to family and system	

Source: Adapted from Sadeghi, Brooks, Stagg-Peterson, and Goldstein (2013).

the implications of low health literacy and clarifies the challenges associated with various demographic populations. A search for systematic reviews on health literacy in Medline and Cumulative Index to Nursing and Allied Health Literature (CINAHL) from 2012 to 2017 revealed approximately 50 publications. The effects of diminished health literacy as well as the benefits of adequate health literacy are well documented (Sadeghi, Brooks, Stagg-Peterson, & Goldstein, 2013). Box 11-1 summarizes many of these effects. However, research about how to close the health literacy gap with evidence-based applicable interventions and tools, as well as what types of tools are most effective when educating low literacy patients, is varied.

Existing studies have collected a variety of demographic information, including race, ethnicity, age, marital status, place of residence, financial and employment status, educational level, smoking and alcohol use, medications, length of time with chronic illness, and the client's health literacy level. Several studies purposefully selected research participants from varying education levels and professions, while others incorporated the clients' family support level and measured whether this was a help or hindrance to chronic disease management.

A search using the keywords *health literacy* and *best practices* in PubMed from 2012 to 2017 revealed more than 40 publications. Despite the depth of information, no definitive indication of best practices exists across the current body of research. Additional research focused on implications of and linkages between specific evidence-based educational topics and outcomes would be of great benefit. However, tailored approaches for different populations are being explored (Cohn et al., 2018; Hasnain-Wynia & Wolf, 2010). Regardless of the method of communication or type of teaching materials, the CDC and AHRQ have developed print and online resources for creating easy-to-read and easy-to-understand written materials. The CDC Clear Communication Index is a research-based tool that can help nurses develop and assess communication materials (CDC, 2015). AHRQ developed the Patient Education Materials Assessment Tool (PEMAT) and User's Guide to assist with a way to evaluate systemically the understandability and actionability of patient education materials (AHRQ, 2017).

RECOMMENDATIONS FOR PRACTICE

The development of health literacy skills occurs over a lifetime through various health experiences and across different contexts. For clients living with chronic conditions such as heart failure, enhanced health literacy can help them adjust and develop self-management skills and may even provide foresight of future risks and adjustment of life plans (Edwards et al., 2012). Health care is often provided in a fashion that is most convenient for the clinician, health-care system, or payer. To foster the person-centered approach necessary to improve health literacy, nurses must spearhead systemic change by implementing health literacy interventions into nursing practice (Parnell, 2014). Health literacy should be addressed for every patient, every time, and in every health-care encounter, to help mitigate the untoward consequences of low health literacy, as well as patient and system outcomes (Loan et al., 2018). The American

BOX 11-2 Nursing Health Literacy Practice Recommendations

Encourage use of a health literacy universal precautions approach.

- Advocate that all patients are at risk for not understanding health information.
- Integrate person-centered nursing practice strategies that encourage patient engagement and health literacy across all interprofessional practice models.
- Promote shame-free environments where health literacy can flourish.
- Use plain language and teach-back in all patient communications.

Source: Adapted from American Academy of Nursing Policy Brief (2018, January–February). *Call for action: Nurses must play a role to enhance health literacy.*

Academy of Nursing recently endorsed health literacy policies, strategies, and initiatives across three domains: practice, health system, and partnerships. Box 11-2 lists suggested nursing recommendations specific to the practice domain in an effort to achieve health literacy practice goals (Loan et al., 2018).

FEASIBILITY OF APPLYING THE EVIDENCE

As the population continues to age and the system requires patients to have increased individual responsibility in chronic disease management, it is vital to provide patient-centered intervention practices that can be implemented at both the systems and patient levels. Nurses can use a "universal precautions" approach and not assume the health literacy skills of their clients. Incorporating each client's religious, spiritual, and cultural preferences into the plan of care and ensuring all clients have access to an interpreter when necessary can enhance effective communication and person-centered care. Speaking in plain language or everyday terms and incorporating teach-back to assess respectfully for understanding are essential components that will help clarify any misunderstandings.

With the understanding that addressing health literacy is essential to providing safe, person-centered care, an increasing number of health-care organizations are emphasizing a focus on system-level factors to ensure that everyone can access, navigate, understand, and use information and services to take care of their health (Brach, Keller, et al., 2012). Nurses can have a vital role in ensuring successful implementation and maintenance of the attributes of a health literate organization.

Health literacy is dynamic and complex, with many factors having an impact on the skills of individuals and systems as they relate to enhancing health outcomes and promoting health and wellness. Nurses can create a culture of health literacy in their practice settings by integrating components of effective communication into all patient safety and quality measures. Performing organizational health literacy assessments; ensuring compliance with regulatory standards for health literacy, patient education, language, and communication access services; and identifying best practices and benchmarking of data assist in the provision of a health literate organization for all (Parnell, 2014).

Key Stakeholders for Evidence-Based Practice Changes

Engaging key stakeholders is a vital part of assessing, planning, implementing, evaluating, and sustaining a culture of health literacy in all areas of nursing practice. "Health care organizations should be structured to make all interactions between health care teams and patients as productive as possible" (Koh, Brach, Harris, & Parchman., 2013, p. 358). Improving health outcomes depends on fully engaging patients in prevention, decision making, and all self-management activities.

Establishing goals and outcome measures to monitor strategies for health literacy and patient engagement can assist both organizations and health-care professionals in improving their ability to meet all patients' health literacy needs. Additional research is needed to determine the most beneficial ways to educate and train all health-care professionals and how to incorporate and sustain health literacy strategies with limited time and resources (Koh et al., 2013).

Promoting health requires more than providing patients with information and tools to make healthy choices. While this is a beginning, we must also partner with key stakeholders in all community sectors because social, economic, and environmental factors all influence health (National Prevention Council, 2011). Health literacy and health promotion are affected by many aspects of society and require multiple stakeholders and a multifaceted approach to lessen the burden of chronic illness and disease self-management, thus encouraging all patients to be empowered and engaged in their health care and health promotion activities. Table 11-2 describes suggested community stakeholders that may be considered for inclusion in a health literacy program.

Table 11-2 Suggested Health Literacy Community Stakeholders

STAKEHOLDER	HEALTH LITERACY ACTIVITIES	GOALS
Health-care providers	Improve patient-provider communication, and patient understanding and compliance; foster policies to support health literacy	Decrease the health literacy related demands on people and improve overall health outcomes and the provision of safe person-centered health care
Health-care systems & Insurers	Improve patient-provider communication, and patient understanding and compliance; comply with federal standards	Improve access to health-care services and health insurance, understand how to use health insurance to promote health and well-being
Nonprofit, voluntary, advocacy, and professional associations	Inform and educate consumers about their rights and responsibilities, help educate health-care providers about the need to communicate health information clearly, give providers tools to improve their communication skills, publish evidence-based decision aids and guides for diverse audiences	Help consumers use health-care services more effectively, provide information and services on health literacy practices to consumers and health-care professionals
Public health agencies	Wide range of activities that connect directly to health literacy, include health literacy in strategic plans and all educational initiatives	Population-based approach, promote and protect the health of everyone
State, tribal, local, and territorial governments	Collaborate with communities to implement policies and programs	Improve coordination, collaboration, and opportunities for engaging community leaders and members
Medical interpreters	Instrumental in helping patients and families navigate the health-care system	Promote health communication and cultural competence
Public libraries	Provide access to easy-to-reach health information, support basic literacy training programs, teach computer skills and provide access to public internet	Promote community awareness of health literacy
Adult education programs	Provide health literacy instruction programs, participate in health literacy partnerships with other organizations, provide tools that help people navigate and access health-care services	Improve learner understanding of oral and printed information
Literacy organizations	Participate in regional consortia and partnerships, may train volunteers	Help learners improve their functional literacy
Social workers	Advocate for patient needs and resources	Empower patients to navigate the health-care system
Community-based social service organizations	Help clients access, navigate, and understand and communicate with local health-care systems	Support to vulnerable populations within the health-care system; empower people to be involved in their health
Health writers and editors	Write in simple language; make public aware of health literacy needs and resources; many learn about health issues from television, magazines, and other public sources	Raise awareness; promote clear accurate, health information to consumers

Source: Adapted from U.S. Department of Health and Human Services (2010b); National Prevention Council (2011).

Interprofessional Health Education Implications

Patient education, effective communication, and enhancement of health literacy are vital roles of the nursing profession. While agencies and organizations support mandates to teach nurses about health literacy, research by Torres and Nichols (2014) revealed little evidence that nursing programs are educating their students with the knowledge and skills necessary to meet the health literacy needs of a diverse patient population. The national Bachelor of Science in Nursing (BSN) program study by Scott (2016) reported 63 percent of the 54 participants educated students in the nursing curriculum regarding the importance of health literacy. However, while 63 percent reported health literacy inclusion in the curricula, 69 percent of the students stated that none of the faculty members were identified as an authority on health literacy (Scott, 2016).

It is important that nurses understand health literacy, its prevalence across all segments of society, and the implications for health outcomes because they have a vital role in providing health information and education to patients across a variety of settings (Speros, 2005). But research shows that nurses tend to overestimate their patient's health literacy more often than they underestimate it, which may contribute to hospital readmission rates and poorer health outcomes (Dickens, Lambert, Cromwell, & Piano, 2013).

Nursing must respond to the call of creating a health literate society by participating in health literacy promotion, education, and research. It is imperative that nurses understand the breadth and depth of health literacy and its prevalence and implications. Healthcare providers must collaborate in an interdisciplinary effort to integrate health literacy strategies into all person-centered care and health promotion activities.

USEFUL RESOURCES

Books

- Bastable, S. B. (2016). *Essentials of patient education* (2nd ed.). Sudbury, MA: Jones & Bartlett.
- Nielsen-Bohlman, L. Panzer, A. M., & Kindig, D. A. (Eds.). (2004). *Health literacy: A prescription to end confusion*. Washington, DC: National Academies Press.
- Doak, C. C., Doak, L. G., & Root, J. H. (1996). *Teaching patients with low literacy skills* (2nd ed.). New York, NY: Lippincott, Williams & Wilkins.
- Jeffreys, M. R. (2015). *Teaching cultural competence in nursing and health care* (3rd ed.). New York, NY: Springer.
- Parnell, T. A. (2015). *Health literacy in nursing: Providing person-centered care*. New York, NY: Springer.
- Schwartzberg, J. G., VanGeest, J. B., & Wang, C. C. (Eds.). (2005). *Understanding health literacy: Implications for medicine and public health*. Chicago, IL: American Medical Association.
- Papalois, V. E., and Theodospoulou, M. (Eds.). (2018). *Optimizing health literacy for improved clinical practices*. Hersey, PA: IGI Global.

Web Sites

- Agency for Healthcare Research and Quality (AHRQ): https://www.ahrq.gov/qual/literacy/
- Center for Health Care Strategies: https://www.chcs.org/resource/health-literacy-fact-sheets/
- Centers for Disease Control and Prevention (CDC): https://www.cdc.gov/healthliteracy
- Harvard School of Public Health: https://www.hsph.harvard.edu/healthliteracy/resources/
- Health Resources and Services Administration (HRSA): https://www.hrsa.gov/about/organization/bureaus/ohe/health-literacy/index.html
- The National Academies of Sciences, Engineering and Medicine: Roundtable on Health Literacy: http://nationalacademies.org/hmd/Activities/PublicHealth/HealthLiteracy.aspx
- National Action Plan to Improve Health Literacy: http://www.health.gov/communication/HLActionPlan/
- The National Network of Libraries of Medicine: https://nnlm.gov/initiatives/topics/health-literacy
- The Health Literate Care Model: https://health.gov/communication/interactiveHLCM/
- National Patient Safety Foundation (NPSF)—Ask Me 3: https://www.npsf.org/?page=askme3
- The Joint Commission: https://www.jointcommission.org/

KEY POINTS

- Health literacy, a necessary skill to function in health-care environments and everyday life, is described as the ability to obtain, process, and understand health information and make appropriate decisions based on this information.
- Clinical research has clearly established a link between limited health literacy and poor health outcomes.
- The impact of low health literacy in the United States disproportionately affects ethnic minorities, individuals who do not speak English, low-income **households**, and the elderly.
- Nurses and other providers engaged in primary and secondary levels of health care must provide clients with relevant, easy-to-understand health **information** about diagnoses, conditions, and treatments.

- Health-care organizations can help improve the literacy levels and outcomes of their clients by setting goals and outcome measures for a health **literacy** program.

Check Your Understanding

1. The best way for a nurse to determine how well a patient understood the discharge instructions provided would be to:
   A. Ask the patient a few open-ended questions about the instructions
   B. Ask the patient if he or she has "any questions about the instructions?"
   C. Ask the patient to write down the discharge instructions and review them together
   D. Ask the patient to tell you how he or she will explain the information to their sister, who was not present but who will be caring for him or her at home
2. While low health literacy can affect everyone, low health literacy is often greater among:
   A. Older adults
   B. People with less education and lower socioeconomic status
   C. LEP people and those from cultural minorities
   D. People with physical and mental disabilities
   E All of the above
3. Which of the following would be strategies to use when communicating in "plain language"?
   A. Provide need-to-know information using common, everyday words
   B. Ask the patient how many years of education she or he completed so you could teach at an appropriate level
   C. Always begin with anatomy and physiology so the patient has a fundamental understanding of her or his disease process
   D. All of the above
4. Implementing a health literacy "universal precautions" approach includes:
   A. Always wash your hands before beginning to teach your patient
   B. Reviewing all patients' demographic intake for number of years of education and learning barriers
   C. Never assuming any patient's health literacy level and use plain language and teach-back with all patients
   D. Always providing more advanced instructions with medical terms for patients who are college educated or professionals
5. Several implications of low health literacy include the following:
   A. Poor health outcomes
   B. Increased hospitalizations
   C. Increased health-care costs
   D. Poor management of chronic illness
   E. All of the above

See "Check Your Understanding" at the end of the book for answers.

REFERENCES

Ad Hoc Committee on Health Literacy. (1999). Health literacy: Report of the Council on Scientific Affairs. *Journal of the American Medical Association, 281*, 552–557.

Agency for Healthcare Research and Quality. (2017, April). The patient education materials assessment tool (PEMAT) and user's guide. Rockville, MD: Author. Retrieved from http://ww.ahrq.gov/professionals/prevention-chronic-care/improve/self-mgmt/pemat/index.html

Baker, D. W. (2006). The meaning and the measure of health literacy. *Journal of General Internal Medicine, 21*(8), 878–883.

Baker, D. B., DeWalt, D. A., Schillinger, D., Hawk, V., Ruo, B., Bibbins-Domingo, K., . . . Pignone, M. (2011). Teach to goal: Theory and design principles of an intervention to improve heart failure self-management skills of patients with low health literacy. *Journal of Health Communication. 16*(S3), 73–88.

Berkman, N. D., Davis, T. C., & McCormack, L. (2010). Health literacy: What is it? *Journal of Health Communication. 15*(Suppl 2), 9–19.

Berkman, N. D, Sheridan, S. L., Donahue, K. E., Halperin, D. J., & Crotty, K. (2011). Low health literacy and health outcomes: An updated systemic review. *Annals of Internal Medicine, 155*, 97–107.

Betancourt, J. R., Renfrew, M. R. Green, A. R., Lopez, L., & Wasserman, M. (2012). *Improving patient safety systems for patients with limited English proficiency: A guide for hospitals.* Rockville, MD: Agency for Healthcare Research and Quality; AHRQ Publication No. 12-0041.

Brach, C., Dreyer, B., Schyve, P., Hernandez, L. M., Baur, C., Lemerise, A. J., Parker, R. (2012, January). *Attributes of a health literate organization: NAM perspectives.* Discussion Paper, National Academy of Medicine, Washington, DC.

Brach, C., Keller, D., Hernandez, L. M., Baur, C., Parker, R., Dreyer, B., . . . Schillinger., D. (2012, June). *Ten attributes of health literate health care organizations: NAM perspectives.* Discussion Paper, National Academy of Medicine, Washington, DC. doi:10.31478/201206a

Centers for Disease Control and Prevention. (2015). The CDC clear communication index. Retrieved from https://www.cdc.gov/ccindex/index.html

Centers for Disease Control and Prevention. (2016). *Health literacy.* Retrieved from https://www.cdc.gov/healthliteracy/learn/

Centers for Disease Control and Prevention. (2018). *About chronic diseases*. Retrieved from https://www.cdc.gov/chronicdisease/about/index.htm

Chen, A. M. H., Yehle, K. S., Plake, K. S., Murawski, M. M., & Mason, H. L. (2011). Health literacy and self-care of patients with heart failure. *The Journal of Cardiovascular Nursing*, *26*(6), 446–451. doi:10.1097/JCN.0b013e31820598d4

Cohn, W., Lyman, J., Broshek, D., Guterbock, T., Harman, D., Kinzie, . . . Garson, A. (2018). Tailored educational approaches for consumer health: A model to address health promotion in an era of personalized medicine. *American Journal of Health Promotion*, *32*(1), 188–197.

Coulter, A. (2012). Patient engagement: What works? *Journal of Ambulatory Care Management*, *35*(2): 80–89. https://doi.org/10.1097/JAC.0b013e318249e0fd

Dickens, C., Lambert, B. L., Cromwell, T., & Piano, M. R. (2013). Nurse overestimation of patient's health literacy. *Journal of Health Communication. 18*, 62–69.

Driscoll, A., Davidson, P., Clark, R., Huang, N., & Aho, Z. (2009). Tailoring consumer resources to enhance self-care in chronic heart failure. *Australian Critical Care*, *22*(3), 133–140.

Edwards, M., Wood, F., Davies, M., & Edwards, A. (2012). The development of health literacy in patients with a long-term health condition: The health literacy pathway model. *BioMed Central Public Health*, *12*(130). Retrieved from http//www.biomedcentral.com/1471-2458/12/130.

Farris, C. (2015). The teach-back method. *Home Health Care Now*, *33*(6), 344–345.

Freedman, D. A., Bess, K. D., Tucker, H. A., Boyd, D. L., Tuchman, A. M., & Wallston, K. A. (2009). Public health literacy defined. *American Journal of Preventive Medicine*, *36*(5), 446–450.

Hasnain-Wynia, R., & Wolf, M. S. (2010). Promoting health care equity: Is health literacy the missing link? *Health Services Research*, *45*, 897–903.

Hossain, W. A., Ehtesham, M. W., Salzman, G. A., Jenson, R. & Calkins, C. F. (2013). Healthcare access and disparities in chronic medical conditions in urban populations. *Southern Medical Journal*, *106*(4), 246–254.

Institute of Medicine. (2004). *Health literacy: A prescription to end confusion*. Washington DC: National Academies Press.

Institute of Medicine. (2011a). *The future of nursing: Leading change, advancing health*. Washington, DC: National Academic Press.

Institute of Medicine. (2011b). *Promoting health literacy to encourage prevention and wellness: Workshop summary*. Washington, DC: National Academies Press.

The Joint Commission. (2010). *Advancing effective communication, cultural competence, and patient and family centered care: A roadmap for hospitals.* Oakbrook Terrace, IL: Author.

Karnick, P. M. (2016). Sorting it out: Cultural competency and healthcare literacy in the world today. *Nurse Science Quarterly*, *29*(2), 120–121.

Koh, H. K., Berwick, D., M., Clancy, C. M., Baur, C., Brach, C., Harris, L. M., & Zerhusen, E. G. (2012). New federal policy initiatives to boost health literacy can help the nation move beyond the cycle of costly crisis care. *Health Affairs*, *31*(2), 434–443. doi:10.1377/hlthaff.2011.1169.

Koh, H. K., Brach, C., Harris, L. M., & Parchman, M. L. (2013). A proposed health literate care model would constitute a systems approach to improving patients' engagement in care. *Health Affairs*, *32*(2), 357–367.

Loan, L. A., Parnell, T. A., Stichler, J. F., Boyle, D. K., Allen, P., VanFosson, C. A., Barton, A. J. (2018, January–February). Call for action: Nurses must play a critical role to enhance health literacy. *Nursing Outlook*, *66*(1): 97–100. Retrieved from https://doi.org/10.1016/j.outlook.2017.11.003

McNaughton, C. D., Cawthon, C., Kripalani, S., Liu, D., Storrow, A. B., & Roumie, C. L. (2015). Health literacy and mortality: A cohort study of patients hospitalized for acute heart failure. *Journal of the American Heart Association*, *4*, e001799.doi: 0.1161/JAHA.115.001799.

National Prevention Council. (2011). *National prevention strategy*. Washington, DC: US Department of Health and Human Services, Office of the Surgeon General.

National Quality Forum. (2009). *Cultural competency: An organizational strategy for high performing delivery systems.* Washington, DC: National Quality Forum. Retrieved from https://www.qualityforum.org/Publications/2009/04/Cultural_Competency__An_Organizational_Strategy_for_High-Performing_Delivery_Systems.aspx

Nutbeam, D. (2000). Health literacy as a public goal: A challenge for contemporary health education and communication strategies into the 21st century. *Health International*, *15*, 259–267.

Ortman, J. M., Velkoff, V. A., & Hogan, H. (2014). An aging nation: The older population in the United States. *Current Population Reports.* Retrieved from https://www.census.gov/prod/2014pubs/p25-1140.pdf

Pandya, C., Batalova, J., & McHugh, M. (2011). *Limited English proficient individuals in the United States: Number, share, growth, and linguistic diversity*. Washington, DC: Migration Policy Institute.

Parnell, T. A. (2014). Nursing leadership strategies, health literacy and patient outcomes. *Nurse Leader*, *12*(6), 49–52. doi:org/10.1016/j.mnl.2014.09.005

Parnell, T. A. (2015). *Health literacy in nursing: Providing person-centered care.* New York, NY: Springer.

Peterson, P. N., Shetterly, S. M., Clarke, C. L., Bekelman, D. B., Chan, P. S., Allen, L..A., . . . Masoudi, F. A. (2011). Health literacy and outcomes among patients with heart failure. *Journal of American Medical Association*, *305*(16), 1695–1701.

Robinson, S., Moser, D. A, Pelter, M. M., Nesbitt, T., Paul, S. M., & Dracup, K. (2011). Assessing health literacy in heart failure patients. *Journal of Cardiac Failure*, *17*(11), 887–892.

Rootman, I., & Gordon-El-Bihbety. D. (2008). *A vision for a health literate Canada: Report of the expert panel on health literacy.* Canadian Public Health Association. Retrieved from http://www.cpha.ca/uploads/portals/h-l/report_e.pdf

Rosland, A. M., Heisler, M., Choi, H. J., Silveira, M. J., & Piette, J. D. (2010). Family influences on self-management among functionally independent adults with diabetes or heart failure: Do family members hinder as much as they help? *Chronic Illness*, *6*(1), 22–33.

Rudd, R. (2010). Improving Americans' health literacy. *New England Journal of Medicine*, *363*(24), 2283–2285.

Sadeghi, S., Brooks, D., Stagg-Peterson, S., & Goldstein, R. (2013). Growing awareness of the importance of health literacy in individuals with COPD. *Journal of Chronic Obstructive Pulmonary Disease,10*, 72–78.

Scott, S. (2016). Health literacy education in baccalaureate nursing programs in the United States. *Nursing Education Perspectives, 37*(3), 153–159.

Shaw, S. J., Armin, J., Torres, C. H., Orzech, K. M., & Vivian, J. (2012). Chronic disease self-management and health literacy in four ethnic groups. *Journal of Health Communication, 17*(0 3), 67–81. doi: 10.1080/10810730.2012.712623

Short, J., McCormack, J., & Copley, A. (2014). The current practices of speech-language pathologists in providing information to clients with traumatic brain injury. *International Journal of Speech-Language Pathology, 16*(3), 219–230.

Smith, B. H., Fitzpatrick, J. J., & Hoyt-Hudson, P. (Eds.). (2011). *Problem solving for better health: A global perspective*. New York, NY: Springer.

Somers, S. A., & Mahadevan R. (2010). *Health literacy implications of the Affordable Care Act*. Washington, DC: Center for Health Care Strategies.

Speros, C. (2005). Health literacy: Concept analysis. *Journal of Advanced Nursing, 50*(6), 633–640.

Sudore, R. L., & Schillinger, D. (2009). Interventions to improve care for patients with limited health literacy. *Journal of Clinical Outcomes Management, 16*, 20–29.

Torres, R., & Nichols, J. (2014). Health literacy knowledge and experiences of associate degree nursing students: A pedagogical study. *Teaching and Learning in Nursing, 9*, 84–92.

U.S. Department of Education. (2006). National Center for Education Statistics. The health literacy of America's adults: Results from the 2003 National Assessment of Adult Literacy. Retrieved from http://nces.ed.gov/pubs2006/2006483.pdf

U.S. Department of Education. (2012). National Center for Education Statistics, Program for the International Assessment of Adult Competencies (PIAAC), U.S. PIAAC 2012/2014; Organization for Economic Cooperation and Development, PIAAC.

U.S. Department of Health and Human Services (2010a). *Healthy people 2020. Topics and objectives. Health communication and health information technology*. Retrieved from http://www.healthypeople.gov/2020/topics-objectives/topic/health-communication-and-health-information-technology

U.S. Department of Health and Human Services. (2010b). Office of Disease Prevention and Health Promotion. *National action plan to improve health literacy*. Washington, DC: Author.

World Health Organization. (1998). Division of Health Promotion, Education and Communications, Health Education and Health Promotion Unit. *Health promotion glossary*. Geneva, Switzerland: Author.

World Health Organization. (2006). *Constitution of the World Health Organization* (45th ed.). Retrieved from http://www.who.int/governance/eb/who_constitution_en.pdf?ua=1

Wu, J. R., Holmes, G. M., DeWalt, D. A., Macabasco-O'Connell, A., Bibbins-Domingo, K., Ruo, B., . . . Pignone, M. (2013). Low literacy is associated with increased risk of hospitalization and death among individuals with heart failure. *Journal of General Internal Medicine, 28*(9), 1174–1180.

Yin, H. S., Jay, M., Maness, L., Zabar, S., & Kalet, A. (2015). Health literacy: An educationally sensitive patient outcome. *Journal of General Internal Medicine, 30*(9), 1363–1368.

Chapter 12

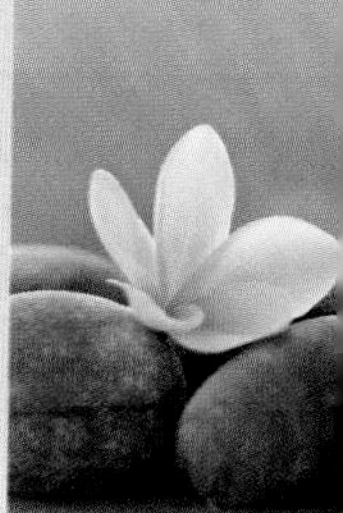

Planning Effective Ways to Help Clients Learn About Health

Marilyn Frenn

LEARNING OBJECTIVES

After completing this chapter, the student will be able to:

1. Develop a PICOT question for health education.
2. Differentiate best practices to facilitate learning from less effective approaches.
3. Discuss issues important to applying health education evidence in practice.
4. Describe ways to evaluate health education.

INTRODUCTION

Much of our health promotion work as nurses involves education, motivation, counseling, and helping clients develop self-management skills. Clients' preferences for information, self-management skill development, and support with providers' delivery of care are associated with greater client satisfaction, treatment adherence, and clinical outcomes (Cogan & Carlson, 2018; Cvengros, Christensen, Cunningham, Hillis, & Kaboli, 2009; Schoeb & Bürge, 2012).

Especially when a global pandemic threatens personal and family health, clients need to be consulted about their preferences (Iqbal, Warner, Paleri, Kovarik, & Kelly, 2020). However, many clients face barriers to participating in shared decision making about their health care (Joseph-Williams, Elwyn, & Edwards, 2014). Clients may believe that they should not ask questions, that providers are too busy for their questions, or that they should just do as they are told because providers know best. As we try to address health education needs for leading health issues and indicators (Government of Canada, 2018; U.S. Department of Health and Human Services [USDHHS], 2018), participation is enhanced when we seek to understand client preferences; adherence and outcomes are better when treatment is congruent with those preferences (Kiesler & Auerbach, 2006; Langbecker, Janda, & Yates, 2013). The COVID pandemic has led to many more telephonic and video consultations (Symonds, Trethewey, & Beck, 2020), but patients share less in these encounters than when they are face-to-face with a clinician (Hammersley et al., 2019). This chapter addresses evidence-based approaches to facilitate learning using multiple approaches to improve health outcomes.

BRIEF HISTORY OF CURRENT THEORIES AND RELATED EVIDENCE

In planning educational interventions, just as with other approaches to health promotion, use of a theoretical framework can help ensure comprehensive and effective implementation and evaluation. As one example, the PRECEDE-PROCEED model guides educational development by assessing needs and defining the priority competencies for learners (Millery, Hall, Eisman, & Murrman, 2014). Educational objectives were informed by specific learner challenges. Hypotheses about how to address the learning needs were developed and innovative approaches considered. The educational program was then delivered and evaluated. Theoretical models help guide development of in-person, print, and online education (Steadman, Chao, Strong, Maxwell, & West, 2014). *E-health* is a common term for interactive computer-based technologies that promote learning designed to foster health through social media, Web sites, and mobile apps (Stellefson et al., 2018). As e-health approaches expand, it is important to note who uses them and how much they interact using the technology, because greater use is associated with improved health outcomes (Price-Haywood, Qingyang, & Monlezun, 2018).

Whether health education takes place in person or via technology, a number of theories can be used to guide learning (Curran, 2014). Evidence supports use of learner-centered approaches (Papadakos et al., 2014). Major components of these approaches include letting people know why they are asked to learn and self-directing education based on prior experience (Brown, 2018). A constructivist approach builds on clients' prior learning (Tamim & Grant, 2017). Nurses should ask clients what they know and what they are interested in learning more about as the first step in health education. People remember and use what is meaningful for them, so engaging them in discussion and affirming what they know and have tried while listening for information about challenges are key. After providing information, asking clients to say or show what they understood helps to determine areas that are unclear.

Principles of Effective Teaching

When helping clients build their health promotion skills, we must be aware that people learn in different ways (Brady, 2013). Awareness of learning styles (Nick, 2014) means that health education should include options for visual learners to understand ways they can promote their health more effectively. Incorporating discussion allows auditory-verbal learners to make the information meaningful. Creating opportunities to practice motor skills solidifies learning for tactile and kinesthetic learners.

These considerations are part of seven principles of effective teaching, which include:

1. High expectations
2. Effective contact
3. Prompt feedback
4. Cooperation among learners
5. Active learning
6. Spending time on the task
7. Respect for various ways of learning (Chickering & Gamson, 1987; Sowan & Jenkins, 2013)

Universal design for instruction principles takes these recommendations further to include multiple flexible approaches to make learning more accessible (Levey, 2018).

Domains of Learning

The cognitive, psychomotor, and affective domains of learning identified by Bloom, Engelhart, Furst, Hill, and Krathwohl (1956) should be considered in planning health education. Moving from simple to complex concepts within the domain is recommended for nurse educators (Luparell, 2014), and the same applies to client learners.

Cognitive

In the cognitive domain, clients start by remembering information, which we can support by asking what they recall about the health issue and helping them understand and apply the information. For example, once clients know the risk factors for obesity, we can ask them to identify which risks may apply to them and their families. By sharing evidence-based approaches to reduce risks identified by clients, we can help them analyze and evaluate the information pertinent to improving their health (Byrne et al., 2018). Clients move to the highest level of cognitive learning by creating a plan to improve their health. Establishing trust, providing support, simplifying information, and assessing understanding are important components in helping clients and their families use health information effectively (Lau et al., 2012).

We can best help clients learn health promotion by engaging them in the process and tailoring the information we provide to their capabilities and communication preferences (Lee, Sulaiman-Hill, & Thompson, 2013). Consider culture when developing health promotion activities. For example, a small-group, experiential learning approach for self-analysis of family history regarding cardiovascular disease was effective in educating African American college students about their risks (Holland, Carthron, Duren-Winfield, & Lawrence, 2014). A group approach was also helpful in an efficacy-building education program for parents of children with chronic illnesses (Kieckhefer et al., 2014). Participants found the sharing of ideas among parents to be the most helpful component of the program.

Psychomotor

When teaching a new skill in the psychomotor domain, demonstrating and having clients perform the skill is the first step. Frequent repetition can help clients adapt their performance to environmental constraints and influences. For example, environmental constraints that clients may encounter can be included in a physical activity program along with group problem solving about continuing the activity safely. Competition with other schools and self-directed programming was useful in teaching high school students cardiopulmonary resuscitation and use of an automatic external defibrillator (Vetter, Haley, Dugan, Iyer, & Shults, 2016). Simulation was helpful in studying children's food choice behavior. Even though they knew what was healthier, they chose based on taste, so parents can facilitate nutritious choices by helping their children develop a taste for healthy foods (Heard, Harris, Liu, Schwartz, & Li, 2016). Moving unhealthy foods out of the optimal locations at the front of the store, where children readily see them, and placing healthy foods there is another important strategy tested with simulation (Wong et al., 2015). The fact that cognitive and affective domains are included in simulated learning argues favorably for including this modality in client education.

Affective

Attitudes, values, beliefs, and emotions affect the information a client can learn and incorporate in his or her lifestyle to improve health. We must first understand their perspectives and then incorporate them in our teaching (Abbass-Dick et al., 2018). Counseling and coaching are two evidence-based approaches for successful affective communication with clients.

Counseling

Counseling is an approach to health education in which health-care providers help clients and families clarify their values and feelings about issues in improving their health. Encouraging reflection is one way to foster growth. As clients and families set goals, nurses model positive changes and provide opportunities for mastery with feedback and personal attention (Fazio-Griffith & Ballard, 2016). Quitline counseling was more effective for smokers referred with a staff phone sign-up (warm handoff) from their hospital room compared to a faxed referral on discharge (Mussulman et al., 2018).

Mindfulness-based therapies have been found particularly helpful for groups who have experienced racism or disenfranchisement (Witkiewitz, Greenfield, & Bowen, 2013). Awareness of moment-to-moment experience and acceptance without judgment characterize mindfulness therapies. For example, these interventions have been helpful for people with chronic conditions both in person and through electronic delivery (Chadi et al., 2018; Mikolasek, Berg, Witt, & Barth, 2018).

Coaching

To improve client knowledge and reduce costs, evidence from randomized-control trials (RCTs) supports coaching with a client decision aid such as a checklist of questions (Stacey et al., 2013). Coaching was defined through a concept analysis to include "a goal-oriented, client-centered partnership that is health-focused and occurs through a process of client enlightenment and empowerment" (Olsen, 2014, p. 18). Personalized content was central to effective online coaching in a review of studies (Lentferink et al., 2017). Recent examples of effective coaching include:

- E-health coaching for lifestyle change (Brandt, Søgaard, Clemensen, Søndergaard, & Nielsen, 2018)
- Helping mothers with occupational performance while addressing family needs (Graham, Rodger, & Ziviani, 2014)
- Encouraging increased activity among those with chronic low back pain (Iles, Taylor, Davidson, & O'Halloran, 2014)
- Encouraging increased activity among those with rheumatoid arthritis (Nessen, Opava, Martin, & Demmelmaier, 2014)
- Discussing sexual concerns (Britton & Bright, 2014)
- Improving readiness to engage in worksite wellness activities (Mettler et al., 2014)

Further research is needed to examine effectiveness and cost of coaching across primary-care client outcomes (Ahluwalia, de Silva, Kumar, Viney, & Chana, 2013). Balancing the pursuit of health outcomes with client autonomy is important, yet it may be challenging to sustain in the role of health coach if clients choose not to work toward health outcomes (Howard & Ceci, 2013; Leahy, 2014).

DISCUSSION OF THE EVIDENCE

Organizing evidence into options for clients to consider helps them engage actively in their own health promotion (Elwyn et al., 2013). The U.S. Preventive Services Taskforce (USPST) (2018b) regularly examines and ranks evidence on a number of health issues, including client education and counseling. These materials are commonly referred to as decision aids, and their ability to clarify client values can be evaluated using international criteria to promote transparency and avoid conflicts of interest among providers, clients, families, and communities (Fagerlin et al., 2012; International Patient Decision Aids Standards [IPDAS] Collaboration, 2019).

Decision Aids

Decision aids help people know their options, thus allowing them to clarify their personal values (Stacey et al., 2014). Nurses and coaches can promote health beyond the clinic setting at community locations frequented by clients (Luque, Ross, & Gwede., 2014). Effective print health education materials should allay concerns with clear, accurate portrayal of risks and benefits (Bishop & Salmon, 2013). Design elements for effective print cancer-related education with Latin groups have been developed (Buki, Salazar, & Pitton, 2009). To develop more appropriate materials, the community of interest needs to be involved in the design, diversity among Latin cultures must be acknowledged, and cultural health beliefs and appropriate language need to be incorporated in the design of the materials.

Videos

Video health education has been found effective for prostate cancer screening, sunscreen adherence, HIV testing, breast self-examination, self-care in patients with heart failure, and female condom use (Tuong, Larsen, & Armstrong, 2014). The authors of the systematic review indicated that the modeling demonstrated in the videos may be a particularly helpful component of learning. Videos were not effective, however, for health education about substance abuse unless the information was specifically tailored to the audience.

Online Media

An online approach directed toward physicians improved shared decision making and reduced prostate screening (Feng et al., 2013). Online diabetes health education was most successful when it included goal setting, interactive feedback, personalized coaching, and peer support. A longer duration of intervention and a strong theoretical framework contribute to effectiveness (Ramadas, Chan, Oldenburg, Hussein, & Quek, 2018). Computer-tailored approaches, in which feedback is given based on client characteristics such as sex or stage of change, were more effective than nontailored interventions (Nikoloudakis et al., 2018). Social media such as Twitter (Jackson, Gettings, & Metcalfe, 2018), YouTube, Facebook, and blogs are increasingly used to target health education, but it is important to evaluate the effectiveness of these approaches for each group and type of behavior (Hsu, Rouf, & Allman-Farinelli, 2018). Interactive games can help sedentary youth and older adults become more physically active (Lee, Xiang, & Gao, 2017; Zhang & Kaufman, 2016).

Avatars are online images of a person used to enact situations, such as those found in adopting healthier behaviors. For example, interventions involving avatars have been helpful with substance abuse and intimate partner violence treatment, although further randomized controlled trials are needed (Easton, Berbary, & Crane, 2018). Avatars also have been useful in helping people remember to take health supplements (Fang, Bjering, & Ginige, 2018) and to reduce college student drinking, especially among heavy drinkers (Earle, LaBrie, Boyle, & Smith, 2018).

Mobile phones are widely used even among historically underrepresented cultural and age groups, and they are potentially better candidates to assist with health behavior change, including influenza vaccine reminders among low-income pregnant women (Stockwell et al., 2014) and addressing cardiovascular risk factors among those with mental health disorders (Abroms, Padmanabhan, & Evans, 2012; Baker et al., 2018; Stockwell et al., 2014). Such applications have also been shown effective in reducing children's sugar-sweetened beverage intake (Nezami, Ward, Lytle, Ennett, & Tate, 2018). Culturally targeted messages may be more acceptable than generic messages. For example, text messages were helpful in promoting condom use and sexually transmitted disease screening among Native American and Alaska Native youth (Yao et al., 2018), as well as with young men who have sex with men and transgender women with HIV (Tanner et al., 2018).

Active Learning

Whether health education is done in person or through other means, principles that facilitate learning are paramount. Active learning improved health literacy, memory, gait, balance, physical activity, and diet in older adults (Uemura, Yamada, & Okamoto, 2018). Community-based participatory research principles were used to involve members of the community in focus groups about educational materials, the plan for screening, and integration into the life of the faith community for a successful HIV education and screening program (Derose et al., 2014). The latter approach requires relationship building with client communities but may yield more successful health promotion in the long term.

Active learning was more effective in changing nursing students' attitudes about their role in screening and intervening for drug use compared with narrated slideshows (Knopf-Amelung et al., 2018). Effective active learning strategies in professional education include team-based learning (Branney & Priego-Hernández, 2018), role playing (McNaughton, Cowell, & Fogg, 2014), games (Adams, Burger, Crawford, & Setter, 2018; Hnatyshyn, 2018), and use of multimedia (Krautscheid & Williams, 2018). Active learners outperform passive learners (Mitchell, Lucas, Charlton, & McMahon, 2018). These evidence-based approaches can be used to construct client and caregiver learning opportunities for more effective application of health knowledge (Cruz-Oliver, Parikh, Wallace, Malmstrom, & Sanchez-Reilly, 2018; Estrada, Rodríguez, & Meléndez, 2018). When active learning approaches were compared with didactic approaches for diabetic education, active-learning group clients demonstrated greater understanding of diabetes, their own values, and guideline-derived target goals (Naik, Teal, Rodriguez, & Haidet, 2011).

EVALUATING LEARNING OUTCOMES

Outcome measures should be determined as part of the educational program planning. Evaluating the context within which health education takes place is likewise important because context can affect learning outcomes. For example, in evaluating an individually based nutrition and physical activity intervention in churches, Harmon, Blake, Thrasher, and Hébert, (2014) conducted a content analysis of the origin and content of print messages on church bulletin boards and newsletters. Barriers to education for those with diabetes were evaluated across 10 studies using a variety of methods, including focus groups, one-on-one interviews, semi-structured interviews, surveys, and a randomized-controlled trial (Yuncken, 2014).

Virtual interventions increasingly show improved health behavior outcomes; for example, choosing water rather than alcohol in a virtual environment resulted in reduced alcohol intake (Wang, Christensen, Jeong, & Miller, 2019). Diet behaviors and anthropometric outcomes were most improved with community-based interventions, intensive nutrition education, and continued communication among stakeholders (Andrade, Lotton, & Andrade, 2018).

Taking into account the client's perspective—including pediatric clients—in evaluating his or her need for health information and the amount, time, and way the information was delivered is imperative because including these aspects can affect a patient's health outcomes (Peña & Rojas, 2014). Indeed, the Centers for Medicare and Medicaid Services evaluate communication about new medications based on patients' answers about the purpose and side effects as a hospital performance measure (Thompson, 2014).

When a health promotion program is based on assessment of need, outcomes flow naturally from resolving that need. For example, a mosque-based intervention tailored to Muslim women effectively increased both intention and completion of mammography in a group with low screening rates (Padela et al., 2018). Client satisfaction with the way information was presented, timing and organization of the presentation and written materials, and perceived level of understanding should also be evaluated (Mkandawire-Valhmu et al., 2018). Once effective programs have been developed, structured education for important health issues can be implemented and outcomes evaluated (Piacentine, Robinson, Waltke, Tjoe, & Ng, 2018).

PATIENT, INTERVENTION, CONTROL, OBSERVATION, AND TIME (PICOT) QUESTION AND EVIDENCE TABLES: PRINT AND E-HEALTH AIDS

In stating your PICOT question, consider the client conditions you see frequently in your practice setting, where providing the best available evidence could make an important improvement in health for many of your clients. Whether your health education program relates to the PICOT question below or to another topic, evaluating learning outcomes is essential to determining whether provided education is addressing client learning needs.

The following is an example of an initial PICOT question comparing health education approaches for print and e-health aids to African American men regarding prostate cancer.

P: For African American males who are 40–69 years old,
I: does an educational brochure,
C: compared to a computer-based program,
O: improve shared decision making regarding prostate cancer screening
T: over a 1-year period?

This PICOT question seemed important given that prostate cancer is the most frequently diagnosed cancer in African American men and that mortality in African Americans is twice that of Caucasians (American Cancer Society, 2016). According to the review of guidelines, the limited benefits and substantial harms of screening with prostate-specific antigen assay (PSA) should be clearly discussed. Risks for prostate cancer are higher in those who are older, are African American, and have a family history of prostate cancer. The USPST (2018a) recommended with a Grade C that men 55 to 69 considering screening discuss the risks and small potential benefit for some men with their clinician, and that providers screen only those requesting it. Grade D was given by the USPST to instances in which PSA should not be used for screening, for example, for men over age 70. Table 12-1 shows the USPST evidence grading system.

African American men tend to develop prostate cancer younger than other groups do, sometimes before age 45; to be diagnosed with more advanced cancer, which is less amenable to treatment; and to request screening less often than do Caucasians (Ivlev, Jerabkova, Mishra, Cook, & Eden, 2018; Nettey et al., 2018). Readers are encouraged to stay abreast of new studies as well as modifications to guidelines because professional groups vary in their recommendations, and further research including African Americans is crucially needed (Ivlev et al., 2018). Some advocate screening guidelines that recommend prostate screening at a younger age for African American men than for men of other races (Reddy, Roberts, Shenoy, Packianathan, Giri, & Vijayakumar, 2018).

Clinicians should be keenly aware of the various perspectives and include them when preparing health education materials. Shared decision making was shown to increase patients' knowledge of the risks of screening and the likelihood of prostate cancer and death from prostate cancer, but results pertaining to African Americans were not described (Martínez-González, Neuner-Jehle, Plate, Rosemann, & Senn, 2018). Subsequent to this review, including studies last completed in 2015, prior screening or discussion of pros and cons of screening were found predictive of screening in African American men, who have lower rates of screening than Caucasian men (Roberts, Wilson, Stiel, Casiano, & Montgomery, 2018). Only studies pertinent to the PICOT question not included in reviews are included in Table 12-2.

Prostate Cancer Screening Decision Aids

Many high-quality decision aids are available for prostate cancer screening and treatment at http://decisionaid.ohri.ca/AZlist.html. Although specific decision aids for patients were not used, integration into the electronic health record (EHR) improved provider-reported shared

Table 12-1 U.S. Preventive Services Evidence Grade System

Grade	Definition	Suggestions for Practice
A	The USPSTF recommends the service. There is high certainty that the net benefit is substantial.	Offer or provide this service.
B	The USPSTF recommends the service. There is high certainty that the net benefit is moderate or there is moderate certainty that the net benefit is moderate to substantial.	Offer or provide this service.
C	The USPSTF recommends selectively offering or providing this service to individual patients based on professional judgment and patient preferences. There is at least moderate certainty that the net benefit is small.	Offer or provide this service for selected patients depending on individual circumstances.
D	The USPSTF recommends against the service. There is moderate or high certainty that the service has no net benefit or that the harms outweigh the benefits.	Discourage the use of this service.
I	I statement: The USPSTF concludes that the current evidence is insufficient to assess the balance of benefits and harms of the service. Evidence is lacking, of poor quality, or conflicting, and the balance of benefits and harms cannot be determined.	Read the clinical considerations section of USPSTF Recommendation Statement. If the service is offered, patients should understand the uncertainty about the balance of benefits and harms.

Source: From U.S. Preventive Services Taskforce. (2018b). *U.S. Preventive Services Task Force Grade Definitions*. Retrieved from https://www.uspreventiveservicestaskforce.org/Page/Name/grade-definitions

Table 12-2 Evidence-Based Health Education Appraisal*

What is your PICOT question? For African American males (40 to 69 years old), does an educational brochure, compared to a computer-based program, improve shared decision making (SDM) regarding prostate cancer screening over a 1-year period?

What database(s), years, and keywords will be searched?
CINAHL last 10 years: Prostate cancer screening; cancer screening; prostatic neoplasms AND decision aids.
Medline last 10 years: Prostatic neoplasms; prostate cancer screening; prostate-specific antigen AND decision support techniques; patient decision aids.

Citation†	Subjects	Method	Results	Rigor of Evidence	Applicable?	Cost?
Aminsharifi et al. (2018)	94 of 106 providers reported SDM for prostate cancer screening in 30% African American patient group.	Descriptive.	Algorithm based on guidelines integrated in EHR leads to increase in reported SDM and increase in PSA screening.	Low.	Yes, because clinicians need to use guidelines pertinent to client group.	EHR facilitates discussions by organizing information to reduce time. No costs reported, although cost of integration in EHR noted.
Boulay (2018)	Two church leaders in a largely African American church were taught about benefits and problems with prostate cancer screening and held monthly meetings with parishioners, sought consent, and provided before and after knowledge test.	Doctor of Nursing Practice project.	Nonsignificant improvement in scores was noted following training with brochures and videos from Institute on Aging, American Cancer Society, Centers for Disease Control and Prevention.	Author designed pre- and posttest.	Much larger randomized controlled study would be needed to use results, including an instrument with acceptable estimates of reliability and validity. Showed some feasibility of potentially useful venue to reach men at risk.	Stated low cost, but no cost figures provided.
Ivlev et al. (2018)	18 studies, including decision aids for prostate cancer screening in men 40 years or older: data on screening intention for approximately 8,400 men and screening for 2,385 men.	Systematic review and meta-analysis through April 2018.	Low-quality evidence showed use of decision aids in any print format reduced screening and seemed congruent with men's values. Further research is needed, but discussion soon after use of decision aid was recommended because men did not act on their intention within the first year after using the decision aid.	High.	Only two studies addressed use of decision aids in African American men.	PSA testing is not cost effective, so if decision aids reduce screening, this may reduce costs.

(*continued*)

Table 12-2 Evidence-Based Health Education Appraisal*—cont'd

Citation†	Subjects	Method	Results	Rigor of Evidence	Applicable?	Cost?
Martínez-González et al. (2018)	Four RCTs comparing SDM to usual care: RCTs included 1,760 men.	Systematic review and meta-analysis.	SDM improved knowledge of the risks of prostate cancer and death from prostate cancer, but was no different than usual care in PSA screening or decisional conflict.	Moderate.	Not many studies, no specification of race/ethnicity except percentage Caucasian, appropriate methods used.	Not specifically addressed.
Saver et al. (2017)	27 men (4% African American).		Preferences for avoiding prostate screening changed significantly after viewing the video, but not after reading the print decision aid. Although intended to foster SDM, intention to discuss screening with their physician decreased significantly. Videos were engaging based on focus groups in diverse communities.	Moderate.	Small sample with few African Americans. Based on 2012 UPSTF recommendation to forgo prostate screening.	NI
Stamm et al. (2017)	329 patients were randomly assigned to usual care, decision aid, or SDM plus decision aid.	RCT	Knowledge was improved in SDM plus decision aid compared to the control, but the decision aid alone resulted in a lower level of knowledge and more frequent prostate antigen screenings.	Moderate.	Only 3.6% were African American, the knowledge instrument was not validated, and there may have been variability in the usual care.	NI
Owens, Friedman, Brandt, Bernhardt, and Hébert (2016)	39 African American men (38 to 66 years old) recruited in community settings, such as churches and barbershops.	Focus groups and 45-item survey.	Men generally had knowledge about prostate cancer screening, but few engaged in SDM with their physician, who they saw as a main source of information. Technologic decision aids were acceptable, and men readily used phones and computers. Avatars were seen as acceptable if they were African American but were reported to be potentially unacceptable to older men. Gas stations were suggested as a place to have kiosk information because not all men go to church. Sports or an attractive woman were suggested to catch attention.	Moderate.	Men were all at least high school educated and most had already had prostate screening. Women are often a source of health information for African American men, but they were not included in the study.	NI

Table 12-2 Evidence-Based Health Education Appraisal*—cont'd

Citation†	Subjects	Method	Results	Rigor of Evidence	Applicable?	Cost?
Sandiford and D'Errico (2016)	50 African American men aged 30–75 in two California churches.	Pretest, posttest decision aid question-and-answer workshop, including a video intervention.	Men had a high level of knowledge at the beginning, which increased slightly after the workshop. Forty-three had at least some college, 38 had prior prostate cancer screening. Thirty-one proceeded with PSA that day, even though authors acknowledged that 1 in 22 African Americans will die from prostate cancer, 1 in 1,000 will avoid death because of screening, and 30 to 40 will be harmed by screening and treatment.	Low.	Investigator developed test, no psychometrics provided, although it was reviewed by experts. No control group. Topics in workshop were well developed. This is an important site for such intervention. Less-educated men need to be included in future studies.	NI
Starosta, Luta, Tomko, Schwartz, and Taylor (2015)	Men aged 45 to 70 (56.2% Caucasian, 39.9% African American) were randomly assigned to a print decision aid (n = 630), a Web decision aid (n = 631), or usual care (n = 632).	RCT	Phone interviews baseline, one month and 13 months after intervention assessed prostate screening pros and cons. Higher baseline cons predicted lower screening for both print and Web decision aids than for usual care. If the limitations of screening were not important at baseline, those men were more likely to get screened after the decision aid. If the limitations of screening were important, the decision aid made no difference. Thus, in both cases it amplified men's initial views.	High.	Large sample, including African American men related to PICOT question. Sample included those with less than high school education through college and low- as well as middle- and high-income men.	NI
Miller (2014)	Participants included African American men ages 30–45 years.	Descriptive.	Men had awareness of risk factors (e.g., race, smoking, first-degree relative with prostate cancer, high-fat diet, low physical activity) but underestimated their risk of developing prostate cancer and their knowledge was uneven. Those with higher education and income demonstrated greater knowledge	Instruments were theory based and had acceptable estimates of reliability.	Has relevance for anticipatory guidance because discussion about prostate cancer being the most commonly diagnosed cancer (39%) in African American men may help improve evidence-based decisions.	NI

(*continued*)

Table 12-2 Evidence-Based Health Education Appraisal*—cont'd

Citation†	Subjects	Method	Results	Rigor of Evidence	Applicable?	Cost?
Miller et al. (2014)	Female partners of 231 African American men.	RCT women given CDC brochure alone or with brochure encouraging partner to initiate discussion with provider.	Message groups did not differ on taking active steps to engage in provider discussion. High-monitoring partners may be effective in influencing their mates to initiate provider discussion, particularly when tailored messaging is provided.	Yes.	Yes, compared two types of brochures, but not computer-based approach.	NI
Berry et al. (2013)	Participants included 494 men with localized prostate cancer who had not made a treatment decision. Nonwhite included, but numbers were not included in report.	RCT in four cities. Measures at baseline, 1 month and 6 months, comparing Internet-based client decision aid with usual education alone.	Decisional conflict resulting from inadequate information was associated with clinical site, being older, being nonwhite, having less income, having more trait anxiety, plus baseline measures of inadequate information and support. Lack of values clarity was associated with clinical site, less income, minimal pre-enrollment use of the Internet, and baseline lack of values clarity and inadequate support. Conflict related to perceived support significantly decreased as men were further from biopsy by number of weeks, with the largest decrease between 1 and 2 weeks, plus associations with clinical site, nonwhite race, and baseline support scores. Being an effective decision maker was associated only with baseline support scores.	Yes, although information on sample characteristics would help with interpretation of results for practice.	Yes, even though this study does not deal with screening, the subgroups needing information and values clarification are important to note.	NI
Gash and McIntosh (2013)	Participants included women (n = 84, 74.3%), African American (n = 61, 53.5%), 3 African American men, 48 (42.1%) Caucasian.	Survey: convenience sample at a health fair.	African American women report different beliefs about prostate cancer screening than do men. African American and Caucasian beliefs were not significantly different.	OK	Yes, because other studies recommend including regarding prostate cancer screening.	NI

Table 12-2 Evidence-Based Health Education Appraisal*—cont'd

Citation†	Subjects	Method	Results	Rigor of Evidence	Applicable?	Cost?
Han et al. (2013)	Participants included 3,427 men age 50 to 74 years.	Survey in nationally representative sample.	64.3% reported no SDM, 27.8% reported discussion of one to two elements only, 8.0% reported full SDM, 44.2% reported no PSA screening, 27.8% reported less-than-annual screening, 25.1% reported nearly annual screening. Greater SDM was associated with higher PSA screening.	High.	Useful; SDM may not be helpful in reducing PSA screening. Community-based screening programs or decision aids may be considered.	
Ilic, Neuberger, Djulbegovic, and Dahm (2013)	Five RCTs with a total of 341,342 participants, but race not included in report.	Systematic review and meta-analysis.	Prostate cancer screening did not reduce deaths in 50- to 69-year-old men and risks are associated with PSA screening, with or without DRE. No studies were found examining DRE alone	High.	Yes, evidence does not support PSA screening, but missing subgroup analysis makes results more difficult to interpret for this PICOT question.	NI
Jimbo et al. (2013)	29 studies, including decision aids for prostate cancer screening, but no data related to race or culture of subjects were examined.	Systematic review years 2000–2012, including decision aids for prostate cancer screening and other cancers.	Studies on decision aids for prostate cancer screening seldom used theoretical frameworks. All provided knowledge (which was increased in all but five, in which there was no difference, and two, in which knowledge was not measured), including on the decision not to screen, information on decision making and on communication. Four included values clarification, 1 provided information on when to stop screening, 3 led to increased screening, 3 led to decreased screening, and 14 led to a more negative attitude about screening.	High.	Yes, the review included many relevant studies.	Only one study examined cost, reporting a $2 cost for the decision aid.
Johnson, Chang, Sun, Miyake, and Rosser (2013)	Participants included 168 primary-care providers in central Florida in 2008.	Survey: convenience sample, 22% response rate.	68% recommend prostate cancer screening to more than 75% of their patients over the age of 50 years, up from 47% in 2006 ($p < 0.001$); 74% felt screening was effective. Knowledge scores were not associated with screening attitudes and behaviors. Despite evidence, provider screening attitudes have changed little over the past 5 years.	OK	Somewhat, in that clients may have gotten conflicting advice from providers without regard to the evidence.	NI

(*continued*)

Table 12-2 Evidence-Based Health Education Appraisal* —cont'd

Citation†	Subjects	Method	Results	Rigor of Evidence	Applicable?	Cost?
McDowell, Occhipinti, and Chambers (2013)	Participants in Australia included 207 men with prostate cancer in first-degree relative and 239 men without this family history.	Path analysis.	Predictors of greater lifetime PSA testing were similar for those with prostate cancer in a relative and without. PSA testing increased with age and a greater number of acquaintances with prostate cancer. For those without a relative, having spoken to a doctor about prostate cancer was associated with increased PSA testing. Perceived risk was not a significant predictor of PSA testing for either sample.	Yes, careful attention to sampling and analysis were reported.	Yes, men with a family history have more than double the risk of prostate cancer, but age, acquaintances, and speaking with a physician influence decision making.	NI
Patel et al. (2013)	Participants included 104 African American men, 45 years and older, who had not been screened for prostate cancer with a PSA and/or DRE within the past year.	Community-based participatory research, three focus groups, individual discussions.	PSA screening was increased.	Rigor was addressed according to the study methods.	Yes, the approach is useful, and African Americans are at higher risk for prostate cancer.	NI
Taylor et al. (2013)	Participants included 1,893 culturally diverse men.	Random assignment to print decision aid, Web-based interactive decision aid, or usual care.	Both decision aids resulted in significantly improved knowledge and reduced decisional conflict compared with usual care up to 13 months later, but they did not affect actual screening rates. Print was initially more appreciated than Web-based, and both were more appreciated than the usual care, but differences were not significant at 13 months.	High.	Yes.	NI
Volk et al. (2013)	Participants included 246 members of American Academy of Family Physicians in 2006 through 2008.	Survey: convenience sample, 57.7% response.	"Physicians who discussed harms and benefits with patients and then let them decide (47.7%) were more likely to endorse beliefs that scientific evidence does not support screening, that patients should be told about the lack of evidence, and that patients have a right to know the limitations of screening. They were also less likely	OK	May be useful in understanding issues in provider behavior.	NI

Table 12-2 Evidence-Based Health Education Appraisal*—cont'd

Citation†	Subjects	Method	Results	Rigor of Evidence	Applicable?	Cost?
			to endorse the belief that there was no need to educate patients because they wanted to be screened. Concerns about medicolegal risk associated with not screening were more common among physicians who discussed the harms and benefits and recommended screening than among physicians who discussed screening and let their patients decide" (from abstract).			
Wilkes et al. (2013)	Participants included 120 physicians in five group practices and 712 male patients aged 50 to 75 years.	Cluster RCT.‡ Web-based educational program on SDM for intervention physicians and patient activation program for one I group of patients (none for other I group) compared with C brochures from the CDC.	Patients' ratings of SDM did not differ between groups. I-activated patients reported that physicians had higher prostate cancer screening discussion rates (p <.01). Standardized patients reported that I physicians were more neutral during prostate cancer screening recommendations (p <.05). Eighty percent had previous PSA tests.	Rigorous design with sample determined through power analysis, randomization, blinding of subjects, and standardized patients.	Yes, there was no difference in online plus print compared to print alone intervention for patients.	NI
Williams et al. (2013)	Participants included 543 men, 61% African American.	RCT booklet decision aid compared with usual care control.	Those getting the booklet decision aid had improved knowledge and less decisional conflict at 2 months compared to usual care.	Yes.	Yes, booklets can be used prior to clinician visits.	NI
Kassan et al. (2012)	Participants included 531 men: average age 57 years (SD = 6.8), 37% African American, 92% had Internet access.	Report of online portion of three-arm RCT.	Of the 256 (only half) who accessed the Web site, they were more likely to be white, to be previously screened, have Internet access, and use the Internet daily. Reported use was overestimated. Eighty-four percent used values clarification tool, and more than 50% viewed each video testimonial based on Web tracking. Baseline	Yes.	Yes, Internet is seen as a viable option, but it was not highly accessed by African American men.	NI

(continued)

Table 12-2 Evidence-Based Health Education Appraisal*—cont'd

Citation†	Subjects	Method	Results	Rigor of Evidence	Applicable?	Cost?
			screening preference was associated with values clarification tool responses and Web site feedback. Older adults used the site, although previous literature has suggested that would not be a useful approach.			
Çapık and Gözüm (2012)	Participants included 73 men over age 40 in Turkey, where prostate cancer is the second highest cause of cancer-related deaths in men.	Pretest/posttest. No control group. Convenience sample followed 3 and 6 months.	Interactive online intervention increased DRE 9.3% to 19.1%, and the PSA measurement rate increased from 6.7% to 31.4%. Perceived susceptibility increased.	Sample provided adequate power. Prostate cancer incidence in Turkey is considerably less than in the United States, so limits reason for study.	Intervention modality worked to increase screening, so it might also be designed to decrease prostate cancer screening, for those who support that approach.	NI
Allen and Berry (2011)	Review of literature, including culturally diverse populations.	Review.	May be premature to declare multimedia decision aids superior to other formats. More research is needed with racially and ethnically diverse samples.	Not a systematic review.	Studies were analyzed for inclusion and focus on diverse samples.	NI
Ferrante, Shaw, and Scott (2011)	Participants included 64 mainly white men in New Jersey in 2009 and 2010.	Grounded theory.	None discussed potential risks of prostate cancer screening with physicians. They received their health information through lay media, friends, or family members, which may facilitate SDM with their health-care provider.	Rigor was addressed as pertinent to the method.	OK, although not with African Americans.	NI
Heyes, Harrington, and Paterson (2011)	Nine studies related to men's experience of prostate cancer screening.	Literature review.	Men experienced embarrassment, confusion, and pain.	Studies were carefully critiqued.	Yes, information may be useful in SDM discussions.	NI

Table 12-2 Evidence-Based Health Education Appraisal* —cont'd

Citation†	Subjects	Method	Results	Rigor of Evidence	Applicable?	Cost?
Myers et al. (2011)	Participants included 313 men eligible for screening.	RCT; before meeting with their physician, all subjects had a phone survey and mailed brochure. I men had a nurse-led "decision counseling" session. C men completed a practice satisfaction survey.	Nurse-mediated decision counseling increased participant prostate cancer screening knowledge, informed decision making, and reduced screening.	Yes.	Yes.	NI
Carter, Tippett, Anderson, and Tameru (2010)	Participants included 76 in focus groups; 405 completed the educational program (166 women, 239 men).	Focus groups and 2-hour PowerPoint with educational brochure and educational program conducted by nine trained community members in churches and community settings. No control group in the Black Belt of Alabama.	After attending the education session, 48% (n =105) were screened who had not been screened within the last 12 months. Screening was paid if had no insurance, but most had insurance.	Weak design, but at-risk group included.	Approach is expensive but somewhat effective to increase screenings if warranted in an at risk group.	Forty-five-dollar incentive to attend educational session.
Holt et al. (2009)	Participants included 49 men ages 45 to 90.	Two-church cluster RCT: 16-page booklet for informed decision making regarding prostate cancer screening, including or not including spiritual messages.	Knowledge increased in the spiritual message group. Decisions about screening did not change in either group.	Instruments had low internal consistency; sample was small without statistical power to detect differences.	Yes, the interventions were acceptable to the participants.	NI

(continued)

Table 12-2 Evidence-Based Health Education Appraisal*—cont'd

Citation†	Subjects	Method	Results	Rigor of Evidence	Applicable?	Cost?
McCormack et al. (2009)	Participants included 376 men (no information on race).	Quasi-experimental longitudinal design with intervention to increase knowledge about prostate cancer screening alone, as part of overall health messages, and a control group.	Knowledge increased most for information in the context of other men's health issues, but it also increased for the prostate cancer screening information compared to the control.	Weak quasi-experimental design without information on race composition of sample.	Presentation of information about overall health may be useful.	NI
Sheehan (2009)	Participants included 123 Caucasian men, ages 45 to 75 years.	One group, pretest/posttest design.	Six-minute video resulted in higher knowledge, rating their personal risk of developing prostate cancer correctly, and intent to discuss prostate cancer screening with their primary-care provider.	Weak design without control.	Video approach may be helpful.	NI
Wray et al. (2009)	Seventy-nine participants.	Needs assessment, focus groups, and process evaluation for prostate screening among African Americans.	Controversy and long-standing distrust of health providers make messages of "talk with your provider" more complicated. Community partners prefer "get screened" messages, contrary to guidelines.	Rigor addressed according to methods.	Yes, cultural and community perspectives need to be considered in planning screening education.	NI

Strength of overall evidence: Good. There are several systematic reviews and meta-analyses, and RCTs, but few detailing subgroup analyses with African American men. Descriptive, qualitative, and community-based approaches with African American men do not offer evidence that is as rigorous, and many use language that screening should be increased rather than advocate decision making by clients with a trend toward less screening for prostate cancer included in national guidelines.

Recommendation: Although computer-based approaches appear to offer more opportunities for tailoring and active learning, not all population groups use them as often as they use print decision aids. Community-based approaches may work best with African American men and other at-risk groups.

* RCT = randomized controlled trial; I = intervention; C = control; NI = no information provided by authors; PSA = prostate-specific antigen; DRE = digital rectal examination; CDC = Centers for Disease Control and Prevention.

† Studies were organized alphabetically, with most recent years first.

decision making based on client characteristics and the various guidelines available (Aminsharifi et al., 2018). These authors reported an increase in screening for both African Americans and Caucasians with use of the algorithm in the EHR, but they also cited an increase in aggressive cancers when screening rates previously dropped.

Computer-based decision aids offer the greatest potential for targeting material to your client, but they are used less often than print materials, especially in studies including African American men. Poor, historically under-represented groups, and rural clients have less access to broadband, reducing access to health information and health-care provision online (Tomer, Fishbane, Siefer, & Callahan, 2020), as well as reducing opportunities for education and work from home in the COVID pandemic. Asking clients to use a decision aid without discussion is not recommended (Stamm et al., 2017). Community-based approaches at churches, barbershops, and other places where men may congregate can effectively reach this at-risk population with decision aids to help them accurately understand their risk for prostate cancer as well as the risks of screening and treatment. Involving community health workers, clinic staff members, and nurses in providing decision aids prior to clinic visits offers the optimal chance for fruitful and time-effective interprofessional shared decision making (Stacey & Legare, 2015).

College-educated African American men tend to have information on prostate cancer screening, so carefully developed decision aids to promote shared decision making are especially needed by those with less education (Sandiford & D'Errico, 2016). In a larger trial including culturally diverse, well-educated men, one-page written decision aids did not reduce use of screenings, including PSA, that likely produce limited benefits. Personalized, multi-level decision aids are likely needed to help people reach decisions different from their prior behavior (Bakan & Erci, 2018). Even with college-educated people, numeracy and ability to understand graphs also needs to be assessed as decision aids are developed and used (Nayak et al., 2016).

APPLYING THE EVIDENCE IN PRACTICE

As new health promotion evidence is considered, it must become part of health education materials and client decision aids. Advocating for national and state funding as well as funding through foundations invested in health will foster development of effective health education materials as the underlying science develops. We also need to consider risks and costs in terms of the benefits of applying what we do know in practice.

Strengths and Limitations of the Body of Evidence

Although a number of meta-analyses, systematic reviews, and RCTs provide the highest quality evidence for health education, specifically client decision aids, they nevertheless have limitations. Studies often lacked a theoretical framework, which limits accuracy in applying the health education program, evaluation of outcomes across studies, and approaches to evaluating whether the program will work in clinical practice rather than in the controlled conditions of the RCT.

Study reports and subject selection criteria often neglect at-risk population subgroups. Studies focused on or including these subgroups often used less rigorous designs or had too limited a sample for statistically significant results. Best practices were not clearly indicated across studies; rather, a compilation of ideas to consider in planning health education was provided.

To make best use of the resources, clinicians are encouraged to compile online resources for issues and client groups regularly seen in their practice setting. For example, online materials have been useful for reducing the risk of hypertension in young African American females (Staffileno, Tangney, & Fogg, 2018). Providing these materials through e-mail or online communications, in waiting rooms, or during the time clients spend with nurses can increase access and use, allowing providers to optimize one-on-one time spent with clients. Print materials should be considered for community-based distribution in places where people can readily find and read them.

Areas for Further Research

Working with professional groups focused on specific health education priorities can permit development of new health education resources that include assessment of client and provider preferences and effectiveness of delivery. Study subjects need to include sufficient numbers of race, culture, income, and gender subgroups for analysis. The cost-effectiveness of health education materials has seldom been included in studies, but it is an increasingly important issue. Health outcomes as well as satisfaction and uptake of the recommendations must be included in evaluation (Sieverink, Kelders, & van Gemert-Pijnen, 2017).

Risks, Costs, and Benefits of Applying the Evidence

The economic aspects of health promotion and preventing illness have always been a challenge. Cost and benefit determinations take place in systems, where the main drivers are the perspectives of those managing budgets, using services, and experiencing health outcomes. Recent examples of these analyses have been reported in the following:

- Weight management for adults comparing online and in-person services (Rollo et al., 2018)
- Child physical activity promotion (Lee et al., 2017)
- Management of child constipation (Sandweiss et al., 2018)
- Prostate cancer screening (Sanghera, Coast, Martin, Donovan, & Mohiuddin, 2018)

We can assume that the health risks relevant to those studies are high, but despite the costs of implementing evidence-based health education, the studies demonstrate risk amelioration and improved health outcomes. Thus, we next consider how to implement evidence-based health education feasibly within our own systems.

Feasibility and Systems Issues

Health promotion can require analysis of systemic and economic influences, such as with obesity prevention and amelioration. We have discussed specific system issues important in applying evidence related to health education and client decision aids in this chapter. Using venues in community settings that clients frequent and preparing materials using culturally tailored, universal design modalities should be considered. Information should be concise and appealing and should allay concerns with accurate portrayal of risks and benefits. Online materials should be organized and presented in formats that clients can readily access, perhaps by e-mail, on waiting room computers, or through mobile apps.

Engaging stakeholders is essential to effective change toward evidence-based practice in any setting. Recent examples related to health education include:

- School-based sexual health promotion (Layzer, Rosapep, & Barr, 2014)
- Improving oral health (Ramsdale & Landes, 2014)

These successful models for engaging stakeholders can be applied in other settings and for other health education initiatives. Important central themes are to engage stakeholders early; listen carefully; summarize key thoughts and evidence; and create a plan including a time line, identifiable outcome evaluations, and cost analyses to be evaluated for sustaining the health education program.

Analysis of local media reports concerning the health issue may be critical to understanding prevailing perspectives and concerns to be addressed (Casciotti et al., 2014). Consider how stakeholders will best be helped when they want to learn how to develop health-promoting organizations and realistically evaluate outcomes.

KEY POINTS

- In this chapter, we have discussed principles of effective teaching for use in helping clients and families learn more about health promotion.
- We have described how to facilitate learning in the cognitive, psychomotor, and affective domains and effectively use counseling and coaching.
- Decision aids were presented along with a discussion of the evidence for print, online, and phone formats.
- Each of these approaches can be used to facilitate active learning, which improves outcomes.
- A case was presented, along with a PICOT question, to integrate these approaches.

Check Your Understanding

1. An advanced practice nurse uses knowledge of population demographic statistics to:
   A. Begin assessing primary sources in the community for likely health risks
   B. Tell community members they need a program on a specific health risk
   C. Seek funding to address population risks
   D. Evaluate resources for health promotion
2. Using a constructivist approach to client health education means:
   A. Starting with learning objectives based on Healthy People 2020
   B. Developing a pamphlet at the fifth-grade reading level
   C. Assessing client knowledge and learning goals
   D. Advocating for additional health education materials
3. The advanced practice nurse needs an outcomes measurement tool for a new client decision aid; first, he or she:
   A. Reviews the literature for instruments with acceptable estimates of reliability and validity
   B. Determines the key outcomes to be measured based on stakeholders' priorities
   C. Writes some questions for the tool over lunch because it needs to be done soon
   D. Uses Google to find tools that look appropriate and are not very long

4. Client learning styles are best addressed by:
   A. Using online modalities because these are the emerging technology
   B. Developing a DVD, incorporating a game, and printing a list of useful Web sites
   C. Giving a lecture as clients arrive for their appointment
   D. Placing brochures in the waiting area
5. To address a common health issue, the advanced practice nurse implements:
   A. Focus groups including staff members, clients, and family members to understand how care can be improved
   B. A literature search to understand the scope of the problem, best practices, and outcomes
   C. The guideline from U.S. Preventive Health Services Taskforce
   D. A video found on the Healthy Canadians Web site
6. A client indicates interest in a healthier diet; the advanced practice nurse:
   A. Gives the client a brochure and asks that she or he read it before the next visit
   B. Says a plan for the client will be developed based on the most recent guidelines
   C. Asks what foods the client is interested in and what the client may have already tried in eating healthier
   D. Says that, for consultation to be paid through insurance, obesity must be present
7. An effective way of working with a culturally diverse patient population when a needs assessment identifies learning needs is to:
   A. Prepare a brochure on common misperceptions in the cultures commonly seen in the health-care setting
   B. Invite members of the client community and staff members to review potential client decision aids for relevance
   C. Explain that, even though studies on which guidelines were developed did not include analyses for their group, they should be followed
   D. Use a translation service to read existing guidelines to clients from diverse populations
8. Recalling the principles of learning theory, the advanced practice nurse considers that clients likely will:
   A. Be interested if the lecture is well organized
   B. Have different preferences and learning needs
   C. Not know much about the topic at hand
   D. Prefer community-based rather than health-setting-based options

See "Reflections on Check Your Understanding" at the end of the book for answers.

REFERENCES

Abbass-Dick, J., Brolly, M., Huizinga, J., Newport, A., Xie, F., George, S., & Sterken, E. (2018). Designing an eHealth breastfeeding resource with indigenous families using a participatory design. *Journal of Transcultural Nursing, 29*(5), 480–488. doi:10.1177/1043659617731818

Abroms, L. C., Padmanabhan, N., & Evans, W. D. (2012). Mobile phones for health communication to promote behavior change. In S. M. Noar & N. G. Harrington (Eds.), *eHealth applications: Promising strategies for behavior change* (pp. 147–166). New York, NY: Routledge.

Adams, V., Burger, S., Crawford, K., & Setter, R. (2018). Can you escape? Creating an escape room to facilitate active learning. *Journal for Nurses in Professional Development, 34*(2), E1–E5. doi:10.1097/NND.0000000000000433

Ahluwalia, S., de Silva, D., Kumar, S., Viney, R., & Chana, N. (2013). Teaching GP trainees to use health coaching in consultations with patients: Evaluation of a pilot study. *Education for Primary Care, 24*(7), 418–426.

Allen, J. D., & Berry, D. L. (2011). Multi-media support for informed/shared decision-making before and after a cancer diagnosis. *Seminars in Oncology Nursing, 27*(3), 192–202. doi:10.1016/j.soncn.2011.04.004

American Cancer Society. (2016). Cancer facts and figures for African Americans 2016–2018. Retrieved from https://www.cancer.org/content/dam/cancer-org/research/cancer-facts-and-statistics/cancer-facts-and-figures-for-african-americans/cancer-facts-and-figures-for-african-americans-2016-2018.pdf

Aminsharifi, A., Schulman, A., Anderson, J., Fish, L., Oeffinger, K., Shah, K.,... Polascik, T. J. (2018). Primary care perspective and implementation of a multidisciplinary, institutional prostate cancer screening algorithm embedded in the electronic health record. *Urologic Oncology: Seminars and Original Investigations, 36*(11), 502.e501–502.e506. doi:https://doi.org/10.1016/j.urolonc.2018.07.016

Andrade, J., Lotton, J., & Andrade, J. (2018). Systematic review: Frameworks used in school-based interventions, the impact on Hispanic children's obesity-related outcomes. *Journal of School Health, 88*(11), 847–858. doi:10.1111/josh.12693

Bakan, A. B., & Erci, B. (2018). Comparison of the effect of trainings based on the transtheoretical model and the health belief model on nurses' smoking cessation. *International Journal of Caring Sciences*, 213–224.

Baker, A. L., Turner, A., Beck, A., Berry, K., Haddock, G., Kelly, P. J., & Bucci, S. (2018). Telephone-delivered psychosocial interventions targeting key health priorities in adults with a psychotic disorder: Systematic review. *Psychological Medicine, 48*(16), 2637–2657. doi:10.1017/S0033291718001125

Berry, D. L., Halpenny, B., Hong, F., Wolpin, S., Lober, W. B., Russell, K. J.,... Swanson, G. (2013). The Personal Patient Profile-Prostate decision support for men with localized prostate cancer: A multi-center randomized trial. *Urologic Oncology, 31*(7), 1012–1021.

Bishop, F. L., & Salmon, C. (2013). Advertising, expectations and informed consent: The contents and functions of acupuncture leaflets. *Acupuncture in Medicine, 31*(4), 351–357. doi:10.1136/acupmed-2013-010416

Bloom, B. S., Engelhart, M. B., Furst, E. J., Hill, W. H., & Krathwohl, D. R. (1956). *Taxonomy of educational objectives: The classification of educational goals.* New York, NY: David McKay.

Boulay, S. M. (2018). Church-based intervention on prostate cancer screening for African-American men. (Doctoral Dissertation) UMI Order AAI10745939 *Church-Based Intervention On Prostate Cancer Screening For African-American Men*, 1-1.

Brady, C. L. (2013). Understanding learning styles: Providing the optimal learning experience. *International Journal of Childbirth Education, 28*(2), 16–19.

Brandt, C. J., Søgaard, G. I., Clemensen, J., Søndergaard, J., & Nielsen, J. B. (2018). Determinants of successful eHealth coaching for consumer lifestyle changes: Qualitative interview study among health care professionals. *Journal of Medical Internet Research, 20*(7), 76–85. doi:10.2196/jmir.9791

Branney, J., & Priego-Hernández, J. (2018). A mixed methods evaluation of team-based learning for applied pathophysiology in undergraduate nursing education. *Nurse Education Today, 61*, 127–133. doi:10.1016/j.nedt.2017.11.014

Britton, P., & Bright, S. R. (2014). "Extraordinary" sex coaching: An inside look. *Sexual & Relationship Therapy, 29*(1), 98–108. doi:10.1080/14681994.2013.864385

Brown, V. (2018). Infusing adult education principles into a health insurance literacy program. *Health Promotion Practice, 19*(2), 240–245. doi:10.1177/1524839917700369

Buki, L. P., Salazar, S. I., & Pitton, V. O. (2009). Design elements for the development of cancer education print materials for a Latina/o audience. *Health Promotion Practice, 10*(4), 564–572. doi:10.1177/1524839908320359

Byrne, J. L. S., Cameron Wild, T., Maximova, K., Browne, N. E., Holt, N. L., Cave, A. J.,... Ball, G. D. C. (2018). A brief eHealth tool delivered in primary care to help parents prevent childhood obesity: A randomized controlled trial. *Pediatric Obesity, 13*(11), 659–667. doi:10.1111/ijpo.12200

Çapık, C., & Gözüm, S. (2012). The effect of web-assisted education and reminders on health belief, level of knowledge and early diagnosis behaviors regarding prostate cancer screening. *European Journal of Oncology Nursing, 16*(1), 71–77. doi:10.1016/j.ejon.2011.03.007

Carter, V. L., Tippett, F., Anderson, D. L., & Tameru, B. (2010). Increasing prostate cancer screening among African American men. *Journal of Health Care for the Poor & Underserved, 21*(3), 91–106. doi:10.1353/hpu.0.0366

Casciotti, D. M., Smith, K. C., Andon, L., Vernick, J., Tsui, A., & Klassen, A. C. (2014). Print news coverage of school-based human papillomavirus vaccine mandates. *Journal of School Health, 84*(2), 71–81. doi:10.1111/josh.12126

Chadi, N., Kaufman, M., Weisbaum, E., Malboeuf-Hurtubise, C., Kohut, S. A., Locke, J., & Vo, D. X. (2018). Comparison of an in-person vs. eHealth mindfulness meditation-based intervention for adolescents with chronic medical conditions: A mixed methods study. *Journal of Adolescent Health, 62*, S12–S12. doi:10.1016/j.jadohealth.2017.11.026

Chickering, A. W., & Gamson, Z. (1987). Seven principles for good practice in undergraduate education. *AAHE Bulletin, 39*(7), 3–7.

Cogan, A. M., & Carlson, M. (2018). Deciphering participation: An interpretive synthesis of its meaning and application in rehabilitation. *Disability & Rehabilitation, 40*(22), 2692–2703. doi:10.1080/09638288.2017.1342282

Cruz-Oliver, D. M., Parikh, M., Wallace, C. L., Malmstrom, T. K., & Sanchez-Reilly, S. (2018). What did Latino family caregivers expect and learn from education intervention "Caregivers Like Me"? *American Journal of Hospice & Palliative Medicine, 35*(3), 404–410. doi:10.1177/1049909117709550

Curran, M. K. (2014). Examination of the teaching styles of nursing professional development specialists, Part I: Best practices in adult learning theory, curriculum development, and knowledge transfer. *Journal of Continuing Education in Nursing, 45*(5), 233–240. doi:10.3928/00220124-20140417-04

Cvengros, J. A., Christensen, A. J., Cunningham, C., Hillis, S. L., & Kaboli, P. J. (2009). Patient preference for and reports of provider behavior: Impact of symmetry on patient outcomes. *Health Psychology, 28*(6), 660–667. doi:10.1037/a0016087

Derose, K. P., Bogart, L. M., Kanouse, D. E., Felton, A., Collins, D. O., Mata, M. A.,... Williams, M. V. (2014). An intervention to reduce HIV-related stigma in partnership with African American and Latino churches. *AIDS Education & Prevention, 26*(1), 28–42. doi:10.1521/aeap.2014.26.1.28

Earle, A. M., LaBrie, J. W., Boyle, S. C., & Smith, D. (2018). In pursuit of a self-sustaining college alcohol intervention: Deploying gamified PNF in the real world. *Addictive Behaviors, 80*, 71–81. doi:10.1016/j.addbeh.2018.01.005

Easton, C. J., Berbary, C. M., & Crane, C. A. (2018). Avatar and technology assisted platforms in the treatment of co-occurring addiction and IPV among male offenders. *Advances in Dual Diagnosis, 11*(3), 126–134. doi:10.1108/ADD-03-2018-0003

Elwyn, G., Lloyd, A., Joseph-Williams, N., Cording, E., Thomson, R., Durand, M.-A., & Edwards, A. (2013). Option grids: Shared decision making made easier. *Patient Education and Counseling, 90*(2), 207–212. doi:http://dx.doi.org/10.1016/j.pec.2012.06.036

Estrada, L., Rodríguez, E., & Meléndez, A. (2018). Healthy choices with problem-based learning. *JOPERD: The Journal of Physical Education, Recreation & Dance, 89*(1), 55–57. doi:10.1080/07303084.2018.1393229

Fagerlin, A., Pignone, M., Abhyankar, P., Col, N., Feldman-Stuart, D., Gavaruzzi, T.,... Whitteman, H. (2012). Clarifying and expressing values. In R. Volk & H. Llewellyn-Thomas (Eds.), *Update of the International Patient Decision Aids Standards (IPDAS) Collaboration's Background Document.* Retrieved from https://decisionaid.ohri.ca/ipdas.html *International Patient Decision Aid Standards (IPDAS) Collaboration website*

Fang, K. Y., Bjering, H., & Ginige, A. (2018). Adherence, avatars and where to go from here: Health Informatics Conference, Sydney, Australia, 2018. *Studies in Health*

Technology & Informatics, 252, 45–50. doi:10.3233/978-1-61499-890-7-45

Fazio-Griffith, L., & Ballard, M. B. (2016). Transformational learning theory and transformative teaching: A creative strategy for understanding the helping relationship. *Journal of Creativity in Mental Health, 11*(2), 225–234. doi:10.1080/15401383.2016.1164643

Feng, B., Srinivasan, M., Hoffman, J. R., Rainwater, J. A., Griffin, E., Dragojevic, M.,... Wilkes, M. S. (2013). Physician communication regarding prostate cancer screening: Analysis of unannounced standardized patient visits. *Annals of Family Medicine, 11*(4), 315–323. doi:10.1370/afm.1509

Ferrante, J., Shaw, E., & Scott, J. (2011). Factors influencing men's decisions regarding prostate cancer screening: A qualitative study. *Journal of Community Health, 36*(5), 839–844. doi:10.1007/s10900-011-9383-5

Gash, J., & McIntosh, G. V. (2013). Gender matters: Health beliefs of women as a predictor of participation in prostate cancer screening among African American men. *Diversity & Equality in Health & Care, 10*(1), 23–30.

Government of Canada. (2018). Healthy Canadians. Retrieved from http://www.healthycanadians.gc.ca/index-eng.php

Graham, F., Rodger, S., & Ziviani, J. (2014). Mothers' experiences of engaging in Occupational Performance Coaching. *British Journal of Occupational Therapy, 77*(4), 189–197. doi:10.4276/030802214X13968769798791

Hammersley, V., Donaghy, E., Parker, R., McNeilly, H., Atherton, H., Bikker, A.,... McKinstry, B. (2019). Comparing the content and quality of video, telephone, and face-to-face consultations: A non-randomised, quasi-experimental, exploratory study in UK primary care. *British Journal of General Practice, 69*(684). doi:10.3399/bjgp19X704573

Han, P. K. J., Kobrin, S., Breen, N., Joseph, D. A., Li, J., Frosch, D. L., & Klabunde, C. N. (2013). National evidence on the use of shared decision making in prostate-specific antigen screening. *Annals of Family Medicine, 11*(4), 306–314. doi:10.1370/afm.1539

Harmon, B. E., Blake, C. E., Thrasher, J. F., & Hébert, J. R. (2014). An evaluation of diet and physical activity messaging in African American churches. *Health Education & Behavior, 41*(2), 216–224. doi:10.1177/1090198113507449

Heard, A. M., Harris, J. L., Liu, S., Schwartz, M. B., & Li, X. (2016). Piloting an online grocery store simulation to assess children's food choices. *Appetite, 96*, 260–267. doi:10.1016/j.appet.2015.09.020

Heyes, S., Harrington, A., & Paterson, J. (2011). A thematic review of men's experiences during the waiting period between prostate-specific antigen and prostate biopsy results. *Journal of Radiology Nursing, 30*(4), 158–169. doi:10.1016/j.jradnu.2011.06.002

Hnatyshyn, T. (2018). Teaching pathophysiology using a card set: An active learning strategy. *Teaching & Learning in Nursing, 13*(2), 129–130. doi:10.1016/j.teln.2017.10.001

Holland, C., Carthron, D. L., Duren-Winfield, V., & Lawrence, W. (2014). An experiential cardiovascular health education program for African American college students. *ABNF Journal, 25*(2), 52–56.

Holt, C. L., Wynn, T. A., Litaker, M. S., Southward, P., Jeames, S., & Schulz, E. (2009). A comparison of a spiritually based and non-spiritually based educational intervention for informed decision making for prostate cancer screening among church-attending African-American men. *Urologic Nursing, 29*(4), 249–258.

Howard, L. M., & Ceci, C. (2013). Problematizing health coaching for chronic illness self-management. *Nursing Inquiry, 20*(3), 223–231. doi:10.1111/nin.12004

Hsu, M. S. H., Rouf, A., & Allman-Farinelli, M. (2018). Effectiveness and behavioral mechanisms of social media interventions for positive nutrition behaviors in adolescents: A systematic review. *Journal of Adolescent Health, 63*(5), 531–545. doi:10.1016/j.jadohealth.2018.06.009

Iles, R. A., Taylor, N. F., Davidson, M., & O'Halloran, P. (2014). An effective coaching intervention for people with low recovery expectations and low back pain: A content analysis. *Journal of Back & Musculoskeletal Rehabilitation, 27*(1), 93–101. doi:10.3233/BMR-130424

Ilic, D., Neuberger, M. M., Djulbegovic, M., & Dahm, P. (2013). Screening for prostate cancer. *Cochrane Database of Systematic Reviews*, (1).

International Patient Decision Aids Standards (IPDAS) Collaboration. (2019) Resources. Retrieved from http://ipdas.ohri.ca/resources.html

Iqbal, M. S., Warner, L., Paleri, V., Kovarik, J., & Kelly, C. (2020). De-intensification of treatment in human papilloma virus related oropharyngeal carcinoma: Patient choice still matters for de-escalation and for the COVID era. *Oral Oncology, 105*, 2–3. doi:10.1016/j.oraloncology.2020.104768

Ivlev, I., Jerabkova, S., Mishra, M., Cook, L. A., & Eden, K. B. (2018). Prostate cancer screening patient decision aids: A systematic review and meta-analysis. *American Journal of Preventive Medicine, 55*(6), 896–907. doi:10.1016/j.amepre.2018.06.016

Jackson, J., Gettings, S., & Metcalfe, A. (2018). "The power of Twitter": Using social media at a conference with nursing students. *Nurse Education Today, 68*, 188–191. doi:10.1016/j.nedt.2018.06.017

Jimbo, M., Rana, G. K., Hawley, S., Holmes-Rovner, M., Kelly-Blake, K., Nease Jr, D. E., & Ruffin, M. T. (2013). What is lacking in current decision aids on cancer screening? *CA: A Cancer Journal for Clinicians, 63*(3), 193–214. doi:10.3322/caac.21180

Johnson, K., Chang, M., Sun, Y., Miyake, M., & Rosser, C. J. (2013). Attitudes and knowledge of primary care physicians regarding prostate cancer screening. *Journal of Cancer Education, 28*(4), 679–683. doi:10.1007/s13187-013-0533-6

Joseph-Williams, N., Elwyn, G., & Edwards, A. (2014). Knowledge is not power for patients: A systematic review and thematic synthesis of patient-reported barriers and facilitators to shared decision making. *Patient Education and Counseling, 94*(3), 291–309. doi:http://dx.doi.org/10.1016/j.pec.2013.10.031

Kassan, E. C., Williams, R. M., Kelly, S. P., Barry, S. A., Penek, S., Fishman, M. B.,... Taylor, K. L. (2012). Men's use of an Internet-based decision aid for prostate cancer screening. *Journal of Health Communication, 17*(6), 677–697. doi:10.1080/10810730.2011.579688

Kieckhefer, G., Trahms, C., Churchill, S., Kratz, L., Uding, N., & Villareale, N. (2014). A randomized clinical trial of the Building on Family Strengths program: An education program for parents of children with chronic health conditions. *Maternal & Child Health Journal, 18*(3), 563–574. doi:10.1007/s10995-013-1273-2

Kiesler, D. J., & Auerbach, S. M. (2006). Optimal matches of patient preferences for information, decision-making and interpersonal behavior: Evidence, models and interventions. *Patient Education and Counseling, 61*(3), 319–341. doi:http://dx.doi.org/10.1016/j.pec.2005.08.002

Knopf-Amelung, S., Gotham, H., Kuofie, A., Young, P., Stinson, R. M., Lynn, J.,... Hildreth, J. (2018). Comparison of instructional methods for screening, brief intervention, and referral to treatment for substance use in nursing education. *Nurse Educator, 43*(3), 123–127. doi:10.1097/NNE.0000000000000439

Krautscheid, L., & Williams, S. B. (2018). Using multimedia resources to enhance active learning during office hours. *Journal of Nursing Education, 57*(4), 256–256. doi:10.3928/01484834-20180322-14

Langbecker, D., Janda, M., & Yates, P. (2013). Health professionals' perspectives on information provision for patients with brain tumours and their families. *European Journal of Cancer Care, 22*(2), 179–187. doi:10.1111/ecc.12011

Lau, D. T., Joyce, B., Clayman, M. L., Dy, S., Ehrlich-Jones, L., Emanuel, L.,... Shega, J. W. (2012). Hospice providers' key approaches to support informal caregivers in managing medications for patients in private residences. *Journal of Pain & Symptom Management, 43*(6), 1060–1071. doi:10.1016/j.jpainsymman.2011.06.025

Layzer, C., Rosapep, L., & Barr, S. (2014). A peer education program: Delivering highly reliable sexual health promotion messages in schools. *Journal of Adolescent Health, 54*(S3), S70–S77. doi:10.1016/j.jadohealth.2013.12.023

Leahy, D. (2014). Assembling a health[y] subject: Risky and shameful pedagogies in health education. *Critical Public Health, 24*(2), 171–181. doi:10.1080/09581596.2013.871504

Lee, B. Y., Adam, A., Zenkov, E., Hertenstein, D., Ferguson, M. C., Wang, P. I.,... Brown, S. T. (2017). Modeling the economic and health impact of increasing children's physical activity in the United States. *Health Affairs, 36*(5), 902–908. doi:10.1377/hlthaff.2016.1315

Lee, J. E., Xiang, P., & Gao, Z. (2017). Acute effect of active video games on older children's mood change. *Computers in Human Behavior, 70*, 97–103.

Lee, S. K., Sulaiman-Hill, C. M. R., & Thompson, S. C. (2013). Providing health information for culturally and linguistically diverse women: Priorities and preferences of new migrants and refugees. *Health Promotion Journal of Australia, 24*(2), 98–103. doi:10.1071/HE12919

Lentferink, A. J., Oldenhuis, H. K. E., Groot, M. D., Polstra, L., Velthuijsen, H., Gemert-Pijnen, J. E. W. C. V.,... van Gemert-Pijnen, J. E. (2017). Key components in eHealth interventions combining self-tracking and persuasive eCoaching to promote a healthier lifestyle: A scoping review. *Journal of Medical Internet Research, 19*(8), 1–1. doi:10.2196/jmir.7288

Levey, J. A. (2018). Universal Design for Instruction in nursing education: An integrative review. *Nursing Education Perspectives (Wolters Kluwer Health), 39*(3), 156–161. doi:10.1097/01.NEP.0000000000000249

Luparell, S. (2014). Faciltate learner development and socialization. In L. Caputi (Ed.), *Certified Nurse Educator review book*. Philadelphia, PA: Wolters Kluwer Health.

Luque, J., Ross, L., & Gwede, C. (2014). Qualitative systematic review of barber-administered health education, promotion, screening and outreach programs in African-American communities. *Journal of Community Health, 39*(1), 181–190. doi:10.1007/s10900-013-9744-3

Martínez-González, N. A., Neuner-Jehle, S., Plate, A., Rosemann, T., & Senn, O. (2018). The effects of shared decision-making compared to usual care for prostate cancer screening decisions: A systematic review and meta-analysis. *BMC Cancer, 18*(1) 1–15. doi:10.1186/s12885-018-4794-7

McCormack, L. A., Bann, C. M., Williams-Piehota, P., Driscoll, D., Soloe, C., Poehlman, J.,... Cykert, S. (2009). Communication message strategies for increasing knowledge about prostate cancer screening. *Journal of Cancer Education, 24*(3), 238–243. doi:10.1080/08858190902935498

McDowell, M. E., Occhipinti, S., & Chambers, S. K. (2013). The influence of family history on cognitive heuristics, risk perceptions, and prostate cancer screening behavior. *Health Psychology, 32*(11), 1158–1169. doi:10.1037/a0031622

McNaughton, D. B., Cowell, J. M., & Fogg, L. (2014). Adaptation and feasibility of a communication intervention for Mexican immigrant mothers and children in a school setting. *Journal of School Nursing, 30*(2), 103–113. doi:10.1177/1059840513487217

Mettler, E. A., Preston, H. R., Jenkins, S. M., Lackore, K. A., Werneburg, B. L., Larson, B. G.,... Clark, M. M. (2014). Motivational improvements for health behavior change from wellness coaching. *American Journal of Health Behavior, 38*(1), 83–91. doi:10.5993/AJHB.38.1.9

Mikolasek, M., Berg, J., Witt, C. M., & Barth, J. (2018). Effectiveness of mindfulness- and relaxation-based eHealth interventions for patients with medical conditions: A systematic review and synthesis. *International Journal of Behavioral Medicine, 25*(1), 1–16. doi:10.1007/s12529-017-9679-7

Miller, D. B. (2014). Pre-screening age African-American males: What do they know about prostate cancer screening, knowledge, and risk perceptions? *Social Work in Health Care, 53*(3), 268–288. doi:10.1080/00981389.2013.875503

Miller, S. M., Roussi, P., Scarpato, J., Wen, K.-Y., Zhu, F., & Roy, G. (2014). Randomized trial of print messaging: The role of the partner and monitoring style in promoting provider discussions about prostate cancer screening among African American men. *Psycho-Oncology, 23*(4), 404–411. doi:10.1002/pon.3437

Millery, M., Hall, M., Eisman, J., & Murrman, M. (2014). Using innovative instructional technology to meet training needs in public health: A design process. *Health Promotion Practice, 15*(1), 39S–47S. doi:10.1177/1524839913509272

Mitchell, H., Lucas, C., Charlton, K., & McMahon, A. (2018). Models of nutrition-focused continuing education programs for nurses: A systematic review of the evidence. *Australian Journal of Primary Health, 24*(2), 101–108. doi:10.1071/PY17088

Mkandawire-Valhmu, L., Lathen, L., Baisch, M. J., Cotton, Q., Dressel, A., Antilla, J.,... Hess, A. (2018). Enhancing healthier birth outcomes by creating supportive spaces for pregnant African American women living in Milwaukee.

Maternal & Child Health Journal, 22(12), 1797–1804. doi:10.1007/s10995-018-2580-4

Mussulman, L. M., Faseru, B., Fitzgerald, S., Nazir, N., Patel, V., & Richter, K. P. (2018). A randomized, controlled pilot study of warm handoff versus fax referral for hospital-initiated smoking cessation among people living with HIV/AIDS. *Addictive Behaviors, 78*, 205–208. doi:10.1016/j.addbeh.2017.11.035

Myers, R. E., Daskalakis, C., Kunkel, E. J., Cocroft, J. R., Riggio, J. M., Capkin, M., & Braddock, C. H., III (2011). Mediated decision support in prostate cancer screening: A randomized controlled trial of decision counseling. *Patient Education & Counseling, 83*(2), 240–246. doi:10.1016/j.pec.2010.06.011

Naik, A. D., Teal, C. R., Rodriguez, E., & Haidet, P. (2011). Knowing the ABCs: A comparative effectiveness study of two methods of diabetes education. *Patient Education & Counseling, 85*(3), 383–389.

Nayak, J. G., Hartzler, A. L., Macleod, L. C., Izard, J. P., Dalkin, B. M., & Gore, J. L. (2016). Relevance of graph literacy in the development of patient-centered communication tools. *Patient Education & Counseling, 99*(3), 448–454. doi:https://dx.doi.org/10.1016/j.pec.2015.09.009

Nessen, T., Opava, C. H., Martin, C., & Demmelmaier, I. (2014). From clinical expert to guide: Experiences from coaching people with rheumatoid arthritis to increased physical activity. *Physical Therapy, 94*(5), 644–653. doi:10.2522/ptj.20130393

Nettey, O. S., Walker, A. J., Keeter, M. K., Singal, A., Nugooru, A., Martin, I. K.,... Murphy, A. B. (2018). Self-reported Black race predicts significant prostate cancer independent of clinical setting and clinical and socioeconomic risk factors. *Urologic Oncology: Seminars and Original Investigations, 36*(11), 501.e501–501.e508. doi:https://doi.org/10.1016/j.urolonc.2018.06.011

Nezami, B. T., Ward, D. S., Lytle, L. A., Ennett, S. T., & Tate, D. F. (2018). A mHealth randomized controlled trial to reduce sugar-sweetened beverage intake in preschool-aged children. *Pediatric Obesity, 13*(11), 668–676. doi:10.1111/ijpo.12258

Nick, J. M. (2014). Facilitate learning. In L. Caputi (Ed.), *Certified nurse educator review book: The official NLN guide to the CNE exam.* (pp. 1–30). Philadelphia, PA: Wolters Kluwer.

Nikoloudakis, I. A., Crutzen, R., Rebar, A. L., Vandelanotte, C., Quester, P., Dry, M.,... Short, C. E. (2018). Can you elaborate on that? Addressing participants' need for cognition in computer-tailored health behavior interventions. *Health Psychology Review, 12*(4), 437–452. doi:10.1080/17437199.2018.1525571

Olsen, J. M. (2014). Health coaching: A concept analysis. *Nursing Forum, 49*(1), 18–29. doi:10.1111/nuf.12042

Owens, O. L., Friedman, D. B., Brandt, H. M., Bernhardt, J. M., & Hébert, J. R. (2016). Digital solutions for informed decision making: An academic-community partnership for the development of a prostate cancer decision aid for African American men. *American Journal of Mens Health, 10*(3), 207–219. doi:https://dx.doi.org/10.1177/1557988314564178

Padela, A. I., Malik, S., Ally, S. A., Quinn, M., Hall, S., & Peek, M. (2018). Reducing Muslim mammography disparities: Outcomes from a religiously tailored mosque-based intervention. *Health Education & Behavior, 45*(6), 1025–1035. doi:10.1177/1090198118769371

Papadakos, C. T., Papadakos, J., Catton, P., Houston, P., McKernan, P., & Jusko Friedman, A. (2014). From theory to pamphlet: The 3Ws and an H process for the development of meaningful patient education resources. *Journal of Cancer Education, 29*(2), 304–310. doi:10.1007/s13187-013-0600-z

Patel, K., Ukoli, F., Liu, J., Beech, D., Beard, K., Brown, B.,... Hargreaves, M. (2013). A community-driven intervention for prostate cancer screening in African Americans. *Health Education & Behavior, 40*(1), 11–18. doi:10.1177/1090198111431275

Peña, A. L. N., & Rojas, J. G. (2014). Ethical aspects of children's perceptions of information-giving in care. *Nursing Ethics, 21*(2), 245–256. doi:10.1177/0969733013484483

Piacentine, L. B., Robinson, K. M., Waltke, L. J., Tjoe, J. A., & Ng, A. V. (2018). Promoting team-based exercise among African American breast cancer survivors. *Western Journal of Nursing Research, 40*(12), 1885–1902. doi:10.1177/0193945918795313

Price-Haywood, E. G., Qingyang, L., & Monlezun, D. (2018). Dose effect of patient-care team communication via secure portal messaging on glucose and blood pressure control. *Journal of the American Medical Informatics Association, 25*(6), 702–708. doi:10.1093/jamia/ocx161

Ramadas, A., Chan, C. K. Y., Oldenburg, B., Hussein, Z., & Quek, K. F. (2018). Randomised-controlled trial of a web-based dietary intervention for patients with type 2 diabetes: Changes in health cognitions and glycemic control. *BMC Public Health, 18*(1), 716–716. doi:10.1186/s12889-018-5640-1

Ramsdale, M. P., & Landes, D. P. (2014). Evaluation of an oral health promotion pilot in County Durham and Darlington. *International Journal of Health Promotion & Education, 52*(2), 60–67. doi:10.1080/14635240.2013.858531

Reddy, A., Roberts, R., Shenoy, D., Packianathan, S., Giri, S., & Vijayakumar, S. (2018). Prostate cancer screening guidelines for African American veterans: A new perspective. *Journal of the National Medical Association*. doi:https://doi.org/10.1016/j.jnma.2018.10.010

Roberts, L. R., Wilson, C. M., Stiel, L., Casiano, C. A., & Montgomery, S. B. (2018). Prostate cancer screening among high-risk Black men. *Journal for Nurse Practitioners, 14*(9), 677–682. doi:10.1016/j.nurpra.2018.07.005

Rollo, M. E., Burrows, T., Vincze, L. J., Harvey, J., Collins, C. E., & Hutchesson, M. J. (2018). Cost evaluation of providing evidence-based dietetic services for weight management in adults: In-person versus eHealth delivery. *Nutrition & Dietetics, 75*(1), 35–43. doi:10.1111/1747-0080.12335

Sandiford, L., & D'Errico, E. M. (2016). Facilitating shared decision making about prostate cancer screening among African American men. *Oncology Nursing Forum, 43*(1), 86–92. doi:https://dx.doi.org/10.1188/16.ONF.86-92

Sandweiss, D. R., Allen, L., Deneau, M., Harnsberger, J., Pasmann, A., Smout, R.,... Dudley, N. (2018). Implementing a standardized constipation-management pathway to reduce resource utilization. *Academic Pediatrics, 18*(8), 957–964.

Sanghera, S., Coast, J., Martin, R. M., Donovan, J. L., & Mohiuddin, S. (2018). Cost-effectiveness of prostate cancer screening: A systematic review of decision-analytical models. *BMC Cancer, 18*(1), 84. doi:https://dx.doi.org/10.1186/s12885-017-3974-1

Saver, B. G., Mazor, K. M., Luckmann, R., Cutrona, S. L., Hayes, M., Gorodetsky, T.,... Bacigalupe, G. (2017). Persuasive interventions for controversial cancer screening recommendations: Testing a novel approach to help patients make evidence-based decisions. *Annals of Family Medicine, 15*(1), 48–55. doi:https://dx.doi.org/10.1370/afm.1996

Schoeb, V., & Bürge, E. (2012). Perceptions of patients and physiotherapists on patient participation: A narrative synthesis of qualitative studies. *Physiotherapy Research International, 17*(2), 80–91. doi:10.1002/pri.516

Sheehan, C. A. (2009). A brief educational video about prostate cancer screening: A community intervention. *Urologic Nursing, 29*(2), 103.

Sieverink, F., Kelders, S. M., & van Gemert-Pijnen, J. E. W. C. (2017). Clarifying the concept of adherence to eHealth technology: Systematic review on when usage becomes adherence. *Journal of Medical Internet Research, 19*(12), 1–18. doi:10.2196/jmir.8578

Sowan, A. K., & Jenkins, L. S. (2013). Use of the seven principles of effective teaching to design and deliver an interactive hybrid nursing research course. *Nursing Education Perspectives, 34*(5), 315–322.

Stacey, D., Bennett, C. L., Barry, M. J., Col, N. F., Eden, K. B., Holmes-Rovner, M.,... Thomson, R. (2014). Decision aids for people facing health treatment or screening decisions. *Cochrane Database of Systematic Reviews*, (1). doi:10.1002/14651858.CD001431.pub2

Stacey, D., Kryworuchko, J., Belkora, J., Davison, B. J., Durand, M. A., Eden, K. B.,... Street, R. L. (2013). Coaching and guidance with patient decision aids: A review of theoretical and empirical evidence. *BMC Medical Informatics and Decision Making, 13*(Suppl. 2).

Stacey, D., & Legare, F. (2015). Engaging patients using an interprofessional approach to shared decision making. *Canadian Oncology Nursing Journal, 25*(4), 455–469.

Staffileno, B. A., Tangney, C. C., & Fogg, L. (2018). Favorable outcomes using an eHealth approach to promote physical activity and nutrition among young African American women. *Journal of Cardiovascular Nursing, 33*(1), 62–71. doi:10.1097/JCN.0000000000000409

Stamm, A. W., Banerji, J. S., Wolff, E. M., Slee, A., Akapame, S., Dahl, K.,... Corman, J. M. (2017). A decision aid versus shared decision making for prostate cancer screening: Results of a randomized, controlled trial. *Canadian Journal of Urology, 24*(4), 8910–8917.

Starosta, A. J., Luta, G., Tomko, C. A., Schwartz, M. D., & Taylor, K. L. (2015). Baseline attitudes about prostate cancer screening moderate the impact of decision aids on screening rates. *Annals of Behavioral Medicine, 49*(5), 762–768. doi:https://dx.doi.org/10.1007/s12160-015-9692-5

Steadman, M., Chao, M. S., Strong, J. T., Maxwell, M., & West, J. H. (2014). C U L8ter: YouTube distracted driving PSAs use of behavior change theory. *American Journal of Health Behavior, 38*(1), 3–12. doi:10.5993/AJHB.38.1.1

Stellefson, M. L., Shuster, J. J., Chaney, B. H., Paige, S. R., Alber, J. M., Chaney, J. D., & Sriram, P. S. (2018). Web-based health information seeking and eHealth literacy among patients living with chronic obstructive pulmonary disease (COPD). *Health Communication, 33*(12), 1410–1424. doi:10.1080/10410236.2017.1353868

Stockwell, M. S., Westhoff, C., Olshen Kharbanda, E., Vargas, C. Y., Camargo, S., Vawdrey, D. K., & Castaño CastaÃ±o, P. M. (2014). Influenza vaccine text message reminders for urban, low-income pregnant women: A randomized controlled trial. *American Journal of Public Health, 104*(S1), e7–e12. doi:10.2105/AJPH.2013.301620

Symonds, R. F., Trethewey, S. P., & Beck, K. J. (2020). Video consultations in UK primary care in response to the COVID-19 pandemic. *British Journal of General Practice, 70*, 228–229. doi: 10.3399/bjgp20X709505

Tamim, S. R., & Grant, M. M. (2017). Exploring instructional strategies and learning theoretical foundations of eHealth and mHealth education interventions. *Health Promotion Practice, 18*(1), 127–139. doi:10.1177/1524839916646715

Tanner, A. E., Song, E. Y., Mann-Jackson, L., Alonzo, J., Schafer, K., Ware, S.,... Rhodes, S. D. (2018). Preliminary impact of the weCare social media intervention to support health for young men who have sex with men and transgender women with HIV. *AIDS Patient Care & STDs, 32*(11), 450–458. doi:10.1089/apc.2018.0060

Taylor, K. L., Williams, R. M., Davis, K., Luta, G., Penek, S., Barry, S.,... Miller, E. (2013). Decision making in prostate cancer screening using decision aids versus usual care: A randomized clinical trial. *JAMA Internal Medicine, 173*(18), 1704–1712.

Thompson, C. A. (2014). Hospitals' performance at medication communication improved, VBP data suggest... value-based purchasing. *American Journal of Health-System Pharmacy, 71*(4), 270–275. doi:10.2146/news140016

Tomer, A., Fishbane, L., Siefer, A. Callahan, B. (2020). *Digital prosperity: How broadband can deliver health and equity to all communities*. Available at: https://www.brookings.edu/research/digital-prosperity-how-broadband-can-deliver-health-and-equity-to-all-communities/

Tuong, W., Larsen, E., & Armstrong, A. (2014). Videos to influence: A systematic review of effectiveness of video-based education in modifying health behaviors. *Journal of Behavioral Medicine, 37*(2), 218–233. doi:10.1007/s10865-012-9480-7

Uemura, K., Yamada, M., & Okamoto, H. (2018). Effects of active learning on health literacy and behavior in older adults: A randomized controlled trial. *Journal of the American Geriatrics Society, 66*(9), 1721–1729. doi:10.1111/jgs.15458

U.S. Department of Health and Human Services. (2018). HealthyPeople.gov. Retrieved from http://www.healthypeople.gov/2020/default.aspx

U.S. Preventive Services Taskforce. (2018a). Final recommendation statement: Screening for prostate cancer. Retrieved from https://www.uspreventiveservicestaskforce.org/Page/Document/RecommendationStatementFinal/prostate-cancer-screening1

U.S. Preventive Services Taskforce. (2018b). *U.S. Preventive Services Task Force Grade Definitions*. Retrieved from https://www.uspreventiveservicestaskforce.org/Page/Name/grade-definitions

Vetter, V. L., Haley, D. M., Dugan, N. P., Iyer, V. R., & Shults, J. (2016). Innovative cardiopulmonary resuscitation and automated external defibrillator programs in schools: Results from the Student Program for Olympic Resuscitation Training in Schools (SPORTS) study.

Resuscitation, 104, 46–52. doi:10.1016/j.resuscitation.2016.04.010

Volk, R. J., Linder, S. K., Kallen, M. A., Galliher, J. M., Spano, M. S., Mullen, P. D., & Spann, S. J. (2013). Primary care physicians' use of an informed decision-making process for prostate cancer screening. *Annals of Family Medicine, 11*(1), 67–74. doi:10.1370/afm.1445

Wang, L., Christensen, J. L., Jeong, D. C., & Miller, L. C. (2019). Virtual prognostication: When virtual alcohol choices predict change in alcohol consumption over 6 months. *Computers in Human Behavior, 90*, 388–396. doi:10.1016/j.chb.2018.08.025

Wilkes, M. S., Day, F. C., Srinivasan, M., Griffin, E., Tancredi, D. J., Rainwater, J. A.,... Hoffman, J. R. (2013). Pairing physician education with patient activation to improve shared decisions in prostate cancer screening: A cluster randomized controlled trial. *Annals of Family Medicine, 11*(4), 324–334. doi:10.1370/afm.1550

Williams, R. M., Davis, K. M., Luta, G., Edmond, S. N., Dorfman, C. S., Schwartz, M. D.,... Taylor, K. L. (2013). Fostering informed decisions: A randomized controlled trial assessing the impact of a decision aid among men registered to undergo mass screening for prostate cancer. *Patient Education & Counseling, 91*(3), 329–336. doi:10.1016/j.pec.2012.12.013

Witkiewitz, K., Greenfield, B. L., & Bowen, S. (2013). Mindfulness-based relapse prevention with racial and ethnic minority women. *Addictive Behaviors, 38*(12), 2821–2824. doi:http://dx.doi.org/10.1016/j.addbeh.2013.08.018

Wong, M. S., Nau, C., Kharmats, A. Y., Vedovato, G. M., Cheskin, L. J., Gittelsohn, J., & Lee, B. Y. (2015). Using a computational model to quantify the potential impact of changing the placement of healthy beverages in stores as an intervention to "nudge" adolescent behavior choice. *BMC Public Health, 15*(1), 1–7. doi:10.1186/s12889-015-2626-0

Wray, R. J., McClure, S., Vijaykumar, S., Smith, C., Ivy, A., Jupka, K., & Hess, R. (2009). Changing the conversation about prostate cancer among African Americans: Results of formative research. *Ethnicity & Health, 14*(1), 27–43.

Yao, P., Fu, R., Craig Rushing, S., Stephens, D., Ash, J. S., & Eden, K. B. (2018). Texting 4 sexual health: Improving attitudes, intention, and behavior among American Indian and Alaska Native youth. *Health Promotion Practice, 19*(6), 833–843. doi:10.1177/1524839918761872

Yuncken, J. (2014). Barriers to implementing change within diabetes care. *Wound Practice & Research, 22*(1), 50–55.

Zhang, F., & Kaufman, D. (2016). Physical and cognitive impacts of digital games on older adults. *Journal of Applied Gerontology, 35*(11), 1189–1210. doi:10.1177/0733464814566678

Unit 3

Trends

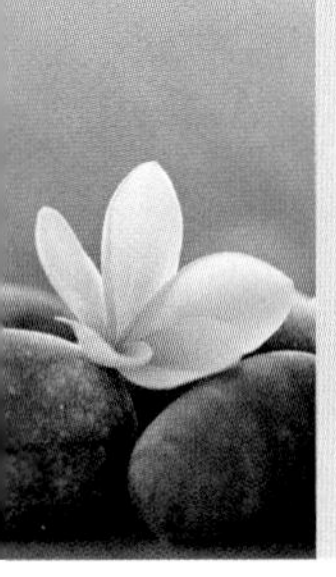

Chapter 13

Applying Health Informatics Concepts and Skills to Health Promotion and Disease Prevention

Ramona Nelson

LEARNING OJBECTIVES

After completing this chapter, the student will be able to:

1. Utilize a wide variety of information resources to support professional practice related to health promotion and disease prevention.
2. Apply informatics-based theories, models, processes, and tools in promoting health and preventing health problems.
3. Analyze the D-W model as a framework to guide the use of informatics tools, procedures, and methods as they apply to health promotion and the prevention of health problems.
4. Analyze current developments in health informatics and their implications for health promotion and disease prevention.

INTRODUCTION

For more than 30 years, the Healthy People initiative has set nationwide health improvement priorities with the vision of supporting a society in which all people live long, healthy lives. Health information technology (IT) and health communication are recognized as integral parts of the implementation and success of Healthy People 2020. Efforts to achieve the Healthy People 2020 vision include building and integrating the public health IT infrastructure in conjunction with the Nationwide Health Information Network (USDHHS Office of Disease Prevention and Health Promotion, n.d.).

The discipline of health informatics focuses on the use of health IT to create a society in which the Healthy People 2020 vision of health and well-being for all members is realized. This chapter explains the major theoretical and foundational concepts of the discipline. Principles of information literacy are then used to explore primary informational resources for health promotion and disease prevention.

Next, the chapter describes the creation of health IT infrastructure in conjunction with the Nationwide Health Information Network, beginning with early efforts to automate and manage patient health data electronically. While electronic management of health data is imperative to the vision of a society with health care for all, it is the individual who must assume responsibility for managing his or her own health. Evidence of this responsibility is demonstrated each time a patient signs a consent form. That person signing the consent form has the ultimate authority and is giving the health-care provider permission to care for him or her. Health-care providers and patients are increasingly recognizing the need to prepare patients for this responsibility. The final section of the chapter discusses the use of informatics tools for client empowerment.

DEFINITION AND SCOPE OF PRACTICE

Health informatics is both an interdisciplinary professional area of specialization and a scientific discipline that integrates the health sciences, computer science, information science, and other analytic sciences with the goal of managing and communicating data, information, knowledge, and wisdom in the provision of health care for individuals, families, groups, and communities (Nelson & Staggers, 2018). Because health informatics deals with all aspects of health-care delivery, a wide range of other analytic sciences are used in the practice of informatics. Some examples of the wide range of sciences include cognitive science, complexity theory, data science, sociology, and linguistics.

When analyzing this definition of health informatics, consider the following key points:

- As an interdisciplinary professional specialty, health informatics includes various health professions, such as dentistry (dental informatics), medicine (medical informatics), and nursing (nursing informatics).
- As a discipline, health informatics covers areas of health care such as public health (public health informatics), acute and chronic care (clinical informatics), and consumer health (consumer health informatics).
- Within this definition, "the provision of health care for individuals, families, groups, and communities" includes not just the treatment of health problems and the use of preventative measures but also the promotion of general well-being.
- Health, computer, and information science as well as other analytic sciences provide processes, tools, methods, and procedures used within the practice of health informatics, but these tools do not define the scope of practice.
- The scope of practice is defined by the data to wisdom (D–W) continuum and the interactions and interrelationships between the megaconcepts inherent in the model. Megaconcepts are overarching structures that incorporate several overlapping and interrelated abstract concepts. For example, the term *bird* reflects a basic concept, referring in a general sense to the many different types of birds. On the other hand, an example of a megaconcept would include love, freedom, or happiness. Megaconcepts are much more abstract and include several other basic concepts. The megaconcepts that make up the D–W continuum and their interrelationships are presented in Figure 13-1.

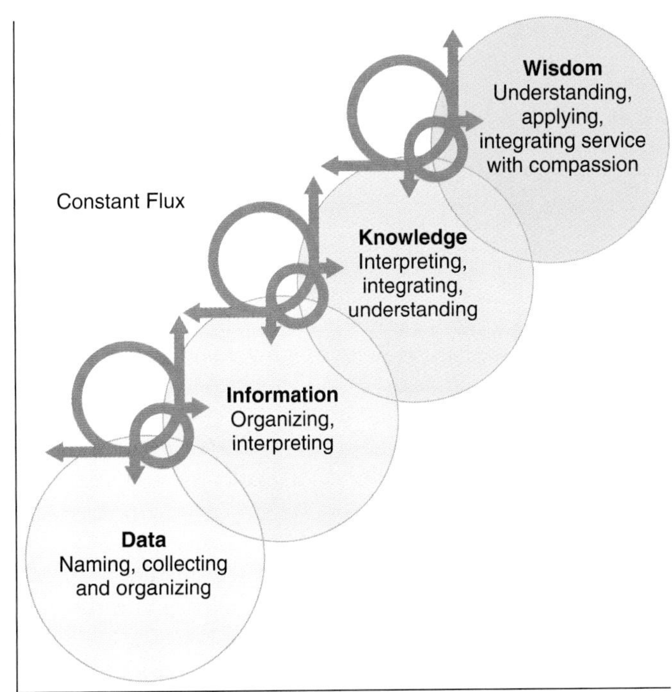

FIGURE 13–1 The Nelson D-W Continuum.
Source: Printed with the permission of Ramona Nelson (Ramona Nelson Consulting). All rights reserved.

Evolution of the Nelson D–W Continuum

The concepts of data, information, and knowledge within the practice of informatics were first introduced by Blum (1986) in the 1980s. Blum defined data as uninterpreted elements such as a person's name, weight, or age. He defined information as a collection of data that have been processed and then displayed as information, such as weight over time. In Blum's model knowledge results when data and information are identified and the relationships between the data and information are formalized. In their classic article "The Study of Nursing Informatics," Graves and Corcoran (1989) used Blum's definitions of the concepts of data, information, and knowledge to explain the study of nursing informatics. This article is considered the foundation for most definitions of nursing informatics.

In 1989, Nelson extended the Blum and Graves and Corcoran data-to-knowledge continuum by including wisdom (Nelson & Joos, 1989). The initial publication provided only brief definitions of the concepts, but later publications included a comprehensive model (Nelson, 2002). The introduction of the concept of wisdom gained professional acceptance in 2008 when the American Nurses Association (ANA) (2008) included this concept and the related Nelson D–W model in *Nursing Informatics: Scope and Standards of Practice*. Over time, the model has been modified to acknowledge more effectively the inter- and intra-environmental factors that influence movement across and within the D–W continuum. Figure 13-1 demonstrates the most current version of this model.

Key Concepts in the Nelson D–W Continuum

By definition, data elements are uninterpreted and therefore meaningless. For example, an annual income of $20,000 could be interpreted as inadequate for meeting basic needs. However, if the person in question is a teenager who is earning extra spending money, the significance of the income is very different. A weight of 140 pounds may be that of an individual who is underweight, overweight, or of normal weight depending on other factors such as age and height.

Data elements are descriptive and/or measurable and, as such, serve as the building blocks for information. Because it is impossible to collect every data element related to any event or problem, assessment of a health-care need begins with a carefully considered decision about what data should be collected based on the information that may be needed.

When data are processed to produce meaning using techniques such as calculating, classifying, graphing, organizing, sorting, and summarizing, information is created. For example, a health promotion Web site written at a graduate level may be meaningless data to the reader with limited health literacy. When the content is translated to the literacy level of the reader, it becomes meaningful—now it provides information. A list of crime rates by itself would be meaningless, but if these data were used to create a graph, information about a community's safety would emerge. Data processing can also create new data elements, such as an average overall crime rate.

When data are processed into information and the relationships between the data and the resulting information are formalized, knowledge is created. For example, understanding how health literacy can affect health-care outcomes requires an understanding of several types of literacy, models of health promotion, and measures for determining health status as well as an understanding of how these different concepts interrelate. The greater the knowledge base used to interpret data, the more information that can be disclosed from that data. For example, the more you know about crime statistics in different age groups and circumstances related to these crimes, the more information you can obtain from a series of statistics.

Collecting an individual's demographic data can provide clues about his or her opportunity to purchase healthy food options. Gathering additional demographic data at the community level improves the interpretation of information available. This is one reason why interdisciplinary health informatics teams can be so much more effective than individual health-care providers.

No current consensus exists about types of knowledge and how they should be classified. Mantzoukas and Jasper (2008) used a secondary qualitative analysis to identify five types of knowledge guiding nursing care of hospitalized patients: (1) personal practice knowledge used in therapeutic relationships; (2) theoretical knowledge about relevant facts; (3) procedural knowledge with ready-made answers for completing nursing-care-related activities; (4) cultural knowledge, comprising written and unwritten norms, rules, and values for care in this setting; and (5) reflexive knowledge that is context-specific and developed through synthesis of the other four types of knowledge through experience.

Lechasseur, Lazure, and Guilbert (2011) used qualitative methods to research the mobilization of knowledge within the critical thinking process of nursing students. They identified nine types of knowledge: intrapersonal, interpersonal, perceptual, moral/ethical, experiential, practical, scientific, contextual, and combinational constructive knowledge. Combinational constructive knowledge was described as "a new type of knowledge, created from a simultaneous combination of all types of knowledge in function of a specific situation" (p. 1936).

The synthesis of different types of knowledge leads to higher levels of thinking with increased complexity, interactions, and interrelationships. At this point of synthesis, knowledge begins to overlap with wisdom. Wisdom is the appropriate use of knowledge in managing or solving human problems, including managing health conditions and promoting health. Wisdom requires synthesizing different types of knowledge and applying this synthesis to real-life situations. For example, a public health nurse may have substantial knowledge about preventing health disease at the community level. Knowing when and how to use that knowledge in working with a community group to change the health status of that community requires a level of wisdom that can be achieved only with experience.

Defining Nursing Informatics

In 1992, ANA recognized nursing informatics as a specialty within the profession of nursing as well as an area of specialty within the discipline of health informatics (ANA, 2001). Over the years the definition has evolved to the current ANA definition: "Nursing Informatics (NI) is the specialty that integrates nursing science with multiple information and analytic sciences to identify, define, manage, and communicate data, information, knowledge, and wisdom in nursing practice" (ANA, 2015, pp. 1–2). Note the relationship between this definition and the definition of health informatics previously presented; both are built on the same concepts.

This section of the chapter has explored the megaconcepts that define and explain the discipline and practice of health informatics. In the next section, the literacies that form the bedrock for the study and application of health informatics are described. Together, these two sections provide the foundation for applying health informatics–based theories, models, processes and tools to health promotion and disease prevention.

INFORMATICS-RELATED LITERACIES AND IMPLICATIONS FOR HEALTH PROMOTION

Effective use of informatics tools and techniques by both health-care consumers and professionals necessitates a level of digital health literacy. Digital health literacy requires the synthesis of (1) basic literacy, (2) computer literacy, (3) information literacy, (4) digital literacy, and (5) health literacy. The interrelationship between these literacies is shown in Figure 13-2.

Basic literacy is more than the ability to read and write; it is formally defined as "the ability to identify, understand, interpret, create, communicate and compute, using printed and written materials associated with varying contexts. Literacy involves a continuum of learning in enabling individuals to achieve their goals, to develop their knowledge and potential, and to participate fully in their community and wider society" (UNESCO, 2004, p. 13). Chapter 12 further explores assessing learning needs and health literacy.

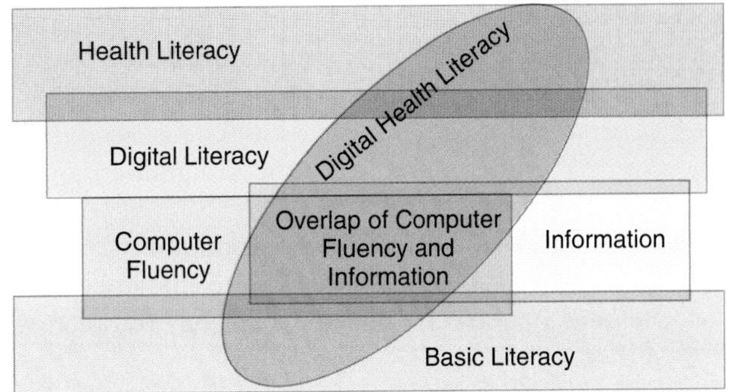

FIGURE 13–2 Overlapping Relationship of Technology-Related Literacies and Basic Literacy. *Source: Printed with the permission of Ramona Nelson (Ramona Nelson Consulting). All rights reserved.*

Computer literacy encompasses (1) contemporary skills for navigating and using computer applications, such as search engines and operating systems; (2) an understanding of foundational concepts of information technology that provides insight into the opportunities and limitations of social media and other information technologies; and (3) intellectual capabilities such as applying information technology to actual problems and challenges of everyday life. (Committee on Information Technology Literacy: National Research Council, 1999).

Information literacy is defined as "the set of integrated abilities encompassing the reflective discovery of information, the understanding of how information is produced and valued, and the use of information in creating new knowledge and participating ethically in communities of learning" (Association of College and Research Libraries, 2016).

Digital literacy includes a set of interrelated competencies:

- The technical competency to operate digital devices such as cameras, e-readers, smartphones, computers, tablets, video game consoles, and so on. This does not mean that one can pick up a new device and automatically be able to use it without direction. Rather, technical competency means one can learn to use the device effectively with the help of the owner's manual and a bit of trial and error.
- The conceptual knowledge to understand the interrelated functionality of digital tools.

- The ability to use these devices to access, manipulate, evaluate, and apply data, information, knowledge, and wisdom in activities of daily living.
- The ability to use emotional intelligence in collaborating and communicating in a digital environment with others.
- The ethical values and sense of community responsibility to use digital devices for the enjoyment and benefit of society (Nelson & Carter-Templeton, 2016).

Health literacy is the ability to access, evaluate, and apply information to health-related decisions. A detailed discussion of health literacy is included in Chapter 11. Resources to support advanced practice nurses working in health literacy can also be found in the Agency for Healthcare Research and Quality (AHRQ) Health Literacy Universal Precautions Toolkit currently located at https://www.ahrq.gov/health-literacy/quality-resources/tools/literacy-toolkit/index.html.

Digital health literacy incorporates each of these skills and abilities to access, understand, appraise, and communicate health information and engage with the demands of different health contexts to promote and maintain good health across the life span. Each of the literacies in this model focuses on a different aspect of literacy, but they overlap and are interrelated. Weakness in any area affects competency in other areas, while improving knowledge and augmenting skills in an area facilitates improvement in other areas.

ACCESSING, EVALUATING, AND USING EVIDENCE-BASED ONLINE RESOURCES FOR HEALTH PROMOTION AND DISEASE PREVENTION

Advanced practice nurses incorporate each of the literacy skills discussed above to collect data and information to complete assessments, develop a plan using evidence-based interventions to meet the needs identified in the assessment, and use standardized measures to evaluate the effectiveness of these interventions. Finding high-quality data and information begins by identifying the scope and organization of the information desired, both of which inform where and how to search for data and information resources. When considering health promotion and disease prevention, three factors can be used to determine the scope and organization of the resources of interest: (1) the concepts of health promotion and disease prevention, (2) the determinants of health, and (3) the concept of client.

The Concepts of Health Promotion and Disease Prevention

Health promotion comprises interventions that improve a client's overall health in pursuit of optimal well-being, as well as interventions to prevent disease. Disease prevention is divided into three levels: primary, secondary, and tertiary prevention. Figure 13-3 defines these concepts and demonstrates the overlap between the concepts of health promotion and disease prevention.

The information resources for promotion and prevention may be organized in terms of health promotion or in terms of the three levels of prevention included in Figure 13-3. Fitness tracking m-health apps are a common example of health promotion tools that improve general wellness. They are not focused on a specific disease but rather on an overall commitment to improving health and fitness. The term *m-health* is derived from the concept of mobile health as a general term in medical care to depict the use of mobile phones and other wireless technology.

Information resources for each of the levels of prevention are not usually organized by levels of prevention but instead in terms of specific diseases. For example, the Centers for Disease Control and Prevention's (CDC's) National Diabetes Prevention Program (National DPP) is a partnership of public and private organizations working to reduce the growing problem of prediabetes and type 2 diabetes with a one-year CDC approved curriculum. Additional information is located at https://www.cdc.gov/diabetes/prevention/index.html.

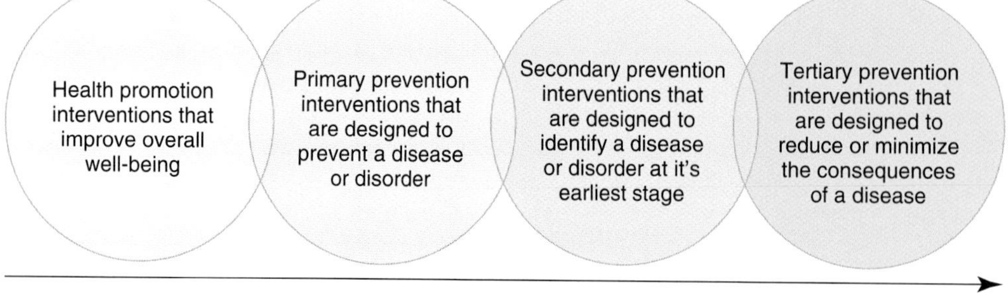

Health promotion interventions that improve overall well-being

Primary prevention interventions that are designed to prevent a disease or disorder

Secondary prevention interventions that are designed to identify a disease or disorder at it's earliest stage

Tertiary prevention interventions that are designed to reduce or minimize the consequences of a disease

FIGURE 13–3 Health Promotion and Disease Prevention Continuum. *Source: Printed with the permission of Ramona Nelson (Ramona Nelson Consulting). All rights reserved.*

This is a primary prevention program, but the information about this program exists under the heading of diabetes.

Health information is also rarely organized around specific interventions because any one intervention might be used at any point in the continuum. For example, exercise might be used to promote well-being, to prevent heart disease, as a screening technique for heart disease, or as part of a cardiac rehabilitation program.

The CDC's approach to organizing information about the prevention of chronic disease provides an excellent example of how information resources related to health promotion and levels of disease prevention are usually organized. "With non-communicable conditions accounting for nearly two-thirds of deaths worldwide, the emergence of chronic diseases as the predominant challenge to global health is undisputed. In the USA, chronic diseases are the main causes of poor health, disability, and death, and account for most of health-care expenditures" (Bauer et al 2014). The CDC works to prevent chronic diseases and their risk factors through four domains, as demonstrated in Box 13-1 (CDC, 2019.

Specific chronic disease prevention programs are then organized by disease, as demonstrated in Table 13-1. Table 13-1 provides examples of resources that can be used by advanced practice nurses in assessing risk and in preventing a wide range of specific health problems.

The Determinants of Health

The second factor that influences the organization of health promotion and disease prevention resources is the identification of factors that determine health status. Almost every characteristic of a society can have

BOX 13-1 How We Prevent Chronic Diseases and Promote Health

Just as many of the same risk factors can cause or worsen most chronic diseases, many of the same approaches can prevent them or reduce their severity. National Center for Chronic Disease Prevention and Health Promotion (NCCDPHP) promotes chronic disease prevention efforts in four key areas, or domains. This approach to preventing chronic diseases and promoting health can help achieve NCCDPHP's vision of healthy people in healthy communities.

Domain 1: Epidemiology and Surveillance: Measuring how many Americans have chronic diseases or chronic disease risk factors

CDC uses dozens of surveillance systems to collect data on chronic diseases and their risk factors. These systems—often the only source of such data—help epidemiologists understand how chronic diseases affect Americans.

Surveillance and epidemiology guide us in putting our resources to the best use. Without them, our prevention and control efforts would be guesswork.

Domain 2: Environmental Approaches: Improving environments to make it easier for people to make healthy choices

Healthy environments promote health and support healthy behaviors in community settings such as schools, child care programs, and worksites. Approaches that improve the environment reach more people, are more cost-effective, and are more likely than individual approaches to have a lasting effect on population health.

Domain 3: Health-Care System Interventions: Strengthening health care systems to deliver prevention services that keep people well and diagnose diseases early

The right health-care system interventions can improve the use and quality of clinical preventive services. These services can help prevent disease or catch it early, reduce risk factors, and manage complications. Giving people better access to quality preventive services can reduce health disparities.

Domain 4: Community Programs Linked to Clinical Services: Connecting clinical services to community programs that help people prevent and manage their chronic diseases and conditions

By linking people who have chronic diseases or chronic disease risk factors to community resources, CDC can help them improve their quality of life, prevent or slow down the disease, avoid complications, and reduce the need for more health care. Improved links between the community and clinical settings often mean that clinicians can refer patients to proven programs, ideally with community organizations and lay providers getting reimbursed by health insurance.

Source: CDC. (2019, July 30). *How We Prevent Chronic Diseases and Promote Health*. Retrieved from https://www.cdc.gov/chronicdisease/center/nccdphp/how.htm.

Table 13-1 Health Promotion and Disease Prevention Programs

Provided By . . .	Program Name and Focus	URL
National Center for Chronic Disease Prevention and Health Promotion (part of the CDC)	Chronic program sites and resources • Cancer • Community health • Diabetes • Heart disease and stroke • Nutrition, physical activity, and obesity • Oral health • Population health • Preventing chronic disease (PCD) journal • Reproductive health • Smoking and tobacco use • Tribal resources	https://www.cdc.gov/chronicdisease/index.htm
National Center for Injury Prevention and Control (The Injury Center, part of the CDC)	The mission of The Injury Center is to prevent injuries and violence through science and action.	https://www.cdc.gov/injury/index.html
The National Center for HIV/AIDS, Viral Hepatitis, STD, and TB Prevention (NCHHSTP, part of the CDC)	NCHHSTP consists of four divisions, each of which is defined by the diseases it addresses: • Division of HIV/AIDS Prevention • Division of STD Prevention • Division of Tuberculosis Elimination • Division of Viral Hepatitis	https://www.cdc.gov/nchhstp/default.htm
The Office of Disease Prevention and Health Promotion (ODPHP, part of the Department of Health and Human Services)	The ODPHP maintains the following Web sites: • health.gov—the home of ODPHP and an essential resource for health information • HealthyPeople.gov—tools and resources for professionals about Healthy People 2020 health objectives • healthfinder.gov—evidence-based, actionable health guidance for consumers	https://health.gov/about-us/
U.S. Preventive Services Task Force (USPSTF)	The Task Force makes evidence-based recommendations about clinical preventive services such as screenings, counseling services, and preventive medications. All recommendations are published on the Task Force's Web site and/or in a peer-reviewed journal.	https://www.uspreventiveservicestaskforce.org/Page/Name/home

an impact on the health of its citizens and can therefore be considered a health determinant. Because everything in a society could be a health determinant, agencies such as Health Canada and the World Health Organization (WHO) have focused on identified key health determinants that deserve special attention (Association of Faculties of Medicine of Canada [AFMC], n.d.)

While there is not a generally accepted international classification or list of key health determinants, the lists created by major organizations demonstrate substantial overlap. Table 13-2 provides examples of these lists from major health-care organizations. The URL for the source of each list is provided in the table, and readers are encouraged to explore these sites and note the specific determinants and how they are classified and measured.

In response to this variation in specific determinants, the Canadian Council on Social Determinants of Health (CCSDH) published *A Review of Frameworks on the Determinants of Health* (Social Determinants of Health Framework Task Group, 2015). The task group identified 36 frameworks from around the world and classified them by type, as follows:

- Explanatory frameworks list determinants followed by a definition and explanation of each determinate.

Table 13-2 Examples of Social Determinants as Identified by Different Health-Related Organizations

Name of the Organization	Determinants of Health	URL
World Health Organization http://www.who.int/en/	• The social and economic environment • The physical environment • The person's individual characteristics and behaviors	https://www.who.int/social_determinants/sdh_definition/en
HHS: Office of Disease Prevention and Health Promotion, part of the Department of Health and Human Services: HealthyPeople.gov https://www.healthypeople.gov/	• Policy making • Social factors • Health services • Individual behavior • Biology and genetics	https://www.healthypeople.gov/2020/about/foundation-health-measures/Determinants-of-Health
Public Health Agency of Canada www.publichealth.gc.ca	• Income and social status • Social support networks • Education and literacy • Employment/working conditions • Social environments • Physical environments • Personal health practices and coping skills • Healthy child development • Biology and genetic endowment • Health services • Gender • Culture	http://www.phac-aspc.gc.ca/ph-sp/determinants/index-eng.php#determinants

- Interactive frameworks identify points of interaction and show relationships between determinants of health. They do not offer strategies.
- Action-oriented frameworks focus on decision- or policy-making processes. They also provide a framework to help identify priority issues and evaluate the potential success of potential interventions (Social Determinants of Health Framework Task Group, 2015).

The frameworks are also grouped by their primary area of focus, as follows:

1. Policy development and decision making
2. Practice approach: population health, health reporting, community development
3. Issue focus: ecosystems and environment, living and working conditions
4. Population focus: gender, aboriginal peoples, children, rural
5. Broad focus

In some references, the terms *determinants of health* and *social determinants of health (SODH)* are used interchangeably (Solberg, 2017). While the term *determinants of health* encompasses all factors that could influence health, social determinants of health are specifically nonmedical factors such as social disadvantages, risk exposure, and inequities that play a fundamental causal role in poor health outcomes (Bharmal, Derose, Felician, & Weden, 2015).

In this chapter, we use the CDC definitions of these terms. The CDC's definition for the term *determinants of heath* includes the social determinants of heath as well as other determinants. It is derived from WHO (World Health Organization, 1946) and Healthy People 2020 (U.S. Department of Health and Human Services, 2009). The CDC's definition for the term *social determinants of health* is derived from the WHO Commission on Social Determinants of Health (CSDH) (2008). See Box 13-2 for both definitions.

Although the importance of SDOH has long been considered in Canada, Great Britain, and other European countries, this recognition is relatively recent in the United States, likely because of the difference in health-care delivery systems (Solberg, 2017). "Changes in the health care landscape, including value-based reimbursement, increased health system and provider accountability, and the addition of millions of people to the health insurance rolls, have created incentives and demand for addressing social determinants of health"

BOX 13-2 CDC Definitions: Determinants of Health and Social Determinants of Health

DETERMINANTS OF HEALTH

Factors that contribute to a person's current state of health that may be biological, socioeconomic, psychosocial, behavioral, or social in nature. Scientists generally recognize five determinants of health of a population:

- Biology and genetics. Examples: sex and age.
- Individual behavior. Examples: alcohol use, injection drug use (needles), unprotected sex, and smoking
- Social environment. Examples: discrimination, income, and gender
- Physical environment. Examples: where a person lives and crowding conditions
- Health services. Examples: access to quality health care and health insurance

SOCIAL DETERMINANTS OF HEALTH

The complex, integrated, and overlapping social structures and economic systems that are responsible for most health inequities. These social structures and economic systems include the social environment, physical environment, health services, and structural and societal factors. Social determinants of health are shaped by the distribution of money, power, and resources throughout local communities, nations, and the world.

Source: CDC: NCHHSTP. Social Determinants of Health: Definitions. March 2014. Retrieved from https://www.cdc.gov/nchhstp/socialdeterminants/definitions.html.

(DeMilto & Nakashian, 2016, p. 5). One example of the increased U.S. interest in SDOH is the Institute of Medicine (IOM) publications identifying specific social determinants of health to include in the electronic health record (EHR). "Substantial empirical evidence of the contribution of social and behavioral factors to functional status and the onset, progression, and effective treatment of disease has accumulated over the past four decades. Yet efforts to improve health care, advance population and public health, and develop and apply social and behavioral research remain largely separate from one another" (Institute of Medicine, 2014). The specific social determinants of health that are recommended for EHR inclusion by the IOM are listed in Box 13-3.

In the United States, the Census Bureau, which attempts to count every U.S. resident every 10 years, is the most important source of population data (United States Census Bureau, 2015). As part of their work gathering population data, they collect several data elements that help determine the population's overall health status and track the determinants of health identified by Healthy People 2020 (U.S. Department of Health and Human Services, 2015a). The Census Bureau partners with many other government agencies to provide an innovative range of databases available for public download and exploration; examples are included in Table 13-3. Table 13-4 shows an example of data from an interactive Excel spreadsheet that allows users to analyze and present poverty rates over time at the national, state, and county levels.

Census Bureau statistics are organized by topic. As shown in Table 13-3, one topic area is health, under which the following data are included:

- Disability: These are statistics about people who have difficulty doing ordinary activities because of physical, mental, or emotional conditions.
- Expenses and investments: These are statistics on how health-care establishments collect funds and spend money, from expenses for day-to-day operations to investments in long-term infrastructure.
- Fertility: These statistics show, for example, a historical perspective of the cumulative fertility experience of women, participation in the labor force, and maternity leave. It should be noted, however, that the National Center for Health Statistics (NCHS), considered the primary source for the number of births, percentage of unmarried mothers, and more.
- Health insurance: The Census Bureau includes data on both private coverage and government coverage, including plans provided through an employer or a union or purchased by an individual from a private company; government health insurance plans include Medicare, Medicaid, military health care, and the Children's Health Insurance Program (CHIP); and individual state health plans.
- HIV/AIDS: The HIV/AIDS Surveillance is updated annually and includes data from population groups in developing countries, information from the medical and scientific literature, presentations at international conferences, and information gathered by the press.
- Small Area Health Insurance Estimates (SAHIE): SAHIE is the only source of single-year estimates of health insurance coverage for states and all counties. SAHIE releases estimates of health insurance coverage by age, sex, race, Hispanic origin, and selected income categories.

BOX 13-3 IOM Recommended Social Determinants of Health for Inclusion in the EHR

SOCIODEMOGRAPHIC DOMAINS

- Sexual orientation
- Race and ethnicity
- Country of origin/U.S. born or non-U.S. born
- Education
- Employment
- Financial resource strain: food and housing insecurity

PSYCHOLOGICAL DOMAINS

- Health literacy
- Stress
- Negative mood and affect: depression and anxiety
- Psychological assets: conscientiousness, patient engagement/activation, optimism, and self-efficacy

BEHAVIORAL DOMAINS

- Dietary patterns
- Physical activity
- Tobacco use and exposure
- Alcohol use

INDIVIDUAL-LEVEL SOCIAL RELATIONSHIPS AND LIVING CONDITIONS DOMAINS

- Social connections and social isolation
- Exposure to violence

NEIGHBORHOODS AND COMMUNITIES

- Neighborhood and community compositional characteristics

Source: Institute of Medicine. (2014). Capturing social and behavioral domains and measures in electronic health records: Phase 2. Washington, DC: National Academies Press.

For an advanced-level nurse supporting health promotion and disease prevention, deciding what data to collect begins by identifying the specific determinants of health important to the question at hand. The frameworks and definitions presented here provide a conceptual context for the advanced practice nurse in developing a systematic approach for identifying the specific determinants of health that may be of concern to the question at hand. They help to answer the question: "What data elements do I need to collect for this specific project or issue?" Table 13-3 provides resources for collecting these data.

The Concept of Client

The third factor that influences how promotion and prevention resources are organized is the concept of client, consumer, and patient. Within health care, these terms can refer to a community, group, family, or individual. In addition, the terms *community* and *group* can overlap and are sometimes used interchangeably. For example, either term can refer to a group as large as the international community (United Nations, 2009) or to a group as small as a subgroup of inmates at a local prison. The term *family* recognizes the wide variation of interrelations and structures that define the concept of family in modern society.

When applied to individuals, the terms *client*, *consumer*, and *patient* reflect the varying relationships that exist between an individual and the health-care system. For example, an individual researching health insurance may have a client relationship with a navigator as she or he determines which product best meets her or his needs. When buying the product, this person becomes a consumer. In using the product that this person has purchased, she or he may function in the role of patient, family, and/or caretaker.

With this framework in mind, we begin by identifying data sources that can be used to support the assessment process when the client is a community. The goal of the assessment is to determine a community's primary health problems and the resources available to promote health and prevent disease within that community. When considering what data should be collected about a country or group of countries, one should consider both data related to the health status of the country and data related to the determinants of health, especially the social determinants. Social determinants of health will be determined by and reflected in the distribution of money, power, and resources throughout local communities, nations, and the world (CSDH, 2008).

At the international level, *community* may refer to a country or a group of countries. Table 13-5 lists data sources that can be used to collect data for determining the health status, social determinants of health, and primary health-related problems within the international community.

The principal source of health statistics for the United States is the NCHS, which is maintained by the CDC

Table 13-3 Data Resources for Social Determinants of Health

Data Source	Types of Data Available	URL
U.S. Census Bureau	Census Bureau statistics are organized by topic. Examples include: • Business: information about businesses in the community. • Education: range of topics, from educational attainment to school districts, costs and financing. • Employment: the official source of statistical data tracking national employment, including employment and unemployment levels, weeks and hours worked, occupations, and commuting. • Families and living arrangements: trends in household and family composition, characteristics of the residents of housing units and how they are related. • Health: insurance coverage, disability, fertility, and other health issues are increasingly important in measuring the nation's overall well-being. • Housing: homeownership rates, statistics on the physical and financial characteristics of our homes. • Income and poverty: cover poverty, income, and wealth. • Population: population statistics cover age, sex, race, Hispanic origin, migration, ancestry, language use, veterans, as well as population estimates and projections.	http://www.census.gov/en.html, then click on Topics
CDC: Sources for Data on Social Determinants of Health	• Chronic disease indicators: state and selected metropolitan-level data for chronic diseases and risk factors. • Community Health Status Indicators (CHSI 2015): primary and associated indicators that affect health outcomes and population health in various domains (e.g., health-care access and quality, health behaviors, social factors, and physical environment) for every state and county and the District of Columbia. • Health Indicators: warehouse provides access to national, state, and local health indicators. Users can query multiple dimensions of population health, health care, and health determinants; view data (in map, chart, or table form); and download indicator data. • Interactive atlas of heart disease and stroke: online county-level mapping of heart disease and stroke by race/ethnicity, gender, and age group. Maps show social and economic factors and health services for the United States, specific states, or territories. • National Center for HIV/AIDS, Viral Hepatitis, STD, and TB Prevention: atlas provides interactive maps, graphs, tables, and figures showing geographic patterns and time trends of the reported occurrence of the following diseases: HIV, AIDS, viral hepatitis, tuberculosis, chlamydia, gonorrhea, and primary and secondary syphilis. • National Environmental Public Health Tracking Network: a system of integrated health, exposure, and hazard maps, tables, and charts with data about environmental indicators. • The Social Vulnerability Index: uses U.S. census variables at tract level to help local officials identify communities that may need support in preparing for hazards or are recovering from disaster. • Vulnerable Populations Footprint Tool: creates maps and reports that identify geographic areas with high poverty rates and low education levels.	https://www.cdc.gov/socialdeterminants/data/index.htm
Healthy People 2020	This site provides a search engine to search for data concerning the 11 Healthy People objectives dealing with the social determinants of health.	https://www.healthypeople.gov/2020/leading-health-indicators/2020-lhi-topics/Social-Determinants

Table 13-4 An Example of Data Available from the U.S. Census Bureau

			Demographic Group		Uninsured				Insured			
Year	**ID**	**Name**	**Number**	**MOE**	**Number**	**MOE**	**%**	**%MOE**	**Number**	**MOE**	**%**	**%MOE**
2013	01000	Alabama	4,008,475	0	636,216	14,701	15.9	0.4	3,372,259	14,701	84.1	0.4
2013	02000	Alaska	658,020	0	137,170	5,322	20.8	0.8	520,851	5,322	79.2	0.8
2013	04000	Arizona	5,473,619	0	1,093,575	21,161	20.0	0.4	4,380,044	21,161	80.0	0.4
2013	05000	Arkansas	2,433,909	0	458,560	11,936	18.8	0.5	1,975,350	11,936	81.2	0.5
2013	06000	California	32,978,809	0	6,382,717	67,813	19.4	0.2	26,596,092	67,813	80.6	0.2
2013	08000	Colorado	4,517,639	0	722,071	16,225	16.0	0.4	3,795,568	16,225	84.0	0.4
2013	09000	Connecticut	2,961,410	0	323,606	11,067	10.9	0.4	2,637,803	11,067	89.1	0.4
2013	10000	Delaware	755,663	0	82,412	4,932	10.9	0.7	673,251	4,931	89.1	0.7
2013	11000	District of Columbia	540,391	0	40,951	3,752	7.6	0.7	499,440	3,752	92.4	0.7
2013	12000	Florida	15,538,084	0	3,775,449	40,008	24.3	0.3	11,762,634	40,008	75.7	0.3
2013	13000	Georgia	8,542,785	0	1,806,594	26,991	21.1	0.3	6,736,190	26,991	78.9	0.3
2013	15000	Hawaii	1,172,629	0	89,341	7,687	7.6	0.7	1,083,288	7,687	92.4	0.7
2013	16000	Idaho	1,361,561	0	255,932	8,800	18.8	0.6	1,105,629	8,800	81.2	0.6
2013	17000	Illinois	10,894,034	0	1,587,714	23,452	14.6	0.2	9,306,319	23,452	85.4	0.2
2013	18000	Indiana	5,487,008	0	885,240	17,669	16.1	0.3	4,601,768	17,669	83.9	0.3
2013	19000	Iowa	2,531,557	0	243,546	7,946	9.6	0.3	2,288,011	7,945	90.4	0.3
2013	20000	Kansas	2,423,120	0	340,965	9,580,	14.1	0.4	2,082,155	9,580	85.9	0.4
2013	21000	Kentucky	3,650,161	0	613,811	14,315	16.8	0.4	3,036,351	4,315	83.2	0.4
2013	22000	Louisiana	3,893,624	0	745,580	16,013	19.1	0.4	3,148,044	16,013	80.9	0.4

Source: United States Census Bureau.

(CDC, 2019). NCHS produces data on a wide range of health indicators. Examples include:

- Births, such as teen, multiple, preterm, and low-birth-weight births
- Diseases and health conditions such as obesity, diabetes, hypertension, cancer, and heart disease
- Other health status measures, including injuries, disabilities, and environmental exposures
- Health-related behaviors such as smoking, physical activity, and alcohol use
- Nutrition and growth charts
- Preventive services such as immunizations and cancer screening
- Reproductive health, including fertility, contraceptive use, and sexual behaviors
- Health insurance coverage and access to care
- Health-care use and services delivered by hospitals, hospital emergency, and outpatient departments and other health-care sites
- The health-care system, including the use of health information technology and electronic medical records, medications prescribed, and complications of care
- Deaths, leading causes of death, fetal deaths, and infant mortality

By using tools provided by NCHS, much of these data can be aggregated at a variety of levels, including tract, city, county, region, and state. While the quality of data from the CDC is usually well respected, exceptions do exist. For example, the estimated maternal mortality rate (per 100,000 live births) for 48 states and Washington, DC, excluding California and Texas,

Table 13-5 Data Sources for National and International Community Assessment

Name	Description	URLS
CDC, Division of Global Migration and Quarantine (DGMQ)	The division within the CDC that "reduce[s] morbidity and mortality among immigrants, refugees, travelers, expatriates, and other globally mobile populations, and . . . prevent[s] the introduction, transmission, and spread of communicable diseases through regulation, science, research, preparedness, and response."	https://www.cdc.gov/ncezid/dgmq/index.html, then click on Travel's Health, then click on Search
Central Intelligence Agency (CIA)	The CIA Factbook provides information on the history, people, government, economy, energy, geography, communications, transportation, military, and transnational issues for 267 world entities. In addition, several health- and education-related fields are included in the People and Society category.	https://www.cia.gov/library/publications/resources/the-world-factbook/
Sheldon Margen Public Health Library	The Sheldon Margen Public Health Library is a division of the library at the University of California at Berkeley.	http://www.lib.berkeley.edu/PUBL/IntHealth.html
The United Nation Children's Fund (UNICEF)	UNICEF is an agency of the UN Economic and Social Council that works for a more equitable world by fighting for the rights of its future: children. (UNESCO, 2004)	http://www.data.unicef.org/. Note the data at this site is organized by health topic or country.
The United Nations Development Programme (UNDP)	The major health concerns of UNDP include AIDS, maternal and child nutrition, and maternal mortality.	http://www.undp.org/content/undp/en/home.html
UNdata	UNdata is a database interface providing access through a single entry point to the major UN databases as well as a comprehensive array of international and national databases.	http://data.un.org/
University of Michigan Library	Global Health Information and Resources: Global Data and Statistics	http://guides.lib.umich.edu/c.php?g=282776&p=1884201
World Bank	The World Bank is like a cooperative and is made up of 188 member countries with a mission to ending extreme poverty and promote shared prosperity.	http://data.worldbank.org/topic/health
World Health Organization (WHO)	WHO is a specialized division within the United Nations whose objective is the attainment by all peoples of the highest possible level of health.	https://www.who.int/data/gho http://www.who.int/countries/en/ http://www.who.int/whosis/en/

increased by 26.6%, from 18.8 in 2000 to 23.8 in 2014. California showed a declining trend, whereas Texas had a sudden increase in 2011 and 2012. California, whose death rate decreased during the period of the analysis and Texas, whose death rate after 2010 doubled within a 2-year period to levels unseen in other U.S. states, were excluded from the analysis for methodology reasons (MacDorman, Declercq, Cabral, & Morton, 2016). In an article summarizing the results of the MacDorman research, a second study, and the editorial published in the 128th volume of the journal *Obstetrics and Gynecology* (pages 427–428, 440–446, and 447–455) Phillips (2016) pointed out that these rates are significantly higher than those the CDC published in the January 2015 issue of *Obstetrics and Gynecology*. This discrepancy in estimated maternal mortality rates suggests that advanced practice nurses need to evaluate carefully the source and quality of *all* data used in the assessment process. The greater the number of data sources and the more consistency that exists from different sources, the more confidence one can have in the information gleaned.

State health departments are another key source of community health data, such as those provided online by Pennsylvania at http://bit.ly/2keKFhp. Table 13-6 includes additional primary sources that can be used to collect data for determining the health status, social determinants of health, and primary health-related problems for communities within the United States. Both health-care professionals and the public can expect

Table 13-6 Additional Data Sources for Federal, State, and Local Community Assessment

Name	Description	URLS
DATA2020 Search	This site provides an interactive data tool that allows users to explore data and technical information related to Healthy People 2020. The tool is structured by 2020 Objectives.	http://www.healthypeople.gov/2020/data-search/Search-the-Data
The County Health Rankings and Roadmaps program	This resource, which is a collaboration between the Robert Wood Johnson Foundation and the University of Wisconsin Population Health Institute, measures several vital health factors, including obesity, smoking, unemployment, access to healthy foods, the quality of air and water, and teen births in nearly every county in America	http://www.countyhealthrankings.org/
America's Health Rankings®	This site provides two yearly reports. The Annual Report uses a variety of health data benchmarks such as smoking and obesity rates to measure and rank the nation's health on a state-by-state basis. The rankings are published jointly by United Health Foundation, the American Public Health Association. and Partnership for Prevention. The Senior Report provides state-by-state data on a variety of health data benchmarks for individuals over age 65.	http://www.americashealthrankings.org/

that these sources will become even more accurate and comprehensive with the continuing implementation of EHR systems and the development of the national Health Information Exchange (HIE).

EHRS

The existence of interoperable electronic health information requires the effective implementation of an EHR system in all health-care settings. The U.S. Department of Health and Human Services notes:

> Public health entities require interoperable electronic health information to detect, track, and manage illness outbreaks. Improved and coordinated access to information from inside and outside the formal delivery system among public health entities and home- and community-based supports increases their ability to analyze population health trends, identify at-risk populations, address local social and health determinants, pursue proactive illness prevention and health promotion strategies, and promote healthy choices for all populations and diverse communities. (U.S. Department of Health and Human Services Office of the National Coordinator for Health Information Technology (ONC), n.d., p. 21)

The concept of maintaining individual health-related data within automated systems started to evolve within the health-care professions in the 1960s. As health information systems were introduced in hospitals in the 1970s, providers and administrators began to consider the benefits of electronic patient records. In 1991, IOM issued a report titled *Computer-Based Patient Record* (CBPR) calling for the development of and providing a framework for an EHR; (Dick, Steen, & Detmer, 1997) however, the document used the term *patient record*. It is important to note the title focused on the patient and did not use the term *medical record*. Since then, other terms commonly used, often interchangeably, have included *electronic medical record (EMR)* and *electronic health record (EHR)*. However, these terms have very different meanings. Consensus on their definitions did not begin to develop until 2009 with the passage of the Health Information Technology for Economic and Clinical Health (HITECH) Act. The correct terminology and definition from the Office of the National Coordinator (ONC) for Health Information Technology and accepted by most health-care professionals are included in Table 13-7.

While a few large academic medical centers experimented with EHRs, the IOM report had no real impact on EHR development due to a number of financial, technical, and social-cultural factors. Except for billing, most of the health-care systems continued to function in a paper-based world (Collen, 1995).

Slow but steady progress began to change on April 27, 2004, when President George W. Bush addressed the topic in his State of the Union address: "... an electronic health record for every American by the year 2014 ... by computerizing health records, we can avoid dangerous medical mistakes, reduce costs and improve care" (Bush,

Table 13-7 Definitions: EMR, EHR, and PHR

Name	Definition	Key Characteristics
Electronic medical record (EMR)	An EMR is a digital version of the historical paper chart maintained in a clinician's office. It contains the medical data and treatment history of a patient, and it is used by clinicians mainly for diagnosis and treatment.	An EMR is more beneficial than a paper chart because using it makes it easier for providers to track data over time. It also provides alerts for scheduling preventive care and treatment follow-up visits, and monitors progress against parameters, such as vaccinations and blood pressure readings. However, the information stored in EMRs is not easily shared with providers outside a practice. It can also be difficult to import data from outside the practice.
Electronic health record (EHR)	An EHR is more comprehensive that an EMR because it focuses on the total health of the patient. It goes beyond the standard clinical data collected in a single provider's office because it can import data to and from a variety of other health-care settings such as hospitals, clinics, nursing homes, and so on. It may also include patient-generated data provided directly by patients.	An EHR is not limited to one setting or provider; rather, it contains data provided by all clinicians involved in a patient's care. EHRs also share information with other health-care providers, such as laboratories and specialists. The interpretational functionality of an EHR depends on a national consensus on technology and terminology standards. All health-care institutions involved in the patient's care are responsible for ensuring the privacy and confidentiality of the data.
Personal health record (PHR)	A PHR can contain much of the same information as an EHR—diagnoses, medications, immunizations, family medical histories, and provider contact information—but they are set up, accessed, and managed by the patient or the responsible caregiver. A PHR can also contain patient-generated data as well as health-care goals and plans for reaching these goals.	The key characteristic of a PHR is that the patient maintains control. As a result, the patient controls who has access to these data. Because the patient is the one consistent factor throughout the life span, a PHR has the potential to be more comprehensive, accurate and current.

Sources: USDHHS: Office of the National Coordinator for Health Information Technology, 2016, and U.S. Department of Health and Human Services, 2015c.

2004). President Bush followed the announcement with an executive order creating the ONC for Health Information Technology under the U.S. Department of Health and Human Services.

However, a significant change in the rate of implementation of EHRs did not begin until the ONC was legislatively mandated in the HITECH Act of 2009 under President Obama. The HITECH Act (1) financially incentivized health providers to adopt EHRs, (2) achieved meaningful use (MU) of these EHRs, and (3) supported the exchange of health information. The concept of MU rested on the five pillars of health outcomes policy priorities:

- Improve quality, safety, and efficiency, and reduce health disparities.
- Engage patients and families in their health.
- Improve care coordination.
- Improve population and public health.
- Ensure adequate privacy and security protection for personal health information (CDC, 2017).

Each of these pillars plays a major role in using health information technology to support health promotion and well-being. The framework for achieving these goals and the approaches for achieving them are illustrated in Figure 13-4.

In implementing the HITECH Act, the federal government determined that improving health-care delivery required changes in providers' behavior and methods of practice. The MU program, administrated through the Centers for Medicare & Medicaid Services (CMS) in cooperation with the ONC, provides monetary incentives for eligible providers (EPs) and eligible entities

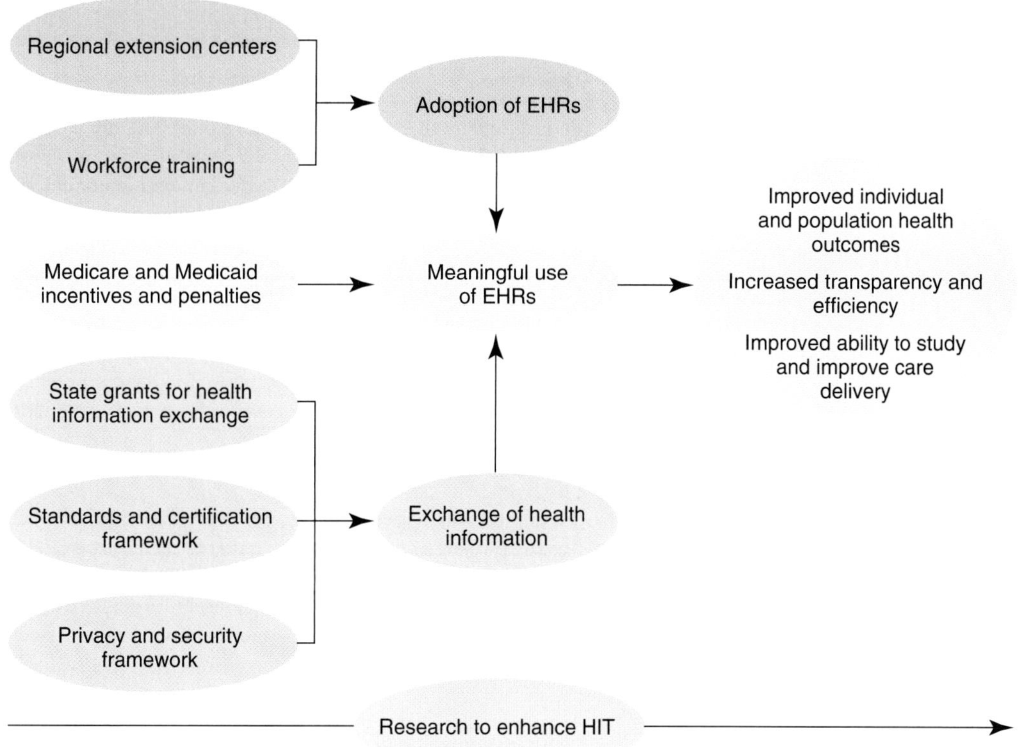

FIGURE 13–4 The HITECH Act's Framework for MU of EHRs. *Source: Blumenthal, 2010.*

(EEs) who effectively use EHRs in providing patient care. The HITECH Act defines an EP as a doctor of medicine or osteopathy legally authorized to practice medicine and surgery, a doctor of dental surgery, a doctor of podiatric medicine, a doctor of optometry, or a chiropractor. EEs include all licensed hospitals that are reimbursed based on the prospective payment system and all critical access hospitals (CAHs). To obtain the Medicare payments, the EP or entity is required to meet MU criteria for certified EHRs (Madison, 2018). The MU program was implemented in three stages, with the EP or EE required to demonstrate specific measurable criteria based on nine MU objectives to receive the monetary incentives.

Table 13-8 describes the focus of each stage and provides a sample objective and measurable criteria. The dates on the table overlap. EPs and EEs can start on different dates and move through the stages at different rates. Some adjustments have been made to the MU objectives with each stage, and additional modifications can be expected. Key objectives are described below.

The stage 3 MU objectives include the following:

1. Protection of patient health information
2. Clinical decision support
3. Computerized provider order entry (CPOE)
4. Electronic prescribing
5. Health Information Exchange (HIE)
6. Patient-specific education
7. Medication reconciliation
8. Patient electronic access to health information
9. Public health reporting (CDC, 2017)

Objective 9 is of special interest to disease prevention and health promotion. It has four measures:

- Measure 1—Immunization Registry Reporting: The eligible hospital or CAH is in active engagement with a public health agency to submit immunization data.
- Measure 2—Syndromic Surveillance Reporting: The eligible hospital or CAH is in active engagement with a public health agency to submit syndromic surveillance data.
- Measure 3—Specialized Registry Reporting: The eligible hospital or CAH is in active engagement to submit data to a specialized registry.
- Measure 4—Electronic Reportable Laboratory Result Reporting (ELR): The eligible hospital or CAH is in active engagement with a public health agency to submit ELR results. (CDC, 2017)

Table 13-8 Example of Criteria for each MU Stage*

Stage	Focus	Objective	Criteria
Stage 1, 2011–2018	Electronically capturing health information in a standardized format.	Send reminders to patients per patient preference for preventive and follow-up care.	More than 20% of all unique patients 65 years or older or 5 years old or younger were sent an appropriate reminder during the EHR reporting period.
Stage 2, 2014–2020	More rigorous health information exchange (HIE).	Use clinically relevant information to identify patients who should receive reminders for preventive and follow-up care and send these patients the reminders, per patient preference.	More than 10% of all unique patients who have had 2 or more office visits with the EP within the 24 months before the beginning of the EHR reporting period were sent a reminder, per patient preference, when available.
Stage 3, 2017–2021	Improving quality, safety, and efficiency, leading to improved health outcomes.	The EP provides patients (or the patient-authorized representative) with timely electronic access to their health information and patient-specific education.	For more than 80% of all unique patients seen by the EP, (1) the patient (or the patient-authorized representative) is provided timely access to view online, download, and transmit his or her health information, and (2) the provider ensures that the patient's health information is available for the patient (or patient-authorized representative) to access using any application of their choice that is configured to meet the technical specifications of the application programming interface (API) in the provider's certified EHR.

* For updated information, check the Web site at https://www.cms.gov/Regulations-and-Guidance/Legislation/EHRIncentivePrograms/index.html

The HITECH Act has had a major impact on the rate of automation within health care. In 2008, fewer than 14% of non-federal acute care hospitals were using at least a basic EHR. By 2015, 96% of these hospitals possessed a certified EHR technology (Henry, Searcy, & Patel, 2016). As of 2015, nearly 9 in 10 of office-based physicians had also adopted at least a basic EHR.

Stage 3, the final phase for the MU incentive program, is in the process of being replaced by the Medicare Access and Children's Health Insurance Program Reauthorization Act (MACRA) of 2015. MACRA, which passed with strong bipartisan support in both the House of Representatives and the Senate, was signed into law on April 16, 2015, by President Obama. The legislation includes the Quality Payment Program, thus making significant changes in how Medicare pays health-care providers. (Quality Payment Program Service Center, n.d.). In contrast to the HITECH Act, in this legislation a health-care provider is defined as a physician, physician assistant, nurse practitioner, clinical nurse specialist, or certified registered nurse anesthetist. The legislation provides meaningful support for and progress toward paying health-care providers for value or the quality of the care provided and not for the volume of care provided (Madison, 2018). To achieve this goal, the program offers two options for health-care provider payment (CMS, 2016):

- The Merit-based Incentive Payment System (MIPS): MIPS replaces three Medicare reporting programs: (1) Meaningful Use of a Certified EHR, (2) the Physician Quality Reporting System, and (3) the Value-Based Payment Modifier with a single payment system. The single program contains four performance categories: quality, advancing care information, improvement activities, and cost. A health-care provider's performance in these four categories determines his or her performance score and payment rate for the care he or she has provided. The reporting requirements for each of these four areas change year to year as health-care providers are provided with a flexible process for changing their practice. It is anticipated that more than 90% of health-care providers will select this option.

- Alternative payment models (APMs): APMs offer incentives to clinicians who provide high-quality and cost-efficient care to specific patient groups. APMs can apply to a specific clinical condition, a care episode, or a population. Examples include the oncology care model (OCM) or next generation accountable care organization (ACO) Model. A variation of this option is the advanced APM, in which the health-care practitioner can earn more for taking on some of the financial risk related to patient outcomes (American Academy of Family Physicians, 2016).

  For example, a neurologist who is part of an advanced APM might agree to a set payment for the initial treatment for a patient with a new diagnosis of epilepsy. Payments for this phase of the patient care would cover initiation of a treatment protocol, all office visits and communication, and care management for a patient for six months. Established criteria would measure the quality of care provided. If the actual cost of providing this treatment is more than the agreed payment amount, the neurologist is forced to provide the care at a loss. On the other hand, if the neurologist can provide the care at a lower cost, she or he can realize a financial gain (American Academy of Neurology, 2018).

With each of these approaches, the practice must be prepared to analyze population data as it transitions from quantity-based care provided to individuals to quality-based care provided to patient populations. The foundational requirement for capturing, aggregating, and analyzing these data are the MU of a certified EHR. Also required are health-care consumers who are equipped, enabled, empowered, and engaged in decisions about their health and health care (Okun & Caligan, 2018).

CONSUMER INFORMATICS AND THE E-PATIENT

Over the last several decades, the role of patient has evolved from a passive recipient of health care to an informed, empowered and engaged consumer, often referred to as an e-patient. New online communication technologies have increased opportunities for individuals to function as cohesive groups and provided increased access to information and knowledge. At the same time, several parallel, interrelated driving forces within health-care delivery and society have encouraged the emergence of today's engaged e-patient: efforts to control and shift health-care costs, the ever-increasing expectation of health-care consumers, and the emergence of powerful health-focused technology companies (Nelson, 2017, June 26). Arising from these events has been the establishment of consumer informatics as a new specialty within health-care informatics (Nelson, 2016; Nelson & Joos, 2012).

The interrelated concepts of consumer/patient engagement and the specialty of consumer informatics include a wide range of subtopics with the common theme of patients and/or consumers playing an active role in decisions related to their health care. For the purposes of this book, we will limit the discussion of consumer informatics and the e-patient to health promotion and disease prevention. The terms used in discussing these topics often have multiple and sometimes overlapping meanings. Table 13-9 provides sources and definitions for common terminology.

Consumer/Patient Engagement

Patient engagement has been defined as the actions an individual takes to obtain the greatest possible benefit from available health-care services. Engagement requires the patient to synthesize robust information and professional advice with his or her own needs, preferences, and abilities to promote health by preventing, managing, and curing disease (Center for Advancing Health, 2010). In this chapter, we are limiting the discussion mainly to patient engagement with the health-care system for the purposes of health promotion and disease prevention. However, patients are also engaging with others besides health-care providers via social media. Awareness is growing among patients and providers that social media–based peer networks of patients such as PatientsLikeMe and Caring Bridge provide valuable information and support for patients with a new or existing disease (Volpp & Mohta, 2017). Thirty percent of adults report they are likely to share information about their health on social media sites with others (ReferralMD, 2018).

Table 13-10 includes guidelines from several professional nursing associations for the professional use of social media in general. Box 13-4 includes tips for professional communication with patients on social media sites. The professional literature discussing consumer/patient engagement and the health-care system can be divided into three areas of focus, which we discuss in the following subsections.

Table 13-9 Key Terms Related to Consumer Informatics and the E-Patient

Term	Definition	Source
Activated patients	Patients who believe they have important roles to play in self-managing care, collaborating with providers, and maintaining their health. Such patients know how to manage their condition, maintain functioning, and prevent health declines; and they have the skills and behavioral repertoire to manage their condition, collaborate with their health providers, and maintain their health functioning as well as access appropriate and high-quality care.	Hibbard, J. H., Stockard, J., Mahoney, E. R., & Tusler, M. (2004). Development of the Patient Activation Measure (PAM): Conceptualizing and measuring activation in patients and consumers. *Health Services Research, 39*(4), 1005–1026.
Consumer-driven health-care plan (CDHP)	A three-tier, health-care payment system consisting of a savings account, out-of-pocket payments, and an insurance plan. The first tier is a pretax account that allows employees to pay for services using pretax dollars. The funds from this account can be used to satisfy the insurance plan deductible. The second tier is the difference, or the coverage gap, between the amount of money in the individual's pretax account and the deductible. The amount that is not covered by the pretax account must be covered by the insured. If health-care expenses exceed the deductible amount, then the third tier, the high-deductible health insurance plan, kicks in.	Yi, Song G. (2010). Consumer-driven health care: What is it, and what does it mean for employees and employers? Washington, DC: U.S. Bureau of Labor Statistics. Retrieved from https://www.bls.gov/opub/mlr/cwc/consumer-driven-health-care-what-is-it-and-what-does-it-mean-for-employees-and-employers.pdf
Digital health	Includes categories such as mobile health (m-health), health information technology (IT), wearable devices, telehealth and telemedicine, and personalized medicine.	U.S. Food and Drug Administration. (2017, January 5). Digital health. Retrieved from https://www.fda.gov/medicaldevices/digitalhealth/
E-health	An emerging field at the intersection of medical informatics, public health, and business. The term refers to health services and information delivered or enhanced through the internet and related technologies. In a broader sense, the term characterizes not only a technical development but also a state of mind; a way of thinking; an attitude; and a commitment for networked, global thinking to improve health care locally, regionally, and worldwide by using information and communication technology.	Eysenbach, G. (2001). What is e-health? *Journal of Medical Internet Research, 3*(2), e20. http://doi.org/10.2196/jmir.3.2.e20. Retrieved from https://www.ncbi.nlm.nih.gov/pmc/articles/PMC1761894/
M-health (also called connected health)	The use of mobile and wireless devices to improve health outcomes, health-care services and health research. Also, mMedical and public health practice supported by mobile devices, such as mobile phones, patient monitoring devices, personal digital assistants (PDAs), and other wireless devices. M-health is a component of e-health.	World Health Organization. (2011). M-health: New horizons for health through mobile technologies. Geneva, Switzerland: World Health Organization. Retrieved from http://www.who.int/goe/publications/goe_mhealth_web.pdf
Patient engagement	The process of taking action to obtain the greatest benefit from the health-care services available to an individual. Using this process, a person harmonizes robust information and professional advice with his or her own needs, preferences, and abilities in order to prevent, manage and cure disease.	Center for Advancing Health. (2010). A new definition of patient engagement: What is engagement and why is it important? Retrieved from http://www.cfah.org/pdfs/CFAH_Engagement_Behavior_Framework_current.pdf

Table 13-9 Key Terms Related to Consumer Informatics and the E-Patient—cont'd

Term	Definition	Source
Patient-generated health data	Patient-generated health data (PGHD) are health-related data created, recorded, or gathered by or from patients (or family members or other caregivers) to help address a health concern. Examples of PGHD include health history, treatment history, biometric data, symptoms, and lifestyle choices. PGHD are distinct from data generated in clinical settings and through encounters with providers in two important ways: 1. Patients, not providers, are primarily responsible for capturing or recording these data. 2. Patients decide how to share or distribute these data to health-care providers and others.	USDHHS ONC. (2017, April 5). Consumer ehealth: Patient-generated health data Retrieved from https://www.healthit.gov/policy-researchers-implementers/patient-generated-health-data
Patient portal	A secure Web site where patients can access their medical history and often certain information from their EHR. Using patient portals, patients can typically complete forms online, communicate with providers, request prescription refills, pay bills, review lab results, and schedule appointments.	The Patient Engagement Playbook. https://www.healthit.gov/playbook/pe/introduction/
Telehealth	The use of electronic information and telecommunications technologies to support and promote long-distance clinical health care, patient and professional health-related education, public health and health administration. Technologies include videoconferencing, the internet, store-and-forward imaging, streaming media, and terrestrial and wireless communications.	U.S. Health Recourses and Services Administration. (2015). Telehealth programs. Retrieved from https://www.hrsa.gov/rural-health/telehealth/index.html

Table 13-10 Professional Nursing Associations and Social Media Guidelines

Association or Publication	Document Title	URL
American Nurses Association (ANA)	ANA's Principles for social networking and the nurse	https://www.nursingworld.org/~4af4f2/globalassets/docs/ana/ethics/social-networking.pdf
Spector, N., & Kappel, D., Online Journal of Issues in Nursing	Guidelines for using electronic and social media: The regulatory perspective.	http://ojin.nursingworld.org/MainMenuCategories/ANAMarketplace/ANAPeriodicals/OJIN/TableofContents/Vol-17-2012/No3-Sept-2012/Guidelines-for-Electronic-and-Social-Media.html
Registered Nurses' Association of Ontario	Social media guidelines for nurses	http://rnao.ca/news/socialmediaguideline
Nursing and Midwifery Council (NMC)	Social networking site guidance	http://www.nmc-uk.org/Nurses-and-midwives/Advice-by-topic/A/Advice/Social-networking-sites/
Nurse.org	Must-read social media advice for nurses	https://nurse.org/articles/nurses-social-media/

BOX 13-4 Communication Tips for Social Media

1. When creating an account on a social media site take the time to review the Terms and Conditions as well as the Privacy Statements documents. These documents are actually formal contracts. If you click "I accept this," it is the same as signing a formal contract.
2. Begin exploring a new social media site by checking the Help section. Before you actually start to use the site, be sure you understand how to configure your settings—especially the privacy-related settings for your site. After you have used the site and are comfortable with how the site actually operates, review the privacy settings again. At this point, you will have a better understanding of these settings and can configure them more effectively.
3. Be honest but do not be exposed. Do not set up false accounts. It can be illegal to set up a false identity on a social media site. This is because sexual predators and other scammers like to use false identities. However, one should refuse to use a site if you must publicly post personally identifiable information such as your birthday, gender, address or phone number. Set up a free e-mail account that does not include your name as your user name or other identifying information to use on social media sites.
4. Remember that *everything* posted on the internet is public and permanent. Marking something private does not guarantee it will remain private. For example, both Facebook and Google have paid substantial fines to the Federal Trade Commission (FTC) for failure to maintain the privacy of data they had promised to protect.

   The FTC has accepted as final a settlement with Facebook resolving charges that Facebook deceived consumers by telling them they could keep their information on Facebook private, and then repeatedly allowing it to be shared and made public. (FTC, 2012a)

   Google Inc. has agreed to pay a record $22.5 million civil penalty to settle Federal Trade Commission charges that it misrepresented to users of Apple Inc.'s Safari Internet browser that it would not place tracking "cookies" or serve targeted ads to those users, violating an earlier privacy settlement between the company and the FTC (FTC, 2012b)

5. Social media accounts can be established for social as well as professional reasons. Maintain your professional identity by not mixing business and pleasure. When you establish an account, think carefully about the following questions: Why do I have this account? Who do I hope to interact with on this social media site? You may have a social media account for interacting with patients and consumers such as an online support group. You may have another account in a different social media setting for interacting with professional colleagues. You may establish a third site for interacting with friends and family.
6. Remember that, when you collaborate on professional sites, you don't have to like the people to work with them. As in your face-to-face professional life, it is important to manage personal conflict so that avoidable conflict does not get in the way of the progress of the group. If you start to feel that conflict is developing, try to ask nonthreatening questions that help to explore an issue rather than be confrontational in stating your position.
7. Successful social media collaboration depends on the full participation of group members. Social media collaboration relies on multiple ideas and perspectives. While you work to understand the views of others, do not hold back from putting forward your view with tact and a clear rationale.
8. Always consider online coursework related to group projects and collaboration as part of your professional life. Relationships established with classmates, faculty members, staff members, and administrators can become an important part of your professional network throughout your career.
9. Learn how to say goodbye when leaving a social media site. Social media sites and social media are rarely lifelong commitments. If you have not used a specific social media site for some time, you should consider making the account inactive or canceling the account. Over time, social media sites can include a collection of contacts you are no longer involved with, or you may need to reorganize who are your professional contacts and who are your personal contacts. A short note explaining, for example, that you are limiting your Facebook page to mainly family and very close friends but would like to keep in touch with professional colleagues via LinkedIn can be more effective than just disappearing. A short note explaining to an online support group that you have another work assignment and will no longer be part of the group is much more professional than just disappearing.

Source: Federal Trade Commission (FTC) (2012a). Press Release: FTC Approves Final Settlement With Facebook. Retrieved from http://www.ftc.gov/opa/2012/08/facebook.shtm. Federal Trade Commission (FTC) (2012b) Press Release: Google Will Pay $22.5 Million to Settle FTC Charges It Misrepresented Privacy Assurances to Users of Apple's Safari Internet Browser. Retrieved from http://ftc.gov/opa/2012/08/google.shtm.

Patient Engagement Research

A large and growing body of research focuses on patient engagement, with an emphasis on the term *patient*. Within this literature, the patient is characterized as a person with a health problem for which he or she is most likely seeking treatment and support from the health-care delivery system. For example, the focus may be on engaging patients in the active management of a chronic disease such as diabetes or making decisions about which medically acceptable treatment option is most appropriate for their personal situation.

Giving patients both access to their health information and electronic tools for using that information can better position them to participate more fully in their care: to self-manage their conditions, coordinate care across multiple providers, and improve communication with their care teams—those directly involved in their care (Ricciardi, Mostashari, Murphy, Daniel, & Siminerio, 2013).

Many studies discuss the benefits of patient engagement and methods or approaches to encourage active engagement effectively. Informatics tools are invaluable for analyzing patient engagement data and delivering effective interventions. For example, a Web-based shared decision guide can be very helpful for a breast cancer patient who must decide between having a mastectomy and a lumpectomy. Data on how this tool is used in real-life situations can provide feedback for improving its effectiveness.

Consumer Engagement Research

The second area of focus within the health-care literature deals with the patient as a health-care consumer, including the purchase of health insurance or the direct purchase of health-care services. In 2015, 90.9% of the U.S. population had health insurance for at least part of the year. Most were covered by private health insurance (67.2%), with the remainder (37.1%) covered by public programs such as Medicare (Barnett & Vornovitsky, 2016). In 2015, the EBRI/Greenwald & Associates Consumer Engagement in Health Care Survey (CEHCS) reported that:

- Thirteen percent of the privately insured individuals were enrolled in a consumer-driven health plan (CDHP).
- Eleven percent were enrolled in a high-deductible health plan (HDHP).
- Seventy-six percent were enrolled in more traditional coverage (Fronstin & Elmlinger, 2015).

Definitions for these different types of insurance plans are provided in Box 13-5.

The availability of insurance options appears to have a positive influence on the level of consumer engagement in health promotion:

- CDHP enrollees were more likely than traditional plan enrollees to report that they had the option to participate in a variety of wellness programs.

BOX 13-5 Common Health Insurance Plans, with Definitions

NAME	DESCRIPTION
Consumer-driven health plans (CDHPs)	Combine a high-deductible health policy that provides protection from catastrophic medical expenses with a tax-favored account that pays routine health-care expenses such as those for prescription medications and doctors' visits.
High-deductible health plans (HDHPs)	Usually feature a higher deductible and lower insurance premiums than those of traditional health plans. The plans include catastrophic coverage to protect against large medical expenses, but the insured is responsible for routine out-of-pocket expenses up until she or he meets the plan deductible.
Traditional plans	Provide a specific package of health benefits in return for a set premium paid to private insurance carrier. Participants may: • choose any provider, • be limited to providers within an established network such as an exclusive provider organization (EPO) or • receive services outside the network but generally at higher costs in an arrangement called a preferred provider organization (PPO)

Source: U.S. Department of Labor: Bureau of Labor Statistics, Office of Compensation and Working Conditions, 2016.

- CDHP enrollees were more likely than traditional plan enrollees to participate in health-risk assessments and biometric screenings (Fronstin & Elmlinger, 2015).

However, it is still unclear how CDHP will affect consumer engagement in health promotion. Studies indicate some reduction in the use of medical services, but the impact that these reductions will have on long-term health outcomes and total medical spending is unclear (Health Policy Commission of Massachusetts, 2013).

The role and impact of CDHP programs on the behavior of intermediaries and provider organizations is currently not well understood (Health Policy Commission of Massachusetts, 2013). For example, health promotion activities often involve a long-term commitment. When a person changes jobs, he or she typically also changes insurance policies. As a result, insurance companies may be reluctant to provide health promotion and preventive services for customers in group employer plans because the coverage provided may be for a limited period. In the future, the data mining of comprehensive longitudinal EHRs may help us understand how different approaches to financing health-care services can influence consumer engagement in health promotion and disease prevention.

Engaging customers who pay directly for services requires providing patients a clear, understandable cost and quality comparison. To make informed health-care decisions, consumers need data on prices and quality of health-care services displayed in a clear and meaningful way. Providing this information can be an effective strategy for encouraging consumers within traditional health insurance benefit plans to seek care from more efficient providers (America's Health Insurance Plans: Center for Policy and Research, 2015). Research has shown that, when the cost and quality information is reported side by side in an easy-to-understand format, consumers made high-value choices. However, this type of information can be very difficult to obtain. (Hibbard, Greene, Sofaer, Firminger, & Hirsh, 2012).

Not only is this information difficult to obtain, but also the information that is available to patients and providers alike reflects costs in a fee-for-service, disease-focused health-care system. For example, the cost of treating a specific condition such as knee joint replacement as well as the quality of the treatment provided by different providers can be analyzed using fee-for-service data. An example of this type of analysis can be seen on a Web site established by ProPublica. Using Medicare data, ProPublica adjusted for differences in patient health, age, and hospital quality and then calculated death and complication rates for individual surgeons performing one of eight elective procedures (ProPublica, 2015). Currently, it is impossible to determine the cost of health promotion activities that could have prevented the need for these surgeries. We hope that, in the future, this type of health promotion information will be made available by (1) collecting data from EHRs that are aggregated via a national wide information system and (2) applying techniques for doing predictive analytics based on big data.

Health Promotion Research

In many ways, literature concerning the use of informatics tools for engaging patients and consumers in health promotion is just beginning to emerge. Table 13-11 shows data from a screen clip of a literature search on Medline. All articles in Medline are indexed using MESH as the standard language or subject term. *Consumer engagement* and *patient engagement* are not subject terms and are not used to index articles in the MESH classification system. However, any term that is used in the title and/or abstract is considered a key term. The first two searches in Table 13-11 were done

Table 13-11 Medline Literature Search Articles Discussing Informatics, Health Promotion, and Patient/Consumer Engagement

☐	#▲	Searches	Results
☐	1	consumer engagement.mp	84
☐	2	patient engagement.mp	827
☐	3	Public Health Informatics/ or Informatics/ or Medical Informatics Computing/ or Dental Informatics/ or Medical Informatics Applications/ or informatics.mp or Medical Informatics/ or Nursing Informatics	20746
☐	4	health promotion.mp or Health Promotion/	73665
☐	5	1 or 2	902
☐	6	3 and 4 and 5	0

Source: Medlineplus.gov

as key term searches. Searches 3 and 4 are subject term searches. Search 5 combines into one database all the articles from searches 1 and 2. As can be seen in search 6, none of the articles in the Medline database that are indexed on the MESH terms *informatics* and *health promotion* include the terms *patient engagement* and *consumer engagement* in their title or abstract.

M-HEALTH

Although current research is limited, smartphone apps and activity trackers for the purposes of health promotion are a rapidly growing sector of health care. A survey conducted by InCroud, a Boston-based mobile technology company, found that 95% of nurses who responded to the survey owned a smartphone, and 88% of them used their smartphone apps in daily nursing work. Bedside access to drug interactions data dominated nurses' smartphone use, with 73% looking up drug information on that device. Some 72% used smartphone apps to look up diseases and disorders (Leventhal, 2015). This would suggest that most nurses are somewhat experienced in using m-health apps, but they are not yet using these apps to engage with patients for health promotion and disease prevention. While there is growing interest in using chronic disease management apps to engage patients in actively managing their health problems, the majority of available m-health apps are concentrated in the areas of wellness, diet, and exercise, as demonstrated in Figure 13-5.

Mobile apps can "help people manage their own health and wellness, promote healthy living, and gain access to useful information when and where they need it" (U.S. Food and Drug Administration, 2015). Examples of these potential and actual benefits include:

- There is immediate feedback on the impact of exercises and other activities.
- A longitudinal record of key data points, such as pulse rate, can be tracked and shared with others, including health-care providers.
- Data collected with m-health apps can be combined with other data to provide a more comprehensive picture of overall fitness. For example, dietary data can be combined with activity data to give a more comprehensive picture of total calories consumed and utilized.
- Well-designed feedback screen can guide an individual in modifying fitness-related activities.

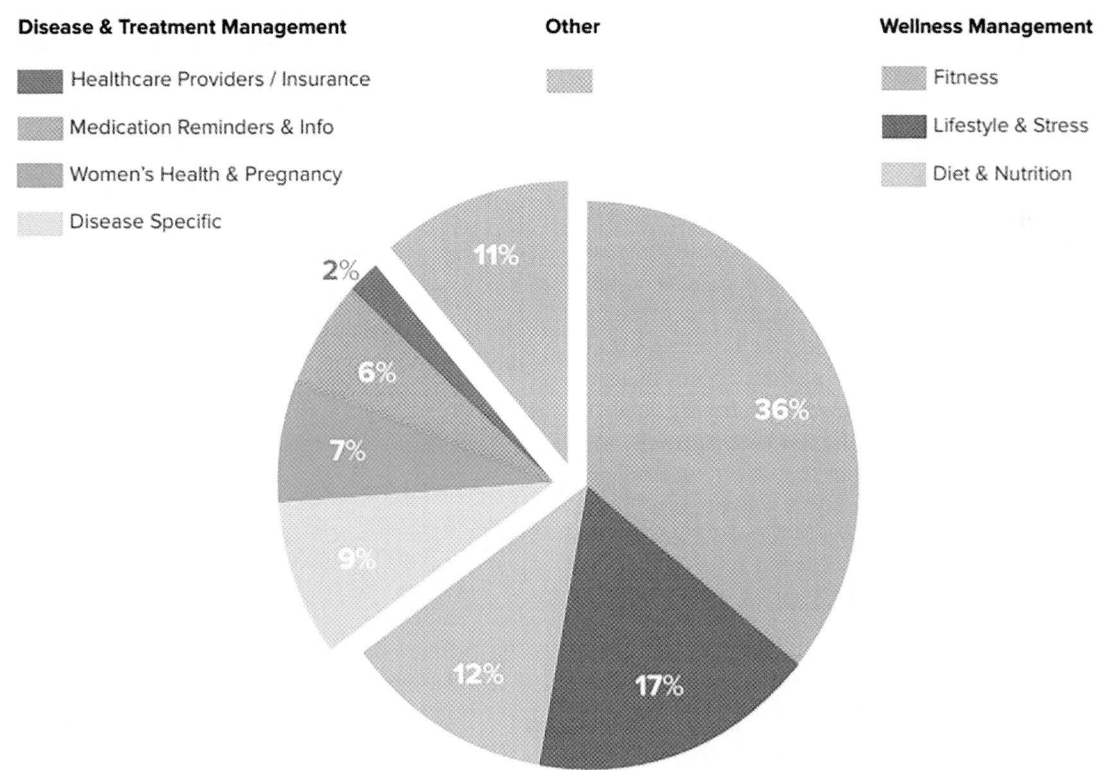

FIGURE 13–5 Classification of M-Health Apps. *Source: The IQVIA Institute for Human Data Science. Used with permission.*

A major challenge of using m-health apps, either to support the care process in an acute setting or to engage patients in health promotion, is the reality that these apps vary greatly in quality. Most m-health apps are created and sold with little to no research or regulation. This issue was noted by the American Medical Association (AMA) in their statement of *Principles to Promote Safe, Effective mHealth Applications*: "Mobile health apps and associated digital health devices, trackers and sensors can vary greatly in functionality, accuracy, safety and effectiveness" (AMA, 2016).

In the United States, very few m-health apps are regulated by the Food and Drug Administration (FDA) as medical devices and therefore most are not required to meet FDA standards. "The FDA is taking a tailored, risk-based approach that focuses on the small subset of mobile apps that meet the regulatory definition of 'device' and that: (1) are intended to be used as an accessory to a regulated medical device, or (2) transform a mobile platform into a regulated medical device" (U.S. Food and Drug Administration, 2015). As can be anticipated from this definition, apps that focus on health promotion and disease prevention are not likely to be regulated. Additional information and examples of m-health apps that are and are not regulated can be found at https://www.fda.gov/MedicalDevices/DigitalHealth/default.htm.

Paul Wicks and Emil Chiauzzi, (2015), in an article aptly titled *Trust but Verify: Five Approaches to Ensure Safe Medical Apps*, discussed several examples of current apps to demonstrate that this is an international problem. Using their five approaches as a starting point, they offer the following suggestions:

1. Educate consumers (and health professionals) on how to make good decisions when selecting and using m-health apps.
2. Identify and share potential harms and problems associated with specific apps in a public online forum.
3. Establish a nonprofit independent agency charged with establishing standards and certifying achievement of these standards by individual apps.
4. Require companies that manufacture and sell m-health apps to demonstrate a process of active medical review before releasing products on the open market.
5. Require FDA approval of all m-health related apps.

Finally, it is important to note that m-health apps are creating a two-way street between EHRs and personal health records (PHRs). Historically the goal was to download data from a variety of EHRs and EMRs to PHRs. With the advent of m-health apps, patients are requesting to upload data into the EHR. For example, a patient being treated for obesity may want to upload information on calories consumed and tracking data related to activity level. The introduction of patient-generated health data (PGHD) into the EHR creates a whole new set of opportunities and challenges for health professionals and institutions.

PHRS

The primary difference between a PHR and an EHR is that the patient owns and controls the PHR, while the EHR is owned by the health-care provider or institution. Patients have a legal right to access most EHR data even though the system itself is purchased and managed by the provider. Most health-care providers establish a procedure through which patients can access data maintained in select sections of the EHR. One of the most common methods is the use of a patient portal. Patient portals often provide secure messaging with health-care providers, medication refills, and appointment scheduling along with limited access to the EHR that can serve as a tethered PHR. Automatic data entry from the EHR is a major advantage for patients. The main disadvantage is that the tethered PHR is linked only to one specific health-care provider or health-care system. In addition, while these systems may include the ability to enter a health history or other questionnaire, a patient's opportunity to enter his or her own data is often highly controlled.

Untethered PHRs may be installed and maintained on the person's personal computer or electronic device, or they may exist as a Web-based system separate from the EHR. The main advantage is that the patient has complete control over the record and can enter data from all providers. However, with the current status of electronic health data, this responsibility can become a major disadvantage because the person is responsible for accessing and transferring all data from her or his various providers' system to the untethered PHRs. Each report, lab result, or other data must be individually transferred, and often there is not an easy interface for this purpose.

Although it doesn't yet exist, the ideal PHR would be a comprehensive networked system that could download and integrate data from multiple sources, including primary and specialty health-care providers, health plans, laboratories, and m-health apps. Users could sign in once and gain access to comprehensive, integrated data. As with EHRs, the development of comprehensive, integrated PHRs depends on the wide implementation

FIGURE 13–6 The Blue Button. *Source: https://www.healthit.gov/patients-families/blue-button/about-blue-button*

of data representation and data exchange standards to create interoperable records (Gibson & Charters, 2018). The ideal PHR would also include artificial intelligence (AI) features, such as customized guidance and alerts that would enable patients to manage their health problems proactively and seek optimal wellness.

The Blue Button initiative, which originated at the Veterans Administration, is the beginning of such a system. The Blue Button (Figure 13-6) is a standard symbol on a patient portal that a patient can click to download his or her own EHR securely. Via the Blue Button Pledge Program, more than 450 organizations are providing Americans with access to their personal health data. The ONC maintains a Web site (https://www.healthit.gov/topic/health-it-initiatives/blue-button) that provides a search function to determine if your health-care provider or service participates in the program (U.S. Department of Health and Human Services, 2015b).

In conclusion, health promotion and disease prevention programs focus on keeping individuals, families, and communities and other groups healthy in each of their human dimensions: physical, social, intellectual, occupational emotional, environmental, and spiritual. WHO defines health promotion as "the process of enabling people to increase control over, and to improve, their health. It moves beyond a focus on individual behavior towards a wide range of social and environmental interventions" (WHO, n.d.)

Certainly, it takes a village to strive for health promotion and disease prevention programs that empower societies to achieve this vision. But the work of achieving such a vision cannot even be conceived of without the health information technology, tools, and processes utilized in health informatics. Nursing is just beginning to use these health informatics concepts and tools to achieve this vision. As health-care providers and patients, consumers, and clients, (including individuals, facilities, and groups) become a village working together to achieve the vision of health promotion and disease prevention, the tools underlying this work will be based in the discipline of health informatics.

KEY POINTS

- The discipline of health informatics is focused on the use of health information technology to create a society in which all people live long, healthy lives.
- Health informatics is both an interdisciplinary professional area of specialization and a scientific discipline that integrates the health sciences, computer science, information science, and other analytic sciences with the goal of managing and communicating data, information, knowledge, and wisdom in the provision of health care for individuals, families, groups, and communities (Nelson & Staggers, 2018).
- Within the profession of health informatics, the scope of practice is defined by the D–W continuum and the interactions and interrelationships between the megaconcepts inherent in the model.
- Effective use of informatics tools and techniques by both health-care consumers and professionals necessitates a level of digital health literacy. Digital health literacy requires the synthesis of (1) basic literacy, (2) computer literacy, (3) information literacy, (4) digital literacy, and (5) health literacy.
- When considering health promotion and disease prevention, three factors can be used to determine the scope and organization of the resources of interest: (1) the concepts of health promotion and disease prevention, (2) the determinants of health, and (3) the concept of client.
- The U.S. Census Bureau, which counts every resident every 10 years, is the most important source of population data. The principal source of health statistics for the United States is maintained by the CDC.
- Public health entities require interoperable electronic health information systems to detect, track, and manage illness outbreaks. The existence of these interoperable electronic public health information systems requires the effective implementation of an EHR system in all health-care settings.
- Patient engagement and consumer engagement includes the actions that an individual takes to obtain the greatest possible benefit from available health-care services at the most reasonable cost. Engagement requires the patient to synthesize robust information, professional advice, and his or her own resources with his or her personal needs, preferences, and abilities to promote his or her health by preventing, managing, and curing disease.

- Full patient engagement requires untethered PHRs to download and integrate comprehensive data from multiple sources, including primary and specialty health-care providers, health plans, laboratories, and m-health apps.

Check Your Understanding

1. Synthesizing the different types of knowledge and applying that synthesis to real-life situations describes the concept of:
   A. Data collection
   B. Knowledge creation
   C. Decision making
   D. Wisdom

2. The ability to use emotional intelligence in collaborating and communicating in a digital environment with others is part of:
   A. Basic literacy
   B. Computer literacy
   C. Information literacy
   D. Digital literacy
   E. Digital health literacy

3. Which of the following statements about the organization of information resources to promote health and prevent health problems is NOT correct?
   A. Three factors that are often used to organize informational resources concerning health promotion and disease prevention are (1) the concepts of health promotion and disease prevention, (2) the determinants of health, and (3) the concept of client.
   B. Information about promoting well-being and levels of prevention is often organized around interventions such as exercise.
   C. Information about m-health applications such as devices tracking fitness is not usually organized by a specific disease but rather around an overall commitment to improving health and fitness.
   D. CDC information resources concerning programs focused on the three levels of prevention for chronic disease is usually organized by specific diseases.

4. Which of the following statements correctly clarifies the difference between the terms *determinants of health* and *social determinants of health*?
   A. The term *determinants of health* is a much more comprehensive term that encompasses all factors that could influence health.
   B. The term *social determinants of health* is a much more comprehensive term that encompasses all factors in society that could influence health.
   C. The terms *determinants of health* and *social determinants of health* have the same meaning and can therefore be used interchangeably.
   D. IOM has recommended that social determinants of health not be included in the EHR because they do not encompass specific health-related data.

5. In the United States, the primary information resource for health statistics is the:
   A. Census Bureau
   B. ONC for information technology
   C. National Library of Medicine
   D. CDC

6. Which of the following is NOT part of the criteria to determine MU as defined by the HITECH Act?
   A. Engaging patients and families
   B. Reducing health disparities
   C. Improving population and public health
   D. Reducing administrative costs for insurance companies

7. Patient engagement is best described as:
   A. The process of harmonizing robust information resources and professional advice with one's own needs, preferences, and abilities in order to prevent, manage, and cure disease
   B. The process of seeking health information from various sources and using that information for decision making about health care activities and services
   C. The process of managing health decisions based on information obtained from the internet, social media sites, activity trackers, and other information resources
   D. The process of preparing for doctor visits by doing research, collecting data points and developing a specific list of questions

8. Research has shown that, when cost and quality information is reported side by side in an easy-to-understand format:
   A. Consumers are not interested because they prefer to follow a physician's advice.
   B. Consumers are often confused by the complexity of the information.
   C. Consumers make high-value choices.
   D. Consumers do not trust the information if it comes from their insurance provider.

9. The primary difference between a PHR and an EHR is that:
   A. The patient owns and controls the PHR, while the EHR is owned by the health-care provider or institution.
   B. The PHR is more comprehensive because the patient can include patient-generated data.
   C. The PHR is easier to maintain because one does not need permission from a health-care provider to access the information.
   D. The PHR is the patient's view of her or his health-care data, whereas the EHR is the health-care provider's view of the same data.

10. The MacDorman, Declercq, Cabral, and Morton (2016) journal article discussing recent increases in the U.S. maternal mortality rate demonstrated which of the following principles related to evaluating the quality of information from different sources?
   A. U.S. government sources are the most reliable sources of health data and should be trusted more than any other data source.
   B. Because there are no generally accepted definitions of terms such as *maternal mortality rate*, health-care providers should expect to find wide variation in the rates reported by different sources.
   C. University-based researchers are the most reliable source of health data and should be trusted over any other data source.
   D. The greater the number of data sources and the more consistency that exists from different data sources, the more confidence one can have in these data.

See "Reflections on Check Your Understanding" at the end of the book for answers.

REFERENCES

American Academy of Family Physicians. (2016, November 11). *Executive summary of the MACRA final rule*. Retrieved from http://www.aafp.org/dam/AAFP/documents/advocacy/payment/medicare/ES-MACRAFinal-102416.pdf

American Academy of Neurology. (2018). *Advanced alternative payment models*. Retrieved from https://www.aan.com/tools-and-resources/practicing-neurologists-administrators/quality-payment-program/advanced-alternative-payment-models-apms/

American Medical Association. (2016, November 16). Press release. AMA adopts principles to promote safe, effective mHealth applications. Retrieved from https://www.ama-assn.org/ama-adopts-principles-promote-safe-effective-mhealth-applications

American Nurses Association. (1994). *Scope of practice for nursing informatics*. Silver Spring, MD: Nursesbooks.org.

American Nurses Association. (2008). *Nursing informatics: Scope and standards of practice*. Silver Spring, MD: Nursesbooks.org.

American Nurses Association. (2015). *Nursing informatics: Scope and standards of practice* (2nd ed.). Silver Spring, MD: Nursesbooks.org.

America's Health Insurance Plans: Center for Policy and Research. (2015). *Health plan tools empowering consumers with provider price information*. Retrieved from https://www.ahip.org/wp-content/uploads/2015/08/ConsumerTools_IssueBrief.8.24.15-2.pdf

Association of College and Research Libraries. (2016, January 11). *Framework for information literacy for higher education*. Retrieved from http://www.ala.org/acrl/sites/ala.org.acrl/files/content/issues/infolit/Framework_ILHE.pdf

The Association of Faculties of Medicine of Canada. (n.d.). Determinants of health and health inequities. In *AFMC primer on population health: A virtual textbook on public health concepts for clinicians* (Chapter 2: The public health educators' network (PHEN)). Retrieved from https://afmc.ca/AFMCPrimer.pdf?ver=1.1

Barnett, J. C., & Vornovitsky, M. S. (2016). *Health insurance coverage in the United States: 2015*. Washington, DC: U.S. Government Printing Office. Retrieved from https://www.census.gov/content/dam/Census/library/publications/2016/demo/p60-257.pdf

Bauer, U., Briss, P., Goodman, R., & Bowman BA . . . (2014). Prevention of chronic disease in the 21st century: Elimination of the leading preventable causes of premature death and disability in the USA. *Lancet, 384*(9937), 45–52. Retrieved from http://www.thelancet.com/journals/lancet/article/PIIS0140-6736(14)60648-6/fulltext

Bharmal, N., Derose, K. P., Felician, M., & Weden, M. M. (2015). *Understanding the upstream social determinants of health: A working paper*. RAND Health. Retrieved from http://www.rand.org/pubs/working_papers/WR1096.html

Blum, B. (1986). *Clinical information systems*. New York: Springer-Verlag.

Blumenthal, D. (2010, February 4). Launching HITECH. *New England Journal of Medicine, 362*(5), 382–385. Retrieved from http://www.nejm.org/doi/full/10.1056/NEJMp0912825#t=article

Bush, G. (2004, April). The 2004 State of the Union address. Retrieved from http://www.washingtonpost.com/wp-srv/politics/transcripts/bushtext_012004.html

Center for Advancing Health. (2010). A new definition of patient engagement: What is engagement and why is it important? Retrieved from http://www.cfah.org/pdfs/CFAH_Engagement_Behavior_Framework_current.pdf

Center for Medicare & Medicaid Services. (2016, October 14). The Quality Payment Program: Overview fact sheet. Retrieved from https://qpp.cms.gov/docs/Quality_Payment_Program_Overview_Fact_Sheet.pdf

CDC. (2017, June 1). *Chronic Disease Prevention and Health Promotion*. Retrieved from https://www.cdc.gov/chronicdisease/about/prevention.htm

CDC Center for Surveillance, Epidemiology, and Laboratory Services. (2017, January 18). *Meaningful Use*. Retrieved from https://www.cdc.gov/ehrmeaningfuluse/introduction.html

CDC: National Center for Health Statistics. (2019). *NCHS Information Sheet: Overview*. CDC. Retrieved from https://www.cdc.gov/nchs/data/factsheets/nchs_overview.pdf

Centers for Disease Control and Prevention. (2014, March 10). Social determinants of health: Definitions. Retrieved from http://www.cdc.gov/socialdeterminants/Definitions.html

Centers for Disease Control and Prevention. (2017, January 18). Meaningful use. Retrieved from https://www.cdc.gov/ehrmeaningfuluse/introduction.html

Centers for Disease Control and Prevention. (2019). NCHS information sheet: Overview. Retrieved from https://www.cdc.gov/nchs/data/factsheets/nchs_overview.pdf

Collen, M. F. (1995). *A history of medical informatics in the United States: 1950 to 1990*. Washington, DC: American Medical Informatics Association.

Commission on Social Determinants of Health. (2008). Closing the gap in a generation: Health equity through action on the social determinants of health. Geneva: World Health Organization. Retrieved from http://whqlibdoc.who.int/publications/2008/9789241563703_eng.pdf

Committee on Improving the Patient Record. (1991, revised edition 1997). In R. S. Dick, E. B. Steen, & D. E. Detmer (Eds.). *The computer-based patient record: An essential technology for health care*. Washington, DC: National Academy Press. Retrieved from https://www.nap.edu/catalog/18459/computer-based-patient-record-an-essential-technology-for-health-care

Committee on Information Technology Literacy: National Research Council. (1999). *Being fluent with information technology*. Washington, DC: National Academy Press. Retrieved from https://www.nap.edu/catalog/6482/being-fluent-with-information-technology

DeMilto, L., & Nakashian, M. (2016). *Using social determinants of health data to improve health care and health: A learning report*. Retrieved from http://www.rwjf.org/en/library/research/2016/04/using-social-determinants-of-health-data-to-improve-health-care-.html

Fronstin, P., & Elmlinger, A. (2015). Findings from the 2015 EBRI/Greenwald & Associates Consumer Engagement in Health Care Survey. Retrieved from https://www.ebri.org/pdf/briefspdf/EBRI_IB_421.Dec15.CEHCS.pdf

Gibson, B., & Charters, K. (2018). Personal health records. In R. Nelson & N. Staggers (Eds.)., *Health informatics: An interprofessional approach* (2nd ed., pp. 241–254). St. Louis, MO: Elsevier.

Graves, J., & Corcoran, S. (1989). The study of nursing informatics. *Image, 21*(4), 227–230.

Health Policy Commission of Massachusetts. (2013). A report on consumer-driven health plans: A review of the national and Massachusetts literature. Retrieved from http://www.mass.gov/anf/docs/hpc/health-policy-commission-section-263-report-vfinal.pdf

Henry, J. P., Searcy, T., & Patel, V. (2016, May). Adoption of electronic health record systems among U.S. non-federal acute care hospitals: 2008–2015: ONC Data Brief 35. Retrieved from https://dashboard.healthit.gov/evaluations/data-briefs/non-federal-acute-care-hospital-ehr-adoption-2008-2015.php

Hibbard, J., Greene, J., Sofaer, S., Firminger, K., & Hirsh, J. (2012, March). An experiment shows that a well-designed report on costs and quality can help consumers choose high-value health care. *Health Affairs, 31*(3), 560–568.

Institute of Medicine. (2014). *Capturing social and behavioral domains and measures in electronic health records: Phase 2*. Washington, DC: The National Academies Press. Retrieved from https://www.nap.edu/catalog/18951/capturing-social-and-behavioral-domains-and-measures-in-electronic-health-records

Lechasseur, K., Lazure, G., & Guilbert, L. (2011, September). Knowledge mobilized by a critical thinking process deployed by nursing students in practical care situations: A qualitative study. *Journal of Advanced Nursing, 67*(9), 1930–1940.

Leventhal, R. (2015, June 10). Survey: Most nurses use smartphones in clinical workplace. Retrieved from https://www.healthcare-informatics.com/news-item/survey-most-nurses-use-smartphones-clinical-workplace

MacDorman, M., Declercq, E., Cabral, H., & Morton, C. (2016, September). Recent increases in the U.S. maternal mortality rate: Disentangling trends from measurement issues. *Obstetrics & Gynecology, 128*(3), 447–455. Retrieved from https://d279m997dpfwgl.cloudfront.net/wp/2016/08/MacDormanM.USMatMort.OBGYN_.2016.online.pdf

Madison, M. P. (2018). The Health Information Technology for Education and Clinical Health Act, Meaningful Use, and Medicare Access and CHIP Reauthorization Act of 2015. In R. Nelson & N. Staggers, (Eds.), *Health informatics, An interprofessional approach* (pp. 455–473). St. Louis, MO: Elsevier.

Mantzoukas, S., & Jasper, M. (2008). Types of nursing knowledge used to guide care of hospitalized patients. *Journal of Advanced Nursing, 62*, 318–326.

Nelson, R. (2002). Major theories supporting health care informatics. In S. Englebardt & R. Nelson (Eds.), *Health care informatics: An interdisciplinary approach*. (pp. 3–27). St. Louis, MO: Mosby.

Nelson, R. (2016, September 13). Informatics: Empowering epatients to drive health care reform: Part I. *OJIN: The Online Journal of Issues in Nursing, 21*(3). Retrieved from https://bit.ly/2IL2b6c

Nelson, R. (2017, June 26). Informatics: Empowering epatients to drive healthcare reform: Part II. *OJIN: The Online Journal of Issues in Nursing, 22*(3). Retrieved from https://ojin.nursingworld.org/MainMenuCategories/ANAMarketplace/ANAPeriodicals/OJIN/TableofContents/Vol-22-2017/No3-Sep-2017/Informatics-Empowering-ePatients-Part-II.html

Nelson, R., & Carter-Templeton, H. D. (2016). The nursing informatician's role in mediating technology related health literacies. In W. Sermeus, P. M. Procter, & P. Weber (Eds.), *Nursing informatics 2016* (Vol. 225, pp. 237–241). Amsterdam, The Netherlands: IOS Press. Retrieved from https://www.ncbi.nlm.nih.gov/pubmed/27332198

Nelson, R., & Joos, I. (1989, Fall). *On language in nursing: From data to wisdom*. PLN Visions, 6.

Nelson, R., & Joos, I. (2012). An introduction: Social media and the transitional roles and relationships in health care. In R. Nelson & I. W. Joos (Eds.), *Social media for nurses*. New York, NY: Springer Publishing Company.

Nelson, R., & Staggers, N. (2018). An introduction to health informatics. In R. Nelson & N. Staggers (Eds.), *Health informatics: An interprofessional approach* (2nd ed., pp. 1–9). St. Louis, MO: Elsevier.

Okun, S., & Caligan, C. (2018). The evolving epatient. In R. Nelson & N. Staggers (Eds.), *Health informatics: An interprofessional approach* (2nd ed., pp. 204–219). St. Louis, MO: Elsevier, Inc.

Phillips, D. (2016, August 8). *Maternal mortality rates on the rise in most US states*. Retrieved from http://www.medscape.com/viewarticle/867225#vp_1

ProPublica. (2015, July 15). Surgeon scorecard. Retrieved from https://projects.propublica.org/surgeons/

The Quality Payment Program Service Center. (n.d.). Quality payment program. Retrieved from https://qpp.cms.gov/

ReferralMD. (2018). 24 outstanding statistics & figures on how social media has impacted the health care industry: 2018 Update. Retrieved from https://getreferralmd.com/2013/09/healthcare-social-media-statistics/

Ricciardi, L., Mostashari, F., Murphy, J., Daniel, J., & Siminerio, E. (2013). A national action plan to support consumer engagement via e-health. *Health Affairs, 2*, 376–384. Retrieved from https://bit.ly/2FYe0bA

Social Determinants of Health Framework Task Group. (2015). *A review of frameworks on the determinants of health*. Retrieved from http://ccsdh.ca/images/uploads/Frameworks_Report_English.pdf

Solberg, S. M. (2017). The social determinants of health: An expanded conceptual framework for nursing. In J. M. Morse (Ed.), *Analyzing and conceptualizing the theoretical foundations of nursing* (pp. 545–568). New York, NY: Springer Publishing Company.

UNESCO. (2004). The Plurality of Literacy and its Implications for Policies and Programmes. Retrieved from UNESCO Education Sector Position. UNESCO: http://bit.ly/1So9eSo

United Nations. (1999, Sept 19). Secretary-General examines 'meaning of international community' in address to dpi/ngo conference. Retrieved from http://www.un.org/press/en/1999/19990915.sgsm7133.doc.html

U.S. Census Bureau. (2015, April 21). About the bureau: What we do. Retrieved from http://www.census.gov/about/what.html

U.S. Department of Health and Human Services. (n.d.). Office of the National Coordinator for Health Information Technology (ONC Federal health IT strategic plan 2015–2020. Retrieved from https://www.healthit.gov/sites/default/files/9-5-federalhealthitstratplanfinal_0.pdf

U.S. Department of Health and Human Services. (n.d.). Framework: The vision, mission and goals of Healthy People 2020. Retrieved from: https://www.healthypeople.gov/sites/default/files/HP2020Framework.pdf

U.S. Department of Health and Human Services. (2009). Healthy People 2020 draft. Washington, DC: U.S. Government Printing Office. Retrieved from https://www.cdc.gov/nchhstp/socialdeterminants/definitions.html

U.S. Department of Health and Human Services. (2015a, June 30). Healthy People 2020: Determinants of health. Retrieved from http://www.healthypeople.gov/2020/about/foundation-health-measures/Determinants-of-Health#social

U.S. Department of Health and Human Services. (2015b, October 29). HealthIT.gov: About the Blue Button movement. Retrieved from https://www.healthit.gov/patients-families/about-blue-button-movement

U.S. Department of Health and Human Services, Office of the National Coordinator for Health Information Technology (May 2, 2019) What are the differences between electronic medical records, electronic health records, and personal health records? Retrieved from https://www.healthit.gov/faq/what-are-differences-between-electronic-medical-records-electronic-health-records-and-personal

U.S. Department of Labor: Bureau of Labor Statistics | Office of Compensation and Working Conditions. (2016, April 21). National Compensation Survey: Glossary of Employee Benefit Terms. Retrieved from https://www.bls.gov/ncs/ebs/glossary20152016.htm

U.S. Department of Labor. (2016, April 21). National compensation survey: Glossary of employee benefit terms. Retrieved from https://www.bls.gov/ncs/ebs/glossary20152016.htm

U.S. Food and Drug Administration. (2015, September 22). Medical devices. Retrieved from https://www.fda.gov/MedicalDevices/DigitalHealth/MobileMedicalApplications/ucm255978.htm

Volpp, K. G., & Mohta, N. S. (2017). Patient engagement survey: Social networks to improve patient health. Retrieved from https://catalyst.nejm.org/survey-social-networks-patient-health/

Wicks, P., & Chiauzzi, E. (2015, September). Trust but verify: Five approaches to ensure safe medical apps. Retrieved from https://bmcmedicine.biomedcentral.com/articles/10.1186/s12916-015-0451-z

World Health Organization. (n.d.). WHO: Topics. Retrieved from http://www.who.int/topics/health_promotion/en/

World Health Organization. (1946). Preamble to the constitution of the World Health Organization as adopted by the International Health Conference, N.Y., 19–22 June 1946; New York: WHO. Retrieved from https://www.ncbi.nlm.nih.gov/pmc/articles/PMC2567708/pdf/12571728.pdf

World Health Organization Commission on Social Determinants of Health. (2008). Closing the gap in a generation: Health equity through action on the social determinants of health: Final report. Geneva: WHO. Retrieved from http://www.who.int/social_determinants/thecommission/finalreport/en/

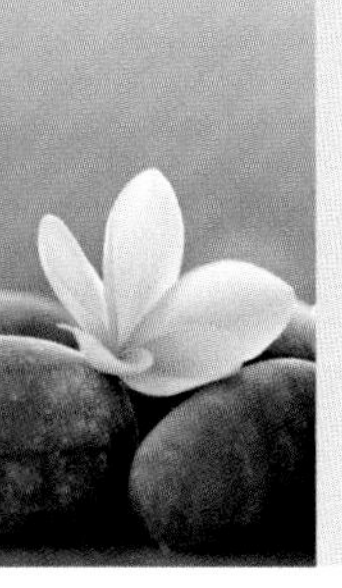

Chapter 14

Cultural Humility in Health Promotion

Denise Saint Arnault

LEARNING OBJECTIVES

After completing this chapter, the student will be able to:

1. Describe the importance of a systematic approach for addressing culture in clinical practice.
2. Critique health-care training models for addressing culture in health care.
3. Explain what culture is and the various components of culture.
4. Describe the cultural humility approach and give the rationale for its components.
5. Explain how patient-centered interviewing and partnership can be achieved in the health-care encounter.
6. Compare and contrast reflexivity and self-awareness.
7. Describe how to carry a culturally centered assessment.

INTRODUCTION

Once comprised of a predominantly non-Hispanic white population, the United States has gradually become a more diverse nation. In the 2010 Census, which was the first time that respondents could provide multiple racial or ethnic categories to describe themselves, just over one-third of the U.S. population reported their race and ethnicity as something other than non-Hispanic white alone (i.e., "minority"), representing an increase of 29% since 2000. Between 2000 and 2010, the Hispanic population grew by 43%. This data reveals that nonwhites represent substantial portions of the U.S. population, including 16% who identify as Hispanic and 13% who identify as African American. It is projected that the portion of U.S. citizens in nonminority categories will decrease to 44% by 2016 at the current growth rates (Colby & Ortman, 2015; Humes, Jones, & Ramirez, 2011).

The single largest non-Caucasian populations in Canada are the 1.5 million First Nations people. In 2011, Canada had a foreign-born population of about 6.5 million, about 20.6% of the total population. This is the highest proportion of immigrants among the G7 countries, many from a diverse array of European countries. Asia, primarily China, is the largest source of immigrants; 7.9 million Canadians speak a primary language other than English or French (Statistics Canada, 2017).

As minority populations increase, so do concerns about health inequities (Anderson, 2012; Isaacson, 2014). Cultural diversity poses many substantial challenges to health services and consumers. Culture influences the experiences, expressions, course, and outcome of health problems, help-seeking strategies, and adherence to interventions (Kirmayer, Guzder, & Rousseau, 2015; U.S. Department of Health and Human Services [DHHS], 2001; World Health Organization, 2016). The clinical encounter aims to address the whole person adequately, but innumerable differences between patient and clinician create challenges.

To mitigate these challenges, clinicians must accurately assess the needs of patients and accommodate diverse worldviews into treatment planning; however, many feel ill-prepared to do so. Despite the efforts to provide cultural sensitivity and cultural competence training in health care in nursing and other health-care fields for more than 25 years, the range of cultural differences in each health-care encounter can make it daunting to address culture in the provider setting. Cultural differences may be rooted in different life experiences, cultural knowledge and identity, social position, social power, differences in language and religion, and a host of other factors. Finally, cultural beliefs, values, and processes influence the provision of health care at the system level as well. The ideals and values of the dominant culture are held within the policies, expectations, practices and procedures of the health-care system, regulating the problems that are assessed and the ways that sociocultural differences are addressed (Kirmayer, 2012).

UNDERSTANDING AND DEFINING CULTURE FOR NURSING EDUCATION AND PRACTICE

Culture refers to integrated patterns of human behavior that include the language, thoughts, communications, actions, customs, beliefs, values, and institutions of racial, ethnic, religious, or social groups (Saint Arnault, 2018). Culture is a system-level phenomenon because it exists outside individuals and groups. However, individuals adopt or accept aspects of culture, hold beliefs and values, and perform behaviors consistent with systemic culture. Therefore, one can say that culture exists both outside and inside individuals and groups at the same time, which makes understanding the concept of culture elusive. However, it also demonstrates how central culture is to our thinking, our feelings, our motivations, and our behavior.

Culture is the interaction of three overlapping domains or dimensions. The first is the group's ideations, which encompass the group members' beliefs, values, religion, myths, symbols, ethnic categories, and worldviews. The ideological domain of culture contains meanings about what is important, preferred, good, right, and normal. It contains meanings about the world and our place within it.

Another domain or dimension of culture is the political and economic patterns of consumption and exchange, wealth and influence, technology, infrastructure, policies, and institutional organization. The political/economic domain of culture includes ways that ideation guides the organization of social structures in society, including how families, groups, and institutions acquire and distribute resources. The political/economic dimension of culture also includes social control, which is how those in power define, regulate, and enforce proper conduct and behavior.

Finally, the practice dimension includes the traditional behaviors, spatial organization, and interpersonal behaviors that are enacted by people and groups. The practice domain includes the traditional rituals, manners of dress, gender relations, child rearing and socialization, etiquette, communication, preferred foods and nutrition practices, and illness prevention and care. The practice aspect of culture includes both power and ideals, but the emphasis is on the power of practice to uphold and embody ideals (sometimes referred to as praxis). Practice is the historical embodiment of tradition (Saint Arnault, 2018).

The "problem" of culture in health care has garnered national attention, both in regard to tracking the role of culture in disparities in health outcomes and emphasizing the necessity of equitable health-care delivery. Research has shown that even when we remove barriers to access to care, such as insurance, racial and ethnic minorities still experience a lower quality of health services and are less likely to receive even routine medical procedures (Anderson, 2012; Bustamante, Morales, & Ortega, 2013). The IOM (2002) report *Unequal Treatment* used federal racial and ethnic categories to understand and document disparities and propose processes in health care that could remedy them (Nelson, 2002). While much of the report emphasizes access issues (language, system expectations, navigation issues, referral patterns, fragmentation of services, and other structural barriers to quality care), it also addressed the complexities of navigating cultural differences in the health-care arena. Referring to these patient-level variables, the IOM report emphasizes attention to patients' values, hopes and fears, trust and doubts, and comfort with the effectiveness and relevance of interventions. While the report recommends engaging patients in culturally relevant care as part of a patient-centered treatment team, it cautions providers to avoid reliance on stereotypes to guide their assessment and planning processes (Bustamante et al., 2013).

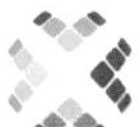

Case Illustration

Li "Edna" Chao immigrated to the United States as an only child with her parents at the age of 10 in 1950. Her family lives in San Francisco. She is Chinese by birth, but she and her parents actively embraced American culture. Her father tried to learn English in the early years, but her mother found it harder because she lived and worked in a Mandarin-speaking community, so she had limited opportunities to converse with English speakers. However, she understood quite a bit of English and watched both Chinese and American TV. Edna was the only one who was fluent in English and also spoke excellent Mandarin.

Edna and her family tried hard to live "the American Dream." She remembers many hard times financially and socially, experiencing discrimination in the schools. In the height of the "sock hop" era, she was criticized for the way she looked and dressed, and even though she tried to fit in, she couldn't seem to escape the expectation that "everyone should look and talk and act the same way." She knew this was true even more for her parents, who seemed to have to struggle for every penny they had and began to keep to themselves and their Chinese community more and more. Even though Edna saw the civil rights activism on TV during her teen years, the changes didn't seem to touch the Chinese immigrant community. She decided that the easiest way to have a social life was to remain mostly in the rapidly growing Chinatown. She grew up feeling "less than," "not quite right," and somewhat disappointed in the promise of America. Nevertheless, she was intelligent, motivated, sensitive, and eager to make a life for herself.

In the early 1970s, everything seemed to turn on its head. In her college in Iowa, where she studied health communication, she was one of a handful of immigrants, making her "stick out" physically. However, she was suddenly very popular in a way. People called her appearance exotic. She was frequently asked about her culture and whether she celebrated Chinese New Year. People said they wished they could come to her house to have "authentic Chinese food." People would touch her hair and comment on how "cool" her eyes were. Somehow, her Chinese-ness became her most valued attribute in the eyes of others. She found herself longing to be just "one of the girls." She also noticed that she felt that being singled out or labeled as "Oriental" or "Asian" felt like people were telling her she wasn't American. On the other hand, it gave her a uniqueness that helped her social life. Besides, she was Chinese and should be proud of it. It would be a betrayal to her parents and the community back home to reject that part of herself. Still, references to her hair and her food choices felt uncomfortable and minimizing.

PATIENT, INTERVENTION, CONTROL, OBSERVATION, AND TIME (PICOT) STATEMENT

In the diverse health-care population (P), how does the cultural humility model (I), compared to other cultural intervention models (C), affect patient and provider satisfaction, improve quality, and reduce health disparities (O) for the current diverse US population (T)?

Movements in Health Care to Address Diversity

Nursing education has embraced several models of culture to frame practitioner education, including multiculturalism, Leininger's (1991) culture care theory, intersectionality and microaggressions, intercultural sensitivity, and cultural competence (Leininger, 1991; Leininger & McFarland, 2006). These models have been criticized and adapted over time, and the model of cultural humility presented below was developed from these critiques. Below we present a sample of these models and related criticisms of each.

Multiculturalism

Early in American history, we embraced the idea of the melting pot, which was the notion that cultural groups who come to the United States would embrace American language, values, norms, and customs. By the 1980s, this idea was replaced by multiculturalism: the ideal that members of different cultures can retain their differences and still live peacefully alongside each other. Assimilation of American values and norms was no longer necessary or even desirable. Multiculturalism promoted maintaining the distinctiveness of multiple cultures rather than older ideals such as social integration, cultural assimilation, and racial segregation.

Multiculturalism has been described as a salad bowl and as a cultural mosaic. From a sociological point of view, multiculturalism is a national value of tolerance and accommodation. A related concept is cultural pluralism, a term used when smaller groups within a larger society maintain their unique cultural identities, and their values and practices are accepted by the wider culture provided they are consistent with the laws and values of the wider society.

In health care, the concept of cultural relativism has been used. This principle holds that others should understand an individual's beliefs and activities in terms of that individual's own culture. Multiculturalism, cultural pluralism, and cultural relativism aim for understanding and unity. In practice, however, people struggle with the ideal of tolerance. On the majority side, people may tend to perceive or even emphasize otherness, exaggerating or stereotyping people and groups who are different from themselves. From the minority side, there is a growing recognition and frustration that multiculturalism leaves the prevailing imbalance of power unchallenged (Hollinger, 2006; Prato, 2016).

Leininger's Culture Care Theory

Leininger was a theorist who applied anthropological concepts specifically to the field of nursing. She proposed the culture care theory and refined it to include a sunrise model in the mid-1970s. This prolific writer went on to create the Transcultural Nursing society in 1983.

The culture care theory aims to define the application of cultural concepts to nursing, urging nurses to assist, support, and facilitate tailoring interventions to the cultural values of the individuals or groups. Leininger defines culturally congruent care as part of the nurse-patient relationship, in which:

> . . . [the] nurse and the client creatively design a new or different care lifestyle for the health or well-being of the client. This mode requires the use of both generic and professional knowledge and ways to fit such diverse ideas into nursing care actions and goals. Care knowledge and skill are often repatterned for the best interest of the clients. (Leininger, 1991, p. 44)

This approach has been highly successful, and it details the steps for assessing the cultural lifeways relevant to nursing care; however, this approach focuses on differences between cultures without explicitly addressing issues of power. The culture care theory clearly recognizes that every person is a product of culture and that everyone has culture. However, clarity on the power dynamics in the relationships of the nurse and the patient and of the minority group with the dominant health-care field are not addressed by this theory.

Intersectionality and Microaggressions

The issues of power and culture have become critical in understanding health and health care. As noted earlier, the dynamics of culture are that it exists both at the system level, influencing policies and practices, and at the individual level, influencing what individuals expect and value. These expectations are held both on the patient side and on the provider side of the relationship. However, the provider is empowered by affiliation with the system to focus on certain issues and not others, to address cultural values and beliefs or not, and to provide or withhold resources. Issues of power in intercultural relationships have been analyzed from the perspective of intersectionality: the awareness that social categorizations such as class, race, and gender are interconnected, overlapping, and interdependent systems of advantage, privilege, and power, as well as the source of discrimination or disadvantage.

Intersectionality is the idea that multiple identities intersect to create a whole that is different from the component identities. This concept emphasizes the concept of identity, maintaining that social identities are the intersection of gender, race, social class, ethnicity, nationality, sexual orientation, religion, age, mental disability, physical disability, mental illness, and physical illness (Shohat & Stam, 2014). From the perspective of intersectionality, concepts of multiculturalism are challenged as simplistic and stereotypical. In addition, the complex intersecting of identities influences any encounter between any two people. This influence in turn affects how communication occurs, how people behave, and the expectations each has for themself and each other.

One of the central concepts in the application of intersectionality to health-care practice is the concept of microaggressions, a term that refers to "brief, everyday exchanges that send denigrating messages to people of color because they belong to a racial minority group" (Sue, 2010). Microaggressions are different from overt, deliberate acts of bigotry because usually the people perpetrating microaggressions intend no offense and are often unaware they are causing harm (Perez Huber & Solorzano, 2017). This analysis illuminates the subtle ways that culture and power influence health-care delivery (Collins, 2015; Murib & Soss, 2015).

Intercultural Sensitivity

Emerging from multiculturalism is cultural sensitivity. It was one of the early approaches to address culture in health care. The key to cultural sensitivity was the development of intercultural communication skills. Through sensitive communication, learners could discern and address cultural differences. Sensitivity of individuals is viewed along a developmental continuum that moves from ethnocentrism (in which the cultural view of the learner is the focus) to cultural relativism. Learners at the earlier stages of the continuum may deny difference, defend against difference, or minimize the importance of difference. Later stages accept, adapt to, and ultimately integrate cultural difference into one's worldview (Majumdaret, Browne, Roberts, & Carpio, 2004).

As noted earlier, this method has several problems. First, like many other models, the cultural sensitivity model focuses on cultural differences rather than acknowledging and helping providers understand that all people are products of culture. It emphasizes development of awareness, which is a useful perspective, but it assumes that this development occurs in a logical and progressive manner. In fact, cultural awareness is not a linear process; it emerges from life experiences, exposure to unfamiliar ways of living, and many other sources. Finally, this approach does not examine power critically. From the perspective of power and privilege, health-care providers who examine power as part of all human interaction must confront their own power and privilege, whether it is earned or unearned. They also have to develop ways of sharing power. A critical analysis of culture would emphasize similarities and differences, the importance of identity as the product of a variety of sources, and the importance of power dynamics in health care (Meydanlioglu, Arikan, & Gozum, 2015).

Cultural Competence

The late 1980s saw an emerging dissatisfaction with U.S. training for health-care providers and a growing concern that the "softer skills" of the clinical encounter were less amenable to tracking and measurement in a traditional medical or nursing school setting. The health-care system was undergoing efforts to manage costs, holding providers accountable for documentation of their skills. Cultural competence emerged as a framework for addressing diversity and inequality in the United States (Betancourt, Green, Carrillo, & Ananeh-Firempong, 2003).

In some articles, cultural competence is a broad term that refers to everything from cultural sensitivity and cross-cultural skills to the specific and measurable outcomes of communication and assessment skills in educational programs (Tervalon & Murray-Garcia, 1998). Models of cultural competence have been widely promoted in textbooks and training materials as strategies to improve the skills of clinicians, health-care services, and systems to address ethnic and cultural diversity (Kirmayer, 2012; Qureshi, Collazos, Ramos, & Casas, 2008).

Cross, Bazron, Dennis, and Isaacs (1989) emphasize that cultural competence is at the individual and the system levels, saying that cultural competence is "a set of congruent behaviors, attitudes, and policies that come together in a system, agency, or among professionals and enable that system, agency, or those professionals to work effectively in cross-cultural situations" (Cross et al., 1989, p. iv). Others have described cultural competence as the requirement that health-care professionals be sensitive to the vast differences among people, differences that include culture, sexual orientation, and socioeconomic status, to provide culturally congruent care (Isaacson, 2014).

The cultural competence movement has been criticized in recent years. Some believe that the literature treats cultures as groups and describes people as "members of a culture" rather than people who hold or share cultural values. This approach assumes that members of any different cultural group share values, beliefs, or attitudes that influence their behaviors within the clinical encounter and that those values, behaviors, or traits can be reliably cataloged and predicted (Kirmayer, 2012). For example, Racher and Annis (2007) wrote that cultural competence implied that one knows or has mastered another's culture, and this "knowing can lead to decreased efforts to learn" (p. 265). While this is consistent with the multiculturalism perspective, it is inconsistent with the intersectionality approach. This notion gives the provider a false sense of security and promotes the tendency to stereotypes groups. It also creates the impossible task of studying many lifeways and cultural traditions and practices represented in our complex health-care constituency. As stated earlier, it ignores the effects of power. Therefore, contemporary practice has turned to new models and metaphors that may help us understand and navigate the cultural encounters of patients and providers.

Cultural Humility

Cultural humility is an emerging field that addresses the multilayered definitions of culture provided above, the fact that all providers are on a developmental trajectory with regard to cultural sensitivity, the fact that power and privilege are critical to address in the health-care arena, and the importance of intersectionality in identity formation. Cultural humility is the "ability to maintain an interpersonal stance that is other-oriented (or open to the other) in relation to aspects of cultural identity that are most important to the [person]" (Hook, Davis, Owen, Worthington, & Utsey, 2013, p. 2).

Cultural humility has been likened to a journey characterized by three factors (Tervalon & Murray-Garcia,

1998). The first factor is the lifelong commitment to self-evaluation and self-critique. This philosophical stance poses that we are never done learning and will always be developing new knowledge and understanding. Like any public servant, nurses must therefore assume the stance of being humble, aware that life is full of a great many things to learn. We also adopt a stance of flexibility, knowing that we are very likely to need to change course as new information reveals itself. Cultural humility takes the position that "we don't know what we don't know," and when we discover that we were in error, we gracefully stand corrected.

The second philosophical position of cultural humility is the earnest desire to learn about power and privilege and to hold the moral position that it is within our scope of practice to interrupt and perhaps repair imbalances where they exist. This is a social justice position that situates health-care practitioners in a position to rectify inequities and power imbalances whenever and wherever they find them. This power may be held within oneself as a function of earned and unearned privilege and may also exist within the routine health-care system within which they practice.

Finally, cultural humility is the attitude, knowledge, and skill set necessary to form alliances. It is the attitude that health care is a partnership and that partnerships evolve through trust and familiarity. This partnership approach requires attention and maintenance, and one's actions of humility and trustworthiness can achieve the therapeutic alliance necessary to traverse the cultural and power differences in the health-care arena (Tervalon & Murray-Garcia, 1998).

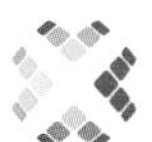

Case Illustration

Edna began to experience a subtle but noticeable decline in her energy and motivation. She felt tired and achy, slept poorly, felt withdrawn, had bouts of anxiety, and experienced anger and resentment. She finished college and went back to San Francisco to live with her parents while she sorted out her feelings. She decided to go to a health clinic and discovered an emergence of facilities founded to serve Asian American patients. At one of these facilities, Edna made an appointment with a female doctor from Vietnam. All the facility's signs were in several languages. Her doctor prescribed counseling, vitamins, and acupuncture for her fatigue. She didn't like the idea of counseling because she wanted to be strong and "take care of things on her own." She also didn't want her parents to think something was wrong with her. She had no interest in acupuncture, even though she knew the treatment was popular among many in her community.

Her experience with the clinic was interesting to her. She liked finally being considered as an American. She even liked the idea of Asian American as an identity. But, somehow, again, her Chinese heritage was the focus of her treatment. Still, this seemed like a positive development overall because people like her parents could finally get care in their own language when the Chinese doctors were working. She wondered whether the Vietnamese doctor would understand her parents' culture, but maybe there was such a thing as Asian culture that could help treat the ever more diverse populations coming to San Francisco. She considered volunteering at the clinic while she recovered. She knew she could translate some of the pamphlets into Chinese for the clinic.

Over the years, Edna noticed that the clinic's population included immigrants from many countries as well as refugees and that many of these individuals required social services as well as health services. In the waiting room on any given day, she might see women in sari or wearing hijab, people from Laos, and people who were Hmong.

Discussion of the Evidence

Studies that evaluate the impact of the practitioner's skills in caring for those of other cultures are difficult to summarize because of the wide range of outcome measures used. For example, Truong, Paradies, and Priest (2014) carried out a meta-review of nineteen systematic reviews that evaluated the impact of cultural competency training. The included reviews covered a variety of health-care settings to examine patient, provider, and health-care access and utilization data. These reviews generally found moderate evidence of provider, access, and health-care utilization outcomes. Unfortunately, evidence that these skills had a direct impact on patient outcomes is weaker (Truong et al., 2014).

Evidence for the value of cultural competence on the outcomes of psychotherapy for minorities is mixed. A systematic review defined cultural competence as ethnic minority-focused treatments and found that incorporating culturally tailored strategies can be efficacious. But there is less support for cultural competence as a useful supplement to standard treatment (Huey, Tilley, Jones, & Smith, 2014). Research is needed to measure specific skills and attitudes across a variety of patient groups.

At the program level, one systematic review examined five system-level interventions: culturally diverse staff, use of interpreter services, cultural competency training, the use of linguistically and culturally appropriate health education materials, and health-care settings for specific cultural groups. Unfortunately, the review found little evidence of the effectiveness of these interventions, but it attributed the lack of findings to the fact that these studies did not examine outcomes that the reviewers deemed critical to system improvement, such as client satisfaction, health status improvement, or racial or ethnic disparities (Anderson et al., 2003). Truong et al. (2014) found that no study on cultural competency examined long-term effects (one year or more) and generally found some evidence that interventions to improve cultural competency can improve patient/client health outcomes. This review also found that many studies did not have objective evidence of intervention effectiveness (Truong et al., 2014).

Cultural humility is a newer approach. In a set of four studies, Hook et al. (2013) demonstrated reliability and construct validity of a client-rated measure of a therapist's cultural humility. They also demonstrated that client perceptions of their therapist's cultural humility are positively associated with developing a strong working alliance and were positively associated with improvement in therapy (Hook et al., 2013).

Recommendations for Practice

The model of cultural humility prescribes attitudes and behaviors that help the practitioner to be open to similarities and differences in culture during each health-care encounter. The primary behaviors are a humble attitude accompanied by personal self-reflection and the development of the professional skill of reflexivity. Next, this mindset is operationalized in the clinical encounter by using the skill of patient-centered interviewing. This facilitates the provider's ability to discern what aspects of culture are relevant to the health-care encounter and will result in optimal patient care.

Humble Attitude

Humble practitioners do not make assumptions, easily admit what they do not know when they truly do not know, and search for resources to enhance their knowledge. They realize they are continually evolving, considering what they know as a hypothesis to test in the current and in future situations. And they know that all knowledge is subject to falsification by the client. For example, providers may begin with an assumption that the patient who is a first-generation immigrant with a first language other than English may have a stronger adherence to his or her birth culture. To be sure of this, however, they would need to ask the patient about his or her values and beliefs rather than relying on the initial assumption.

Self-Reflection

Self-reflection is a realistic and ongoing self-appraisal. Adopting a self-reflective practice requires patience, practice, and effort. It requires a critical evaluation of who you are as a person and as a practitioner and of your reactions in the practice setting. Everybody has assumptions about what constitutes health, who you are and should be in the clinical encounter, how a clinical encounter should go, what constitutes success and why, and what constitutes failure and why. These assumptions and beliefs form the background of every encounter, no matter what cultural differences exist between provider and client. These come from training, personality, educational experiences, and a host of other sources. Facing them can be difficult, especially when they are at odds with the values and expectations of self-reflective, patient-centered, culturally humble practice. Therefore, it is helpful to have prompts or questions that you can ask yourself as you move through your development as a practitioner. Self-reflection can be done through journaling, talking with a friend or colleague, in small-group discussions, in a supervised setting, in leadership training, or even while relaxing in the bathtub after a rough day.

Reflexivity

Reflexivity is a term used in research to refer to a personal, critical analysis of intersectionality. It is attention to power and privilege in any encounter, whether it be the researcher and their participants or the provider and their patients. Reflexivity focuses attention on the matrix of domination and power (Murib & Soss, 2015). The reflexive skill is to bring to consciousness often ill-defined and multidimensional cultural identities and backgrounds, both in oneself and others. Power matrices are situational and fluid, sometimes shifting many times in a day. Context can dramatically shift a power matrix. A full professor of neurosurgery has much more power in a surgical arena than she or he would in a field hospital in remote Kenya, where almost no one speaks English. Therefore, one must watch how power dynamics shift as people of different races, ethnicities, classes, linguistic capabilities, sexual orientations, physical abilities, genders, educational backgrounds, and migration histories move in and out of contexts or fields.

Patient-Centered Interviewing

Patient-centered interviewing signals to the patient that the practitioner values the patient's agenda and perspectives through a more engaged and interactive and less controlling style. Only the patient is uniquely qualified to help health-care providers understand his or her identity and clarify the relevance and importance of factors such as race, ethnicity, religion, and class on the present illness or wellness experience (Tervalon & Murray-Garcia, 1998).

LEARN Framework

The LEARN framework is a mnemonic developed by Berlin and Fowkes (1983) to facilitate patient-centered interviewing in clinical training. The letters LEARN stand for the following:

- ***Listen.*** Hear what the person is describing and help him or her explain his or her mindset if needed. If you need to ask questions or probe more deeply, do so after the person explains. In addition, narrate these steps to the patient as they take place and let the patient know you are doing so to develop your understanding fully.
- ***Explain.*** Explain everything. Explain why you are asking the questions you ask. Explain the things you think are happening with the client's health.
- ***Acknowledge.*** Acknowledge the patient's feelings and perceptions as well as confusion or difficulties. Acknowledge your own efforts to understand and acknowledge that you know many things from your training and that you are trying to make sure that this is what is best for the patient but that the patient is the expert when it comes to the patient. Thus, you want to hear from the patient every step of the way. Also, acknowledge that she or he may not understand everything she or he is told, but that you can provide the necessary skills and information to help the patient achieve this understanding.
- ***Recommend.*** Treatments are recommendations with supporting rationale. You are trying to give patients your best advice, but as things change or progress, the best treatment protocol may change and evolve.
- ***Negotiate.*** Health care is a negotiation about what is needed, wanted, and acceptable. This is critical in health care because it is the set of behaviors that demonstrates that the provider accurately understands the patient's perspective, has clearly explained their own clinical judgement, and that the provider emphasizes that their clinical relationship should be viewed as a partnership (Berlin & Fowkes, 1983).

Culture-Centered Interviewing

Culture influences an individual's health beliefs, practices, values, and expectations for and access to health care. Culture affects how people communicate, understand, and respond to health information and how they interact with health professionals. By exploring culture and health, health professionals can learn about their clients' understanding of their health concerns, explore the broader contexts influencing their clients' health and wellness, and enhance their capacity to develop respectful and collaborative working relationships with clients.

Simple models can help health professionals guide cross-cultural conversations and learn about and understand their clients' views, values, and beliefs about their health. Each model enhances understanding between health professionals and clients and can be used during assessments and during the development and management of care plans. These models are consistent with adopting a cultural humility perspective. A cultural humility perspective acknowledges that culture is complex, diverse, and dynamic and therefore the most useful way to approach a client is with genuine curiosity, openness to learn, and a willingness to reflect on what a person is bringing to the encounter from his or her own background.

The following focused questions can help the provider understand the client's perception of his or her problems and the expectations and desires for healing (Kleinman, 2015; Kleinman, Eisenberg, & Good, 1978):

- **What do you call your problem? What name do you give it?** This helps you refer to the problem using the client's words and creates an understanding of how the patient views the health issue intellectually, socially, and emotionally.
- **What do you think has caused it?** This helps you understand what the client thinks caused the health issues and begins to reveal what he or she thinks can and should be done about it.
- **Why did it start when it did?** This is similar to the routine clinical questions about illness course, but it adds a dimension about precipitating events or conditions. These are usually related to causes but also include elements such as stress, life changes, vulnerability, fatigue, or other conditions that make illness possible in a client's worldview.
- **What does your sickness do to your body? How does it work inside you?** This area is called ethnophysiology and helps the practitioner understand how the client understands his or her inner workings. It also helps the practitioner identify areas for additional teaching about pathophysiology.

- **How severe is it? Will it get better soon or take longer?** This question gets at the client's illness expectations. Here, the practitioner learns about how the illness affects functioning, and how the client usually performs self-care when symptoms are present.
- **What are the chief problems your sickness has caused for you (personally, with family members, with work colleagues, etc.)?** This question connects to severity and function but adds the elements of social network, social support, and other resources that the person needs and from his or her environment.
- **What do you fear most about your sickness?** This can reveal the emotional impact that the illness has had on the client and the worries he or she associates with it. Often, the client will talk about another time when he or she had the same illness, someone else who had it, or things he or she has heard about the illness. This is also an important place for education if fears can be allayed or new treatments introduced.
- **What kind of treatment do you think you should receive? What are the most important results you hope to receive from the treatment?** This question gets at expectations and desires for the health-care encounter and helps the client summarize what she or he knows and what she or he fears, hopes for, and thinks is needed.

CULTURAL HUMILITY AND HEALTH-CARE POLICY

The concept and processes that support addressing culture in health care are consistent with the training and procedures outlined in national practice and policy guidelines. For example, the cultural dimensions of health care are defined in the Think Cultural Health (TCH) model advanced by the Office of Minority Health (U.S. DHHS, 2014). TCH is dedicated to advancing health equity at every point of contact. This program responds to the need of the underserved and the providers who care for them by explaining how providers can respond to diversity and measure the impact of that response.

For example, program and quality improvement is addressed by Standard 1 of the National Enhanced Culturally and Linguistically Appropriate Services (CLAS) standards. The Principal Standard is to: "Provide effective, equitable, understandable, and respectful quality care and services that are responsive to diverse cultural health beliefs and practices, preferred languages, health literacy, and other communication needs." Agencies are expected to train students, preceptors, and providers to be aware of their own cultural beliefs, how to assess and respond to the cultural beliefs of their patients, and how to change beliefs and attitudes that will translate into better health care. The aim of the CLAS Standards, especially Standard 1, is twofold: to provide patients with assurances that disrespect or discrimination of any kind is intolerable and, with reasonable assistance, to overcome language, cultural, physical, or communication barriers.

Effective care and services are "those that successfully restore an individual to his/her desired health status and help to protect his/her future health. An essential part of ensuring that care and services are effective is to ensure that they are culturally and linguistically appropriate" (Smedley, Stith, & Nelson, 2009). Cultural and linguistic competency allows providers to navigate the cultural and linguistic factors that affect trust, rapport, communication, and adherence (Ngo-Metzger & Fund, 2006).

Equitable care and services are those that apply to all individuals and groups regardless of their cultural identity, race, education, health literacy, age, sexual orientation, ethnicity, religion, physical or mental disability, language, gender, gender expression, gender identity, income, class, and access to care (National Partnership for Action to End Health Disparities, 2011).

Understandable care and services include the clear exchange of information between providers and patients. They assist individuals to comprehend available treatment options and what they need to stay well.

Respectful care and services are those that foster an environment in which individuals from diverse backgrounds feel comfortable discussing their needs. The concept of cultural humility is a framework that is consistent with, supports, and enables the manifestation of the CLAS standards in routine practice.

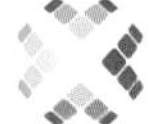

Case Illustration

Now in her 50s, Edna is married, with two children of her own, living a middle-class life in San Francisco. She works in a medical communication firm as a translator and serves on the board of a policy group providing education and advocacy for the very large Asian population in her city. She also cares for her aging parents. She never really got over her fatigue, pain, bouts of anxiety, or bitterness about American society letting her down. She felt misunderstood, marginalized, stereotyped, and frustrated by the mistreatment and poverty in the Asian communities she served.

Finally, after trying hard to keep up with the demands of her busy life, she decided that her feelings needed attention and that she would try going back to a health-care provider. The Asian clinics really seemed set up for different communities now, and the emphasis was on health-care needs different from her own, so she ventured to a clinic outside her local community. She was assigned to a family nurse practitioner (NP), a soft-spoken but direct fellow who made her feel welcome. After getting the picture about the initial reason for her visit, he began to ask her about her history with health care, her life in general, and some of her values about health. Edna decided to bring up her dissatisfaction with her care in the past, and her NP responded, "You know, I don't know much about what it must be like coming from a different country at such a young age. I guess, growing up where I did, we met lots of people from different walks of life, but I can't really make any assumptions about what you think, what you believe, or your experiences. Maybe, as we learn about each other, I might ask some simple questions, but I just want to understand how you understand your world, and how these feelings you are having fit into that." He began to ask her questions about her symptoms in detail, probing about how she understood them and what she wanted as a result of her visit. After some time, he summarized all that Edna had said and told her about some of the possibilities for testing that could help figure out her symptoms, including bloodwork, and a more thorough analysis of the heart murmur he detected.

At the end of the visit, the NP said, "Well, this was a good beginning, but health care is a partnership, you know? We have to keep trying to get at the bottom of these long-lasting feelings you have had and find a plan that works for you. You mentioned that you still hold on to some of the values and practices taught to you by your parents, but you also really want to be recognized as an American. Please challenge me if I make assumptions along the way. For now, let's keep moving toward getting you feeling 'peppy' again!"

As Edna walked away from the visit, she felt somehow like a door had opened. The NP didn't have all the answers, but she wanted to talk about herself and her struggles. She never thought about having a health-care partner before, but having one now suited her very well. Edna found herself actually looking forward to her next appointment.

CONCLUSION

Heath-care systems have been engaged in training the workforce in cultural skills for decades. The cultural humility proposal shifts the attention to different aspects of cultural skills, but it does not itself add to the risks, costs, or benefits of training. It is entirely feasible and somewhat simpler to use this approach in training. However, it requires a fundamental shift in the way practitioners approach patient care, so in some ways it requires a "culture shift" in training models. Therefore, systems and supervisors are critical to the success of these programs and must model these approaches in both routine care and supervision. Cultural humility can also foster interprofessional practice quality because it is a stance toward mutual understanding and partnership in all interactions, benefiting patients and interprofessional interactions alike.

USEFUL RESOURCES

Cultural Humility: People, Principles and Practices. YouTube four-part video series. https://www.youtube.com/watch?v=_Mbu8bvKb_U. Chavez, V. (2012). Cultural humility: People, principles and practices. San Francisco State University. YouTube.

Culturally Connected Online Training: https://culturallyconnected.ca/cultural-humility/

American Medical Association. (2007). Incorporating universal communication principles. Adapted from Reducing the risk by designing a safer, shame-free health care environment.

Center for Linguistic and Cultural Competency in Health Care: https://minorityhealth.hhs.gov/omh/browse.aspx?lvl=2&lvlid=34

KEY POINTS

- There is an ever-increasing need to address the diversity of beliefs, values, and lifestyles in our health-care system.
- Efforts in the 1980s focused on multiculturalism and cultural sensitivity, but these approaches have since been criticized for neglecting cultural diversity within populations and for ignoring power differentials between the majority and minority groups.
- Mandates for health-care standards were introduced in the late 1980s that emphasized skill and competency, but these were criticized for creating stereotypes about groups and disregarding power issues in health care.

- The relatively new concept of intersectionality helps providers attend to the ways that diverse identities such as class, culture, and religion overlap to create matrices of power, and helps them to consider the broad, diverse identities of both patients and providers and how these influence the health-care encounter.
- Cultural humility is an approach that promotes a humble attitude of flexibility and a stance that one is always learning about others, and emphasizes how culture influences health care in general and how power influences the health-care encounter. With this approach, the provider and the patient are considered partners in a therapeutic alliance that integrates the perspectives and expectations of the provider and the patient into a collaborative treatment plan.

Check Your Understanding

1. Multiculturalism in health care has been criticized because it:
   A. Aims for tolerance and unity between groups of diverse people
   B. Categorizes people in large groups, ignoring intracultural differences
   C. Emphasizes diversity instead of assimilation
   D. Leads to political unrest
2. The goals of cultural competence are to:
   A. Recognize and address power differences between people
   B. Learn about cultural differences
   C. Address cultural differences in treatment planning
   D. Both B and C
3. Intersectionality is the recognition that people from different cultures have different ways of interacting.
   A. True
   B. False
4. Microaggressions are generally intentional bigotry.
   A. True
   B. False
5. Cultural humility can be considered:
   A. A philosophical position
   B. A therapeutic approach
   C. A set of values
   D. All of the above
6. Cultural humility differs from cultural competency because cultural humility:
   A. Recognizes the need for continuous learning
   B. Develops treatment plans based on distinct cultural patterns
   C. Helps practitioners to adopt a position of flexibility
   D. Both A and C

See "Reflections on Check Your Understanding" at the end of the book for answers.

REFERENCES

Anderson, L. M., Scrimshaw, S. C., Fullilove, M. T., Fielding, J. E., Normand, J., & Services, Task Force on Community Preventive Services. (2003). Culturally competent healthcare systems: A systematic review. American Journal of Preventive Medicine, *24*(3), 68–79.

Anderson, K. M. (Ed.). (2012). How far have we come in reducing health disparities?: progress since 2000: workshop summary. Washington, DC: National Academies Press.

Berlin, E. A., & Fowkes, W. C., Jr. (1983). A teaching framework for cross-cultural health care: Application in family practice. *Western Journal of Medicine*, *139*(6), 934.

Betancourt, J. R., Green, A. R., Carrillo, J. E., & Ananeh-Firempong, O., 2nd (2003). Defining cultural competence: A practical framework for addressing racial/ethnic disparities in health and health care. *Public Health Reports*, *118*(4), 293.

Bustamante, A., Morales, L., & Ortega, A. (2014). Racial and ethnic disparities in health care. In G.F. Kominski (Ed.) Changing the US health care system: Key issues in health services policy and management (4th ed. pp. 103–134). Hoboken , NJ: Jossey-Bass.

Colby, S. L., & Ortman, J. M. (2015). Projections of the size and composition of the US population: 2014 to 2060: Population estimates and projections. Retrieved from https://mronline.org/wp-content/uploads/2019/08/p25-1143.pdf.

Collins, P. H. (2015). Intersectionality's definitional dilemmas. *Annual Review of Sociology*, *41*, 1–20.

Cross, T., Bazron, B., Dennis, K., & Isaacs, M. R. (1989). *Towards a culturally competent system of care*. Washington, DC: Georgetown University Child Development Center.

Hollinger, D. A. (2006). *Postethnic America: Beyond multiculturalism*. New York, NY: Basic Books.

Hook, J. N., Davis, D. E., Owen, J., Worthington, E. L., Jr., & Utsey, S. O. (2013). Cultural humility: Measuring openness to culturally diverse clients. *Journal of Counseling Psychology*, *60*(3), 353.

Huey, S. J., Jr, Tilley, J. L., Jones, E. O., & Smith, C. A. (2014). The contribution of cultural competence to evidence-based care for ethnically diverse populations. *Annual Review of Clinical Psychology*, *10*, 305–338.

Humes, K., Jones, N. A., & Ramirez, R. R. (2011). Overview of race and Hispanic origin, 2010: US Department of Commerce, Economics and Statistics Administration, US Census Bureau.

Isaacson, M. (2014). Clarifying concepts: Cultural humility or competency. *Journal of Professional Nursing*, *30*(3), 251–258.

Kirmayer, L. J. (2012). Rethinking cultural competence. *Transcultural Psychiatry, 49*(2), 149.

Kirmayer, L. J., Guzder, J., & Rousseau, C. (Eds.). (2015). Cultural consultation: Encountering the other in mental health care. New York: Springer Science & Business Media.

Kleinman, A. (2015). Supplementary module 1: Explanatory model. *DSM-5® handbook on the cultural formulation interview*, 56.

Kleinman, A., Eisenberg, L., & Good, B. (1978). Culture, illness, and care: Clinical lessons from anthropological and cross-cultural research. *Annals of Internal Medicine, 88*, 251–288.

Leininger, M. M. (1991). The Theory of Culture Care Diversity and Universality. In Culture care diversity and universality: A theory of nursing (pp. 5–67). New York: National League for Nursing Press.

Leininger, M. M., & McFarland, M. R. (2006). Culture care diversity & universality: A worldwide nursing theory. Sudbury, MA: Jones & Bartlett Learning.

Majumdar, B., Browne, G., Roberts, J., & Carpio, B. (2004). Effects of cultural sensitivity training on health care provider attitudes and patient outcomes. *Journal of Nursing Scholarship, 36*(2), 161–166.

Meydanlioglu, A., Arikan, F., & Gozum, S. (2015). Cultural sensitivity levels of university students receiving education in health disciplines. *Advances in Health Sciences Education, 20*(5), 1195–1204.

Murib, Z., & Soss, J. (2015). Intersectionality as an assembly of analytic practices: Subjects, relations, and situated comparisons. *New Political Science, 37*(4), 649–656.

National Partnership for Action to End Health Disparities. (2011). *National stakeholder strategy for achieving health equity.* Rockville, MD: U.S. Department of Health & Human Services, Office of Minority Health.

Nelson, A. (2002). Unequal treatment: Confronting racial and ethnic disparities in health care. *Journal of the National Medical Association, 94*(8), 666.

Ngo-Metzger, Q., & Fund, C. (2006). *Cultural competency and quality of care: Obtaining the patient's perspective.* New York: Commonwealth Fund.

Pérez Huber, L., & Solorzano, D. G. (2015). Racial microaggressions as a tool for critical race research. *Race Ethnicity and Education, 18*(3), 297–320.

Prato, G. B. (2016). *Beyond multiculturalism: Views from anthropology*. London: Routledge.

Qureshi, A., Collazos, F., Ramos, M., & Casas, M. (2008). Cultural competency training in psychiatry. *European Psychiatry, 23*, 49–58.

Racher, F. E., & Annis, R. C. (2007). Respecting culture and honoring diversity in community practice. *Research and Theory for Nursing Practice, 21*(4), 255–270.

Saint Arnault, D. M. (2018). Defining and theorizing about culture: The evolution of the cultural determinants of help seeking-revised. *Nursing Research, 67*(2), 161–168.

Shohat, E., & Stam, R. (2014). *Unthinking eurocentrism: Multiculturalism and the media*. New York: Routledge.

Smedley, B. D., Stith, A. Y., & Nelson, A. R. (2009). *Unequal treatment: Confronting racial and ethnic disparities in health care (with CD).* Washington, DC: National Academies Press.

Statistics Canada. (2015). Immigration and Ethnocultural Diversity in Canada. Retrieved from https://www12.statcan.gc.ca/nhs-enm/2011/as-sa/99-010-x/99-010-x2011001-eng.cfm.

Sue, D. W. (2010). *Microaggressions in everyday life: Race, gender, and sexual orientation*. Hoboken, N.J.: Wiley.

Tervalon, M., & Murray-Garcia, J. (1998). Cultural humility versus cultural competence: A critical distinction in defining physician training outcomes in multicultural education. *Journal of Health Care for the Poor and Underserved, 9*(2), 117–125.

Truong, M., Paradies, Y., & Priest, N. (2014). Interventions to improve cultural competency in healthcare: A systematic review of reviews. *BMC Health Services Research, 14*(1), 99.

U.S. Department of Health and Human Services. (2001). Mental health: Culture, race and ethnicity: A supplement to mental health: A report to the Surgeon General. Rockville, MD: Public Health Service, Office of the Surgeon General.

U.S. Department of Health and Human Services. (2014). Office of Minority Health Fact Sheet: National Standards for Culturally and Linguistically Appropriate Services in Health and Health Care, National CLAS Standards. Retreived from https://minorityhealth.hhs.gov/omh/browse.aspx?lvl=2&lvlid=53.

World Health Organization. (2016). Social determinants of health Retrieved from http://www.who.int/social_determinants/en/

Interprofessional Health Promotion

Patricia W. Underwood

LEARNING OBJECTIVES

After completing this chapter, the student will be able to:

1. Describe the salient components of patient-centered interprofessional collaborative practice.
2. Discuss the existing evidence supporting interprofessional collaborative practice as a strategy to promote health and achieve the Triple Aim.
3. Identify the types of data needed to evaluate the outcomes of interprofessional practice.
4. Compare the questions to be considered in joining or starting a patient-centered interprofessional collaborative practice.
5. Devise strategies for addressing barriers to interprofessional practice.

INTRODUCTION

The movement to improve the quality of health care came to prominence with the release of two major reports by the Institute of Medicine (IOM): *To Err Is Human: Building a Safer Health System* (IOM, 2000) and *Crossing the Quality Chasm: A New Health System for the 21st Century* (IOM, 2001). The direction of this reform was further delineated with the promulgation of the Triple Aim for health care by the Institute for Healthcare Improvement (IHI) calling for improving the experience of care, improving the health of populations, and reducing per capita costs of health care (Berwick, Noland, & Whittington, 2008).

Basing care on evidence is viewed as a key element in improving population health, but that evidence must be applied within the context of the complexity of the patient's problems and individual preferences to improve his or her experience. Addressing complex contexts is recognized as a key element in improving and promoting health; however, rarely does one health profession have all the knowledge needed to achieve the desired outcomes regardless of how collaboratively it involves the patient/family. The challenge then becomes how to access the constellation of interprofessional knowledge without unduly increasing the cost of care or adding to the complexity in a manner that increases the likelihood of error.

Patient-centered interprofessional collaborative practice (PCIPCP) is viewed as a strategy for harnessing the multiple sources of knowledge needed and applying them within the context of patient and population differences. It affords the opportunity across settings to apply the standards of best-practice evidence tailored to capitalize on the unique variations in the individual's needs and resources. Earnest and Brandt (2014) eloquently describe PCIPCP, likening it to "creating a stronger whole from disparate parts" by weaving distinct threads "into a tightly knit cloth that will wrap around" patients and families "and guarantee the maximal opportunity for health in all its dimensions" (p. 500).

Regardless of setting, interprofessional collaborative practice (IPCP) as a strategy for increasing the quality of health promotion brings unique challenges. As the complexity of care delivery increases, careful coordination within and external to the health-care team is essential. Potential barriers to effective interprofessional practice (IPP) must be recognized and plans must be developed to address them in order to maximize care quality. This chapter will illustrate how health promotion and achievement of the Triple Aim depends on the application of evidence-based, patient-centered care within the context of effective interprofessional teams. Effective health-care teams collaborate and coordinate care. Collaboration and coordination are grounded in mutual respect, a shared vision, equity in power and responsibility, and effective communication. Without any of these elements, too many disparate players heighten the complexity and opportunities for error and/or costly duplication. Although knowledge of team skills is critical to effective collaboration, the focus of this chapter will be on IPP as a key strategy for health promotion. The nature of IPP merits consideration by nurse practitioners as they develop or join practices within both acute- and primary-care settings.

WHAT IS IPCP?

Several definitions of IPCP are currently used and emphasize different elements of this practice. Freeth, Hammick, Reeves, Koppel, and Barr (2005) defined IPP as two or more professions working as a team bound by the common elements of purpose, mutual respect, and commitment. This definition stresses the minimum participants and elements necessary to constitute IPCP.

The World Health Organization (WHO) (2010), on the other hand, emphasizes the inclusion of the care recipients and focuses on the outcomes when they define IPP as "multiple health workers from different professional backgrounds working together with patients, families, caregivers, and communities to deliver the highest quality of care" (p. 7). Herbert's (2005) definition combines the collaborators and the purpose with attention to process: collaborative patient-centered practice is "the continuous interaction of two or more professionals or disciplines organized into a common effort to solve or explore common issues with the best possible participation of the patient" (p. 1). This definition currently informs the work of the Canadian government–funded collaborative patient-centered practice project (Fox & Reeves, 2015). Although the initiative for patient-centered care has grown out of the consumer rights' and quality assurance movements, Fox and Reeves (2015) suggest that the addition of this concept to IPCP avoid becoming a shift of responsibility to the patient but instead become a concerted effort to share power and involve the patient in decision making and in sharing information, power, and responsibility. Providing patients with access to their electronic health records is one such aspect of sharing information.

In the United States in 2009, the Interprofessional Education Collaborative (IPEC) was formed by six health professions education associations: the American Association of Colleges of Nursing, the American Association of Colleges of Osteopathic Medicine, the American Association of Colleges of Pharmacy, the American Dental Education Association, the American Association of Medical Colleges, and the Association of Schools and Programs of Public Health to encourage the development of interprofessional education (IPE). In the view of IPEC's Expert Panel (2011), IPP was the key to safe, quality, accessible, patient-centered care. To achieve that vision of health care required "the continuous development of interprofessional competencies by health professions students as part of the learning process, so that they enter the workforce ready to practice effective teamwork and team-based care" (p. 1).

In its report *Core Competencies for Interprofessional Collaborative Practice*, IPEC's Expert Panel (2011) adopted the WHO definition of IPCP and made a distinction between interprofessional teamwork and interprofessional team-based care. Interprofessional teamwork focuses on the "levels of cooperation, coordination and collaboration characterizing the relationships between professions in delivering patient-centered care." Interprofessional team-based care, by contrast, refers to "care delivered by intentionally created, usually relatively small work groups in health care, who are recognized by others as well as by themselves as having a collective identity and shared responsibility for a patient or group of patients, e.g., rapid response team, palliative care team, primary care team, operating room team" (p. 2). Interprofessional teamwork focuses more on the process of care, whereas team-based care is defined in structural terms. The reality in health-care delivery is that effective interprofessional collaboration must embody the concepts of effective team collaboration whether these teams are more fixed in caring for a specific population or more fluid, forming, dissolving, and re-forming based on geographic assignment of responsibility, as might occur within an emergency department.

In developing a report on the collaboration of nurse practitioners and family practice physicians, Way, Jones, and Basing (2000) defined IPCP as a "process for communication and decision making that enables the separate and shared knowledge and skills of care providers to synergistically influence the client/patient care provided" (p. 3). This definition clearly values what the different professions are bringing to the relationship and emphasizes the synergy that is created through the shared communication and decision making. What is missing is the involvement of the client/family in that process.

A definition that includes an emphasis on client needs yet surrenders the authority of any one profession was put forward by Masterson (2002), who defined interprofessional collaboration as "a willingness to share and indeed give up exclusive claims to specialized knowledge and authority if other professional groups can meet patient/client needs more efficiently and appropriately" (p. 333). Sharing and giving up traditional authority appear to be critical components of interprofessional collaboration, but a devaluing of specialized professional knowledge may not be an advantage in the long run.

A new definition blending some of the key elements of current definitions might have the advantage of setting the expectations for practice that could be consistently implemented and evaluated in relation to outcomes. A blended definition of PCIPCP might be stated as "a process by which two or more professions synergize their separate and shared knowledge and skills within a context of mutual respect to fully engage patients/families in optimizing their health." Such a process has the potential for achieving the highest quality of care possible. Effective IPCP requires that a common definition be accepted as a basis for a shared team vision.

EVIDENCE OF IPCP OUTCOMES

In determining the evidence supporting interprofessional team care, the patient, intervention, control, observation, and time (PICOT) question would take the following format: In (the patient population), what is the effect of IPCP on (outcomes specified) compared with traditional/non-IPP? The intent would be to look across populations to see what evidence exists that supports the conclusion that varied health professions practicing in a collaborative model could improve health outcomes across acute- and primary-care settings. Findings of systematic reviews would provide guidance for health policy, resource allocation, and pre- and post-licensure education and development. A variety of outcomes could be measured specific to the health-care issue salient to the population of focus but should also include perceptions of the patient's experience and cost-effectiveness.

When the WHO (2010) issued its seminal report *Framework for Action on Interprofessional Education and Collaborative Practice*, a variety of evidence was cited that supported their conclusion that collaborative IPP could strengthen health systems and improve health outcomes in both acute- and primary-care settings. Among the systematic reviews included were two that incorporated a variety of patient populations and four that focused on a specific population (mental health, heart failure, or total parenteral nutrition patients). Two literature reviews and four individual studies were also cited. Six reviews and one study focused more specifically on IPE. Collaborative IPP was seen to improve patient satisfaction and decrease lengths of stay, complications, mortality rates, and clinical errors among hospitalized patients. Positive outcomes for community mental health patients included decreased suicide rates, increased satisfaction and acceptance of treatment, and reduced outpatient visits.

One of the evidence reviews for IPP included in the 2010 WHO report and four others are particularly noteworthy. Three Cochrane Collaboration reviews synthesize evidence from 1999 to 2015. The initial review of research from 1999 to 2006 (Reeves et al., 2009) was followed by a Cochrane review of studies from 2006 to 2011 (Reeves, Perrier, Goldman, Freeth, & Zwarenstein, 2013). The most recently published Cochrane review synthesized studies through 2015 (Reeves, Pelone, Harrison, Goldman, & Zwarenstein, 2017). Mitchell, Tieman, and Shelby-James's (2008) synthesis of five systematic reviews of literature from 1990 to 2006 has been used as a basis for policy development. A final piece of current evidence is provided by Brandt, Lutfiyya, King, and Chioreso's (2014) scoping review of research for the inclusion of evidence supporting the achievement of IHI's Triple Aim outcome.

Cochrane Systematic Reviews

Reeves and colleagues searched the literature for studies that employed randomized control trial (RCT), controlled before and after (CBA), or interrupted time series (ITS) designs that measured patient/health outcomes as a result of the implementation of interprofessional care. In most instances, the interprofessional care was not critically examined, but a program to promote interprofessional care had been implemented. In the first review of literature from 1999 to 2006 (Reeves et al., 2009), only six studies meeting the criteria were found. In a subsequent review (Reeves et al., 2013), an additional nine studies meeting the criteria for consideration as part of the evidence supporting IPCP were located. The total number of studies (15) was still deemed too small and varied for meta-analyses or generalizations. None of the studies compared an interprofessional model of care delivery to the usual model of intraprofessional care, nor did they assess the process of interprofessional care.

In 2017, Reeves et al. completed a third Cochrane review of research on interprofessional collaboration. In this review, their aim was to look for studies that did compare usual care to IPCP intervention and used strong research designs (randomized controlled individual or cluster studies). Although the databases searches were extensive and included publications through 2017, only nine studies met the strict criteria for inclusion in this review. Five studies had been included in previous reviews, and four new studies were added. Again, the number was too small for a meta-analysis. While there was a trend to support the positive influence of IPCP on patient outcomes, the quality of the evidence was low. The trend of support for the positive influence of IPCP on patient/health outcomes and the practices examined in individual studies provides considerations for clinicians as they seek to improve practice delivery in selected settings and with defined populations.

Patient Outcomes in Early Reviews, 1999–2006 and 2006–2011

In five studies, patient outcomes were improved. Three studies focusing on diabetic populations found significant improvements in control of the diabetes (Barcelo et al., 2010; Janson et al., 2009; Taylor, Hepworth, Buerhaus, Dittus, & Speroff, 2007). Among emergency department patients, Campbell et al. (2001) found significant increases in the satisfaction of abused women, while Morey et al. (2002) reported a significant drop in clinical errors. Three studies reported significant improvements in professional behaviors: Helitzer et al. (2011) found increased patient-centeredness, Weaver et al. (2010) related improvements in briefings and information sharing among the team, and Young et al. (2005) cited improved team competencies.

Mixed results for patient outcomes were particularly evident in two studies. Rask et al. (2007) found no differences in fall rates among nursing home residents as a result of IPCP but did report a significant decrease in the use of restraints. Strasser et al. (2008) found that stroke patients who received IPCP care made significant functional gains but experienced no differences in lengths of stay. A third study found mixed results for professional behaviors (R. S. Thompson et al., 2000). Within the emergency department, professionals asked more frequently about domestic violence, but the identification of abuse cases was not increased. The final four studies in the review found no differences in patient satisfaction (Brown, Boles, Mullooly, & Levinson, 1999), adverse patient outcomes (Nielson et al., 2007), improved diabetic testing (Hanbury, Wallace, & Clark, 2009), or positive outcomes among depressed patients (C. Thompson et al., 2000).

Although a slight trend was seen for an increase in positive patient outcomes and professional behaviors following some intervention designed to increase the effectiveness of IPP, the reviewers concluded that the evidence was weak and recommended further research with stronger research designs (Reeves et al., 2013). Reviewers also recommended that steps be taken to examine the process and cost-effectiveness of IPP.

Cochrane 2017 Review

The third systematic review explored the question, Can strategies to improve interprofessional collaboration have a positive impact on the delivery of care to patients? (Reeves et al., 2017, p. 2). Only RCT studies were sought examining publications through November 2015. Five studies from previous reviews and four new studies meeting these stringent criteria were found. Again, the strength of the evidence was generally low, but the reviewers reported some clinically interesting findings. In eight of the studies, an IPP intervention was compared with traditional care.

Reeves et al. (2017) affirmed the observation that "the extent to which different health and social care professionals work well together affects the quality of the care that they provide" (p. 2). Specifically, evidence was found to support the positive influence of IPCP on patient functional status, providers' adherence to recommended practices, and the use of health-care resources. The fact that the forms of IPCP (IPP rounds, IPP meetings, and IP checklists) differ widely complicates the attribution of outcomes to IPCP.

The reviewers were encouraged by the increase in research seeking to measure efforts to improve IPCP and their practice outcomes. They recommend that, in future studies, sufficient time be given for the IPCP to be implemented prior to outcome evaluation and that outcome evaluation occurs over a more extended period of time.

Mitchell, Tieman, and Shelby-James Literature Review

Multidisciplinary (interprofessional) care as a potential moderator of the demands of chronically ill patients on the health system was the focus of five systematic reviews of literature from 1990 to 2006 conducted by Mitchell, Tieman, and Shelby-James (2008). Each review was limited to examining the integration, coordination, and "multidisciplinary" approaches designed to address the health needs associated with one of the following conditions: palliative care, diabetes, stroke, chronic obstructive pulmonary disease, and frail aging (Tieman et al., 2006). For this review, multidisciplinary care was defined as "professionals from a range of disciplines working together to deliver comprehensive care that addresses as many of the patient's health and other needs as possible" (Mitchell, Tieman, & Shelby-James, 2008, p. S61). The literature review was limited to Australia, the United Kingdom, New Zealand, Canada, the Netherlands, and Sweden. Key findings included some support for the positive influence of multidisciplinary care on patient outcomes, but this approach did not necessarily reduce costs. Authors stated, "Effectiveness and implications of system level multidisciplinary approaches and changes have yet to be fully determined" (Tieman et al., 2006, p. 1). Suggestions for further research were made, including the importance of examining both the multidisciplinary and team components of care.

Although the terms *multidisciplinary* and *interprofessional* have commonly been used interchangeably, interprofessional is currently the preferred designation, especially in the United States, to refer to the collaboration of various health professions. *Multidisciplinary* has been used to connote the collaboration of several medical specialties or the collaboration of health-related and non-health-related disciplines. Outside the United States, these terms may be used interchangeably.

Brandt, Lutfiyya, King, and Chioreso Scoping Review

Brandt, Lutfiyya, King, and Chioreso (2014) conducted a scoping review of IPE and IPCP literature from 2008 to 2014 to determine the impact of IPP on the Triple Aim of improving population health, controlling health-care costs, and improving patient outcomes and experience. A scoping review commonly precedes a systematic review and is designed to create a preliminary map of the evidence when the scope of the review is particularly broad. Such a review can help inform the research question for the systematic review.

From 1,176 articles focused on IPE or IPCP, only 133 research studies were found. Of these studies, 75% were conducted within countries having a national health system (much different from the United States), 55% reported a sample size of less than or equal to 50, and 43% focused on care provided by two to four professions. Only 16.5% of the papers included one of the Triple Aims as a study outcome, and 2% (or three papers) included two of the Triple Aims. Despite the fact that 83 studies focused on IPCP as opposed to IPE, none of the studies reviewed looked at the implications of IPCP on health-care costs. The research tended to focus on practice processes rather than outcomes, leading the reviewers to conclude that evidence supporting the belief that IPCP can serve as the catalyst for transforming the health-care system is insufficient. They recommend a research agenda employing a variety of rigorous methods, with Triple Aim outcomes as the dependent variables. Demographic and ecological variables would be examined as covariates to the independent variable of collaborative practice. They further recommend high-quality qualitative research to examine the health-care experience specific to different contexts.

Collective Findings

These reviews clarify that studies focused on IPP have largely examined the outcomes of educational programs designed to promote IPP without critically examining the effectiveness of interprofessional team care as a mediator of patient outcomes. Numerous studies used qualitative and descriptive designs and thus did not meet the rigor necessary for consideration as supporting evidence. Instead, they widen our understanding of the phenomenon of IPCP and the complex considerations that need to be addressed in more controlled studies.

Studies measuring patient outcomes frequently measured patient satisfaction due to the availability of valid and reliable measurement instruments and the accessibility of data collection. Unfortunately, satisfaction instruments are often of limited sensitivity, especially when satisfaction tends to be high, and thus fail to distinguish significantly between traditional and IP models of practice. On the other hand, cost-effectiveness research is more difficult to implement because it requires complex designs. This should not dissuade the practitioner, however, from a commitment to collecting outcome data routinely. At the same time, it is essential to attempt to describe the IPCP model as it is being implemented consistent with outcome data collection to provide future researchers with clues about salient process variables. Regardless of researchers' challenges in developing and evaluating the evidence for IPCP and regardless of practitioners' limitations in applying this evidence, the positive responses of both patients and providers to effective IPCP continue to support the interest in moving health care in this promising direction.

BRINGING TOGETHER RESEARCH AND PRACTICE

The optimization of IPCP in improving patient experience, population health, and cost reduction will require the shared collaboration of researchers and practitioners. RCT designs, the gold standard of evidence, are difficult to achieve in naturalistic settings, but appropriate comparisons can be achieved between traditional care and IPCP, as illustrated in a study by Underwood, Schuiling, and Slager (2003).

IPCP Model

Nurse midwives approached a researcher to help them measure the outcomes of their practice that integrated the professions of midwifery and perinatology. Before engaging in a review of practice outcomes, the nature of the practice was examined from a narrative perspective. Characteristics that exemplified IPCP were evident, including respect for each profession's unique and shared knowledge, trust, and practicing to each profession's full scope. Communication appeared effective, although this was not measured specifically in the context of application of team skills. Shared leadership was apparent as the midwife led the team for patients whose pregnancies and births followed expected patterns, gained the perinatologist's input relative to questions of risk, shared leadership in the presence of pattern deviation, and yielded leadership in the presence of significant complications. In more traditional maternity practices, when pregnancies and births become complicated, the primary provider (midwife or obstetrician) usually releases the care of the patient to the perinatologist. Within the model of IPCP the perinatologist assumed the leadership of the team in these instances, but the midwife remained very much involved in the holistic management of the patient.

Patient Outcomes

The care outcomes of the integrated practice model (IPM) were compared with those of traditional obstetric (TOB) care rendered by obstetricians delivering patients at the same community hospital. A retrospective chart review of mother and baby outcomes as well as an assessment of charges was conducted for all patients (n = 265) delivered within the IPM for a given year and compared to a sample of 347 randomly selected patients delivered through TOB care. The IPM patients were significantly younger, were more racially and ethnically diverse, had higher social risk factors (drugs, alcohol, low socioeconomic status), and experienced more pregnancy and birth complications. Nevertheless, mother and baby outcomes were as good or better than TOB patients and charges were comparable. The TOB patients had twice as many induced labors and significantly more elective cesarean sections ($X^2 = 9.6, p = .003$).

Although the design was not experimental and patient satisfaction was not measured, this study illustrates the ability to measure patient outcomes and at least one component of costs (charges). To transform health care, nurse practitioners must collect data to measure practice outcomes, including patient experience, population outcomes, and cost-effectiveness. In addition, examining and documenting the process of that practice, especially the characteristics of interprofessional collaboration so that appropriate comparisons can be made across practices, is equally important.

THE PROCESS OF IPCP

The effectiveness of IPCP likely accounts for at least some of the variance in the health outcomes achieved. Although few studies have systematically evaluated the process of IPCP, key components of practice efficacy have been widely discussed and barriers have been noted.

Evidence (Schadewaldt, McInnis, Hiller, & Gardner, 2013) from multiple studies of IPCP highlights the critical components of mutual respect; effective communication, including shared language; and a willingness to share power and team leadership based on the primacy of the patient's needs at the moment of care. At an organizational level, limited system change in implementing care models that support cost-effective collaboration, lack of role clarity, and competing visions work as barriers to effective IPCP. Best practices within organizations have been identified (Robert Wood Johnson Foundation [RWJF], 2015). At a global level, variations in scopes of practice and regulatory policies, inequities in reimbursement, professional education that lacks opportunities for meaningful collaborative experiences, and limited exemplars of effective IPCP have been noted as creating obstacles for needed system change.

Facilitators and Barriers

Schadewaldt, McInnis, Hiller, and Gardner (2013) conducted an integrative review of studies from seven countries that focused on the process of collaboration between physicians and nurse practitioners in primary care, including perceived and measured barriers and facilitators. Quantitative, qualitative, and mixed-method studies were included among the final 27 studies published between 1990 and 2012 that met the review criteria. The majority of studies (n = 23) came from the United States, Canada, and the United Kingdom.

Component Identification

Five themes emerged in relation to facilitators of and barriers to collaboration. The most commonly identified barrier (in 56% of the studies) related to a lack of clarity about the nurse practitioner (NP) scope of practice. Lack of clarity led to lack of confidence in NPs' skills and perceived need to engage in supervision, which in turn was viewed as increasing the physician's workload. Mutual confidence in their partner's competence was seen to facilitate collaboration. Role clarity and mutual confidence were essential to recognizing the complementarity of each profession's skills as a basis for functioning as a team. Shared goals were also essential to effective collaboration; however, NPs and physicians did not always ascribe the same meaning to the term *collaboration*. NPs were more likely than physicians to view collaboration in a team sense consistent with IPP.

A second theme related to experience in working together. Physicians who had previously worked with NPs were quicker to achieve a level of trust important to effective collaboration. Three studies suggested that a period of 3 to 6 months working together was needed to support the development of an effective collaborative relationship (Faria, 2009; Legault et al., 2012; Long, McCann, McNight, & Bradley, 2004).

A third theme highlighted power inequities, including a hierarchical structure and limited reciprocity of referrals and consultations (Bailey, Jones, & Way, 2006; Long et al., 2004). Lack of reciprocity was identified as a barrier in nine of the studies reviewed. Although hierarchical power has been consistently identified as a barrier to collaboration, expectations regarding referral and consultation are not so clear due to differing definitions of these terms within and outside a team practice concept. One of the studies (Way, Jones, & Bushing, 2000) specifically indicated that an imbalance of referrals was viewed as evidence of a lack of shared care.

The fourth and fifth themes were traditional and related to legalities and economics. Many physicians studied viewed themselves as legally responsible for the NPs' practice, and an equal number mentioned effective communication as important to mitigating this concern. With regard to economics, many believed NPs were insufficiently reimbursed. Although regulatory and reimbursement issues vary internationally and can be addressed only at a wider systems level, these studies suggested that, at the level of individual practices, NPs and physicians are finding ways to work around them.

Review Limitations

A major limitation of this review was that responses of some NPs and physicians may have been a function of the regulatory context of the country in which the study was conducted. The greatest number of studies was from the United States (41%), however, with another 22% from Canada, which most closely parallels U.S. advanced practice nursing (APN) education. The methodologic quality of the studies also presented a caution, with more than half using qualitative designs. The importance of the review rests on the fact that it is the first integration of evidence coming specifically from NPs. Key findings highlighted the slow development of a collaborative interprofessional relationship and suggested that opportunities for such collaboration within educational programs may further the process.

Affirmation of Facilitators and Barriers

A U.S. study of NPs by Pogbosyan, Norful, and Martsolf (2017) using mixed methods affirmed the findings of the previous review. Effective NP-physician relationships are critical to effective teamwork and take time to develop. In collaborative practices, time and space must be given to allow for such interactions. Administrative and organizational support for NP practice are also important. Disparate access to organizational support, absent advocacy for the NP role, and limitations for actual collaboration are barriers to effective teamwork.

INTEGRATED MODEL OF PCIPCP

Achieving PCIPCP requires a commitment to change as well as an understanding of the complex factors involved at system, organizational, and team levels. It also necessitates an understanding of the differing demands of practice within temporary versus long-term teams. Figure 15-1 is intended to convey the dynamic nature of the interaction of provider and patient systems as they engage to promote health and increase satisfaction with care at the individual level. PCIPCP also has the potential to increase health and improve costs at population levels. NPs wishing to implement PCIPCP must recognize both the collective and individual action needed. Changes at system levels require political action, including the involvement of professional organizations and educational institutions. Although understanding the current status of regulations, standards, and reimbursement issues governing their practice is essential for NPs, they will be most directly involved in change at the level of the organization—whether it is a medical center or a primary-care clinic—and at the point of care.

Organizational Best Practices

In 2014, RWJF conducted a study of organizations involved in PCIPCP in an attempt to identify best practices. The organization was guided by a definition of interprofessional collaboration that is slightly more explicit than the one previously proposed:

> Effective interprofessional collaboration promotes the active participation of each discipline

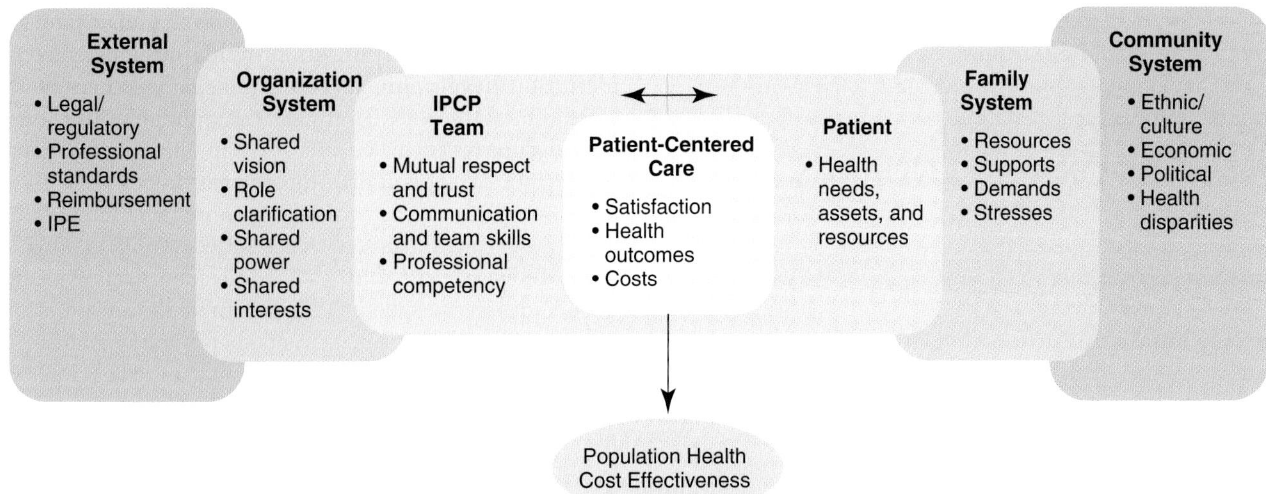

FIGURE 15–1 Model of Patient-Centered Interprofessional Collaborative Practice (PCIPCP) Depicting the Intersection of the Provider and Patient Systems.

in patient care, where all disciplines are working together and fully engaging patients and those who support them, and leadership on the team adapts based on patient needs.

Effective interprofessional collaboration enhances patient- and family-centered goals and values, provides mechanisms for continuous communication among caregivers, and optimizes participation in clinical decision-making within and across disciplines. It fosters respect for the disciplinary contributions of all professionals (RWJF, 2015, p. 1).

Twenty organizations, including hospitals and community health centers, were involved in interviews, and seven were interviewed on site to determine what supported PCIPCP and the outcomes of that practice. It is important to note that each site visited was at a different point in its journey to implement PCIPCP. From these interviews and site visits, six guiding principles for PCIPCP were extracted (RWJF, 2015, p. 3):

1. PCIPCP takes time to develop.
2. Relationships are the building blocks of effective teams.
3. Pockets of IPP already exist in most organizations that can spread.
4. The term *interprofessional collaboration* needs to be embedded in the culture.
5. Start small.
6. Creating a culture of interprofessional collaboration requires multiple reinforcing practices.

Evidence demonstrates that PCIPCP does not happen overnight, but seeing that a small group of committed providers can begin to spread the message with potentially dramatic results is encouraging. When patients feel that their providers are working collaboratively so they do not have to share their stories repeatedly and are not given conflicting information, they are more satisfied with their care. When their providers clearly communicate that the values and preferences of the patient are taken into account, patients may be more motivated to adhere to the mutually developed plan for health promotion. In their assessment of the 20 organizations, the RWJF team identified six promising practices contributing to the advance of PCIPCP (RWJF, 2015, p. 13):

1. Putting the patient first as an organizational vision and team level requirement.
2. Demonstrating leadership commitment to interprofessional collaboration as an organizational priority through words and actions.
3. Creating a level playing field that enables team members to work at the top of their license, know their roles, and understand the value they contribute. (This includes clarifying a shared language.)
4. Cultivating effective team communication.
5. Exploring the use of organizational structure to hardwire interprofessional practice.
6. Training different disciplines together so that they learn how to work together.

These promising practices include factors that are relevant at system, organizational, and team levels, but their individual and collective impact will need to be evaluated through future research.

REGULATIONS AND PROFESSIONAL STANDARDS

The *Consensus Model for APRN Regulation: Licensure, Accreditation, Certification and Education* (NCSBN, 2008) and *The Future of Nursing* report (IOM, 2010) are paving the way to reducing scope of practice issues with respect to advanced nursing practice. Major nursing organizations are collaborating with other health-care entities and foundations to advance the IOM recommendation that scope of practice barriers be removed to enable nurses to practice to the full extent of their education and training. A clear common vision, significant political ability, support from major funders such as RWJF, and collaboration with other health professions are essential to address regulations across state levels. Collaboration with consumer groups such as the American Association of Retired Persons (AARP), who argue in support of removing barriers to practice as a consumer access issue, is also important.

The involvement of NPs in regulatory change and the movement for regulatory consistency across states are critical. This involvement may include direct participation in advocacy activities by speaking with one voice or indirect participation by maintaining membership in one's professional or specialty practice organizations. It is essential that NPs keep up to date regarding the current state of practice regulations so that they can clarify their scopes of practice appropriately and maintain role parity within the interprofessional team.

REIMBURSEMENT EQUITY

PCIPCP increases the likelihood that care will be coordinated across sites and across the life span. Unfortunately, the involvement of several professions engaging in health promotion also creates problems with respect to health-care reimbursement. Traditionally, reimbursement has gone to the primary-care provider, most typically the physician in some form of fee for service. The Affordable Care Act (ACA) of 2010 authorized the Centers for Medicare and Medicaid Services (CMS) to develop new models of interprofessional team practice and payment reform.

It is anticipated that even as governmental regulatory and legislative modifications of health-care payment mechanisms evolve and even in light of reduced costs, reimbursement equity will continue to be a challenge. For example, the Missouri Quality Initiative (MOQI) responded to the CMS Innovation Center call to reduce avoidable hospitalizations among nursing facility residents by developing an IPP model with employed NPs. The MOQI IPP model was implemented in 16 nursing homes in urban areas in the Midwest. Over a 4-year period, hospitalizations were reduced by 40% for all causes and 58% for potentially avoidable causes (Rantz, Birtley, Fleshner, Crecelius, & Murray, 2017). The Medicare expenditures were similarly reduced by 34% and 45%, respectively. Unfortunately, regulations related to the timing of NP visits (before or after an initial physician visit) and the employment status of the NP (employed by the facility versus some type of primary practice) vastly complicate reimbursement.

In 2014, the Care Coordination Task Force, led by the American Nurses Association (ANA) and the American Academy of Nursing (AAN), began a review with the intent of recommending policies that would continue to support the pivotal role of nurses in care coordination. They used the definition of care coordination advanced by the National Quality Forum (NQF; 2014): "the deliberate synchronization of activities and information to improve health outcomes by ensuring that care recipients' and families' needs and preferences for health care and community services are met over time" (p. 2). This definition is consistent with PCIPCP. NQF's primary policy priority recommendation was that "payment should be expanded for consistency across all qualified health professionals delivering high-value care coordination activities" (Lamb et al., 2015, p. 523). The Task Force believed that achieving this policy would actualize an interprofessional workforce to address the needs of people with complex and chronic conditions. This recommendation is consistent with the Department of Health and Human Services' creation of a Health Care Payment Learning and Action Network through the CMS to spread value-based payment models.

IPE

The preparation of health professionals through a system of IPE does much to change the cultural perspective of those entering practice. Although components of IPE have existed since the 1960s, its systematic inclusion as a curricular requirement is more recent, and programs vary widely. Although IPEC has set forward the standards for IPE, it is essential that the implementation of PCIPCP models increase and that educators and practitioners need to collaborate in the planned inclusion of health professions students.

In 2012, with a grant from the Health Resources and Services Administration (HRSA), the National Center for

Interprofessional Practice and Education (NCIPE) was established at the University of Minnesota as a nexus for the development of IPE and IPCP. Additional funding from the Josiah Macy Jr. Foundation, RWJF, the Gordon and Betty Moore Foundation, and the John A. Hartford Foundation has accelerated the development of teamwork and collaboration among the health professions.

Farrell, Payne, and Heye (2015) argue that, from the perspective of NP education, effective IPCP requires an "interprofessional mindset" that is best achieved by moving away from the siloed approach to an inclusion of IPP within the socialization to advanced practice roles. A number of innovative IPE programs are being tested within initial NP education and as fellowships following master's programs.

One example of a nurse practitioner's education program integrating IPE is the collaboration of NP and dental students within the context of a dental clinic (Victoroff et al., 2014). The Collaborative Home for Oral Health, Medical Review, and Health Promotion (CHOMP) provides an opportunity for IPCP in serving an underserved population in the Oral Medicine and Admitting Clinic and the Pediatric Dentistry Clinic. The students collaborate in obtaining a health history, and the NP performs a limited physical examination. The students huddle with their faculty preceptors and then offer needed dental and health promotion services (immunizations, basic diagnostic tests, health promotion, and preventive education). The CHOMP program provides meaningful collaborative practice opportunities that may set the stage for future collaboration within structures such as medical homes.

An example of a NP program following a master's program is the Primary Care ANP Interprofessional Fellowship offered by the West Haven Veterans Administration (VA) facility, which is one of the VA Centers of Excellence in Primary Care. The fellowship was designed to provide postgraduate clinical training, "form interprofessional practice partnerships with physician trainees, and establish a collaborative interprofessional team-based primary care model" (Zapatka, Conelius, Edwards, Meyer, & Brienza, 2014, p. 378). Fellows joined teams of one physician, one NP, three interns, one RN, and a health-care technician. The program was built on four educational domains: shared decision making; interprofessional collaboration; performance improvement; and sustained relationships to achieve patient-centered, continuous, comprehensive, coordinated care for veterans. Evaluation of the program indicated that it was effective in bridging into professional practice, expanding an appreciation of health professionals' roles, and developing a commitment to interprofessional teamwork.

Meaningful clinical IPCP opportunities as part of the education of health-care professionals would be expected to establish a cultural perspective and skills to support IPCP. Consistent with Schadewaldt et al.'s (2013) integrative review, opportunities for physicians to work with NPs, even within an educational program, would help to build respect and confidence in competence, which are essential for forming a future collaborative practice.

ORGANIZATIONAL VARIABLES

The factors discussed in the following subsections have an impact on the implementation of IPCP at an organizational level.

Lack of Shared Vision

Pohl, Hanson, Newland, and Cronenwett (2010) view lack of a shared vision as the major barrier to effective and efficient IPP. In their analysis of NPs' potential to deliver primary care and lead teams, they reflect that, although much overlap in roles and scopes of practice exists among primary-care providers (NPs, physician assistants [PAs], and physicians), conflicting drivers relative to costs and leadership may stand in the way of achieving a common vision of patient-centered care. Achieving a shared vision at the care organization level is facilitated when professional organizations and key stakeholders, such as IOM/Academy of Medicine, RWJF, and the Josiah Macy Jr. Foundation, hold a common definition of PCIPCP.

Role Clarification

Although professional role dimensions and limits are set by regulatory and professional standards, roles need to be clarified to achieve optimal efficiency within care institutions and to achieve care delivery that avoids inappropriate duplication within the organization. The various health-care professions have unique as well as common knowledge. The goal in role clarification is not to create cross-trained professionals but to emphasize the unique and essential contributions of each profession in collaborating with patients to address their complex health needs. It also acknowledges the shared roles and knowledge in relation to health promotion.

Role clarification requires that all professionals are comfortable with their limitations and knowledgeable about other professionals' roles. For example, primary-care physicians and NPs have much shared knowledge to bring to the management of chronically ill populations. Acknowledgment of what physicians offer in relation to management of acute exacerbations of a chronic condition or when complexity and risk are magnified is as important as respecting the special efficacy of NPs in educating and motivating clients and helping them to mobilize support to address their needs from a holistic perspective.

Shared Leadership

A consistent barrier to IPP across studies is a culture in which the physician is automatically the head of the care team. As Pohl et al. (2010) suggest, this often translates into physician-centric language, which extends the barrier to IPP. A culture shift at the organizational level that supports shared leadership is one of the key factors in promoting IPP. This shift may be supported through system-level perspectives such as the Canadian Interprofessional Health Collaborative (CHIC, 2010) model, which includes collaborative leadership as one of its core competencies, the ACA requirement for patient evaluation of both physicians and nurses as a component of reimbursement, and the VA (2010) Centers for Excellence in Primary Care initiative. The purpose of this last initiative is to "foster transformation of clinical education by preparing graduates of health professional programs to work in and lead patient-centered interprofessional teams . . ." (VA, 2010, p. 1). The strongest driver for shared leadership, however, may come from the organizational adoption of a vision of patient-centered care that can transcend multidisciplinary competition.

TEAM FACTORS

At the level of the health-care team, the professional and personal relationships among team members become critical in influencing outcomes. Although the organizational context helps to set the stage for building trust when common values are acknowledged and professional identities are not threatened, the coupling of mutual respect and actual team skills in working with clients and families accounts for effectiveness that can achieve the Triple Aim.

Mutual Respect and Trust

Mutual respect is consistently identified as a core requisite for effective team function. It is facilitated by organizational structures that provide an opportunity for the various professions to learn about each other's roles, are clear in role expectations and responsibilities, and value the unique contributions of each profession. Tubbesing and Chen (2015) performed a qualitative key informant assessment of nine exemplary IPP sites in the University of Washington Medical Center system and found that mutual respect and coordination of care were the primary themes that emerged. Because mutual respect and trust may take time to build, the application of team skills may provide a compensatory advantage in the short term.

Team Skills

Communication and shared language, coordination, cooperation, and conflict resolution are critical team skills in this context. Interprofessional teams may include a constant set of providers delivering care to a designated population or teams that are formed and re-formed from a slightly larger range of providers, such as occurs within a perioperative or emergency department. However teams are defined and described, all team members must share a common language and possess common skills to optimize the function of the team and health outcome achievement. Differences in language that are unrecognized or not addressed create a barrier to achieving desired outcomes.

Language differences are often hidden when two or more professions use the same term but with dissimilar meanings. For example, NPs and physicians may both advocate "sharing," but the NP may mean "exchanging ideas about patient management," whereas the physician may mean "sharing patients" (Schadewaldt et al., 2013, p. 7). Similarly, working together may mean providing advice on the physician's part, while the NP may mean engaging in a reciprocal discussion (Schadewaldt et al., 2013, p. 7). Failure to come to consensus early in any team's formation regarding the meaning of commonly used terms will only compound problems later.

TeamSTEPPS

The Department of Defense and the Agency for Healthcare, Research, and Quality (AHRQ) have collaborated in developing an evidence-based set of skills that are critical to the effective functioning of health-care teams. These team strategies and tools to enhance performance and patient safety are called TeamSTEPPS, and they are available online and through TeamSTEPPS training programs. They include four key principles: leadership, situation monitoring, mutual support, and communication (see Table 15-1). As health-care professionals develop team skills, mutual trust will be enhanced, and they become more likely to achieve a shared mental model and quality care. A shared mental model is a common understanding about the situation and team processes and roles; it is achieved through effective communication (Cannon-Bowers, Tannenbaum, Salas, & Volpe, 1995). It is the hallmark of effective teams and thus a characteristic of effective IPCP.

Table 15-1 Key Principles of TeamSTEPPS

Principle	Definition
Leadership	Coordinating the activities of the team by ensuring that team actions are understood, changes in information are shared, and team members have the necessary resources.
Situation monitoring	Scanning and assessing situational elements to gain information, understanding, or maintain awareness to support team functioning.
Mutual support	Anticipating and supporting other team members' needs through accurate knowledge about their responsibilities and workload.
Communication	Exchanging information among team members clearly and accurately.

Edmondson (2012) has written about "teamwork on the fly," which is especially appropriate to the health-care arena. She describes five behaviors that are critical to successful teaming:

- Speaking up (communicating honestly and directly)
- Experimenting (taking an iterative approach in planning)
- Reflecting (observing, questioning, and discussing processes and outcomes)
- Listening intently (working hard to understand others)
- Integrating (synthesizing different points of view)

These behaviors capture many of the components of TeamSTEPPS (AHRQ, 2010) and help to achieve what Gordon, Mendenhall, and O'Connor (2012) term "team intelligence," which is "the active capacity of individual members of a team to learn, teach, communicate, reason, and think together, irrespective of position in any hierarchy, in the service of realizing shared goals and a shared mission" (p. 10).

PCIPCP CASE STUDY

Health promotion and optimization initiatives ideally occur across the wellness/illness spectrum. Within primary-care settings, these initiatives are still largely intraprofessional, with physicians, NPs, or PAs acting as primary-care providers who consult with specialists as needed. Although this mode of practice makes it easier to address reimbursement issues, it affords limited opportunity to consider how comorbidities and the individual complexity of the patient may be addressed simultaneously rather than adhering to the standard of practice for a single issue. PCIPCP may offer advantages in planning care for patients with complex health issues and modifying those plans when significant health disruptions occur. The primary provider may retain leadership of the team across disruptions, or leadership may shift temporarily according to the nature of the problem. Because these disruptions may result in trips to an emergency department or require hospitalization, IPCP approaches to health promotion have evolved to a greater extent in these settings, but they are finding increasing adoption in accountable care organizations (ACOs), nurse-managed centers (NMCs), patient-centered medical homes (PCMHs), and Veterans Administration system clinics.

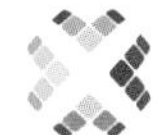

Case Illustration

A primary-care physician is retiring and refers his patients to an office with four primary-care physicians and two Adult NPs (ANPs). The patients are being reassigned to the ANPs because the ANPs are newer to the practice and currently have lower caseloads. JL, a 64-year-old single white male, is one of the patients who will be assigned to an ANP.

JL has an appointment to discuss his concerns about a cough that has persisted for more than three months and that makes it difficult for him to sleep at night. He complains of shortness of breath when awake. Antibiotics and cough medicine have not helped. "His heart aches," and he is so tired that he cannot keep up with his job as a sales manager for four states because it requires long-distance driving Monday through Friday. This has forced him to take a medical leave, and he is being pressured into early retirement.

As an older teen/young adult, JL had abused drugs and alcohol but was able to overcome this "with the help of God" and self-discipline. He continued to be a heavy smoker but has not smoked in the past 12 years. He has some arthritis and frequent lower back pain. Because of his history of drug abuse, he avoids analgesics and sees a chiropractor. JL also has type II diabetes severe enough to require insulin. He monitors his glucose levels closely and controls his blood sugar level with daily injections of a long-lasting insulin that is not currently covered by his health insurance. He states that he attempts to eat a healthy diet.

JL sees a cardiologist for hypertension and follow-up for a prior mild myocardial infarction. He takes numerous medications, including digoxin, a statin, a beta-blocker, an anticoagulant, and an ACE inhibitor.

JL is a staunchly independent man living alone, having divorced 25 years ago. Proximate social support is limited because he has made few geographically close relationships due to traveling throughout the week. Three neighbors, one younger and two older, offer some support. An elderly mother and two younger brothers live more than 900 miles (close to 15 hours) away. He is estranged from his 30-year-old daughter, whom he has not seen in two years.

During the physical assessment, premature ventricular contractions are noted along with rales/rhonchi in the right lower lobe of the lung. Blood pressure appears controlled, although JL complains of occasional dizziness on standing (possible orthostatic hypotension). In response to questioning, JL complains of urinary hesitancy but states that his previous physician told him not to worry as it was simply a sign of aging.

JL maintains that he "knows his body" and wants to be involved in all care decisions. He is intelligent but of limited health literacy and prefers to get information from the internet. He does not have the energy to do much reading. He is very private about most things, does not accept help readily, and does not want outsiders coming to his house. He is very persistent in maintaining his usual way of doing things, including sleeping in his second-floor bedroom, even though accessing it is increasingly difficult.

PCIPCP Reflection

The case illustration about JL is complex from physiologic, psychologic, and social/environmental perspectives. Table 15-2 highlights just a few of the challenges that can occur when several providers are involved in a patient's care and reflects on how they might be ameliorated through PCIPCP. For example, PCIPCP could have helped control JL's growing stress related to the persistent health challenges and changing financial/work status through consistent, clear communications and the opportunity to develop an individualized health promotion plan. It was critical for this patient that he

Table 15-2 PCIPCP for JL in a Primary-Care Setting

Traditional Care	Outcome	Potential PCIPCP	Potential Outcome
Communication among the specialty doctors and primary-care provider was limited to referrals to a specialist, who assumed at least temporary responsibility for a designated health problem, and formal notes from consulting specialists to the primary-care provider detailing the treatment that was administered. The cardiologist has managed anything cardiac-related, and the primary-care provider has assumed responsibility for health promotion, treatment of the diabetes, and any other emerging health problems.	Care fragmentation. Delayed diagnosis of a potentially worsening cardiac situation. Primary emphasis on pharmacologic strategies to manage health deviations. Missed opportunities to engage the patient in proactive self-care strategies.	Collaborative planning for the ongoing management of JL's care might have provided cohesion for the overall management plan, with a better understanding of each profession's sphere of expertise and what observed changes might have an impact on JL's total health and therefore should be shared. For example, the urinary hesitancy might be a by-product of the beta blocker, or it might be something that needed referral to a urologist. Collaboration among providers while engaging the patient in the decision making could potentiate the use of nonpharmacologic strategies for addressing hypertension and glucose management.	Increased patient engagement in appropriate self-care and symptom monitoring. Early diagnosis of alterations in health. Stabilization of health and avoidance of unnecessary hospitalizations or trips to the ER. Increased patient satisfaction due to increased health literacy and support of contribution to care decisions.

Table 15-2 PCIPCP for JL in a Primary-Care Setting—cont'd

Traditional Care	Outcome	Potential PCIPCP	Potential Outcome
		Consistency of communications with the patient can be enhanced, and strategies for increasing JL's health literacy could have been identified.	
The involvement of numerous medical specialists and other providers enhances the opportunities for conflicting communications.	JL at times felt caught in the middle when he received different information from his cardiologist and his primary-care provider (especially in the area of diet management). This increased his anxiety and stress, which had a negative effect on his functioning.	Brief team meetings can accommodate compromise in recommendations consistent with overall health issues (diet for cardiac improvement and glucose control). Enables team members to speak with a consistent voice.	Clear, consistent communication with the patient helps create a sense of control and decreases stress, which can optimize well-being even in situations that are largely outside anyone's control. While not quantifiable in the short-term, this may enhance patient adherence to a plan that he has contributed to developing.
Often providers are unaware of the costs of different drugs. Expectation that the patient will find the resources to pay for recommended treatment.	Consideration was not given to the cost of selected medications or treatments.	Involvement of a medical social worker in planning may contribute to the selection of affordable drugs and treatments. This also might help the patient as circumstances shift from medical leave to retirement. The cost of selected options and resources for payment could have been considered.	Collaborative planning with patient input when prescribed numerous medications can help achieve patient medication adherence and effectiveness and provide affordable choices or identification of financial resources. Holding appropriate expectations in the health situation and knowing what to do or who to call with symptom changes or questions can decrease costly readmissions. The following problems JL identified as important might have been addressed more effectively: 1. Management of his back pain. 2. Managing the cost of his medications beyond what insurance would pay. 3. Being able to get adequate sleep.

have some idea of what to expect in his current health situation, how to manage his health, and who to call if he was unable to manage his health independently. It was also critical to consider both pharmacologic and nonpharmacologic strategies for symptom management within the context of his daily living situation.

One of the arguments against IPCP in primary-care settings is the challenge of engaging providers in team conferences when they are geographically distant. Even when all the critical providers are in the same geographic location, they must overcome barriers of traditional power differentials and a lack of understanding of what each profession can contribute to an evolving plan of care. Relationship building is essential to the development of trust, but it cannot be achieved overnight.

An additional challenge is presented by the ad hoc nature of most teams. Team members may vary across specialties, leading to limited team cohesion. White, Eklund, McNeal, Hochhalter, and Arroliga (2018, pp. 380–381) discuss potential solutions to improve ad hoc team functioning, but team members must value IPCP and make a commitment to its implementation. Even with this commitment, communication problems often create barriers to its achievement and result in inconsistent communications among team members and with the patient. Use of shared terminology; clear and concise statements; and predictable formats such as situation, background, assessment, and recommendations (SBAR) can enhance the building of shared expectations and team rapport.

White et al. (2018) recommend looking at other team members while interacting to enhance comprehension by observing nonverbal communication. Technology increasingly overrides the argument against IPCP due to the difficulty in finding time to assemble in one place. Videoconferencing through third-party providers, Skype, or FaceTime provides options for engaging team members at different locations in a quick conference.

Another challenge of IPCP is that of leadership of the team. NPs are often ideal team leaders or co-leaders because of their holistic perspective not only in the moment but across the trajectory of care. Within an IPCP perspective, leadership doesn't mean simply providing recommendations; it also means bringing all critical voices to the table, including those of the patient and his or her family and making sure they are heard, facilitating the development of an evolving plan, and deciding which team members are most appropriate to address specific patient issues. Although management of what providers view as the major health problem/diagnosis is critical, addressing the problems that the patient views as most important is essential to promoting long-term positive health outcomes.

OPPORTUNITIES FOR IPCP BY NPS

As NPs enter practice, consideration of the factors that influence PCIPCP may be useful in identifying or selecting preferred practice options. Peterson, Phillips, Puffer, Bazemore, and Petterson (2013) estimate that 50% of physician primary-care practices include APNs as part of their team. NPs increasingly join or lead patient care teams within acute-care settings. Practice options are also expanding within primary settings to include more NPs starting their own NMCs and joining PCMHs and ACOs. The opportunity to practice collaboratively, however, does not mean that PCIPCP is reaching a desired level of efficacy. The NP must assess the practice and use leadership and change skills to engage other professionals in practice improvement.

Role Opportunities in Acute-Care Settings

NPs assume pivotal roles in interprofessional collaboration to promote health within acute- and primary-care settings. The three practice models most typically found within acute care are discussed here, with three roles at different stages of evolution within the acute-care setting. Being a member of an ongoing team and practicing with a specialty physician are clearly collaborative. Managing a panel of patients is more independent. NPs in this last role have to work to maintain a vision of IPCP.

Member of an Ongoing Team

In this role, the NP provides care for a group of patients, such as the groups one usually finds in an intensive care unit (ICU). These teams tend to be led by the physician but are truly interprofessional. NPs provide valued input and may be responsible for the handoff of patients who are transferred out of the unit.

Manager of a Patient Panel

In this model, ACNPs manage a panel of patients on non-ICUs in the place of interns and residents. Whether the practice is interprofessional or whether the NP is simply replacing the physician model or assuming an expanded primary nurse function depends on the commitment of the NP to interprofessional collaborative care. Within a PCIPCP vision, the NP can have a major impact on the coordination of care within the hospital and the transitions of care as the patient moves across settings. NPs leading PCIPCP teams can put systems of care in place to reduce readmissions of chronically ill patients that most frequently occur within the 30-day postdischarge period.

The value of this role was supported in a mixed-methods study by Van Soeren, Hurlock-Chorostecki, and Reeves (2011), who examined the role of NPs within the acute-care setting of nine Ontario, Canada, hospitals. Specifically, they focused on "how NPs contribute to enhancing patient care through enactment of their profession-specific role and how they collaborate with colleagues to deliver improved interprofessional care" (p. 245). A purposive sample of 46 practitioners was selected, representing 10% of NPs employed within the nine hospitals. Focus groups included 243 interprofessional colleagues. Quantitative data supported the major role components of patient-focused clinical practice and consultation. Qualitative comments revealed that NPs were valued for their advanced patient knowledge and approachability and "contributed to improvements in patient safety through their capacity to augment care delivery" (p. 248). The majority of NP consultations were with physicians and other nurses who enhanced IPP through collaboration, often assuming responsibility for debriefing the patient care team. In fact, they were seen as the glue that brought the team together. Although it was clear from this study that the NPs were engaged in interprofessional teamwork, the outcomes of this practice were not measured.

Collaborative Practice with a Specialty Physician

A third role that finds NPs functioning within an interprofessional team in the acute-care setting emerges when the NP is in a collaborative practice with a specialty physician. As patients are admitted to the acute-care setting for surgery or to address a major exacerbation of a chronic condition, the team follows the patient and has a major role in planning for transitions of care.

ACO

In some ways the third acute care role is similar to that afforded by an ACO in the care provision across the continuum. Although the term *ACO* was not coined until 2006, it was one of the strategies included in the 2010 ACA. The hallmark of ACOs is the provision of coordinated care to Medicare patients by teams of providers (including hospitals, physicians, and NPs) who assume responsibility for measurably improving health outcomes while reducing the cost of care for a designated population. CMS defines ACOs as "an organization of healthcare providers that agrees to be accountable for the quality, cost, and overall care of Medicare beneficiaries who are enrolled in the traditional fee for service program who are assigned to it" (CMS, 2015).

ACOs are built on three principles:

1. Provider-led organizations with a strong base of primary care that are collectively accountable for quality and total per capita costs across the full continuum of care for a population of patients.
2. Payments linked to quality improvements that also reduce overall costs.
3. Reliable and progressively more sophisticated performance measurement, to support improvement and provide confidence that savings are achieved through improvements in care (McClellan, McKethan, Lewis, Roski, & Fisher, 2010).

The emphasis on teamwork and coordination of care fosters but does not guarantee a vision of IPCP.

Patient-Centered Medical Homes

Also within the primary-care setting, NPs are increasingly welcomed as part of a PCMH, one of the newer models of organizing primary care to achieve the Triple Aim (Berwick, Nolan, & Whittington, 2008) through the involvement of a variety of professions. Reynolds et al. (2015) suggest that the PCMH is designed to "deliver the right care for patients, by the right professional, at the right time, in the right setting, for the right cost" (p. 1013). Whether this model provides interprofessional care or simply "one-stop shopping" depends on the collaborative involvement of various professionals in planning and revising care for patients across the life span. The Commonwealth Fund *Health Care Quality Survey* of 2006 suggested that having a medical home is particularly useful in improving health for vulnerable populations and in addressing racial and ethnic disparities (Beal, Doty, Hernandez, Shea, & Davis, 2007). For the purposes of the survey, a medical home was defined as a setting that provides patients with "timely, well-organized care and enhanced access to providers." Concerted effort has to be made when implementing a PCMH to avoid the criticism that too often it is physician-centric and physician-led (Pohl et al., 2010).

NMC

A final opportunity for NPs to engage in interprofessional health promotion is through the NMC. Sutter-Barrett, Sutter-Dalrymple, and Dickman (2015) describe a hybrid NMC that uses the Bridge Care model to deliver interprofessional care (nursing, medicine, social work, psychology, and nutrition) to low-income and underserved populations. Free care is provided on a temporary basis to individuals who do not have a medical home. The sustainability of this model is enhanced by community partnerships and referrals, affiliation with an academic school of nursing where part of the teaching load of nurse practitioner faculty is practice at the NMC, and early and ongoing evaluation that informs modifications and provides a basis for dissemination of clinic successes. The community participation and academic resources are key in supplementing fundraising and external grant acquisition. In addition to addressing a significant gap in health care, the Bridge Model clinics provide valuable clinical sites for the education of health professionals within the IPP model.

Considerations in Joining or Starting a PCIPCP

As mentioned, although a number of practice opportunities for NPs committed to PCIPCP exist, simple inclusion of providers from several professions does not guarantee that the practice is interprofessional or collaborative. PCMHs, for example, may simply represent the same geographical location of professionals to whom the patient may be referred according to the primacy of the health concern. Several areas to question in determining whether a particular practice fits the NP's expectations and education include vision and goals, evidence of PCIPCP processes, shared power, and reimbursement equity according to responsibility and experience (Table 15-3). Also important is making certain that physicians apply the same meaning to terms such as *collaboration*.

Planned change skills can be used to help move practice protocols in the direction of PCIPCP using strategies such as Kotter's stages of change model (Kotter & Rathgerber, 2005) or the IHI's Plan-Do-Study-Act (PDSA) system (see Table 15-4). In Kotter's model, eight

Table 15-3 Considerations in Joining or Starting a PCIPCP

Joining a PCIPCP	Starting a PCIPCP
1. What are the vision and goals for the practice? 2. What processes are evidence of IPCP versus parallel efforts of autonomous practitioners? 3. How consistent with your expectations is the NP role within the practice? 4. What evidence is there of shared leadership and shared power? 5. How equitable are reimbursement and salary policies? 6. Do team members define critical concepts, such as collaboration, in the same way?	1. Based on your targeted patient population, what professions should be collaborators within the practice? 2. What prior experiences have your proposed collaborators had working with a NP? 3. What IPE experiences have your proposed collaborators had? 4. Can they commit to a vision of PCIPCP? 5. What knowledge and experience do potential collaborators have in relation to team skills? 6. What strategies will need to be implemented to ensure a shared language?

Table 15-4 Useful Resources for Implementing PCIPCP

Name of Organization or Skill Set	Description	Web Site
Agency for Healthcare, Research and Quality	AHRQ's Patient-Centered Medical Home Resource Center includes both evidence and evaluation, as well as tools for implementation. Under the latter area, there is an excellent guide for creating patient-centered team-based primary care.	https://pcmh.ahrq.gov/page/creating-patient-centered-team-based-primary-care
Institute for Healthcare Improvement	Home site for Institute for Healthcare Improvement includes Web-based training related to the Triple Aim and the Plan-Do-Study-Act model to evaluate changes to improve health outcomes and other available programs and tools to improve the quality and safety of health care.	www.ihi.org
National Center for IPP and IPE	NEXUS is the home for the organization that "leads, coordinates and studies the advancement of collaborative, team-based health professions education and patient care" to improve quality, outcomes, and cost of care. Data depository for projects evaluating IPP, measurement tools, publications, implementation tools, and other resources.	www.nexusipe.org
TeamSTEPPS Training	The home site within AHRQ for access to information and free materials related to the TeamSTEPPS training.	www.teamstepps.ahrq.gov
TeamSTEPPS Implementation	Site includes all the guidelines and materials for implementing TeamSTEPPS in healthcare organizations	https://www.ahrq.gov/teamstepps/instructor/essentials/implguide.html

stages of change may be clustered into three phases: setting the stage, deciding what to do, and making it stick. In the first phase, it is important to create a sense of urgency for the change and pull the team together. The second phase involves developing both the vision and strategies for the change, communicating with others to gain buy-in, empowering others to act, producing short-term wins, and (of critical importance) not letting up. In phase three, it is essential to create a new culture with the change integrated. For PCIPCP, this means making the mode of working together and with the patient/family a way of life.

Similar issues should be considered when NPs decide to start their own PCIPCP (see Table 15-3). A theme that presents across studies of IPE and IPCP implementation is the importance of resolving differences in culture and language among professions and clarifying roles at the onset of collaboration. There is a tendency to focus immediately on structure and procedures of practice because they are more tangible. Failure to clarify the less tangible issues of shared culture, goals, and language will only result in emerging barriers as new structures and procedures are implemented. The linchpin in efforts to achieve PCIPCP is open, ongoing, effective communication through which the valuing of all providers and the patient's input can be conveyed; roles, vision/goals, and language clarified; and conflicts resolved. The way may not be easy, but in all likelihood, it will lead to better patient outcomes and increased patient and provider satisfaction.

CONCLUSIONS

Foundations, policy makers, and many providers are committed to the concept of PCIPCP as a promising strategy to promote health and address the Triple Aim of health-care reform. ACA includes provisions that support innovations in health-care delivery and the role of APNs within new systems of care. Governmental entities (CMS, IHI, AHRQ, HRSA) are joined by private foundations in funding promising practices aimed at creating patient-centered care systems and tools to promote team skills and quality care improvements. Major health profession accrediting bodies have required the inclusion of IPE, and the National Center for IPP and IPE has been established.

Although evidence supports the efficacy of PCIPCP, its strength is limited by inadequate measurement of Triple Aim outcomes and the extant process of IPCP and the use of patient satisfaction measures with limited sensitivity. NPs practicing within PCIPCP systems must be conscious of the attributes of that practice and encourage the collection of data to document care effectiveness. Collaborating with researchers, who may help determine the salience of particular system variables on patient outcomes and design measures of cost-effectiveness, is also critical. Prerequisite to documenting processes and outcomes of PCIPCP care delivery, NPs must collaborate interprofessionally in clarifying the vision of PCIPCP and moving their practice toward the actualization of that vision. Table 15-4 highlights resources that may be useful for the implementation and evaluation of IPCP.

Even with the increasing support for PCIPCP among major health policy organizations and health professions and a growing body of evidence supporting achievement of desired health outcomes, NPs must be aware of the potential impact of predicted or actual disruptions to the healthcare system. A predicted disruption is the shortage of primary care physicians coupled with an increasing demand arising from legislation such as the Affordable Care Act. Auerbach, et al. (2013), conducted a study to forecast the need for physicians, NPs, and physician assistants (PA) in 2025, if newer delivery models of patient-centered medical home (PCMH) or nurse-managed center (NMC) were employed compared to the status quo. One of their conclusions was that the physician shortage could be ameliorated through the use of both PCMH and NMC. Their predictions seemed to support the team-based approach to care in the PCMH, particularly if the number of non-physician members of the team increased. Thus, responses to the physician shortage could serve to promote PCIPCP.

An actual health system disruption is exemplified by the Covid-19 pandemic of 2020. The grounding IPCP principles of mutual respect, shared vision, equity in power and responsibility, and effective communication were essential to achieving the best possible health outcomes for the population while retaining an efficiency of effort. An event of this magnitude required not just experts in infection control, virology, and epidemiology, but others who could address health in a more holistic way in order to incorporate considerations such as mental health and economics. Ideally, the guiding team also required input from the various populations affected so that solutions could be appropriately tailored and accepted. It was clear when the balance of input was present (health system integrity was maintained and appropriate attention was given to other major issues effecting health) and when it was not (infected patients were admitted to facilities housing the most vulnerable populations, some hospitals over capacity while others were underused, and virus-free patients with cardiac, renal, or cancer diagnoses going untreated). Hopefully, one of the outcomes of this challenge is the increased acceptance that the vision of IPCP holds the greatest promise in achieving this nation's desired health outcomes.

It is remarkable that in 2020 – the Year of the Nurse – nurses at all levels were so significantly challenged and recognized for their ability to address those challenges. Nurse practitioners can capitalize on this recognition by engaging in and documenting PCIPCP.

Commitment to PCIPCP strengthens the opportunities to practice to the NPs' full scope and highlights the major contribution that NPs can make to health promotion.

KEY POINTS

- PCIPCP can be defined as a process by which two or more professionals synergize their separate and shared knowledge and skills within a context of mutual respect to engage patients and their families fully in optimizing their health.
- The development of evidence regarding Triple Aim outcomes is challenging due to the complexity of the process of PCIPCP implementation across patient populations, care delivery settings, and focal health concerns and the need to employ strong research designs.
- Although the quality of evidence supporting the effectiveness of PCIPCP compared to traditional care is weak, promising trends support the positive influence of IPCP on patient outcomes.
- Effective IPCP must embody the concepts of effective team collaboration, whether implemented in the context of ad hoc or established teams.
- NPs practicing within PCIPCP systems must be able to delineate the specific attributes of team collaboration being implemented and encourage the collection of data to document care outcomes and effectiveness. This critical assessment and documentation must be ongoing and not just at points of designated care review.
- Commitment to PCIPCP requires the identification of potential barriers to that practice and development of plans to address them to maximize care quality and health promotion.
- Organizational best practices to promote IPCP include putting the patient first, leadership commitment to IPCP as an organizational priority, creating a level playing field, cultivating effective team communication, using organizational structure to hardwire IP practice, and training different professions together.

Check Your Understanding

1. The major difference between interprofessional teamwork and interprofessional team-based care is:
   A. Whether teams are ad hoc or ongoing
   B. The focus on process versus structure
   C. Whether the teams have an identity
   D. There is none: the terms may be used interchangeably.
2. All of the following facilitate effective team functioning *except*:
   A. Mutual trust among members
   B. Clarity of role delineation
   C. Consistent team leader for each patient
   D. Practice of team skills by members
3. Developing evidence to support the effectiveness of PCIPCP in enhancing patient outcomes and Triple Aim achievement is most challenging due to the:
   A. Frequent use of qualitative research and the limitations in sample sizes
   B. Need to restrict research to the use of RCT, controlled before and after (CBA), and time series designs
   C. Challenges in measuring the process of IPCP as a mediator of patient outcomes and complexity of cost-effectiveness research
   D. Limitations in randomly assigning patients to different delivery modes and the frequent use of patient satisfaction as the outcome measure
4. The most critical question to answer in joining a PCIPCP is:
   A. What are the vision and goals for the practice?
   B. Is the salary the same for physicians and NPs?
   C. How is time allotted for visits determined?
   D. What professions are included on the team?
5. The most frequently documented barrier to IPCP is the:
   A. Time to communicate among team members
   B. Challenges in working out reimbursement issues
   C. Increased workloads for team members
   D. Lack of understanding about the NP's scope of practice

See "Reflections on Check Your Understanding" at the end of the book for answers.

REFERENCES

Agency for Healthcare Research and Quality. (2010). *TeamSTEPPS* (AHRQ Publication No. 06-0020-2). Washington, DC: Author.

Auerbach, D. I., Chen, P. G., Friedburg, M. W., Reid, R., Lau, C., Buerhaus, P. I., & Mehrotra,A. (2013). Nurse-managed health centers and patient-centered medical homes could mitigate expected primary care physician shortage. *Health Affairs, 32*. Retrieved from: https://doi.org/10.1377/hlthaff.2013.0596

Bailey, P., Jones, L., & Way, D. (2006). Family physician/nurse practitioner: Stories of collaboration. *Journal of Advanced Nursing, 53*, 381–391. doi:10.1111/j. 1365-2648.2006.03734.x

Barcelo, A., Cafiero, E., de Boer, M., Mesa, A. E., Lopez, M. G., Jimenez, R. A., . . . Robles, S. (2010). Using collaborative learning to improve diabetes care and outcomes: The VIDA project. *Primary Care Diabetes, 4*(13), 145–153. doi:10.1016/j.pcd.2010.04.005

Beal, A. C., Doty, M. M., Hernandez, S. E., Shea, K. K., & Davis, K. (2007). *Closing the divide: How medical homes promote equity in health care—results from the Commonwealth Fund 2006 Health Care Quality Survey*. Retrieved from http://www.commonwealthfund.org

Berwick, D. M, Noland, T. W., & Whittington, J. (2008). The Triple Aim: Care, health, and costs. *Health Affairs, 27*, 759–769.

Brandt, B., Lutfiyya, M. N., King, J. A., & Chioreso, C. (2014). A scoping review of interprofessional collaborative practice and education using the lens of the Triple Aim. *Journal of Interprofessional Care, 28*, 393–399. doi:10.3109/13561820.2014.906391

Brown, J. B., Boles, M., Mullooly, J. P., & Levinson, W. (1999). Effect of clinical communication skills training on patient satisfaction: A randomized controlled trial. *Annals of Internal Medicine, 131*, 822–829.

Campbell, J. C., Coben, J. H., McLoughlin, E., Dearwater, S., Nah, G., Glass, N., . . . Durborow, N. (2001). An evaluation of a system-change training model to improve emergency department response to battered women. *Academic Emergency Medicine, 8*, 131–138.

Canadian Interprofessional Health Collaborative. (2010). *A national interprofessional competency framework*. Retrieved from www.chic.ca

Cannon-Bowers, J. A., Tannenbaum, S. I., Salas, E., & Volpe, C. E. (1995). Defining competencies and establishing team training requirements. In R. A. Guzzo, E. Salas, and Associates (Eds.). *Team effectiveness and decision making in organizations*. San Francisco, CA: Jossey-Bass.

Center for Medicare and Medicaid Services. (2015). Accountable Care Organizations. Retrieved from https://www.cms.gov/aco

Earnest, M., & Brandt, B. (2014). Aligning practice redesign and interprofessional education to advance Triple Aim outcomes. *Journal of Interprofessional Care, 28*, 497–500. doi:10.3109/13561820.2014.933650

Edmondson, A. C. (2012, April). Teamwork on the fly: How to master the new art of teaming. *Harvard Business Review*, 72–80. Retrieved from http://www.hbr.org/2012/04/teamwork-on-the-fly-2

Faria, C. (2009). *Nurse practitioner perceptions and experiences of interprofessional collaboration with physicians in primary health care settings*. Master's thesis, Queen's University, Kingston, Ontario, Canada.

Farrell, K., Payne, C., & Heye, M. (2015). Integrating professional collaboration skills into the advanced practice registered nurse socialization process. *Journal of Professional Nursing, 31*, 5–10.

Fox, A., & Reeves, S. (2015). Interprofessional collaborative patient-centered care: A critical exploration of two related discourses. *Journal of Interprofessional Care, 29*, 113–118. doi:10.3109/13561820.2014.954284

Freeth, D., Hammick, M., Reeves, S., Koppel, I., & Barr, H. (2005). *Effective interprofessional education: Development, delivery, & evaluation*. Oxford, UK: Blackwell.

Gordon, S., Mendenhall, P., & O'Connor, B. B. (2012). *Beyond the checklist: What else health care can learn from aviation teamwork and safety*. Ithaca, NY: IRL Press.

Hanbury, A., Wallace, L., & Clark, M. (2009). Use of a time series design to test effectiveness of a theory-based intervention targeting adherence of health professionals to a clinical guideline. *British Journal of Health Psychology, 14*, 505–518.

Helitzer, D. L., Lanoue, M., Wilson, B., de Hernandez, B. U., Warner, T., & Roter, D. (2011). A randomized controlled trial of communication training with primary care providers to improve patient-centeredness and health risk communication. *Patient Education & Counseling, 82*, 21–29.

Herbert, C. (2005). Changing the culture: Interprofessional education for collaborative patient- centered practice in Canada. *Journal of Interprofessional Care, Supplement 1*, 1–4.

Institute of Medicine. Committee on Quality of Health Care in America. (2000). *To err is human: Building a safer health system*. Washington, DC: National Academy Press.

Institute of Medicine. Committee on Quality of Health Care in America. (2001). *Crossing the quality chasm: A new health system for the 21st century*. Washington, DC: National Academy Press.

Institute of Medicine. (2010). *The future of nursing: Leading change, advancing health*. Retrieved from http://books.nap.edu/openbook.php?record_id=12956&page=R1

Interprofessional Education Collaborative Expert Panel. (2011). *Core competencies for interprofessional collaborative practice: Report of an expert panel*. Washington, DC: IPEC.

Janson, S. L., Cooke, M., McGrath, K. W., Kroon, L. A., Robinson, S., & Baron, R. B. (2009). Improving chronic care of type 2 diabetes using teams of interprofessional learners. *Academic Medicine, 84*, 1540–1548.

Kotter, J., & Rathgerber, H. (2005). *Our iceberg is melting*. New York: St. Martin's Press.

Lamb, G., Newhouse, R., Beverly, C., Cropley, S., Kurtzman, E., Rantz, M., . . . Peterson, C. (2015). Policy agenda for nurse-led care coordination. *Nursing Outlook, 63*, 521–530.

Legault, F., Humbert, J., Amos, S., Hogg, W., Ward, N., Dahrouge, S., & Ziebell, L. (2012). Difficulties encountered in collaborative care: Logistics trumps desire. *Journal of the American Board of Family Medicine, 25*, 168–176.

Long, A., McCann, S., McNight, A., & Bradley, T. (2004). Has the introduction of nurse practitioners changed the working patterns of primary care teams? A qualitative study. *Primary Health Care Research & Development, 5*(1), 28–39.

Masterson, A. (2002). Cross-boundary working: A macro-political analysis of the impact on professional roles. *Journal of Clinical Nursing, 11*, 331–339.

McClellan, M., McKethan, A. N., Lewis, J. L., Roski, J., & Fisher, E. S. (2010). A national strategy to put Accountable Care into practice. *Health Affairs, 29*, 982–990. doi:10.1377/hlthaff.2010.0194

Mitchel, G. K., Tieman, J. J., & Shelby-James, T. M. (2008). Multidisciplinary care planning and teamwork in primary care. *Medical Journal of Australia, 188*(8), S61-64.

Morey, J. C., Simon, R., Jay, G. D., Wears, R. I., Salisbury, M., Dukes, K. A., & Berns, S. D. (2002). Error reduction and performance improvement in the emergency department through formal teamwork training: Evaluation results of the MedTeams project. *Health Services Research, 37*, 1553–1581.

National Council of State Boards of Nursing. (2008). *Consensus model for APRN regulation: Licensure, accreditation, certification, and education.* Retrieved from http://www.ncsbn.org/Consensus_Model_for_APRN_Regulation_July_2008.pdf

National Quality Forum. (2014). *Priority setting for healthcare performance measurement: Addressing performance measurement gaps in care coordination.* Retrieved from http://www.qualityforum.org/Publications/2014/08/Priority_Setting_for_Healthcare_Performance_Measurement_Addressing_Performance_Measure_Gaps_in_Care_Coordination

Nielson, P. E., Goldman, M. B., Mann, S., Shapiro, D. E., Marcus, R. G., Pratt, S. D., . . . Sachs, B. P. (2007). Effectiveness of teamwork training on adverse outcomes and process of care in labor and delivery: A randomized controlled trial. *Obstetrics & Gynecology, 109*, 48–55.

Peterson, L. E., Phillips, R. L., Puffer, J. C., Bazemore, A., & Petterson, S. (2013). Most family physicians work routinely with nurse practitioners, physician assistants, or certified nurse midwives. *Journal of the American Board of Family Medicine, 26*, 244–245. doi:10.3122/jabfm.2013.03.120312

Pogbosyan, L., Norful, A. A., & Martsolf, G. R. (2017). Primary care nurse practitioner characteristics: Barriers and opportunities for interprofessional teamwork. *Journal of Ambulatory Care Management, 40*, 77–86.

Pohl. J. M., Hanson, C., Newland, J. A., & Cronenwett, L. (2010). Analysis and commentary unleashing nurse practitioners' potential to deliver primary care and lead teams. *Health Affairs, 29*, 900–905. doi:10.1377/hlthaff.2010.0374

Rantz, M. J., Birtley, N. M., Fleshner, M., Crecelius, C., & Murray, C. (2017). Call to action: APRNs in U.S. nursing homes to improve care and reduce costs. *Nursing Outlook, 65*, 689–696.

Rask, K., Parmelee, P. A., Taylor, J. A., Green, D., Brown, H., Hawley, J., . . . Ouslander, J. G. (2007). Implementation and evaluation of a nursing home fall management program. *Journal of the American Geriatrics Society, 55*, 342–349.

Reeves, S., Pelone, F., Harrison, R., Goldman, J., & Zwarenstein, M. (2017). Interprofessional collaboration to improve professional practice and healthcare outcomes. *Cochrane Database Systematic Review*, 6. doi:10.1002/14651858.CD000072.pub3

Reeves, S., Perrier, L., Goldman, J., Freeth, D., & Zwarenstein, M. (2013). Interprofessional education: Effects on professional practice and healthcare outcomes (update). *Cochrane Database of Systematic Reviews*, 3. doi:10.1002/14651858.CD002213.pub3 Retrieved from http://www.thecochranelibrary.com Retrieved from https://pubmed.ncbi.nlm.nih.gov/23543515/

Reeves, S., Zwarenstein, M., Goldman, J., Barr, H., Freeth, D., Hammick, M., & Koppel, I. (2009). Interprofessional education: Effects on professional practice and health care outcomes. *Cochrane Database of Systematic Reviews*, (1). doi:10.1002/14651858.CD002213.pub2

Reynolds, P. P., Klink, K., Gilman, S., Green, L. A., Phillips, R. S., Shipman, S., . . .Davis, M. (2015). The Patient-Centered Medical Home: Preparation of the workforce, more questions than answers. *Journal of General Internal Medicine, 30*, 1013–1017. doi:10.1007/s11606-015-3229-2

Robert Wood Johnson Foundation. (2015). Lessons from the field: Promising interprofessional collaboration practices. White Paper. Retrieved from www.rwjf.org

Schadewaldt, V., McInnes, E., Hiller, J. E., & Gardner, A. (2013). Views and experiences of nurse practitioners with collaborative practice in primary care: An integrative review. *BioMed Central Family Practice*, 2–11. Retrieved from http://www.biomedcentral.com/1471-2296/14/132

Strasser, D. C., Falconer, J. A., Stevens, A. B., Uomoto, J. M., Herrin, J., Bowen, S. E., & Burridge, A. B. (2008). Team training and stroke rehabilitation outcomes: A cluster randomized trial. *Archives of Physical Medicine & Rehabilitation, 89*, 10–15.

Sutter-Barrett, R. E., Sutter-Dalrymple, C. J., & Dickman, K. (2015). Bridge Care Nurse: managed clinics fill the gap in health care. *The Journal for Nurse Practitioners, 11*, 262– 265. doi:10.1016/j.nurpra.2014.11.012

Taylor, C. R., Hepworth, J. T., Buerhaus, P. I., Dittus, R., & Speroff, T. (2007). Effect of crew resource management on diabetes care and patient outcomes in an inner-city primary care clinic. *Quality & Safety in Health Care, 16*, 244–247.

Thompson, C., Kinmonth, A. L., Stevens, L., Preveler, R. C., Stevens, A., Osler, K. J., . . . Campbell, M. J. (2000). Effects of a clinical-practice guideline and practice-based education on detection and outcome of depression in primary care: Hampshire depression project randomized controlled trial. *Lancet, 355*, 185–191.

Thompson, R. S., Rivara, F. P., Thompson, D. C., Barlow, W. E., Sugg, N. K., Maiuro, R. D., Rubinowice, D. M. (2000). Identification and management of domestic violence: A randomized trial. *American Journal of Preventive Medicine, 19*, 253–263.

Tieman, G.K., Mitchell, J.J., & Shelby-James, T.M. (2008). Multidisciplinary care planning and teamwork in primary care. *Medical Journal of Australia, 188*, 8, S61-64.

Tieman, G.K., Mitchell, J.J., Shelby-James, T.M., Currow, D., Fazekas, B., O'Doherty, L. J., . . . Reid-Orr, D. (2006). Integration, coordination, and multidisciplinary approaches in primary care: A systematic investigation of the literature. *Canberra: Australian Primary Health Care Research Institute.* Retrieved from http:www.anu.edu.au/aphcri/Domain/Multidisciplinary-Teams/Final_25_Currow.pdf

Tubbesing, G., & Chen, F. M. (2015). Insights from exemplar practices on achieving organizational structures in primary care. *Journal of the American Board of Family Medicine, 28*, 190–194. doi:10.3122/jabfm.2015.02.140114

Underwood, P. W., Schuiling, K., & Slager, J. (2003, March). *An evaluation of a partnership model for childbearing care.* Paper presented at the meeting of the Midwest Nursing Research Society, Indianapolis, IN. Virginia Henderson Global Nursing e-Repository Sigma Theta Tau International, October 17, 2011. Retrieved from http://hdl.handle.net/10755/160466

Van Soeren, M., Hurlock-Chorostecki, C., & Reeves, S. (2011). The role of nurse practitioners in hospital settings: Implications for interprofessional practice. *Journal of Interprofessional Care 25*, 245–251. doi:10.3109/13561820.2010.539305

Veterans Administration. (2010). *VA Centers of Excellence in Primary Care Education.* Retrieved from www.va.gov/OAA/docs/CoEPCE_Stage_1_RFP.pdf

Victoroff, K., Savrin, C., Demko, C., Iannadrea, J., Freudenberger, S., & Musacchio, C. (2014). Interprofessional clinical experiences in dental education. *Current Oral Health Reports, 1*, 161–166. doi:10.1007/s40496-014-0021-z

Way, D., Jones, L., & Basing, N. (2000). *Implementation strategies: Collaboration in primary care—family doctors and nurse practitioners delivering shared care.* Toronto, Canada: The Ontario College of Family Physicians. Retrieved from http://www.eicp.ca/en/toolkit/management-leadership/ocfp-paper-handout.pdf

Weaver, S. J., Rosen, M. A., DiazGranados, D., Lazzara, E. H., Lyons, R., Salas E., . . . King, H. B. (2010). Does teamwork improve performance in the operating room? A multileveled evaluation. *Joint Commission Journal on Quality & Patient Safety, 36*, 133–142.

White, B. A. A., Eklund, A., McNeal, T., Hochhalter, A., & Arroliga, A. (2018). Facilitators and barriers to ad hoc team performance. *Baylor Medical Center Proceedings, 31*, 380–384. doi:.org/10.1080/08998280.2018.1457879.

World Health Organization. (2010). *Framework for action on interprofessional education and collaborative practice.* Geneva, Switzerland: WHO Department of Human Resources for Health. Retrieved from http://www.who.int/hrh/nursing-midwifery/en/

Young, A. S., Chinman, M., Forquer, S. L., Knight, E. L., Vogel, H., Miller, A., . . . Mintz, J. (2005). Use of a consumer-led intervention to improve provider competencies. *Psychiatric Services, 56*, 967–975.

Zapatka, S. A., Conelius, J., Edwards, J., Meyer, E., & Brienza, R. (2014). Pioneering a primary care adult nurse practitioner interprofessional fellowship. *Journal for Nurse Practitioners, 10*, 378–386.

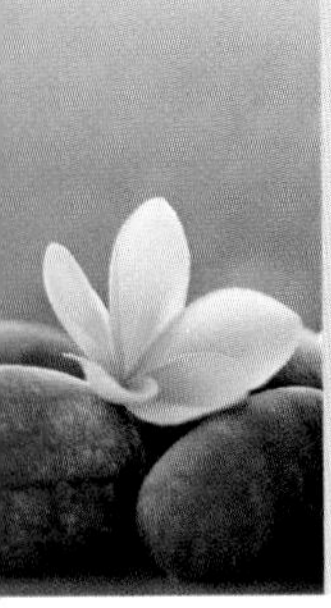

Chapter 16

Ethical Comportment in Promoting Health

Alexandre A. Martins

LEARNING OBJECTIVES

After completing this chapter, the student will be able to:

1. Discuss the ethical values and principles of the nursing profession.
2. Describe the ethical elements of health promotion for patients, families, communities, and populations.
3. Discuss the history and development of the Western ethics tradition and describe how it affects nursing practice.
4. Describe the theoretical foundations that have shaped ethics in nursing practice.

INTRODUCTION

Caring for another person, regardless of the reason he or she needs care, is an art of attention, sensitivity, and compassion. Some affirm that care is an essential part of human existence. Others are even more radical and say that care is the essence of being human (Boff, 2014). People like to be cared for, and it seems that most people like to care for others. If these tendencies hold true, the nursing profession holds a privileged role as caregivers to those who have physical and/or psychological illnesses.

The art of care is part of nursing's mission to promote health. This art is present in the daily activity of a nurse, who, according to the American Nurses Association's (ANA) Code of Ethics, embodies the nursing practice "with compassion and respect for the inherent dignity, worth, and unique attributes of every person" (ANA, 2015, p. v). In nursing practice, the art of care goes beyond the relationship with an individual patient because it extends to families, communities, and populations in a commitment to promote population health and well-being.

In nursing practice, caring for individuals and populations requires certain technical skills. Years of education are necessary to prepare a nurse to care for the sick and promote the health of the community. But the acquisition of technical skills is not enough for a nurse to commit to the art of care. It is also necessary to have motivations grounded on values able to sustain and to promote the dignity of individuals and populations. One of these values, as stressed by the ANA Code of Ethics, is compassion. This value is a movement toward the other who is suffering. Compassion is not a mere emotional feeling but a dynamic feeling that makes someone act to address the other person's need. Based on this feeling, the art of care transforms into actions that empower the inherent dignity of a vulnerable person (such as a patient in a hospital or a client in public health initiatives) through technical skills and ethical comportment. The goal is the optimal well-being of the vulnerable person.

This chapter focuses not on the technical skills needed for the art of care in nursing practice but on the values and principles that support and orient ethical comportment as a fundamental element. Advanced practice nurses must possess the ethical competence to identify and address ethical conflicts in the professional setting. Thus, the goal of this chapter is to offer important elements for ethical advanced practice in promoting care and health for patients, families, communities, and populations.

Studies have suggested that ethical education increases the confidence of nurses, enhances their ability to deal with ethical conflicts, and helps them address moral stress (Laabs, 2012). Ethical education for nurses must begin in undergraduate programs and must be an ongoing personal commitment and a social responsibility through a nurse's entire career. The rapid development of medical technology and sociocultural transformations creates new ethics challenges that necessitate regular and frequent education. The huge pluralism of North American society makes this challenge even bigger as encounters between different cultures and belief systems create more space for potential ethical conflicts, especially in the health-care field. After finishing school, a nursing student must be prepared to deal with this challenge and be aware of the importance of an ongoing ethical education to keep up the ability of promoting health as an art of care.

This chapter provides a historical and theoretical exploration of the Western tradition of ethics from ancient times until the specific development of bioethics in the second half of the 1900s. However, the theoretical perspective is not removed from the reality of nursing practice, and this chapter will also provide tools that nurses can use to address ethical conflicts in practice.

THEORETICAL FOUNDATIONS

Ethics begins when a moral behavior raises questions. Following this logic, a specific behavior becomes questionable when it does not meet major values and beliefs that shape the moral practice of a particular social group. This questionable action is not necessarily evil or wrong, but it is different from habitual actions that most members of a social group automatically recognize as reflecting their values. This questionable action could be anything from an innocent deed because of lack of full understanding of a value to a decision to act against a well-established value. Regardless of the reason, the action causes a social group to think about new ways to express its values or to punish the person who acted against them. Ethics is a study that aims at understanding the morals of a social group and the values, principles, and practices that shape society and progress when new challenges cause questionable actions to occur.

Ethics and *morality* are two words that are often used synonymously. For the purpose of this text, we'll use the understanding of the ANA Code of Ethics that clarifies their meanings: "*Morality* . . . refers to what would be called personal values, character, or conduct of individuals or groups within communities and societies. *Ethics* refers to the formal study of that morality from a wide range of perspectives including semantic, logical, analytical, epistemological, and normative. Thus, ethics is a branch of philosophy or theology in which one reflects on morality" (ANA, 2015, pp. xi–xii).

As a study, ethics aims to help us understand our morality and perfect it by embodying moral practices that reflect our values. This is a dynamic movement; unprecedented situations and challenges almost always produce new ways of embodying values through morality. The health-care field is a clear example of this: The development of new medical technologies challenges health professionals to embody a moral behavior expected of their profession in new and creative ways, without damaging the higher principles of a social group such as inherent human dignity. Here, we move from the ethics study about the philosophical nature of morality to a study of its application in a specific area, which is known as applied ethics.

Virtue Ethics

Bioethics appeared as a specialized ethical discipline when scientific development began to challenge the moral practices of scientists and health professionals. Bioethics is a discussion of these challenges to guarantee that development will benefit human life without sacrificing its dignity or the dignity of vulnerable individuals. Before the arrival of this specialized ethical discipline, ethics was constructed in a long history that formed a consistent tradition that today provides foundations, theories, and approaches to illuminate contemporary bioethical discussion. Ethics as a study of human deeds began in ancient Greece. Perhaps the Socratic-Platonic school was the first to dedicate itself to guiding individuals to act based on ethics. Following his mentor, Socrates, Plato developed an ethic in which the person is guided by a superior good achieved and understood by contemplation. According to Rémi Brague's interpretation, good for Plato is a creative principle that guides moral action (Brague, 2015).

Ancient Greek philosophers were the first to manifest their preoccupation with ethics. Aristotle developed a virtue ethics system that has marked the Western world.

Aristotle's system aims to lead individuals to happiness by encouraging them to embody a rational and political being. Aristotle defined ethics as the "science of ethos," a practical science that searches for understanding individuals' actions as they are organized in society. Ethos is embodied in individuals' morality as reflected by their actions meant to achieve an end. For Aristotle, this end is *eudaimonia*, "the happiness of human beings." An ethos provides values and principles that are translated into virtues for good actions. Through repetition of a virtue such as justice, a person acquires a habit of acting justly. Virtues, then, become a means to achieve happiness. Therefore, a virtuous person is one who forms his or her character as an educational process of absorbing and acting out values and virtues provided by the ethos. Using the virtue of prudence, or discernment, a person creates the ability to make right ethical choices toward happiness.

In the Christian perspective, the human creature is valued as a likeness of God, its creator, which provides more significant values for the human to follow. The concept of person is extremely important for Western bioethics, and many affirm that this concept was created and developed by Christian theology in its search for an explanation of the personhood of Jesus (Bellino, 1997, p. 121). Under this theory, God created the human being with freedom, marked by intrinsic dignity and an inner character as sources of ethical choice and behavior.

Aquinas developed a theological ethics of virtues in which he began with God as creator and ended with a mystical crowning. His theological ethics is based on the Aristotelian notion of virtue, sustained in the paradigm that human beings have a natural and universal desire to achieve the human good (Oliver, 2005). Habit occurs when a virtue becomes part of a person who performs virtuous actions in society. The intellect is the faculty of discernment that makes one do right by acting through virtues.

As discussed above, virtue ethics is focused on moral dilemmas in everyday life, not necessarily those concerning a field of thought such as biotechnology and health care. However, some scholars have used the virtue ethics perspective to reflect on bioethical dilemmas (Devettere, 2010; Keenan, 1999). Virtues are practical in that individuals learn by *doing* to become a moral person. Virtues are more than concepts; they are existential practices. Therefore, in bioethics, a virtue ethics approach expands the vision of health-care professionals and scientists from an ethical discussion when facing a conflict to an ethical comportment that embraces all professional practices. Alastair V. Campbell (2013) says: "VE [virtue ethics] is also relevant to bioethics because of its emphasis on the whole moral life rather than on incidents of moral choice and dilemma" (p. 35).

Autonomy and Duty-Bound Ethics

During the Age of Enlightenment, German philosopher Immanuel Kant raised a new ethical perspective that captured the imagination of the Western world. Kant defined personhood by the presence of autonomous reasoning. From this autonomy, the origin of principles and foundations for moral actions should arise. Kant wanted to create a moral principle, determinant of any ethical value, that could be a universally accepted law. He created a formula, *categorical imperative*, to arrive at moral laws as maximums of unconditional obedience. Categorical imperative is the rule that any action must be uniquely based on a principle of action that can become a universal law. This imperative does not allow exception, regardless of specific contexts or situations, because the possibility of exception would take away the autonomy of moral action. Kantian ethics provided the main foundation for the deontological approach in bioethics, which calls for the avoidance of certain actions that are always immoral regardless of circumstances, good intentions, or favorable consequences (Devettere, 2010, p. 11).

Kant's theory also opened space to accommodate specialized fields, such as applied ethics; these disciplines focus on the application of ethical principles in specific areas rather than on developing a philosophical ethical system of universal character. Some of the main expressions of specialized ethics are professional codes of ethics created for various industries and practitioners. The ANA Code of Ethics as well as the American Medical Association (AMA) Code of Medical Ethics are examples of these professional codes that provide relevant specialized ethics to orient the moral practices of nurses and physicians, respectively.

Although professional codes of ethics have a strong element of duty, an ethical equation cannot sufficiently address ethical conflicts in health care. Codes regulate duties and responsibilities of professionals and present values and principles for the ethical embodiment of the profession. However, the dynamism of health-care practices often raises issues for which one cannot find an objective answer in a code or other deontological system. This requires a moral discernment from the professional to analyze the situation; understand all elements involved in the case, from clinical diagnosis to legislation, to patient's values; and judge the possible ways to address the issue. This moral reasoning process considers the written values and duties of the deontological code but also examines the particulars of each case;

accounts for the resources available; and gives voice to patients, families, and communities.

Modern ethical theories guide health-care professionals as they face ethical challenges. A health-care professional addressing an ethical dilemma must consider the medical, human, and ethical resources available. Medical resources include treatments and associated medical instruments and technology, medication, and appropriate space. Human resources are the health-care professionals needed to perform the treatment, such as physicians, nurses, and professionals to assist with aspects beyond clinical care. Ethical resources are the theories, approaches, and frameworks foundational to analyzing a case and guiding decisions, as well as bioethicists and members of the organization's ethics committee.

Utilitarianism

This theory, also known as consequentialism, bases ethical decision making on the possible consequences of a potential action. The utility of the moral action must bring the greatest benefit possible or benefit the greatest number of people. A famous phrase related to this theory is "the greatest good for the greatest number." Under this theory, a moral action is one that aims at maximizing good consequences; it accepts some suffering as long as the intention is to minimize bad consequences.

Libertarianism

This theory focuses on individual freedom of the individual, grounded on the negative notion of right. Positive right is when individuals have the right to social goods provided by the community, such as health care and education. Negative right is the individual freedom from a superior institution that limits your action or imposes taxes. Libertarians affirm that all individuals must be free from social control. This theory also sustains a "don't harm principle" in which the freedom of an individual does not justify any action against the physical and moral integrity of another. A person's own good does not allow damaging another person. Mutual respect is expected (Campbell, 2013).

Communitarianism

In contrast to libertarianism, communitarianism is based on social good and solidarity and affirms positive rights and a social contract that can distribute goods among citizens. Members of a community are responsible for contributing to the common good that must grow and be distributed to all according to need. Some people contribute more because they can; others receive more because they lack resources and thus need more. This logic is regulated based on social justice and fairness. Campbell (2013) says, "Communitarian ethics can enhance our approach to bioethical issues by stressing the social dimension of our potential solutions, and . . . it has particular force when we are considering justice in health care provision" (p. 40).

THE EMERGENCE OF BIOETHICS

The term *bioethics* appeared for the first time in the work of Van Rensselaer Potter in an article named "The Science of Survival" and then in the book *Bioethics: Bridge to the Future* (Potter, 1971). In the twentieth century, specialized ethical study in the field of health care, primarily to cover medical research and then clinical practice, became an urgent need. Health-care ethics focused on the protection of human subjects, and self-determination of individuals appeared as a response to abuses against the integrity of human persons, especially vulnerable groups. The Nuremberg trials in 1946 to judge the abusive actions of Nazi doctors in their medical experiments on human subjects were a keystone for the origin of bioethics. These trials resulted in one of the first international documents for the protection of individuals' self-determination in participating in medical research, known as the Nuremberg Code. It was the origin of informed consent.

Other historic travesties of ethics also contributed to the development of bioethics. Most notorious was the revelation of abuse during experiments on people infected with syphilis in Tuskegee, Alabama. Medical researchers purposely infected African Americans with syphilis in the course of these experiments and denied them treatment for the disease, even after research found the treatment to be effective. This abuse was revealed in 1972. A commission was created to analyze this case, which resulted in the 1978 Belmont Report. This report outlined three basic principles to be applied to all research with human subjects: respect for individual autonomy, beneficence, and justice.

The rapid development of medical science and technology also raised questions on how to best protect and benefit humanity. The ability to do organ transplants generated new issues. The first renal transplant was in 1954 in Brigham Hospital in Boston. The first heart transplant occurred in 1967 in Cape Town, South Africa. These advancements raised questions about mortality that required a new medical definition of death. Neurological criterion was added to the existing cardiopulmonary criterion to determine whether death has occurred. In 1968, an ad hoc committee at Harvard Medical School developed the definition of brain death. Brain death is the condition in which there is no brain activity, but other physiological functions, such as the heart beating and breathing, can be kept functioning by the support of machines like mechanical ventilators (Butts & Rich, 2016, p. 281).

In addition, new medical technology, such as chronic hemodialysis in 1960 and treatment to address fertility issues by in vitro fertilization in 1978, raised concerns. Policies to regulate some medical practices, like the landmark 1973 case *Roe v. Wade* that gave American women the right to abortion, also raised ethical dilemmas. New medical technologies, treatments, and drugs are constantly in development and are often studied using human subjects. Although improving well-being is the goal, these developments raise new questions that must be addressed to prevent all of us, but especially vulnerable persons and populations, from harm while making the benefits widely available.

The realm of liberal individualism in bioethics, established in the context of the Belmont Report of the National Commission, has influenced one of the most remarkable bioethical frameworks: the ethics of principles, also known as principlism, which is grounded on the principles of autonomy, beneficence, nonmaleficence, and justice. This framework was first proposed by Tom L. Beauchamp and James F. Childress (2013) in their book *Principles of Biomedical Ethics* (the book was first published in 1979). The influence of this work is paradigmatic and impressive because it has become a standard for addressing ethical issues in health care in the United States; it has also been exported to other nations, especially in the Western Hemisphere. Brief definitions of the principles that form the basis for principlism will be provided next.

Autonomy is the self-determination of a human person that is reflected in his or her right to make health-care decisions and volunteer to participate in research. Individuals must be free from coercion and respected in their decisions and values. This principle creates the obligation of clinicians and researchers to provide clear, adequate, precise, and intelligible information for their patients and volunteers in research to empower them to make autonomous decisions. In other words, the principle of autonomy requires the necessity of informed consent from patients and volunteers.

Nonmaleficence simply means the health-care providers' obligation to do no harm. Beneficence originated in the Hippocratic corpus when it stated that the obligation of the physician is to do good for his or her patient. Action toward others must contribute to their welfare. This principle asserts that health-care decisions and actions, as well as research on human subjects, must benefit others. These actions must be in the best interest of patients and populations. The principle of beneficence also embraces actions in public health care for the benefit of families, communities, and populations.

First, the principle of justice in a clinical setting refers to the obligation to treat patients fairly and with equal care. Second, this principle is used in social justice, especially in matters of public health-care strategies, allocation of resources, health-care coverage, and social determinants of health. Many perspectives on justice exist. The ethical theories presented in this chapter, for example, libertarianism and communitarianism, have different perspectives, especially in matters of social justice. But this does not justify neglecting to address inequalities in accessing health care. Therefore, the principle of justice claims fairness in accessing health care but opens the door for societies to find ways to achieve this goal.

Principlism was exported to other countries, including middle- and low-income ones. Initially, these countries, many of which were marked by social injustice and health inequalities, accepted and adopted principlism in the same way that it was used in the United States. But later, especially in Latin America, health-care providers, philosophers, theologians, and others worried about health-care ethics realized that they needed to go beyond principlism to respond to the health-care challenges realistically in their communities (Martins, 2012). This raised new perspectives, ones that also included the social aspect of accessing health care. Some of these new perspectives have the social reality of health inequalities as the starting point of bioethics (Pessini, 2012, p. 147). Even in the United States, new approaches have become part of bioethical debates and decision-making processes, such as the focus on care with quality, respect, and meaning to achieve optimal quality of life (Dall'Agnol, 2014).

In conclusion of this section, we return to the virtue ethics perspective, which focuses primarily on ethics in daily life. In this aspect, it is not a bioethical theory like principlism. Rather, it is a perspective from which a provider tries his or her best to embody ethical behavior in health-care practice, and ethicists and bioethicists address ethical issues in the health-care field. This perspective does not provide answers to all ethical problems but gives us tools to address them: the virtue of moral discernment and prudential reasoning. Therefore, virtue ethics helps us embody the art of care in bioethics and nursing practice in all areas, from clinical practice to actions in public and global health.

CLINICAL ETHICS AND CHALLENGES IN THE LIMITS OF LIFE

The high speed of technological development in the last 100 years has created many possibilities that once were unthinkable, including countless comforts and advantages. Technology has enabled people to cross the ocean in only a few hours in a flight from New York City to Paris. We can talk to and see loved ones and business associates around the world at the push of a button. Many diseases that killed thousands in the past are now easily treated; others have been completely eradicated from some areas of the world. We can give those whose hearts have failed a life-extending transplant. We can help infertile couples conceive biological children. In some regions, life expectancy is over 80 years.

For many, however, these developments are too good to be true. Technological progress is not available to all. While some countries have life expectancy of 80 years, those in other nations do not expect to live beyond 50. While rich nations have resources to transplant hearts, others must live with high rates of child mortality. Many citizens can access medications to treat their diseases, but vulnerable citizens of poor nations are still victims at high risk for their health in experiments of which they are unaware.

The art of care in bioethics is a virtue of looking at the other, especially the vulnerable, with compassion. This other is a proxy, the one a nurse is caring for in her clinical shift. It includes those who are suffering because of lack of access to health care in poor areas throughout the world. And the other is also the earth, the mother who provides resources for all of us. The ethics of care in health care is based on a relationship that values people in their inherent dignity. It is a perspective that does not reduce the individual or community considered "other."

Clinical ethics in nursing practice occurs in the relationship between nurses and their patients and in a context of physical and psychological care. In the context of health care, this relationship extends to the patient's family and community because they are part of his or her universe of values and decisions. Ethical comportment is expected from nurses in their practice, but this behavior does not create clinical immunity from possible ethical conflicts. Such conflicts may happen even in a context of excellent ethical comportment among health-care professionals. Conflicts can arise for many reasons, including different values between professionals or institutions and patients, availability or scarcity of resources, choices of treatments, risks and fears, different cultures, different religious perspectives, and insurance interference. Therefore, ethical comportment must be completed with the ability to make ethical decisions, essential for moral excellence in the professional practice of a nurse (Fry & Johnstone, 2002).

According to the ANA Code of Ethics, "the nurse's primary commitment is to the recipients of nursing and healthcare services—patients or clients—whether individuals, families, groups, communities, or population" (ANA, 2015). This statement stresses the obligations that nurses have toward the recipients of health-care services. This is a broad statement in the sense that it includes public health-care services to communities and populations. In clinical treatments, nurses must look first to the best interest of their patients. To that end, it's important to include patients in the decision-making process about their care. The ANA assumes a dialogical and participatory perspective for processes of decision making. This is also a process of moral reasoning that encourages the virtue of discernment with participation of those who are involved in a clinical case.

Even with the embodiment of this process of moral reasoning and participatory discernment, conflicts might arise. People have different values, beliefs, and perspectives. A nurse is not immune from this reality. He or she also has individual values that may conflict with patients' values and choices. The ANA expects nurses to interact actively with patients to create a relationship based on trust, assist with their decision making, and respect and support their choices. However, the writers of the ANA Code of Ethics are aware that these choices may generate conflicts, so the nurse must strive to perform actions in the best interest of the patient that are also in accordance with the patient's values.

The Concept of Personhood

Sometimes, nurses and patients have a direct conflict because of different values or beliefs. Consider personal beliefs about personhood that may arise in the case of high-risk pregnancy. Some patients or providers may believe that the fetus is not yet a person, so the autonomy of the mother must prevail, even if she chooses to terminate the pregnancy. Another individual may consider the fetus as a person and prioritize the protection of this vulnerable being. This kind of conflict can also be influenced by the values of the treatment institution, such as a Catholic hospital that does not perform abortions. This limits the patient's choices and makes the ethical conflict even more complex. The ANA Code of Ethics clearly states that a nurse is not obliged to go against his or her own beliefs. However, leaving the problem does not solve the case for the patient, the institution, and the other nurse who will take part in the treatment. Moral reasoning and discernment are essential to address the conflict. Part of this reasoning is awareness of each person's values. Although abortion is legal in the United States, ethical conflicts transcend the law. The concept of person is worth considering because it often arises in health care, particularly in relation to beginning-of-life and end-of-life issues.

The ANA Code of Ethics does not define the concept of person, but it does affirm "the inherent dignity, worth, and unique attributes of every person" in Provision 1. This means that dignity is not a mere attribute of a person but an intrinsic value, something unnegotiable. However, who is classified as a person is not addressed in the ANA Code. Perhaps this was a conscious choice made to embrace different concepts of person in a pluralist society such as the United States. Regardless, it is clear that the ANA respects all values and belief systems, a position that makes it even more important for nurses to understand the concept of person in a pluralistic society.

Our age, as in times past, is marked by applied ethics, a result of fragmentation and specialization of this field. Although established ethical codes serve as guides for moral practice, they do not offer objective answers for all ethical dilemmas. We must still think ethically, considering the realities of a situation, the ethical issues at hand, and the values involved. Reflecting on the concept of person is an example of thinking ethically. At the same time, the comprehension of the main lines of this debate provides tools for ethical discussions in decision-making processes in health.

Although divergent opinions exist about what constitutes personhood, this definition serves as the basis for deciding who is considered a person and thus deserves to have his or her dignity respected and promoted. In every debate about issues related to the limits of life, whether at the beginning of life or at its end, the concept of person is key to our understanding of the positions taken with respect to both the human being and the biological organism, particularly regarding those who are vulnerable. While there are many ways to define the concept of person, only two will be discussed here. Together they make it possible to synthesize the broader discussion; Engelhardt describes these two definitions as general secular morality and religious morality (Engelhardt, 1996).

General Secular Morality

From the perspective of general secular morality, not every human being is a person. A distinction is made between biological life and personal life. Biological human life takes precedence over the person because this life is a physiological cellular corpus beyond ethical concern. Regarding the body, one does not speak about the use of reason and will but rather about the process of development common to all living beings. This development begins from a cell and, if all goes as planned, the organism will move to the apex of development. Eventually, it begins to weaken and reaches the end of its biological life, when it is broken down by microorganisms present in nature. For a biological human life to be considered a person, it must have the power to consent and to exercise moral authority. That is, it must be able to participate in a web of relationships with other human beings, in which everyone has an active role as autonomous and self-aware moral subjects, capable of establishing connections, working with others, and setting limits. This forms the basis for holding that person accountable for his or her actions.

This perspective excludes many humans from personhood, including infants, the mentally disabled, and those with dementia. Embryos and fetuses are not considered persons under this definition. Individuals in a coma are not considered persons, although they once were persons and could be again. Those living in a persistent vegetative state (PVS) are not persons and will not return to the state of personhood. According to general secular morality, these human beings do not possess the same rights as those considered persons; any invasive or arbitrary action done to them would not be viewed as immoral. Thus, a moral question would never even be posed because morality itself is understood as the relationship between persons. The only foundation for defending these beings would be reasons of affection or solidarity, such as the relationship of a mother with a fetus that she would never abort, not for moral reasons but because of the affective relationship of love and care that has been established with this unborn being. At the same time, the choice to have an abortion because of an unwanted pregnancy to which no emotional bonds of attachment have been established would not be considered an immoral action. Reasoning based on bonds of affection or solidarity would also protect those with dementia, the mentally disabled, and those in a PVS who are kept alive. In other situations, the issue of affectivity is not as salient. For example, doctors and researchers consider embryos to be in the initial stage of the biological process and therefore view any kind of manipulation to be acceptable.

Legislation tends to protect those individuals who are not technically considered persons by general secular morality. In the case of abortion, the legal basis for this procedure is not whether a fetus is or is not a person but the right that women have over their bodies and the right of confidentiality between women and doctors. In terms of nursing practice, the ethical obligation is to care for those individuals as long as they are under clinical nursing responsibility. This ethical obligation also includes an interactive and respectful relationship with these individuals' surrogates.

Religious Morality

For the perspective of so-called religious morality, we refer to the moral paradigm conceptualized by the Catholic church, which maintains that no separation exists between biological human life and personal human life. Every human is considered a being with a biological, rational, and moral life. The starting point of human life is based not on phenomenological observation but rather on the ontological nature of the human being as revealed in the Bible. For the Catholic church, the human person is endowed with a unique nature willed by God from the time of conception, or even before, because every human being who is conceived has been thought of and willed by the creator. What makes a human being a person is not the ability to exercise reason, human freedom, and relate to other people within a network of moral responsibility. Rather, it is one's very nature stemming from the will of God, a nature that is unique and unchangeable.

Based on this foundation, the Catholic church takes its stance in defense of life in every situation because every person and situation calls for moral responsibility. If someone cannot act morally, he or she does not cease to be a person because his or her nature is willed by God and never changes. Hence, a relationship of moral responsibility exists among people possessing the normal use of reason and will toward people in positions of vulnerability and dependence. Once again, this responsibility is founded upon biblical revelation. It also demands that value of the person, which requires the defense of life and the dignity of the human person always, even in relationships among moral strangers.

Unlike general secular morality, where the foundation used to defend a fetus or someone in a PVS is a matter of affection and solidarity, religious morality asserts that the relationship between two human beings goes beyond affection and solidarity. It is a relationship between personal subjectivities, which possess the same nature. This relationship requires a commitment on the part of those who have more potential to assume greater moral responsibility for protecting the dignity of the vulnerable.

Human dignity is no longer understood as an intrinsic element of human nature. All humans have equal dignity, but each must live according to the contingencies of his or her situation. For example, the manner in which one advances the life and dignity of a person who has mental disabilities is different from the manner used on behalf of a person possessing a normal capacity for reason, consciousness, and will. Nevertheless, both are entitled to have their dignity defended and advanced through the actions, circumstances, and conditions of a decent life. No one grants dignity to others. What happens is that real injustices are done by those who have more power, which prevents the most vulnerable from a dignified life. This goes for biological issues, such as the examples used so far, as well as social factors such as poverty and marginalization. These injustices, when viewed as a biological or social web of existence, prevent others from living with dignity. The situations in which they live, barely on the threshold of human existence, become ever more dramatic in the underworld of injustices, depersonalization, and objectification.

These two moral perspectives exemplify the different sets of morality present in different societies. They are behind people's moral decisions in many health-care situations. Understanding them helps us make decisions and helps nurses deal with moral stress, especially when stress arises from a conflict of perspectives between nurses and patients/surrogates or between nurses and physicians. Handling these conflicts as an art of care allows the nurse to arrive at a final decision and to provide care during the decision-making process, care that is dialogical and includes other professionals (interdisciplinary), patients (or their surrogates), and families and communities (when they are needed and are an important part of the process).

PROPOSED DECISION-MAKING FRAMEWORK

Many frameworks exist for decision making in health care, but it is still impossible to make a perfect decision. Ethical dilemmas and conflicts are as dynamic as human life. The specific circumstances of one case might lead to a different ethical decision than in a similar case. A context of scarcity, for example, provides fewer possible answers to address a problem than a context with an abundance of resources. To be aware of these particularities and limits is part of the decision-making process. The following suggested framework provides an appropriate transition from clinical issues to public and global health issues.

Health-care decision making must begin with a horizon, or objective, and be grounded in a reality. The horizon is health promotion of individuals (patients in treatment) and/or communities and populations (public health care). In a clinical context, the reality is the diagnosis, options for treatments, available human and material resources, time, patients' preferences and choices, values, principles, and legislation. In public and global health, the elements that constitute the reality are not different from the clinical context, but additional elements are determined by the focus of health promotion for the population rather than for an individual patient. Epidemiological studies (including social determinants of health), main health needs, options of preventive actions and primary-care services, knowledge of the public health system in place, possibilities of community-based participation, and local values must be considered as part of the reality of a situation.

Ethical theoretical background provides the essential knowledge and foundation to guide moral reasoning in a process of discernment. This includes identifying the main values generating the conflict. Consider the case of a pregnant woman diagnosed with cancer. Treating the cancer would affect the normal development of the fetus, who then would be at high risk for birth defects or mortality. To protect the fetus, cancer treatment is best postponed until after childbirth. However, this option will make the pregnant woman very weak and sick, with a high risk of dying during delivery. Physicians cannot guarantee that both lives will be saved. They recommend the cancer treatment, saying that abortion will not be provoked, but as an undesired consequence, this risk cannot be controlled. They apply the principle of double effect to justify this recommendation morally. As part of an ethical theoretical background, this principle says that if an action targets a good end, but it may have a second inevitable consequence, this action does not intend to provoke an evil. The second effect is not pursued or desired but is out of control. This unwanted effect is not in itself morally wrong (Butts & Rich, 2016). However, the pregnant woman, motivated by her values and beliefs, prefers to take the risk of dying without receiving the cancer treatment to save the life of her child. Ethical theoretical background helps us understand her values and subsequent choice. Consequently, it provides foundations for dialogue with the patient and those involved in the case, creating a process of discernment for decision with respect, comprehension, and support.

This framework, which suggests a virtue ethics approach of moral discernment, does not affirm that picking one theory would provide enough ethical theoretical background to guide a decision. A process of discernment suggests that health professionals responsible for guiding decision making must also discern which ethical theory is more appropriate to address the case at hand. Experiences have shown that a balance between different theories seems to be most appropriate to illuminate ethical conflicts. Therefore, a nurse must have enough ethical theoretical background and sensitivity to create the best ethical foundations to use to address the case at hand.

Quality of life is connected to what is beneficial for patients, families, communities, and populations. Public health interventions and strategies strive to promote health by restoring people's health conditions and/or by preventing diseases to keep good health status as long as possible. In an ideal situation, treatments and public health strategies are combined with individual and community moral values. But this does not always happen, which creates conflict. Many individuals make sacrifices to maintain their values, as with the pregnant woman in the previous example who risks death to save her child's life. Moral reasoning and discernment require a balance between treatment options and public health strategies, as well as between patient and community values when there is a conflict. In public health, this kind of conflict can be prevented by studies of local communities and targeted populations based on cultural and ethical values. These studies help shape public health policies that already must balance health strategies and community values. Participation of patients, families, and community representatives is also fundamental to define treatment regimens and public health strategies. This participation potentiates health-care effectiveness and prevents ethical conflicts.

Health-care decision making must be democratic in the sense that it includes participation, dialogue, and communal decisions. Health-care decisions based on moral discernment must engage those involved in a dialogue whenever possible. Of course, this dialogue is not absolute in the sense that everybody must participate in all situations. Some cases, such as emergency care, require quick decisions based solely on medical expertise about the best course of action for the patient's health. However, awareness of the circumstances that limit dialogue and participation is part of moral reasoning. Nurses have a great opportunity to advocate for the best interests of their clients by encouraging this type of dialogue in the care setting.

SOCIAL ETHICS AND PUBLIC HEALTH-CARE STRATEGIES

Studies have shown the connection between social factors and health status, a concept called social determinants of health (World Health Organization [WHO], 2011b). Ideally, social factors have a positive impact on the health status of individuals, groups, and populations, with a health-care system that offers accessible services from primary to tertiary care, including health education, to promote well-being and restore health. However, the reality of health care for most countries, communities, and populations is far from this ideal situation. Even high-income countries suffer with social injustices and health disparities that affect the social conditions of minorities, including in the United States, where marginalized, low socioeconomic communities are more vulnerable to illness and struggle to access health-care services (Dickman, Himmelstein, Woolhandler, 2017).

Research affirms an undeniable connection between poverty and ill health (WHO, 2015b). Poor and vulnerable groups are most affected by social inequalities that have a negative impact on health and well-being. The poor are more vulnerable to illness, and without good health, they do not have the necessary conditions to improve their lives because good health is a condition of development (WHO Commission on Macroeconomics and Health, 2003). In other words, poverty causes ill health, which in turn makes people poorer and thus produces a lower health status. This can also result in a structural cycle of violence and injustice against those who have never had the opportunity to change their lives (Farmer, 2003).

This reality shows the necessity of a broad and serious consideration of social justice in public health care. This consideration must be intersectional, involving not only the health-care field but also socioeconomic policies to create opportunities and address health factors while promoting population health and access to health-care services.

Principles and perspectives guide choices for designing or reforming health-care systems as well as for elaborating public health-care strategies at the local, state, and national levels (and internationally in actions of global health). In their role as advocates for the well-being and best care of patients, families, communities, and populations, nurses have the right, responsibility, and duty to participate in the public debate on health-care system and public health-care strategies (ANA, 2015).

The virtue ethics approach for decision making in health care gives first place to the principle of justice in a public health debate. The common good of communities gains priority; therefore, justice becomes social justice to orient public health toward the goal of addressing health disparities and promoting population health. As noted above, principles and perspectives lead choices. Thus, it is important that nurses be aware of and understand public debates in health care to participate; create an atmosphere of dialogue and discernment; and exercise their role as advocates for individuals, communities, and populations.

Nurses' participation in public health debates can be divided into two areas: health-care systems and reforms, and public health-care strategies to promote well-being and health-care delivery. The former is more theoretical and is intended to shape health-care policies at the systemic level. This debate and its subsequent decision making have an impact on health-care coverage and delivery, for example, whether health care is delivered based on a public health system supported by taxpayers or in a market through which people must purchase health-care services. These decisions also shape the allocation of health-care resources. Different countries have chosen distinct approaches and priorities. For instance, Cuba and Canada have a public health-care system financed with public money. Cuba's system has a strong emphasis on primary care. The United States adopted a free-market system in which people must purchase private insurance. This system focuses on tertiary care with high-tech medical services. Some countries, such as Brazil and India, have public health-care systems managed by the government and also allow the existence of private insurance and the offer of private health-care services. In these countries, private systems offer complementary health services for those who want and can afford them.

Health care is subject to ongoing debate. Systems frequently undergo reforms, changes, and even complete transformations. These changes can be driven by political power, structural needs, new diseases, new health-care services, new medications and technologies, outbreaks, epidemics, demographic changes, scarcity, natural disasters, and even revolutions and wars. Specific interest groups with great political influence also affect the health-care debate and decisions. For example, financial groups benefit from a market-based health-care system in which they profit from the promotion of universal coverage.

In the United States, health care has been the subject of political debate among policy makers and the public for decades. Every new federal administration since the market-based approach was established has intended to promote health-care reform. The Obama administration created the Affordable Care Act (McDonough, 2012); the Trump administration wants to repeal it and create a new plan that was promised but the administration failed to deliver. Health-care professionals cannot be absent from this debate. Nurses are advocates for the best interest of individuals', families', communities', and populations' well-being and care.

The second area of participation in public health care relates to strategies and actions to promote health and health-care delivery. This addresses the question of the best type of health-care delivery system for a particular population. The decision-making framework described above can be used to address this question in five steps. Step one is defining the horizon or the objective. In public health, this is connected to one element of step two (reality): epidemiological studies and main health needs. The objective is health and well-being promotion, but concrete targets must be developed for each intervention. For example, epidemiological studies, including demographic understanding of population changes, show evidence of health needs that must be addressed with more urgency in short-term or long-term actions and goals. Evidence-based studies help to define allocation of resources and measure cost-effectiveness. This process occurs on broad levels, such as on the state and national levels. One example is creating strategies to immunize entire populations. A similar process occurs to plan strategies to address health needs on the local level; for instance, evidence-based studies show that the population of a city of approximately 10,000 people is in a steady process of aging. This demands more geriatric and assisted services than the local system can offer on a sufficient scale to address this need. The demographics have changed, but the health system is still the same. Now the health system needs to be adapted to respond to this new reality.

The primary focus of health-care services is also part of public health-care strategies and actions. Together with concrete objectives, this focus determines allocation of resources and availability of health-care services, including who will access these services and how. For example, if the focus is preventive and primary care, strategies will consider resources and actions that can make this kind of care more efficient in achieving the defined concrete objectives. If the choice is to focus on tertiary care, strategies and resources are planned and allocated in order to provide this kind of service.

Principles and values influence the way that health-care services are made available and accessible. These will define, especially at the national level, whether health care will be offered with universal access targeting coverage of the entire population or as a privilege that some individuals and groups can access based on their capacity to purchase these services. Studies and reports have suggested that public systems that focus on primary care and universal coverage have given better results in promoting health and well-being (WHO, 2008; WHO, 2015b). All elements of the framework above must be considered to create a moral discernment in addressing the health needs of communities and populations.

Ethical questions raised by public health care are not only those of justice and health inequalities. Public health-care strategies and actions also raise specific ethical questions regarding the relationship between professionals and clients. Many of these issues are familiar to the clinical context, such as informed consent and the individual autonomy of refusing a public health action. In public health care, nurses have the same ethical duties as nurses working in a clinical context, from respecting self-determination to maintaining confidentiality. However, many ethical issues are raised by public health-care activities targeting full populations or specific groups. They are usually connected to broad programs of health and epidemiological vigilance and control, involving, for example, immunization campaigns, screening programs, behavior modification, and even policies that make it difficult for people to access a harmful product such as cigarettes. The COVID-19 pandemic is also a good example of the need of public health measures to mitigate the spread of the coronavirus, such as mandating social distancing during the pandemic, that raise ethical issues. Tension arises between the rights of individual self-determination and the communal benefits of public health efforts (Holland, 2014). Participation in epidemiological research and collection of data, which is important in defining public health strategies, also raises ethical issues because it involves risk that must be addressed to respect autonomy and individual values. The moral discernment framework alerts us to consider the principles and values of groups and populations when defining public health-care plans. Engaging community members in the decision process is extremely valuable to reduce ethical issues and to address ethical problems properly.

When public health-care actions go beyond national borders, global health begins. The COVID-19 pandemic made clear the existence of health issues that cross borders and the need of global collaboration. In a world marked by inequalities, poverty, and precocious death of thousands of people in low-income countries because of preventable and treatable diseases, global health raises important ethical questions that must be addressed to promote the health and well-being of individuals, families, communities, and populations. The ANA Code of Ethics states: "Nurses understand that the lived experiences of inequality, poverty, and social marginalization contribute to the deterioration of health globally . . . Global health, as well as the common good, are ideals that can be realized when all nurses unite their efforts and energies" (ANA, 2015, pp. 31, 36).

KEY POINTS

- Nursing is an art of care requiring technical and professional competency, compassion, sensitivity, commitment to justice, leadership, and ethical comportment along with the ability to handle conflicts.

- Whether in the clinical context, public health, or global health, the art of care integrates moral reasoning and discernment as part of a virtue ethics approach to guide decision-making processes in health care.
- Bioethics is part of the art of care in health promotion and the well-being of individuals, families, communities, and populations at local, national, and international levels.
- Bioethics and the art of care are not mechanical comportments and practices but rather a dynamic movement of discernment and actions in relationships among people with their cultures, values, beliefs, dramas, fears, sufferings, social and health needs, desires, and hopes.
- This is a complex reality that is also a beautiful challenge when it is seen from the perspective of an art of care that promotes human dignity, justice, health, and well-being.

USEFUL RESOURCES

Alma-Ata Declaration. (1978). http://www.who.int/publications/almaata_declaration_en.pdf

Belmont Report. (1979). http://www.hhs.gov/ohrp/regulations-and-policy/belmont-report/

Code of Ethics of the American Nursing Association. (2015). http://www.nursingworld.org/codeofethics

Code of Medical Ethics of the American Medical Association. (2016). http://www.ama-assn.org/ama/pub/physician-resources/medical-ethics/code-medical-ethics.page

Declaration of Helsinki. (1964). https://www.wma.net/policies-post/wma-declaration-of-helsinki-ethical-principles-for-medical-research-involving-human-subjects/

Hippocratic Oath. http://guides.library.jhu.edu/c.php?g=202502&p=1335752

Nuremberg Code. (1947). https://history.nih.gov/research/downloads/nuremberg.pdf

Rio Political Declaration of the Social Determinants of Health. (2011). http://www.who.int/sdhconference/declaration/en/

Universal Declaration of Human Rights. (1948). http://www.un.org/en/universal-declaration-human-rights/

Universal Declaration on Bioethics and Human Rights. (2005). http://www.unesco.org/new/en/social-and-human-sciences/themes/bioethics/bioethics-and-human-rights/

Check Your Understanding

1. Which choice best defines the word *compassion*?
   A. The love a parent feels for a child
   B. A dynamic feeling that makes one act to address another person's need
   C. A nurse's technical skill
   D. Goodwill for all of humanity

2. Which theory bases ethical decision making on achieving "the greatest good for the greatest number"?
   A. Utilitarianism
   B. Kantian ethics
   C. Virtue ethics
   D. Libertarianism

3. The Nuremberg Code and Belmont Report contributed to what field of study?
   A. Postmodernism
   B. Environmental studies
   C. Bioethics
   D. Stoicism

4. In which case does a treatment institution's values limit the choices of the patient?
   A. A father and daughter who receive medical care through a free clinic
   B. A woman who is considering terminating a pregnancy while she is a patient at a Catholic hospital
   C. A pregnant woman with cancer who decides to delay treatment until after her baby is born
   D. A middle school student who asks the school nurse for a menstrual pad after getting her first period

See "Reflections on Check Your Understanding" at the end of the book for answers.

REFERENCES

American Nurses Association. (2015). *Code of ethics for nurses: With interpretive statements.* Silver Spring, MD: Author.

Beauchamp, T. L., & J. F. Childress. (2013). *Principles of biomedical ethics* (7th ed.). New York: Oxford University Press.

Bellino, F. (1997). *Fundamentos de bioética: Aspectos antropológicos, ontológicos e morais.* Bauru, Brazil: EDUSC.

Boff, L. (2014). *Saber cuidar: Ética do humano—compaixão pela terra* (20th ed.). Petrópolis, Brazil: Vozes.

Brague, Réne. (2015, February). The necessity of the good. *The First Things,* 250, Feb., 47–52.

Butts, J. B., & Rich, K. L. (2016). *Nursing ethics: Across the curriculum and into practice* (4th ed.) Burlington, MA.: Jones & Bartlett Learning.

Campbell, A. V. (2013). *Bioethics: The basics.* New York: Routledge.

Dall'Agnol, D. (2014). Cuidar e respeitar: Atitudes fundamentais na bioética. In L. Pessini, L. Bertachini, & C. de P. Barchifontaine (Eds.), *Bioética, cuidado e humanização: Sobre o cuidado respeitoso* (Vol. II, pp. 201–224) São Paulo, Brazil: Loyola & Centro Universitário São Camilo.

Devettere, R. L. (2010). *Practical decision making in health care ethics: Cases and concepts* (3rd ed.). Washington, DC: Georgetown University Press.

Dickman S. L., Himmelstein, D. U., Woolhandler, S. (2017). Inequality and the health-care system in the USA. *The Lancet, 389* (10077), 1431–1441. Retrieved from http://dx.doi.org/10.1016/S0140-6736(17)30398-7

Engelhardt, H. T. (1996). *The foundation of bioethics* (2nd ed.). New York: Oxford University Press.

Farmer, P. (2003). *Pathologies of power: Health, human rights, and the new war on the poor.* Berkeley, CA: University of California Press.

Fry, S., & Johnstone, M.-J. (2002). *Ethics in nursing practice: A guide to ethical decision making* (2nd ed.). Malden, MA: Blackwell Science.

GBD 2015 SDG Collaborators. (2016). Measuring the health-related Sustainable Development Goals in 188 countries: A baseline analysis from the Global Burden of Disease Study 2015. *The Lancet* 338 (10053), 1813–1850. Retrieved from http://dx.doi.org/10.1016/S0140-6736(16)31467-2

Holland, S. (2014). Public health: IV. Ethics. In B. Jennings (Ed.). *Encyclopedia of bioethics* (4th ed., pp. 2617–2623). New York: Macmillan Reference USA.

Keenan, J. F. (1999). "Whose perfection is it anyway?" A virtuous consideration of enhancement. *Christian Bioethics, 5*(2), 104–120.

Laabs, C. A. (2012). Confidence and knowledge: Regarding ethics among advanced practice nurses. *Nursing Education Perspectives, 22*(1), 10–14.

Martins, A. A. (2012). *Bioética, saúde e vulnerabilidade: Em defesa da dignidade dos mais vulneráveis.* São Paulo, Brazil: Paulus.

McDonough, J. E. (2012). *Inside national health reform.* Berkeley, CA: University of California Press.

Oliver, S. (2005) The sweet delight of virtue and grace in Aquinas's ethics. *International Journal of Systematic Theology*, 7(1), 52–71.

Pessini, L. (2012). Um grito ético por justiça e equidade no mundo da saúde. In A. A. Martins & A. Martini (Eds.). *Teologia e saúde: Compaixão e fé em meio à vulnerabilidade humana* (pp. 145–156). São Paulo, Brazil: Paulinas.

Potter, V. R. (1971). *Bioethics: Bridge to the future.* Englewood Cliffs, NJ: Prentice-Hall.

World Health Organization. (2008). *World health report 2008: Primary health care*. Geneva, Switzerland: WHO Press. Retrieved from http://www.who.int/whr/2008/en/index.html

World Health Organization. (2011a). *Closing the gap: Policy into practice on social determinants of health.* Discussion Paper. Geneva, Switzerland: WHO Press. Retrieved from http://www.who.int/sdhconference/discussion_paper/en/

World Health Organization. (2011b). *World conference on social determinants of health: Meeting report.* Rio de Janeiro, Brazil: WHO Press. Retrieved from http://dssbr.org/site/documentos-de-referencia/

World Health Organization. (2013). *World health report 2013: Research for universal health coverage.* Geneva, Switzerland: WHO Press. Retrieved from http://www.who.int/whr/en/

World Health Organization. (2015a). *Global health ethics: Key issues*. Geneva, Switzerland: WHO Press.

World Health Organization. (2015b). *Health in 2015: From MDGs to SDGs.* Geneva, Switzerland: WHO Press. Retrieved from http://www.who.int/gho/publications/mdgs-sdgs/en/

World Health Organization Commission on Macroeconomics and Health. (2003). *Investing in health: A summary of the findings of the Commission on Macroeconomics and Health*. Geneva, Switzerland: WHO Press. Retrieved from http://www.who.int/macrohealth/infocentre/advocacy/en/

Chapter 17

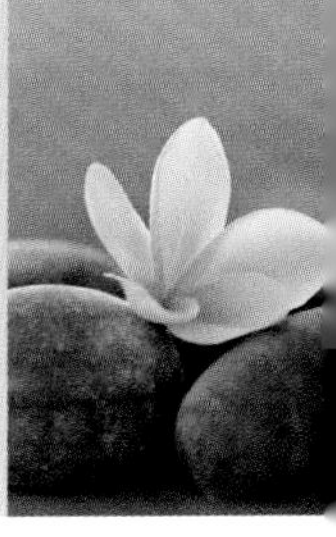

Use of Complementary Therapies for Health Promotion

Ruth Lindquist

LEARNING OBJECTIVES

After completing this chapter, the student will be able to:

1. Describe the background of the use of complementary therapies and integrative health approaches in the United States and the present use of these therapies across the life span by the public and health-care providers.
2. Describe the knowledge base underlying the use of complementary therapies and the need for evidence-based practice, including the strengths and weaknesses of current evidence.
3. Articulate recommendations for the use of complementary therapies in practice.
4. Identify Web sites and other resources to locate credible information about complementary therapies for health promotion.
5. Describe suggested strategies for incorporating complimentary and alternative therapies (CAT) to achieve the goals of Healthy People 2020.
6. Understand graduate competencies of safety and efficacy established by quality and safety education for nurses (QSEN).
7. Identify areas for future research on the use of CAT for health promotion.

INTRODUCTION

Complementary therapies have excellent potential for use in practice for health promotion. Up-to-date information on the use of these therapies by advanced practice nurses and clinical nurse leaders can help clients to achieve their goals for improved health and well-being, thus supporting goals for Healthy People 2020. This chapter presents an overview of complementary and alternative therapies in nursing, particularly as used by advanced practice nurses. The focus of this chapter is on the use of complementary and alternative therapies for health promotion.

This chapter is intended to assist advanced practice nurses and clinical nurse leaders to incorporate, refer, or recommend complementary and alternative therapies in their practice and develop integrative health approaches to advanced nursing practice and the provision of care. Advanced practice nurses and clinical nurse leaders are uniquely positioned to promote health using patient-centered, evidence-based practice by providing accurate and timely information about complementary and alternative therapies to help clients achieve their desired health promotion goals (Sackett, Strauss, Richardson, Rosenburg, & Haynes, 2000). Information provided in this chapter can also be applied to nurses' own self-care. Experiencing these therapies can inspire a broader appreciation for their use across a wide range of practice settings, specialties, and special populations. This chapter gives an overview of CAT as used for health promotion, highlighting selected therapies that are broadly effective for health promotion as well as those that the practitioner may encounter most frequently in practice. Because so many complementary therapies have not been definitively studied, the use of these non-traditional therapies instead of prudent use of allopathic medicine is not advocated in this chapter. The therapies described are considered adjuncts to Western medicine in the delivery of advanced practice nursing care.

TERMS AND DEFINITIONS

Because the focus of this chapter is on complementary and alternative therapies, the language surrounding these terms is also clarified through commonly agreed-upon definitions (Box 17-1). Although many sources for these definitions exist, the most authoritative and accessible definitions will be used wherever possible. The National Center for Complementary and Integrative Health (NCCIH) is a primary, foundational source for definitions and the content of this chapter (NCCIH, 2016a). Complementary therapies are non-mainstream practices used together with conventional medicine, sometimes called Western medicine. In this chapter, we use the term *complementary and alternative therapies (CATs)* rather than complementary and alternative *medicine* to avoid the disciplinary reference to medicine that, for some, would exclude the use of these therapies in the practice of professional nurses. It is also noted that the former National Center for Complementary and Alternative Medicine (NCCAM) was recently renamed the National Center for Complementary and Integrative Health (NCCIH, 2016a).

Definitions of integrative health care are many but all involve bringing conventional and complementary approaches together in a coordinated way. Although the coordination of approaches may benefit clients, the integration of CAT into practice is far from complete in the United States. In this text, we do not focus on integrating therapies but rather on the therapies themselves.

Health promotion goes beyond traditional daily activities such as using sunscreen, eating a nutritious diet, exercising regularly, and taking safety precautions such as using seat belts. A central component to health promotion is health literacy, or one's ability to read and process information and use critical evaluation skills to turn this data into knowledge that can influence good health choices. When used to enhance health, complementary therapies are also part of health promotion, and alternative therapies provide additional treatment options beyond conventional medicine.

BOX 17-1 Selected Chapter Terms and Definitions

alternative therapy: A non-mainstream practice that is exclusive of mainstream health care (Ali & Katz, 2015).

complementary and alternative medicine (CAM): CAM is a broad domain of resources, encompassing health systems, modalities, and practices and their accompanying theories and beliefs beyond those intrinsic to a society's current dominant health system. These resources are associated with positive outcomes by their users (IOM, 2005, p. 19).

complementary therapy: A non-mainstream practice that is used along with conventional medicine (NCCIH, 2016b).

integrative health strategies and *integrative health approaches:* Strategies or approaches that combine conventional and complementary approaches in a coordinated way, which in theory offers the best of both conventional and CAM health-care practices (Ring et al., 2014; Ali & Katz, 2015).

Categories and Types of CAT

The use of CAT can help both providers and clients achieve the goals of Healthy People 2020. However, evidence is needed to assure clients and providers that the time and money invested in therapies is safe and cost-effective. Evidence is also required for insurers to consider payment for CAT. Numerous therapies included on the NCCIH Web site are divided into two subgroups: mind and body practices, and natural products. Mind and body practices include Reiki, therapeutic touch, storytelling, yoga, tai chi, qigong, guided imagery, music intervention, humor therapy, prayer, biofeedback, animal-assisted therapy, massage, relaxation therapies, breathing, healing touch, light therapy, acupressure/acupuncture, reflexology, and magnet therapy. Natural products used for health promotion include a very wide range of products available to the consumer, and they will be further summarized below.

Another category of CAT includes whole systems of care such as naturopathic medicine, homeopathy, Ayurvedic medicine, Tibetan medicine, and traditional Chinese medicine. These provide an encompassing approach to care along with system-relevant therapies.

Generating evidence in the study of whole systems of care is complex and goes beyond the scope of this chapter.

Health Promotion and Self-Care

Health promotion is a broad term that embraces the ability and activities of individuals to exercise control over their own health. Health promotion may be viewed as an essential element of self-care. It encompasses a broad range of social and environmental interventions that can benefit people and improve their health, quality of life, and well-being. It addresses and focuses on the root causes of ill health, not just on its treatment and cure. Beyond traditional daily activities (such as using sunscreen, eating a nutritious diet, getting enough physical activity, avoiding pollution and toxic chemicals, and wearing seat belts and helmets), complementary therapies may be used to enhance health, quality of life, and well-being. Personal engagement and the ability to read, process, and understand health-related knowledge and information to evaluate the effects of remedies selected are essential for health promotion, including use of CAT.

Health promotion is also personally important for nurses. Providing care for others may be stressful, so self-care is needed to safeguard the well-being of this large segment of the health-care workforce. Clients are best served when providers are well, focused, balanced, and relaxed, and nurses are perhaps most effective when they are role models of good health. Self-care involves basic activities such as eating a balanced diet, exercising, getting adequate sleep and rest, praying and/or meditating, keeping a sense of humor, and learning stress mastery skills (Leonard, 2014).

Using integrative approaches to deliver effective evidence-based CAT ensures that the scientific foundations of practice are utilized even while responding to patient needs and preferences. Practicing nurses must understand the evidential foundation of CAT just as they understand the scientific foundations of therapies used in the provision of allopathic health care. The informed use of CAT can expand therapeutic options for health promotion and has the potential to improve outcomes. For these potential benefits to be realized, however, nurses must be well-informed about the use, referrals, and recommendations of CAT for health promotion.

It is reasonable to hypothesize that nurses' knowledge, attitudes, and personal use of CAT would be associated with their referral, recommendation, and use of CAT in their professional practice. We examined this hypothesis by reviewing a national survey of critical-care nurses. Although data from nurses working in critical-care settings do not generally emphasize the use of CAT for health promotion, the importance of nurses' knowledge, attitudes and personal use of CAT as associated with their use in practice is evident. This underscores the purpose of this chapter: to provide background knowledge and evidence for the appropriate, safe, informed, and effective use of CAT in practice for health promotion and for nurse and client self-care.

SUMMARY OF THE EVIDENCE

Before we describe the available evidence underlying the use of CATs for health promotion, let's review the background and history of the use of CAT across the life span in the United States by various providers and in different settings, including current statistics and national initiatives.

Research on CAT: Need for Evidence

NCCIH has systematically amassed substantial evidence about the use of CAT in recent decades, creating an amazing resource for nurses and health professionals around the world. At the link "Health Topics A to Z" on the NCCIH Web site, you'll find descriptions of therapies and summaries of evidence and known efficacy of therapies for given conditions (NCCIH, 2016b). This government resource provides a history of the evolution and use of complementary therapies and describes a broad range of interventions, along with a summary of the evidence for specific conditions.

CAT can make a positive difference in the quality of our care and outcomes. However, making broad generalizations about CATs or even conclusions about the use of specific CATs and their efficacy is difficult. Combining therapies may augment the effectiveness of treatment and achievement of outcomes, but this may also confound efforts to determine which component or CAT was effective. Determining efficacy for CAT for health promotion is also difficult because outcomes are affected (potentially confounded) by numerous simultaneous self-care actions. CATs are typically offered in the context of a trusting therapeutic relationship.

Use of Complementary Therapies in the United States

In 2012, results from a large national survey of U.S. adults found the estimated use of complementary therapies to be around 33% (NCCIH, 2012). Use of CAT by the population and population subgroups has remained relatively consistent over the last couple of decades. What is concerning, however, is that 61.5% of CAT users reported that they did not tell their providers about their use of these therapies (NCCIH, 0000). These numbers suggest significant potential for CAT to interact with prescribed allopathic medications and therapies, raising the risk for adverse outcomes or preventing achievement of the therapeutic intent of either or both types of therapies. Accurate knowledge of the safety and efficacy of CATs as used for specific purposes is needed to inform discussions between clients and providers and thus enable safe and optimal use. This points to an urgent need for evidence related to the safety and efficacy of CATs and their use for specific conditions by specific client populations to ensure safe, cost-effective use.

It is clear from these use statistics that members of society want and demand complementary and alternative therapies, thus requiring health-care practitioners to learn about and discuss these therapies with their clients. Consumer use is significant and has held steady over the years. The available evidence to guide the use of therapies lags behind the public's use of therapies; thus, much more research is needed to identify parameters of safety and to determine whether given CATs are effective for achievement of the intended and desired outcomes. Health professionals need to be informed and knowledgeable about the therapies and the evidence (or lack of evidence) for their use to have informed discussions with clients, guide or recommend CAT use, and refer clients to credible or credentialed CAT providers.

In 1998, the Center for Complementary and Alternative Medicine was founded within the National Institutes of Health in the United States. In 2014, it was renamed the Center for Complementary and Integrative Health (NCCIH, 2016a). Its mission is to define, through rigorous scientific investigation, the usefulness and safety of complementary and integrative health interventions and their roles in improving health and health care, including health promotion and self-care. The NCCIH Web site has a wealth of useful, up-to-date information regarding therapies and the evidence supporting their use for specific conditions and populations. The NCCIH Web site is perhaps the most credible source of information regarding CAT and was a primary source of information for this chapter.

Table 17-1 presents selected mind-body therapies, including yoga, meditation, and massage, that have been found to be effective in achieving selected targeted outcomes of health promotion. These are good general approaches for practitioners to recommend for broad positive changes in a range of salient health promotion outcomes. The selected therapies can be used for diverse patient populations and nontraditional healthy populations.. The therapies included may help individuals manage life's stresses, improve sleep, manage weight, improve mood, and enhance quality of life. These CATs are best integrated into the client's ongoing routines and lifestyle behaviors.

To place these CATs within the client's health promotion routine, the practitioner may employ the counseling interventions recommended in a scientific statement of the American Heart Association (AHA) to promote health-related behaviors related to eating and physical activity (Artinian et al., 2010). Authors of that statement recommended the use of counseling to promote the incorporation of healthy behaviors. They recommended a combination of two or more strategies, including approaches such as establishing a plan to include goal setting, obtaining feedback, and self-monitoring. (Artinian et al., 2010).

Nurse Knowledge, Attitudes, and Use of CAT

In a survey of critical-care nurses (n = 726), investigators found that most nurses used one or more complementary therapies in practice; a majority had some knowledge of more than half of the 28 therapies listed; and a majority desired additional training and increased availability of therapies for patients, patients' families, and nursing staff (Tracy et al., 2005). In this national survey of a random sample of critical-care nurses, most of the 726 respondents reported using one or more complementary therapies in practice—the most common being diet therapy, exercise, relaxation techniques, and prayer. Respondents generally required more evidence to use or recommend conventional therapies than to use or recommend CATs.

In this survey of critical-care nurses, nurses' personal use of CAT was found to be associated with their use in practice (Lindquist, Tracy, & Savik, 2003). A majority of respondents reported use of CAT, with approximately 50% or more of the nurse respondents reporting use of exercise, diet, massage, spiritual direction or prayer, relaxation therapies, and herbal therapies (Lindquist et al., 2005). Nurses' personal use of therapies was also related to knowing more types of therapies, using them more often in practice, and perceiving more therapies as beneficial. It was concluded that educational programs to promote nurses' knowledge and personal use could lead to an increase in appropriate use of therapies in practice to benefit patients and their families.

More than a decade has passed since the last survey in critical care. Personal use of therapies is indeed a significant factor in recommending and referring others. The link between providers' use and their recommendations, referrals, and use in practice is an important one. An increase in knowledge about CAT and evidence for CAT's safe and effective use in practice could provide substantial benefit for client health promotion.

Table 17-1 Selected CATs with Evidence for a Wide Range of Health Promotion Outcomes

Therapy	Selected Health Promotion Outcomes and References
Meditation/mindfulness-based stress reduction	Improved sleep (Gross et al., 2010; Goyal et al., 2014) Reduced stress (van Son, Nyklíček, Pop, & Pouwer, 2012) Reduced anxiety (Bohlmeijer, Prenger, Taal, & Cuijpers, 2010; Gross et al., 2010; Goyal et al., 2014; Sedlmeier et al., 2012; van Son et al., 2012) Reduced depression (Bohlmeijer et al., 2010; Goyal et al., 2014; Hartmann et al., 2012; van Son et al., 2012) Improved diet/eating behaviors (O'Reilly et al., 2014) Improved cognition/brain connectivity (Kilpatrick et al., 2011) Pain (Goyal et al., 2014; Hilton et al., 2016; Morone et al., 2016) Social functioning/self-confidence (Sedlmeier et al., 2012) Physical functioning (Morone et al., 2016) Blood pressure reduction (Bai et al., 2015; Hartmann et al., 2012; Schneider et al., 2005; Schneider et al., 2012) Fatigue (van Son et al., 2012) Quality of life (Hilton et al., 2016; van Son et al., 2012)
Yoga	Improved mood (Hartfiel, Havenhand, Khalsa, Clarke, & Krayer, 2011) Well-being (Hartfiel et al., 2011) Immune functioning (Morgan, Irwin, Chung, & Wang, 2014) Fatigue (Galantino et al., 2012) Depression (Pascoe & Bauer, 2015) Physical functioning (flexibility/balance/strength) (Galantino et al., 2012) Blood glucose (Chimkode, 2015; Okonta, 2012) Blood pressure (Okonta, 2012) Cholesterol (Okonta, 2012) Weight management (Okonta, 2012; Seo et al., 2012) Social functioning/self-confidence (Hartfiel et al., 2011) Reduced stress (Smith, Hancock, Blake-Mortimer, & Eckert, 2007) Cognition (Lee, Moon, & Kim, 2014) Pain (Cramer, Lauche, Haller, & Dobos, 2013) Reduced anxiety (Li & Goldsmith, 2014; Smith et al., 2007). Quality of life (Smith et al., 2007; Lee et al., 2014)
Massage therapy	Improved sleep (Harris, Richards, & Grando, 2012; Nerbass, Feltrim, de Souza, Ykeda, & Lorenzi-Filho, 2010; Richards, 1998) Decreased stress/relaxation (Harris & Richards, 2010) Decreased pain (Chang, Wang, & Chen, 2002; Mok & Woo, 2004; Seyyed-Rasodi, Salehi, Mohammadpoorosi, Goljaryan, & Seyyedi, 2016; Wang & Keck, 2004) Decreased anxiety (Chang et al., 2002; Currin & Meister, 2008; Richardson et al., 2000; Seyyed-Rasodi et al., 2016) Decreased fatigue (Currin & Meister, 2008) Blood pressure (Chen et al., 2013) Quality of life (Williams et al., 2005) Health and well-being (McFeeters, Pront, Cuthbertson, & King, 2016) Weight [gain] in preterm infants (Diego, Fiedl, & Hernandex-Reif, 2014)

State nurse practice acts include specific language regarding CAT, and nurses' scope and standards of practice support the use of CAT in professional practice. However, safe and effective administration of some CATs, such as acupuncture, Reiki, or massage, requires special education and/or certification. A practice guideline for complementary therapies was developed by the College of Nurses of Ontario (CNO; 2014) to clarify the role that CATs have in practice and to guide their use. The document clarifies that an ethical accountability of the nurse must ensure that the client is informed about use and that the nurse understands the CAT to be delivered; the client must be informed, and client consent must be obtained; the nurse must be knowledgeable about the appropriateness of the therapy according to the findings of the initial health assessment; and the nurse must know the risks and desired effects/outcomes of the selected CAT and how to measure them. The nurse must also assess whether she or he has the authority to provide a given CAT as approved or recognized within the practice setting or agency. The nurse must have the technical skills and recognize when additional knowledge and expertise is needed (CNO, 2014).

RECOMMENDATIONS FOR PRACTICE

Pender's Health Promotion Model served as a primary foundation for the work of this chapter (Pender, 1990) and guided the general framework for exploration of the use of CAT in health promotion. This framework comprises the elements of initially assessed health status, an integrative approach to CAT interventions, and health-related outcomes. The model broadly encompasses spiritual, physical, mental/psychological, and emotional outcome dimensions with enough detail to make outcome evaluation more tangible and measurable. The initially assessed health status elements are paired with the corresponding desired outcomes.

In Pender's model, the CATs that are used are discussed, and they are selected by and agreeable to both the client and provider to target the client's need areas (health status, client goals, and disease risks) gathered from the assessment; the selection of the specific CAT is informed by the client's preference and offered concurrently with traditional allopathic therapies used or appropriate for the client for health promotion or disease management. This process includes CAT administration, education, and information sharing about the evidence for efficacy, dose, frequency, and duration; recommendations may be given and referrals made.

AHA's Life's Simple 7 (AHA, 2017) was also examined to identify additional health promotion targets. The targets of the Life's Simple 7 elements include lose weight, don't smoke, reduce blood pressure, control blood sugar, reduce cholesterol, exercise more, and eat better. Instructional content is available at AHA's Web site under "My Life Check—Life's Simple 7."

Finally, the Model for Well-Being (Kreitzer, 2016) was examined for potential conceptual incorporation of dimensions of well-being (purpose, security, community, environment, health, and relationships) into the set of health promotion outcomes. Together, these models informed the selection of the health promotion outcomes identified in Figure 17-1. CATs, as described in this chapter, can be applied within this framework to address initially assessed health status and health-promoting opportunities mutually determined by the client and the advanced practice nurse, clinical nurse leader, or advanced practice nursing student.

CAT Familiarity for Advanced Practice Nurses

Education that includes foundational CAT content would help ensure that advanced practice nurses are prepared to assess clients' appropriate use of CAT, evaluate safety and compatibility with other CATs or allopathic therapies, and recommend CATs or refer clients to specialized CAT practitioners. In addition, educational content would familiarize practitioners with CATs and prepare them for situations outside the comfort zone of usual care. In the case of advanced practice, it is important to know what natural products are used by the client (e.g., herbals, supplements) to make sense of findings from physical assessments and avoid adverse interactions between CATs and allopathic medicines.

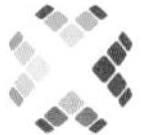

Case Illustration

Dr. Johnson was a new advanced practice nursing (CRNA/DNP) program graduate who had taken a position as a nurse anesthetist at a large metropolitan county hospital soon after graduation. As he came into the office one morning, he encountered a huddle of anesthesia providers discussing a client case. A middle-aged woman had arrived for her biopsy along with her so-called healer. The anesthesia providers were loudly adamant that they could not allow a healer into the operating room during the biopsy procedure, and none would agree to take the case under those conditions. Dr. Johnson, having had content relating to complementary therapies and healing practices woven into the curriculum of his graduate program, was familiar with a wide range of therapies, healing practices, and health-promoting approaches. He interviewed the woman and learned of her desire to have the healer by her side during the biopsy procedure where she could exercise presence and the laying on of hands. Confident about the low risk, familiar with a wide range of healing practices, and aware of his client's preferences, he made the decision to allow the healer in

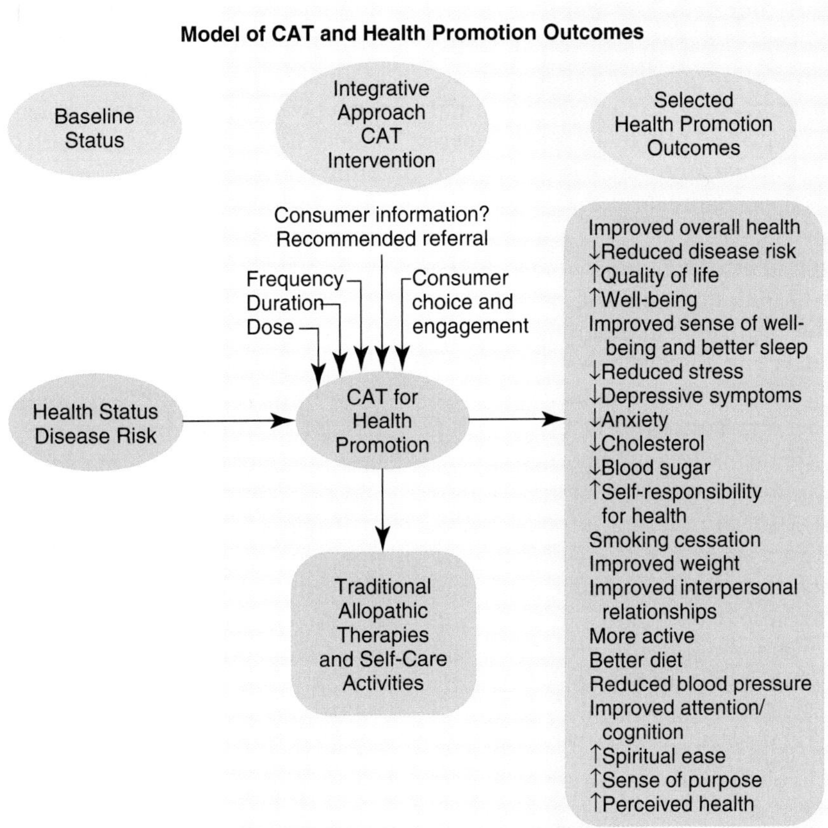

FIGURE 17-1 Model of CAT and Health Promotion Outcomes. *Source: Adapted from Walker et al. (1987); AHA Life's Simple 7 (AHA, 2017); Pender Health Promotion Model (Pender, 2011).*

the operating room and took the case. Because of his exposure to a broad range of complementary therapies, Dr. Johnson accepted the presence of the healer and reported that he had seldom delivered so little anesthesia in a procedure nor had a blood pressure been so well controlled.

Practice Foundations

Several foundational practice components of high-quality nursing care are embraced by CAT, including listening, presence, touch, and the creation of a healing environment (Lindquist, Tracy, & Snyder, 2018). These practice foundations are rooted in the understanding that the health-care provider is a potent healing force in his or her own right. The presence and compassion of the nurse as a healer is a crucial synergistic foundational and adjunct therapy (Drake, 2014). A distinctive characteristic of many who work in health care is that they are not repelled by human suffering but instead seek to be of help, to listen and lean into the story (Maizes & Low Dog, 2011). This characteristic can be demonstrated simply and effectively by bearing witness to someone's story, helping a patient organize and prioritize his or her health concerns, and offering a partnership for disease prevention and health promotion over a life span. These practices establish the trusting relationship in which client needs and goals can be safely expressed and next steps established for health promotion and wellness.

Authentic presence is healing and changes the nature of the nurse-patient relationship (Penque & Snyder, 2014). Presence requires the practice of intentionality: bringing a conscious awareness to the assessment of the patient's body, mind, and spirit (Deary, Roche, Plotkin, & Sahourek, 2011). Consideration is given for age relevancy, life circumstances, patient goals, and willingness to change while being attentive to physiologic disorders and signs of depression or other psychological conditions (Drake, 2014).

Therapeutic listening has long been an essential component of the nursing profession. Reduced anxiety, depression, and hostility and greater satisfaction with care are potential client outcomes of therapeutic listening (Watanuki, Tracy, & Lindquist, 2014). Therapeutic touch can be learned but requires more extensive instruction and has a leveled sequence of credentialing. Healing environments are also foundational to our practice (Kreitzer & Langevin, 2014). Unhurried, quiet, and comfortable waiting rooms and patient areas can generate a more intimate response from the patient, reduce stress, and provide an opportunity for the nurse to listen deeply (Geimer-Flanders, 2009).

Nurses' application of listening, presence, and touch in the context of a healing environment can work in powerful ways to assist the patient in exploring a change from health imbalance and discord toward a higher quality of life and a life free of preventable diseases. The integrative model of care stresses the belief within caregivers that they are themselves an important instrument of healing beyond the immediacy of medications and surgery (Drake, 2014). Promoting provider skills that foster a client-driven encounter where the provider partners with the client may be more valuable in triggering the client's innate capacity for health and well-being and promoting the overarching health promotion and disease prevention goals in the 10-year plan, Healthy People 2020, set by the U.S. Department of Health and Human Services (USDHHS) in 2010. The national plan objectives seek to promote the following overarching goals (USDHHS, n.d.) while closely reflecting the intended and symbiotic nature of CATs:

- Attain high-quality, longer lives free of preventable disease, disability, injury, and premature death.
- Achieve health equity, eliminate disparities, and improve the health of all groups.
- Create social and physical environments that promote good health for all.
- Promote quality of life, healthy development, and healthy behaviors across all life stages.

Selected Mind-Body CATs for Health Promotion

Mind and body therapies included in this chapter are those judged to be the most broadly relevant to health promotion outcomes described in the model (Figure 17-1), with evidence for health promotion outcomes for selected CATs cited in Table 17-1.

Meditation

Evidence exists for the effectiveness of meditation in treating symptoms of chronic diseases including pain, hypertension, anxiety, depression, irritable bowel syndrome, diabetes, cancer, and insomnia (Gross, Christopher, & Reilly-Spong, 2018). Studies of meditation have been done with populations of patients with heart disease, those who have undergone transplant procedures, and veterans of war for post-traumatic stress disorder (PTSD) to reduce symptoms and improve quality of life (Gross, Christopher, & Reilly-Spong,2018).

In our work with women with heart disease, we studied a program of mindfulness-based stress reduction to reduce stress and promote health (Lindquist et al., 2015). Mindfulness-based stress reduction (MBSR) was developed by Jon Kabat-Zinn (2013). The standard program is 8 weeks, and weekly meetings are supplemented with participants' practice of skills, including sitting meditation, body scan, and yoga. In our study, middle-aged women with heart disease completed diaries to record the activity, date, time, length, and response to sessions of meditation. Polar monitors were worn during the practice to record heart rate, meditation effectiveness, and adherence. Qualitative data were gathered and the content was analyzed to examine the range of benefits experienced. In addition to stress reduction, participant-reported benefits included increased strength and flexibility; more energy; and improved self-esteem, interpersonal relationships, posture, sleep, range of motion, and physical functioning (Lindquist et al., 2015).

Transcendental meditation was found to be an effective approach to blood pressure reduction and management (Anderson, Liu, & Kryscio, 2008; Brook et al., 2013; Brook, Jackson, Giorgini, & McGowan, 2015). A literature review on the use of mindfulness-based interventions for obesity-related eating behaviors from the 18 (86%) of the studies that were reviewed found improvements in eating behaviors that were targeted in the studies (O'Reilly, Cook, Spruijt-Metz, & Black, 2014).

Stress is ubiquitous in the daily lives of our clients (Lindquist, Witt, & Crane, 2014). It plays a role in the development, progression, or symptom exacerbation of many if not most human illnesses (Cohen, Janicki-Deverts, & Miller, 2007). Thus, stress management can be considered a cornerstone of health promotion/disease prevention. In a review of 47 trials that included 3,515 participants, authors of one systematic review and meta-analysis concluded that participation in programs of meditation can result in small to moderate reductions of negative dimensions of psychological stress (Goyal et al., 2014).

Yoga

Physical activity is an important aspect of health promotion. Exercise may be construed as a nontraditional or complementary therapy for this purpose. In the innovative research program of Dr. Diane Treat-Jacobson (Treat-Jacobson, Bronas, & Salisbury, 2014), arm exercise is used to improve function and reduce symptoms of persons with peripheral artery disease. Exercise is commonly prescribed for various conditions and is part of the Surgeon General's daily lifestyle recommendations. Yoga can be used to improve mobility and function and reduce arthritic and other types of chronic pain.

Yoga is an ancient form of exercise that can promote health and physical, emotional, and mental well-being (AHA, 2013). Nurses can recommend yoga to clients who want to improve their overall health and well-being and to those with specific goals to improve blood pressure, improve flexibility, reduce joint and skeletal pain, and reduce stress. Yoga can be adapted to address the needs and to accommodate the safety concerns for most client populations (e.g., pregnant women, frail patients, children). A fuller description of the types of yoga can be obtained on the NCCIH Web site (NCCIH, 2013a); Harris (2018) gives a thorough summary in her chapter on massage in the text *Complementary & Alternative Therapies in Nursing* (Lindquist, Tracy, & Snyder, 2018).

Massage therapy

Massage therapy is a broadly effective CAT that can improve quality of life, enhance physical functioning, and reduce stress. It is appropriate for virtually all client populations. The ancient practice of massage has been shown to be effective in treating pain and improving stiffness and function of persons with osteoarthritis of the knee (Perlman, Sabina, & Williams, 2006). A fuller description of the types of massage can be obtained on the NCCIH Web site (NCCIH, 2016e); Harris (2018) gives a thorough summary in a chapter on massage in the text *Complementary & Alternative Therapies in Nursing* (Lindquist, Tracy, & Snyder, 2018).

Natural products

Natural products include herbal medicines (plant-based therapies, botanicals, or phytotherapies), dietary supplements (including mycotherapies), and nutraceuticals (vitamin, mineral, and nutritional therapies) (Plotnikoff & Lillehei, 2018). Even simple multivitamins taken for health promotion fall into the category of natural products. Public awareness of nutrition's health promotion potential has created increased availability of diverse food sources with added nutrients and supplemental ingredients (e.g., nutraceuticals). Products in this category include calcium-fortified drinks, drinks fortified with electrolytes and vitamins, and margarines fortified with plant stanols and sterols to reduce total cholesterol and low-density lipoproteins. Safety of the products and the amount ingested (potential overuse) are important to include in the health assessment, in addition to consideration of the product's potential benefits and client's reason for use. Aromatherapy is also included in this category of CATs (Halcón, 2018).

Two principles are foundational to the use of natural products. First, what is natural is not always good; second, if some is good, more is not necessarily better. Adherence to these principles is critical in a world where consumers are offered promises of good health and vitality through advertising and have unfettered access to over-the-counter products online and in pharmacies and department stores. Indeed, a number of these products are effective, some are safe and yet have not been shown to be effective, and some are ill-advised. From a review of the literature examining the effects of commercially available dietary supplements on resting energy, authors question whether supplement-induced increases in resting energy expenditure are superior to ingestion of regular dietary constituents with similar ingredients (Vaughan, Conn, & Mermier, 2014). For clients seeking advice for health promotion, attention might first be directed to a nutritious, balanced diet (U.S. Preventive Services Task Force [USPSTF], 2017). The type, amount, purpose, and effects of dietary supplements should be evaluated for every client currently taking supplements, and all supplement intake should be examined for safety.

SAFETY CONSIDERATIONS

Even natural therapies that are proven effective can cause harm if they are used incorrectly, if they are overused, or if interactions with prescription medication or other treatments occur. While many products on the market are safe, others include ingredients that can cause organ damage or even death, depending on the dose, length of time taken, and other client-related factors and health conditions. Dietary supplements are available to consumers based on evidence of safety and can be removed from the market only by the Food and Drug Administration (FDA) if proven unsafe (Plotnikoff & Lillehei, 2018). Depending on manufacturing standards, products purchased by the client may be tainted or contaminated. It is good practice to discuss these issues with clients so that they are informed users of these products.

Practitioners must also be concerned about the quality of the products used. A safety mechanism put in place by the U.S. Pharmacopeia (USP) is the voluntary dietary supplement verification program (Frisvold, 2018). Product labels containing the USP-verified mark certify that the product has been tested and audited as a supplement that meets criteria for the label-identified amount and potency, does not contain harmful levels of contaminants, and meets the FDA's good manufacturing practices (Frisvold, 2018).

Taking a comprehensive history that includes intake of natural products and supplements can be challenging for caregivers. The 2012 National Health Interview Survey estimated that more than 40% of clients do not disclose the use of CATs to their providers (Jou & Johnson, 2016). The authors speculated that clients may fear being told that they are not safe or that the provider has discouraged or could discourage them from taking them, they may not believe that the provider needs to know, they may fear a negative provider response or doubt the provider's knowledge of CAT, there may be a real or perceived lack of time during the visit, the provider may not ask, or the client is not *currently* using CAT but has done so in the past (Jou & Johnson, 2016; Merry, 2016). A deliberate, thoughtful, nonjudgmental approach should be used when inquiring about the use of natural products or other forms of CATs. It is advisable to ask and ask again in a different way so that the client understands the whole range of products considered part of the health history. Questions to ask might include: "Are you using any herbs?" "Are you using any vitamins?" "Are you using any dietary supplements?" Follow-up questions could include, "What is the dose?" "What is the source?" "What directions are you following?" "Why are you taking it?" "Are you working with any other health professionals?" (Plotnikoff & Lillehei, 2018, p. 6).

An accurate health history that includes natural products allows the provider to evaluate the safety of the product(s) in light of the patient' condition, assess potential interactions with concurrent prescription medications, and ensure that the therapeutic effects of prescribed therapies may be realized. During the health assessment that includes CATs, the provider also has the opportunity to educate individuals about safe and beneficial use of the products or to advise discontinuance when necessary.

Giving clients evidence-based information is important. Provide educational materials from a credible source as handouts so that clients can refer to them after the visit. Spoken information is often forgotten, so the provider cannot rely on clients to do a thorough follow-up search for product information. You can ask the client to bring the products to a future appointment so that you can evaluate their quality, dose, and appropriateness; evidence of product efficacy (including cost-effectiveness) may also be discussed. Working closely with a pharmacist and building a relationship with the client over time are important to gathering a thorough history and providing advice accordingly.

CAT Use for Health Promotion with Special Populations

Clients in vulnerable populations, including children and adolescents, may benefit from CAT for health promotion, but caution is recommend because few long-term studies have examined CAT use with children, and children are not just small adults. Their metabolism, immune system, digestive system, and central nervous system are still maturing (NCCIH, 2017b).

Examples of specific client populations who might benefit from CATs include those with traumatic brain syndromes; those receiving palliative care, end-of-life care, or cancer care; those undergoing cancer surgery; those with acute coronary syndromes; and those visiting the emergency room. Counseling patients to improve health promotion involves patient-centered care specific to individual priorities and utilizes evidence-based guidelines. Patients who can identify a comprehensive health plan for the promotion of their physical, emotional, and social health will be more able create a template for success as they age.

Important client differences must be considered in applying the evidence in practice. CATs may not be effective for all clients due to individual differences, preferences, gender, and specific conditions. Health-care access and affordability are issues related to the use of CATs for health promotion. Obstacles can also include decreased mobility, lack of insurance, low income level, transportation difficulties, and cultural norms that may prohibit certain CATs or integrative approaches. A study using data from the 2012 National Health Interview Survey on the perceived benefits of using complementary and alternative medicine by race/ethnicity among midlife and older adults found significant differences by race/ethnicity. Minority groups were less likely to use CAT, but those who used these therapies reported perceived greater benefits than white Hispanic users (Johnson et al., 2019).

Evidence Summary and Areas for Future Research

Research evidence related to the use of CATs for health promotions to achieve desired outcomes among diverse populations leaves many questions unanswered. For example, who should administer CATs, and at what frequency and dose? How well can findings of efficacy be generalized across populations, conditions, and settings? Although some evidence is available to support the use of CATs for health promotion, more research is needed to achieve optimal health promotion outcomes. The paucity of research is particularly evident for natural products, where the lack of standardization of products adds additional complexity to the investigation. The users of evidence must be cautious when generalizing findings across populations (e.g., generalizing the findings of adult populations to children or adolescents, generalizing findings of pregnant or lactating women to frail older women, generalizing findings of joint pain relief in normal healthy joints versus pain relief in joints of clients with advanced rheumatoid arthritis). When evidence is not available, practitioners and clients should proceed with caution, balancing costs and potential efficacy with foremost attention to safety.

When evaluating the evidence of efficacy of CATs, we must consider the potential power of the placebo effect. Complete understanding of the placebo effect remains elusive, yet it may be at the heart of the healing professions (Kaptchuk & Miller, 2015). Although the mechanisms that explain the placebo effect are still a matter of speculation, experts think it contributes significantly to the effectiveness of most CATs. Authors suggest that the placebo effect predominantly produces symptom relief rather than modifying pathophysiological aspects of disease conditions. Thus, how a CAT is recommended, referred, or delivered may have an impact on the success of the therapy. Potential placebo effects should be addressed along with reports of the efficacy of CATs.

INTEGRATING CATS INTO PRACTICE

The impetus for integrating CAT approaches for health promotion into practice settings is driven by several key factors. Chronic health conditions associated with lifestyle and modifiable behaviors are the leading cause of morbidity and mortality in the United States (Thompson & Nichter, 2015). Federal health guidelines recommend disease prevention education that is holistic and includes social and physical environments (USDHHS, 2017) as well as the national initiatives toward more team-based care systems that foster increased patient safety and patient-centered care (Quality Safety Education for Nurses [QSEN], 2017).

Lifestyle behavior change is a common goal of providers of conventional medicine and CAT-specific providers. Allopathic medicine and complementary therapies can be provided together. When delivered from an integrative health framework, they are truly complementary in the most genuine sense of the term. The integrative approach combines the Institute of Medicine's (IOM) Triple Aim recommendations for improving patient satisfaction, patient safety, and the efficacious use of health-care resources (Berwick, Nolan, & Whittington, 2008). The holistic approach provides a template for change that promotes longevity, health equity, and healthy environments for individuals and populations across the life span. To integrate CATs into a conventional practice, the patient population, staff members and setting, evidence of therapies, the internal team to champion the integration, evaluation methods, and education and research should be considered.

The first step is to assess and understand the patient population served at the practice and their health determinants. This is key to promoting the best health population outcomes. Health determinants such as the physical environment, social environment, individual behavior, biology and genetics, and access to health services all play a role in health promotion and positive population outcomes.

Identifying Practice Opportunities for Health Promotion

The next step is determining the best opportunities for health promotion utilizing CAT. Options for CAT within health-care settings include provider care from synchronous or asynchronous interprofessional teams, a single provider, CAT-specific or a conventionally trained provider with additional CAT training, or groups and programs or referrals to external providers. CATs may be administered, they may be recommended, or referrals can be made by practitioners within the context of a trusting therapeutic relationship.

Interprofessional Care and CATs for Health Promotion

Health-care providers working within an interprofessional practice model have been shown to increase the practice of safe, high-quality, accessible, patient-centered care desired by patients and providers alike (Interprofessional Education Collaborative, 2016). Community resources can include low-cost and accessible programs for stress reduction, support groups, and integrative approaches including CATs.

CAT use in health-care practice settings is increasing; many larger health systems have services that incorporate CATs, such as acupuncture, massage, and aromatherapy, in their hospital and clinic settings (Can, 2013). Nurses must have in-depth knowledge about the wide array of therapies to apply in practice and to recommend to clients.

Complementary therapies often meet less resistance from conventional practitioners when they are based in health promotion programs (Thompson & Nichter, 2015). Indeed, health promotion and disease prevention are key components of care common across the largest group of CAT providers and their professional organizations, and they are also part of the education and training standards for acupuncture, chiropractic medicine, and naturopathic medicine (Goldblatt et al., 2013).

Group health interventions have been shown to improve disease knowledge, provide greater satisfaction with care, and decrease some health risks (McNeil et al., 2013). These programs can provide evidence-based, low-cost group care in complementary therapies that increase informed patient decision making, self-management, and life skills and enhance the forming of strategic and supportive partnerships with providers (Pechacek, Drake, Terrell, & Torkelson, 2015). Such models currently exist to optimize aging; provide group prenatal care; and offer menopause transition support, group acupuncture, stress reduction therapies, and chronic pain management.

In health promotion, it is essential to consider the pacing and demands of the recommendations for change. All potential relapses in progress can be adjusted as each patient progresses at her or his own pace. Being attentive to the transformative shift in client response and evaluating outcomes following the implementation of CATs is important so that the outcomes may be documented and the use reinforced, discontinued, or replaced with a different type of CAT, as indicated.

To be successful for health promotion, the therapies must be employed as directed.

How do you get these therapies into practice? What models of care delivery can be used? What is the evidence for the effectiveness of CAT, for health promotion? Which health promotion outcome will you target? For example, will you target improved nutritional status, more positive subjective perceptions of health, or increased vitality? Health promotion has numerous dimensions. Goals must be mutually set through the discussion between the provider and client, provider observations, and client preferences for self-care.

CAT Champions

A study by Hawk, Ndetan, and Evans (2012) found that the most effective strategy in reinforcing health promotion and disease prevention was a greater number of patient contacts, or time spent with the patient. To ensure adequate time for patient education and participation with complementary therapists, a six-week course was developed that allowed for conventional and CAT providers to interact and instruct the participants multiple times throughout the course. The team of providers included physicians, advance practice nurses, a psychologist, a functional nutritionist, a massage therapist, a Reiki healer, a health coach, and an acupuncturist.

The health coach facilitating the courses utilized a relationship-based care model that encourages group interaction; participants reported that the group work reinforced an understanding of the midlife aging process and health promotion options. CAT-based care options for health promotion and disease prevention were discussed throughout the course. Topics included developing a restorative practice using breathing techniques and relaxation, optimal nutrition to improve health with aging, the use of acupuncture for common ailments occurring at midlife, and massage techniques for sleep disorders and stress reduction. Participants reported that these options introduced them to a new world of alternative perspectives and resources for common medical concerns (Pechacek et al., 2015)

A series of validated evaluation tools were implemented before and after the program to assess quality of life, symptoms associated with midlife aging, self-advocacy skills, psychological assessments, and preventive screening knowledge. In summary, patients were found to be highly satisfied with the group approach to health promotion facilitated by a health coach that included CAT options and peer support. Complementary perspectives and resources presented by an interprofessional team provided another way of viewing and working with common health concerns and prevention (Pechacek et al., 2015).

Barriers to the Use of CATs

In general, barriers to the use of CATs in practice include the roots of traditional education in scientific method and conventional medicine. The acceptability of CATs can be affected by conflicts between practitioners of complementary and alternative therapies and conventional therapies. Factors affecting acceptance of CATs include lack of knowledge of efficacy, lack of belief in efficacy, lack of consensus about use, lack of evidence base, lack of comfort with therapy, and lack of interest.

Preparation of CAT Practitioners and Providers

Some CATs can be delivered by the practitioner, and instruction for each CAT can be offered to the client in writing and verbally. Some therapies that could benefit clients require referral. Advanced practice nurses who are interested in health promotion may have a range of patient information materials available on various forms of CATs. The primary-care setting is perhaps the best setting for health promotion because providers typically have more interaction with clients over time and thus have potentially developed trusting therapeutic relationships.

Finding a qualified therapist to administer CATs that require credentials can be challenging. It is important to understand practitioner preparation, licensing, credentials, certification, education, and experience. More information about provider qualifications and general guidance about how to identify a qualified provider can be found on the NCCIH Web site. Provide clients with a referral where possible, or recommend that they seek a referral from their insurers; find out as much as possible about the potential provider before receiving treatment; determine whether the CAT provider is willing to work with the conventional-care provider; discuss health conditions and determine whether the provider has worked with others with similar conditions; determine the cost, and don't assume that the practitioners services will be covered by health insurance (NCCIH, 2016h).

USEFUL RESOURCES

Numerous resources are available to support the inclusion of health promotion in evidence-based advanced nursing practice. The resources listed below are readily available from credible sources and are useful for both providers and clients. General and specific information about CATs and content that can contribute to baseline assessments or assessments of outcomes are available on these sites.

Selected Outcome Assessment Tools

- NIH PROMIS® measures: http://www.healthmeasures.net/explore-measurement-systems/promis
- Health-Promoting Lifestyle Profile II (Walker, Sechrist, & Pender, 1987): https://www.brandeis.edu/roybal/docs/Health-Promoting%20Lifestyle%20Profile%20II%20_website_PDF.pdf
- 36-Item Short Form Health Survey (SF-36): https://www.rand.org/health/surveys_tools/mos/36-item-short-form.html
- Perceived Stress Scale (PSS) (Cohen, 1994): http://www.mindgarden.com/documents/PerceivedStressScale.pdf
- PHQ-9 (depression): http://www.phqscreeners.com/
- Health-Related Quality of Life Measures: https://www.cdc.gov/hrqol/methods.htm#2

Client Education Materials for Complementary Therapies

- NCCIH: https://nccih.nih.gov/health/webresources
- Mayo Clinic: http://www.mayoclinic.org/healthy-lifestyle/consumer-health/in-depth/alternative-medicine/art-20045267
- Cleveland Clinic: https://my.clevelandclinic.org/health/articles/complementary-therapy
- Earl E. Bakken Center for Spirituality and Healing, University of Minnesota: https://www.takingcharge.csh.umn.edu

Web Sites

- National Center for Complementary and Integrative Health (NCCIH): https://nccih.nih.gov
- Mayo Clinic: http://www.mayoclinic.org/departments-centers/integrative-medicine-health
- Cochrane Database of Systematic Reviews (search *complementary therapies*): http://www.cochranelibrary.com/cochrane-database-of-systematic-reviews/
- American Botanical Council: http://abc.herbalgram.org/site/PageServer
- American Nutraceutical Association: http://www.americanutra.com
- Natural Standard (Natural Medicines) Databases: https://naturalmedicines.therapeuticresearch.com/databases.aspx
- International Congress for Educators in Complementary and Integrative Medicine: www.icecim.org
- Consortium of Academic Health Centers for Integrative Medicine (CAHCIM): www.cachim.org
- American Academy of Family Physicians (2016), Recommended Curriculum Guidelines for Family Medicine Residents, Health Promotion and Disease Prevention: http://www.aafp.org/dam/AAFP/documents/medical_education_residency/program_directors/Reprint267_Health.pdf
- Agency for Healthcare Research and Quality (AHRQ): https://www.guideline.gov/search?q=complementary+therapies
- Global Conference on Health Promotion; The Helsinki Statement on Health All Policies; World Health Organization, June 2013: http://www.who.int/healthpromotion/conferences/8gchp/8gchp_helsinki_statement.pdf?u a=1.

Nursing Textbook/Reference Resource

- Lindquist, R., Tracy, M. F., & Snyder, M. (2018). *Complementary & alternative therapies in nursing* (8th ed.). New York: Springer.

KEY POINTS

- CAT use continues to be significant in the U.S. population, with estimates of adult use from the 2012 National Health Survey at 33%.
- Advanced practice nurses and clinical nurse leaders will continue to encounter patients using CATs; informed providers in consultation with informed consumers can ensure that CAT use is safe and effective, based on the available evidence. Thus, inclusion of CATs and integrative health approaches in advanced nurse education curricula as well as continuing education is important.
- A practical model for the use of CATs for health promotion identifies numerous targets for health promotion/health promotion outcomes.
- Meditation, yoga, and massage are CATs that address a broad range of potential health promotion outcomes, are largely accessible, and can be recommended for virtually all client populations.
- A thorough, complete, and accurate health history that includes CAT use, especially natural products, can open the door to discussion related to client goals for health promotion and discussion and education regarding safe and effective use of CATs.
- Some evidence is available to support the use of CATs for health promotion; however, more research is needed to achieve optimal health promotion outcomes.

Check Your Understanding

1. Which of the following therapies would be considered a mind and body practice?
   A. Homeopathy
   B. Chemotherapy
   C. Guided imagery
   D. Tibetan medicine
2. According to a 2012 survey by the NCCIH, what percentage of adults in the United States use complementary therapies?
   A. 5%
   B. 33%
   C. 75%
   D. 90%
3. Which of the following is *not* a foundational practice component of high-quality nursing care embraced by CAT?
   A. Listening
   B. Touch
   C. Creation of a healing environment
   D. Mysticism
4. Which definition best describes yoga?
   A. An ancient form of exercise that can promote physical, emotional, and mental well-being
   B. Herbal medicines and dietary supplements
   C. A form of hypnosis
   D. The use of magnetic fields for healing
5. Which government agency in the United States has the authority to remove dietary supplements from the market if they are proven unsafe?
   A. Agency for Healthcare Research and Quality
   B. Food and Drug Administration
   C. Centers for Disease Control and Prevention
   D. National Institutes of Health
6. What do experts suggest may contribute significantly to the success of most CATs?
   A. Use in health promotion programs
   B. Participating in a research study
   C. Television advertising
   D. Word of mouth
7. In Tracy et al. (2005), which of the following is among the most commonly used complementary therapies by the critical-care nurses surveyed?
   A. Diet therapy
   B. Hypnosis
   C. Traditional Chinese medicine
   D. Qigong
8. What does the CNO practice guideline for CATs state is the nurse's accountability with regard to CATs?
   A. Nurses must discourage any alternative therapy use by clients.
   B. Nurses should encourage all clients to use alternative therapies.
   C. Each nurse must assess whether she or he has the authority to provide a given CAT as approved.
   D. Nurses may only administer dietary supplements to clients.

9. Which of the following is a target of the AHA's Life's Simple 7?
   A. Take a multivitamin daily.
   B. Avoid all dairy.
   C. Limit smartphone use.
   D. Control blood sugar.

10. Gross and colleagues (2018) provide evidence of which therapy for treating symptoms of pain, hypertension, and anxiety?
   A. Meditation
   B. Chiropractic medicine
   C. Herbalism
   D. Biofeedback

See "Reflections on Check Your Understanding" at the end of the book for answers.

REFERENCES

Ali, A., & Katz, D. L. (2015). Disease prevention and health promotion: How integrative medicine fits. *American Journal of Preventive Medicine, 49*(5), S230–S240.

American Association of Colleges of Nursing QSEN Education Consortium. (2012). *Graduate-level QSEN competencies-knowledge, skills and attitudes.* Retrieved from http://www.aacn.nche.edu/faculty/qsen/competencies.pdf

American Heart Association. (2013). *Yoga and heart health.* Retrieved from http://www.heart.org/HEARTORG/HealthyLiving/PhysicalActivity/FitnessBasics/Yoga-and-Heart-Health_UCM_434966_Article.jsp#.WWPYPDOZNBw

American Heart Association. (2017). *My life check—Life's Simple 7.* Retrieved from http://www.heart.org/HEARTORG/Conditions/My-Life-Check—Lifes-Simple-7_UCM_471453_Article.jsp#.WUrPeTPMxBw

Anderson, J. W., Liu, C., & Kryscio, R. J., (2008). Blood pressure response to transcendental meditation: A meta-analysis. *American Journal of Hypertension, 21*, 310–316.

Artinian, N. T., Fletcher, G. F., Mozaffarian, D., Kris-Etherton, P., Van Horn, L., Lichtenstein, A. H., . . . Burke, L. E., & American Heart Association Prevention Committee of the Council on Cardiovascular Nursing. (2010). Interventions to promote physical activity and dietary lifestyle changes for cardiovascular risk factor reduction in adults: A scientific statement from the American Heart Association. *Circulation, 122*(4), 406–441.

Bai, Z., Chang, J., Chen, C., Li, P., Yang, K., & Chi, I. (2015). Investigating the effect of transcendental meditation on blood pressure: A systematic review and meta-analysis. *Journal of Human Hypertension, 29*(11), 653–662. doi:10.1038/jhh.2015.6

Berwick, D. M., Nolan, T. W., & Whittington, J. (2008). The Triple Aim: Care, health, and cost. *Health Affairs, 27*(3), 759–769.

Brook, R. D., Appel, L. J. Rubenfire, M., Ogedegbe, G., Bisognano, J. D., Elliott, W. J., . . . Rajagopalan, S. (2013). Beyond medications and diet: Alternative approaches to lowering blood pressure: A scientific statement from the American Heart Association. *Hypertension, 61*, 1360–1383.

Brook, R. D., Jackson, E. A., Giorgini, P., & Mcgowan, C. L. (2015). The when and how to recommend "alternative approaches" in the management of high blood pressure. *The American Journal of Medicine, 128*, 567–570.

Can, G. (2013). Integrating non-pharmacological therapies with Western medicine in cancer treatment. *Evidence-Based Anticancer Complementary and Alternative Medicine, 4*, 252–274.

Centers for Disease Control and Prevention. (2016). Health-related quality of life. Retrieved from https://www.cdc.gov/hrqol/wellbeing.htm

Chang, M. Y., Wang, S. Y., & Chen, C. H. (2002). Effects of massage on pain and anxiety during labour: A randomized controlled trial in Taiwan. *Journal of Advanced Nursing, 38*, 68–73.

Chen, W.-L., Liu, G.-J., Yeh, S.-H., Chiang, M.-C., Fu, M.-Y., & Hsieh, Y.-K. (2013). Effect of back massage intervention on anxiety, comfort, and physiologic responses in patients with congestive heart failure. *Journal of Alternative and Complementary Medicine, 19*, 464–470. doi:10.1089/acm.2011.0873

Cohen, S. (1994). The perceived stress scale. Menlo Park, CA: Mind Garden. Retrieved from http://www.mindgarden.com/documents/PerceivedStressScale.pdf

Cohen, S., Janiki-Deverts, D., & Miller, G. E., (2007). Psychological stress & disease. *JAMA, 298*, 1686–1687.

College of Nurses of Ontario. (2014). *Complementary therapies: A practice guideline*. Pub. No. 41021. Toronto, Ontario: College of Nurses of Ontario. Retrieved from https://www.cno.org/globalassets/docs/prac/41021_comptherapies.pdf

Cramer, H., Lauche, R., Haller, H., & Dobos, G. (2013). A systematic review and meta-analysis of yoga for low back pain. *The Clinical Journal of Pain, 29*(5), 450–460.

Currin, J., & Meister, E. A. (2008). A hospital-based intervention using massage to reduce distress among oncology patients. *Cancer Nursing, 3*, 214–221. doi:10.1097/01.NCC.0000305725.65345.f3

Deary, L., Roche, J., Plotkin, K., & Zahourek, R. (2011). Intentionality and hatha yoga: An exploration of the theory of intentionality, the matrix of healing—a growth model. *Holistic Nursing Practice, 25*(5), 246–253. doi: 10.1097/HNP.0b013e31822a02e0

Diego, M. A., Fiedl, T., & Hernandez-Reif, M. (2014). Preterm infant weight gain is increased by massage therapy and exercise via different underlying mechanisms. *Early Human Development, 90*(3), 137–140. doi:10.1016/j.earlhumdev.2014.01.009

Drake, D. (2014). Integrative nursing management of fatigue. In M. J. Kreitzer, & M. Koithan (Eds.) *Integrative Nursing* (pp. 273–285). New York: Oxford University Press.

Frisvold, M. H. (2018). Functional foods and nutraceuticals. *Complementary & Alternative Therapies in Nursing* (8th ed., pp. 359–374). New York: Springer.

Galantino, M. L., Green, L., Decesari, J. A., Mackain, N. A., Rinaldi, S. M., Stevens, M. E., . . . Mao, J. J. (2012). Safety and feasibility of modified chair-yoga on functional outcome among elderly at risk for falls. *International Journal of Yoga, 5*(2), 146–150.

Geimer-Flanders, J. (2009). Creating a healing environment: Rationale and research overview. *Cleveland Clinic Journal of*

Medicine, 76, Suppl 2, S66–S669. http://doi.org/10.3949/ccjm.76.s2.13Goldblatt E, Wiles M, Schwartz J, Weeks J. Competencies for optimal practice in integrated environments: examining attributes of a consensus interprofessional practice document from the licensed integrative health disciplines. *Explore (NY)*. 2013;9(5): 285–291. doi:10.1016/j.explore.2013.06.006 Goyal, M., Singh, S., Sibinga, E. M., Gould, N. F., Rowland-Seymour, A., Sharma, R., . . . Haythornthwaite, J. A. (2014). Meditation programs for psychological stress and well-being: A systematic review and meta-analysis. *JAMA Internal Medicine*, *174*(3), 357–368. doi:10.1001/jamainternmed.2013.13018

Gross, C. R., Christopher, M. S., & Reilly-Spong, M. (2018). Meditation. In R. Lindquist, M. Tracy, & M. Snyder (Eds.). *Complementary & alternative therapies in nursing* (8th ed., pp. 177–200). New York: Springer.

Gross, C. R., Kreitzer, M. J., Thomas, W., Reilly-Spong, M., Cramer-Bornemann, M., Nyman, J. A., . . . Ibrahim, H. N. (2010). Mindfulness-based stress reduction for solid organ transplant recipients: A randomized controlled trial. *Alternative Therapies in Health and Medicine*, *16*(5), 30–38.

Halcón, L. (2018). Aromatherapy. In R. Lindquist, M. Snyder, & M. F. Tracy (Eds). *Complementary/alternative therapies in nursing* (8th ed., pp. 319–339). New York, NY: Springer.

Harris, M. (2018). Massage. In R. Lindquist, M. F. Tracy, & M. Snyder (Eds.). *Complementary & alternative therapies in nursing* (8th ed., pp. 249–264). New York, NY: Springer.

Harris, M., & Richards, K. C. (2010). The physiological and psychological effects of slow-stroke back massage and hand massage on relaxation in the elderly. *Journal of Clinical Nursing*, *19*, 917–926.

Harris, M., Richards, K. C., & Grando, V. T. (2012). The effects of slow-stroke back massage on minutes of nighttime sleep on persons with dementia in the nursing home. *Journal of Holistic Nursing*, *30*(4), 255–263. doi:10.1177/08980101112455948

Hartfiel, N., Havenhand, J., Khalsa, S. B., Clarke, G., & Krayer, A. (2011). The effectiveness of yoga for the improvement of well-being and resilience to stress in the workplace. *Scandinavian Journal of Work, Environment and Health*, *37*(1), 70–76.

Hartmann, M., Kopf, S., Kircher, C., Faude-Lang, V., Djuric, Z., Augstein, F., . . . Nawroth, P. P. (2012). Sustained effects of a mindfulness-based stress-reduction intervention in type 2 diabetic patients: Design and first results of a randomized controlled trial (the Heidelberger Diabetes and Stress-study). *Diabetes Care*, *35*(5), 945–947.

Hawk, C., Ndetan, H., & Evans, M. W., Jr. (2012). Potential role of complementary and alternative ehalth care providers in chronic disease prevention and health promotion: An analysis of National Health Interveiw Survey data. *Preventive Medicine*, *54*, 18–22.

Hilton, L., Hempel, S., Ewing, B. A., Apaydin, E., Xenakis, L., Newberry, S., . . . Maglione, M. A. (2016). Mindfulness meditation for chronic pain: Systematic review and meta-analysis. *Annals of Behavavioral Medicine*, *51*(2), 199–213. doi:10.1007/s12160-016-9844-2

Institute of Medicine. (2005). *Complementary and alternative medicine in the United States.* Washington, DC: The National Academies Press. Retrieved from https://doi.org/10.17226/11182

Interprofessional Education Collaborative. (2016). *Core competencies for interprofessional collaborative practice: 2016 update.* Washington, DC: Interprofessional Education Collaborative.

Jou, J., & Johnson, P. J. (2016). Nondisclosure of complementary and alternative medicine use to primary care physicians: Findings from the 2012 National Health Interview Survey. *JAMA Internal Medicine*, *176*, 545–546.

Kabat-Zinn, J. (2013). *Full catastrophe living; Revised and updated edition.* New York, NY: Penguin Random House.

Kaptchuck, T. J., & Miller, F. G. (2015). Placebo effects in medicine. *New England Journal of Medicine*, *373*, 8–9. doi:10.1056/NEJMp150402

Kilpatrick, L. A., Suyenobu, B. Y., Smith, S. R., Bueller, J. A., Goodman, T., Creswell, J. D., . . . Naliboff, B. D. (2011). Impact of mindfulness-based stress reduction training on intrinsic brain connectivity. *Neuroimage*, *56*(1), 290–298.

Kreitzer, M. J. (2016). *Taking charge of your health: What is well-being?* Retrieved from https://www.takingcharge.csh.umn.edu/what-wellbeing

Kreitzer M. J., & Langevin, M. (2014). Creating optimal healing environments. In R. Lindquist, M. F. Tracy, & M. Snyder (Eds.). *Complementary & alternative therapies in nursing* (7th ed., pp. 47–63). New York, NY: Springer.

Lee, M., Moon, W., & Kim, J. (2014). Effect of yoga on pain, brain-derived neurotrophic factor, and serotonin in premenopausal women with chronic low back pain. *Evidence-Based Complementary and Alternative Medicine: eCAM*, 203173. doi:10.1155/2014/203173

Leonard, B. (2014). Complementary therapies: Nurses' self-care. In R. Lindquist, M. Tracy, & M. Snyder (Eds.). *Complementary & alternative therapies in nursing* (7th ed., pp. 17–26). New York, NY: Springer.

Li, A. W., & Goldsmith, C. W. (2014). The effects of yoga on anxiety and stress. *Alternative Medicine Review*, *17*(1), 21–35.

Lindquist, R. (2015, Spring). Unanticipated salutary effects of mindfulness on women's lives - implications for practice and research. 2015–2016. Interdisciplinary Women's Health Lecture Series, Deborah Powell Center of Excellence, University of Minnesota, Minneapolis, MN.

Lindquist, R., Tracy, M. F., & Savik, K. (2003). Personal use of complementary and alternative therapies by critical care nurses. *Critical Care Nursing Clinics of North America*, *15*(3), 393–399.

Lindquist, R., Tracy, M. F., & Snyder, M. (2018). *Complementary & alternative therapies in nursing* (8th ed.). New York: Springer.

Lindquist, R., Witt, D., & Crane, L. (2014). Integrative nursing management of stress. In M. J. Kreitzer & M. Koithan, (Eds.), *Integrative Nursing* (pp. 200–2013). New York: Oxford University Press.

Maizes, V., & Low Dog, V. (2010). *Integrative women's health.* New York: Oxford University Press.

McFeeters, S., Pront, L., Cuthbertson, L. & King, L. (2016). Massage, a complementary therapy effectively promoting the health and well-being of older people in residential care settings: A review of the literature. *International Journal of Older People Nursing*, *11*(4), 266–283.

McNeil, D. A., Vekved, M., Dolan, S. M., Siever, J., Horn, S., & Tough, S. C. (2013). A qualitative study of the experience of Centering Pregnancy group prenatal care for physicians. *BMC Pregnancy Childbirth, 13*(Suppl 1), S6. doi:10.1186/1471-2393-13-S1-S6

Merry, C. (2016). Leading causes of CAM nondisclosure. *AHC Media*. Retrieved from https://www.ahcmedia.com/articles/138780-leading-causes-of-cam-nondisclosure

Mok, E., & Woo, C. P. (2004). The effects of slow-stroke massage on anxiety and shoulder pain in elderly stroke patients. *Complementary Therapies in Nursing & Midwifery, 10*, 209–216.

Morgan, N., Irwin, M. R., Chung, M., & Wang, C. (2014). The effects of mind-body therapies on the immune system: meta-analysis. *PLoS One, 9*(7), e100903.

Morone, N. E., Greco, C. M., Moore, C. G., Rollman, B. L., Lane, B., Morrow, L. A., . . . Weiner, D. K. (2016). A mind-body program for older adults with chronic low back pain: A randomized clinical trial. *JAMA Internal Medicine, 176*(3), 329–337. doi:10.1001/jamainternmed.2015.8033

National Institute for Complementary and Integrative Health. (2012). *National Health Interview Survey: Key findings*. Retrieved from https://nccih.nih.gov/research/statistics/NHIS/2012/key-findings

National Institute for Complementary and Integrative Health. (2013a). *High cholesterol and complementary health practices: What the science says.* Retrieved from https://nccih.nih.gov/health/providers/digest/cholesterol-science

National Institute for Complementary and Integrative Health. (2015). *Omega 3 supplements: In depth.* Retrieved from https://nccih.nih.gov/health/omega3/introduction.htm

National Center for Complementary and Integrative Health (2016a). *Complementary, alternative, or integrative health: What's in a name?* Retrieved from https://nccih.nih.gov/health/integrative-health

National Institute for Complementary and Integrative Health. (2016b). *Echinacea*. Retrieved from https://nccih.nih.gov/health/echinacea/ataglance.htm

National Institute for Complementary and Integrative Health. (2016c). *Gingko*. Retrieved from https://nccih.nih.gov/health/ginkgo/ataglance.htm

National Institute for Complementary and Integrative Health. (2016d). *Health topics A to Z.* Retrieved from https://nccih.nih.gov

National Center for Complementary and Integrative Health. (2016e). Home page. Retrieved from https://nccih.nih.gov

National Institute for Complementary and Integrative Health. (2016f). *Massage therapy*. Retrieved from https://nccih.nih.gov/health/massage

National Institute for Complementary and Integrative Health. (2016g). *Melatonin: In depth*. Retrieved from https://nccih.nih.gov/health/melatonin

National Institute for Complementary and Integrative Health. (2016h). *Placebo effect*. Retrieved from https://nccih.nih.gov/health/placebo

National Institute for Complementary and Integrative Health. (2016i). *6 things to know when selecting a complementary health practitioner.* Retrieved from https://nccih.nih.gov/health/tips/selecting

National Center for Complementary and Integrative Health. (2016j). *10 most commonly used therapies among adults.* Retrieved from https://nccih.nih.gov/research/statistics/2007/most-common-cam-therapies-among-adults

National Institute for Complementary and Integrative Health. (2017a). *5 things to know about safety of dietary supplements for children and teens.* Retrieved from https://nccih.nih.gov/health/tips/child-supplements

National Institute for Complementary and Integrative Health. (2017b). *Probiotics: In depth*. Retrieved from https://nccih.nih.gov/health/probiotics/introduction.htm

Nerbass, F. B., Feltrim, M. I. Z., de Souza, S. A., Ykeda, D. S., & Lorenzi-Filho, G. (2010). Effects of massage therapy on sleep quality after coronary artery bypass graft surgery. *Clinics (Sao Paulo), 65*(11), 1105–1110. doi:10.1590/S1807-59322010001100008

Okonta, N. R. (2012). Does yoga therapy reduce blood pressure in patients with hypertension? *Holistic Nursing Practice, 26*(3), 137–141.

O'Reilly, G. A., Cook, L., Spruijt-Metz, D., & Black, D. S. (2014). Mindfulness-based interventions for obesity-related eating behaviors: A literature review. *Obesity Reviews, 15*(6), 453–461. doi:10.1111/obr.12156

Pascoe, M. C., & Bauer, I. E. (2015). A systematic review of randomised control trials on the effects of yoga on stress measures and mood. *Journal of Psychiatric Research*, 68, 270–282.

Pechacek, J., Drake, D., Terrell, C., & Torkelson, C. (2015). Interprofessional intervention to support mature women: A case study. *Creative Nursing, 21*(3), 134–143.

Penque, S., & Snyder, M. (2014). Presence. In R. Lindquist, M. F. Tracy, & M. Snyder (Eds.), *Complementary & alternative therapies in nursing* (7th ed.). New York, NY: Springer.

Pender, N. (1990). Expressing health through lifestyle patterns. *Nursing Science Quarterly, 3*(3), 115–122.

Pender, N. J. (2011). Health promotion model manual. Retrieved from https://deepblue.lib.umich.edu/bitstream/handle/2027.42/85350/HEALTH_PROMOTION_MANUAL_Rev_5-2011.pdf?sequence=1

Perlman, A. I., Sabina, A., & Williams, A-L., et al. (2006). Massage therapy for osteoarthritis of the knee: A randomized controlled trial. *Archives of Internal Medicine, 166*(22), 2533–2538. doi:10.1001/archinte.166.22.2533

Plotnikoff, G. A., & Lillehei, A. S. (2018). Herbal medicines. In R. Lindquist, M. F. Tracy, & M. Snyder (Eds.). *Complementary & alternative therapies in nursing* (8th ed.). New York: Springer.

QSEN Institute. (2014). *QSEN competencies*. Retrieved from http://qsen.org/competencies/pre-licensure-ksas/

Quality and Safety Education for Nurses Institute. (2017). *Competencies for nursing, pre-licensure and graduate.* Retrieved from http://qsen.org/competencies/

Richards, K. C. (1998). Effect of a back massage and relaxation intervention on sleep in critically ill patients. *American Journal of Critical Care*, 7, 288–299.

Ring, M., Brodsky, M., Low Dog, T., Sierpina, S. V., Locke, A., Kogan, M., . . . Saper, R. (2014). Developing and implementing core competencies for integrative medicine fellowships. *Academic Medicine, 89*(3), 421–428. http://dx.doi.org/10.1097/ACM.0000000000000148. [PubMed]

Sackett, D., Strauss, S. E., Richardson, W. S., Rosenburg, W., & Haynes, R. B. (2000). *Evidence-based medicine: How to practice and teach EBM* (2nd ed., p. 1). Edinburgh, Scotland: Churchill Livingstone.

Schneider, R. H., Alexander, C. N., Staggers, F., Orme-Johnson, D. W., Rainforth, M., Salerno, J. W., Sheppard, W., . . .

Nidich, S. I. (2005). A randomized controlled trial of stress reduction in African Americans treated for over one year. *American Journal of Hypertension, 18*(1), 88–98.

Schneider, R. H., Grim, C. E., Rainforth, M. V., Kotchen, T., Nidich, S. I., Gaylord-King, C., . . . Alexander, C. N. (2012). Stress reduction in the secondary prevention of cardiovascular disease: Randomized, controlled trial of transcendental meditation and health education in Blacks. *Circulation: Cardiovascular and Quality Outcomes, 5*(6), 750–758.

Scholle, J. M., Baker, W. L., Talati, R., & Coleman, C. I. (2009). The effect of adding plant sterols or stanols to statin therapy in hypercholesterolemic patients: Systematic review and meta-analysis. *Journal of the American College of Nutrition, 28*(5), 517–524.

Sedlmeier, P., Eberth, J., Schwarz, M., Zimmermann, D., Haarig, F., Jaeger, S., & Kunze, S. (2012). The psychological effects of meditation: A meta-analysis. *Psychological Bulletin, 138*(6), 1139–1171.

Seo, D. Y., Lee, S., Figueroa, A., Kim, H. K., Baek, Y. H., Kwak, Y. S., . . . Han, J. (2012). Yoga training improves metabolic parameters in obese boys. *Korean Journal of Physiology & Pharmacology, 16*(3), 175–180.

Seyyed-Rasodi, A., Salehi, F., Mohammadpoorosi, A., Goljaryan, S., & Seyyedi, A. (2016). Comparing the effects of aromatherapy massage and inhalation aromatherapy on anxiety and pain in burn patients. *Burns, 42*(8), 1774–1780 doi:10.1016/j.burns.2016.06.014

Skarlovnik, A., Janić, M., Lunder, M., Turk, M., & Šabovič, M. (2014). Coenzyme Q10 supplementation decreases statin-related mild-to-moderate muscle symptoms: A randomized clinical study. *Medical Science Monitor, 20*, 2183–2188. doi:10.12659/MSM.890777

Smith, C., Hancock, H., Blake-Mortimer, J., & Eckert, K. (2007). A randomized comparative trial of yoga and relaxation to reduce stress and anxiety. *Complementary Therapies in Medicine, 15*(2), 77–83.

Taylor, B. A., Lorson, L., White, C. M., & Thompson, P. D. (2015). A randomized trial of coenzyme Q10 in patients with confirmed statin myopathy. *Atherosclerosis, 238*(2), 329–335. http://dx.doi.org/10.1016/j.atherosclerosis.2014.12.016

Thompson, J., & Nichter, M. (2015). Is there a role for CAM in preventive and promotive health? *Medical Anthropology Quarterly, 30*(1), 80–99.

Tracy, M. F., Lindquist, R., Savik, K., Watanuki, S., Sendelbach, S., Kreitzer, M. J., & Berman, B. (2005). Use of complementary and alternative therapies: A national survey of critical care nurses. *American Journal of Critical Care, 14*, 404–415.

Treat-Jacobson, D., Bronas, U. G., & Salisbury, D. (2014). Exercise. In R. Lindquist, M. Tracy, & M. Snyder (Eds.). *Complementary & alternative therapies in nursing* (7th ed.). New York, NY: Springer.

Upchurch, D. M., & Rainisch, B. K. W. (2012). Racial and ethnic profiles of complementary and alternative medicine use among young adults in the United States: Findings from the National Longitudinal Study of Adolescent Health. *Journal of Evidence-Based Complementary & Alternative Medicine, 17*(3), 172–179.

U.S. Department of Health and Human Services. (n.d.). Office of Disease Prevention and Health Promotion. *Healthy People 2020: Framework.* Retrieved from https://www.healthypeople.gov/sites/default/files/HP2020Framework.pdf

U.S. Department of Health and Human Services. (2017). Office of Disease Prevention and Health Promotion. *Healthy People 2020: Health-related quality of life and well-being.* Retrieved from https://www.healthypeople.gov/2020/topics-objectives/topic/health-related-quality-of-life-well-being

U.S. Preventive Services Task Force. (2017). Behavioral counseling to promote a healthful diet and physical activity for cardiovascular disease prevention in adults without cardiovascular risk factors: US Preventive Services Task Force Recommendation Statement. *JAMA, 318*(2),167–174. doi:10.1001/jama.2017.7171

van Son, J., Nyklíček, I., Pop, V. J., & Pouwer, F. (2011). Testing the effectiveness of a mindfulness-based intervention to reduce emotional distress in outpatients with diabetes (DiaMind): Design of a randomized controlled trial. *BMC Public Health, 11*, 131.

Vaughan, R. A., Conn, C. A., & Mermier, C. M. (2014). Effects of commercially available dietary supplements on resting energy expenditure: A brief report. *ISRN Nutrition, 2014*(2014), Article ID 650264, 7 pages. http://dx.doi.org/10.1155/2014/650264

Veziari, Y., Leach, M. J., & Kumar, S. (2017). Barriers to the conduct and application of research in complementary and alternative medicine: A systematic review. *BMC Complementary and Alternative Medicine, 17*, vol. 2014. 166. doi:10.1186/s12906-017-1660-0

Walker, S. N., Sechrist, K. R., & Pender, N. J. (1987). The Health-Promoting Lifestyle Profile: Development and psychometric characteristics. *Nursing Research, 36*, 7–81.

Wang, H. L., & Keck, J. F. (2004). Foot and hand massage as an intervention for postoperative pain. *Pain Management Nursing, 5*, 59–65.

Watanuki, S., Tracy, M. F., & Lindquist, R. (2014). Therapeutic listening. In R. Lindquist, M. F. Tracy, & M. Snyder (Eds.). *Complementary & alternative therapies in nursing*, (7th ed., pp. 39–54). New York: Springer.

Williams, A. L., Selwyn, P. A., Liberti, L., Molde, S., Njike, V. Y., McCorkle, R., . . . Katz, D. L. (2005). A randomized controlled trial of meditation and massage effects on quality of life in people with late-stage disease: A pilot study. *Journal of Palliative Medicine, 8*, 939–952.

Unit 4

Risk Identification, Prevention, and Health Promotion with Special Populations

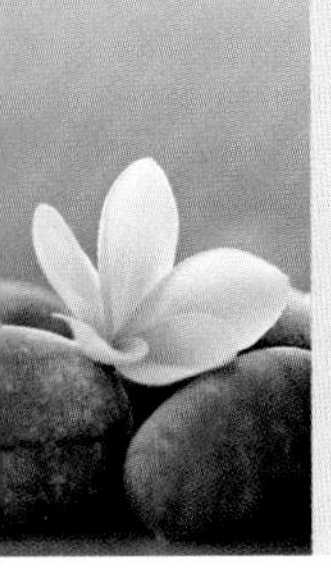

Chapter 18

Health Promotion for Individuals with Disabilities

Veronica Garcia Walker, Janet A. Levey, Tracie Harrison, and Whitney Thurman

LEARNING OBJECTIVES

After completing this chapter, the student will be able to:

1. Describe how health promotion measures can remove barriers to care for those who have disabilities.
2. Describe how health promotion has changed over time to include the specific needs of people who have disabilities.
3. Explain how the concept of universal design diffused to learning environments.
4. Apply universal design and health literacy approaches to health promotion instruction.
5. Discuss current research for measuring training on universal design for health-care providers.
6. Describe the responsibility of educators and advance practice nurses to design and deliver universally accessible health promotion education.
7. Describe the different reasons for universal design and person-centered care for health promotion of people with disabilities.

INTRODUCTION

Health promotion is a central element of the nursing profession. Some nursing scholars argue that promoting health is and has always been the primary goal of professional nursing practice because health—as opposed to illness—has long been identified as the central concern of nursing (Clark, 1993; Smith, 1990). The goal of health promotion is to improve and maintain health, and although this goal seems straightforward, health promotion practice is complex and evolving (Young, 2002), remaining a contested concept within the nursing discipline (Maben & Clark, 1995; Piper, 2009). The complexity of health promotion practice is directly related to long-held values, beliefs, and assumptions about what health means and thus the best ways to promote health. The climbing rates of chronic disease as well as risk factors for disease suggest that in today's health-care context, advance practice registered nurses (APRNs) should engage critically with the question, "What is health promotion?" to advance the health of their patients. People who have disabilities experience disparities in almost all areas of health and health care, so appropriate and tailored health promotion practices become especially important (Krahn, Walker, & Correa-de-Araujo, 2015).

This chapter will provide an overview of the historical understanding of health promotion and the theoretical perspectives that influence contemporary health promotion practice before critiquing the extent to which health promotion interventions adequately consider the realities of people who have disabilities. We integrated the interventions with the intention of providing knowledge on the available health promotion strategies for people with disabilities. Nurses, including APRNs, should understand what health promotion means in the context of disability and feel empowered to engage in health promotion efforts that extend beyond the individual biomedical factors to reach the structural and achievable political factors that wield tremendous influence on the lives of people who have disabilities.

HISTORICAL AND THEORETICAL PERSPECTIVES

Before embarking on our journey through the evolution of health promotion, it is important to consider what we mean by *health*. There is no universally agreed upon definition of *health*, but it is widely accepted that health is different for different people and at different times in their lives and may therefore be viewed on a continuum of subjective perceptions (Ewles & Simnett, 1999). Frequently, health is defined as the absence of illness. Other definitions of health include broader aspects such as functional status, psychological well-being, and global self-perceptions. A commonly cited definition put forth by the World Health Organization (WHO; 1974) defines health as "a state of complete physical, mental, and social well-being and not merely the absence of disease or infirmity." This progression in the understanding of health has significant implications for people with disabilities: a definition of health that goes beyond the absence of illness raises the possibility that *anyone* can be healthy (Becker, 1996). We subscribe to this broader definition of health that moves along an illness orientation to incorporate social and psychological dimensions of well-being.

Current literature suggests that a wide range of theoretical perspectives on health promotion influence nursing practice. This diversity reflects the diversity that is inherent in human experience and that therefore must be inherent in effective health promotion practices. These interventions differ depending on patient circumstances such as economic resources, cultural group, age, gender, or disability. For the APRN, selecting an appropriate intervention for use in particular circumstances requires the practitioner to be able to appraise theories in common usage critically, which in turn requires an understanding of how and why knowledge has evolved in the field (Young, 2002).

Understanding Health Promotion

Health promotion has been defined as any endeavor directed at enhancing the well-being of individuals, families, groups, communities, and/or nations through strategies involving supportive environments, coordination of resources, and respect for personal choice and values (Maville & Huerta, 2002). This seemingly straightforward, albeit broad definition belies the contested nature of this concept and the divergent historical and theoretical perspectives informing nursing's contemporary conceptualizations of what it means to promote health. Although a complete discussion of health promotion in the nursing discipline is beyond the scope of this chapter, a few key developments bear mentioning to challenge assumptions and enable APRNs to use a health promotion philosophy when providing care to people with disabilities.

In 1974, the Canadian government published a discussion paper entitled *A New Perspective on the Health of Canadians* (Lalonde, 1974). The Lalonde Report, as it came to be called, proved to be a seminal document in the field of health promotion. The report was intended to break down the pervasive public belief that health results from medical intervention and argued that future increases in population health status would require efforts to improve the environment, modify risky personal health behavior, and increase knowledge of human biology (MacDonald, 2002). Despite equal emphasis on the importance of environmental and biological influences on health, the Lalonde Report resulted in reinforcing a professional understanding of health promotion as synonymous with disease prevention and health education (MacDonald, 2002). This conflation of terms represents a common misinterpretation because, in theory, health promotion and health education are distinct activities. Health promotion encompasses socioeconomic and environmental determinants of health and includes the narrower concept of health education (Whitehead, 2008). Regardless, the understanding of health promotion as confined to individual-level efforts aimed at behavior and lifestyle modification fostered by the Lalonde Report gained traction around the globe, and the influence is still evident today.

In the United States, the Department of Health, Education and Welfare (USDHEW)—the precursor to the federal Department of Health and Human Services (USDHHS)—produced the *Forward Plan for Health*, which emphasized the importance of improving both the personal health habits of Americans as well as the environment in which they lived and worked (USDHEW, 1976). Subsequently, the federal government set national objectives for disease prevention, health protection, and health promotion in the report *Healthy People: The Surgeon General's Report on Health Promotion and Disease Prevention* (USDHEW, 1979). Healthy People now serves as the blueprint for federal health promotion and disease prevention efforts in the United States, with goals and objectives updated for each subsequent decade since the initial 1979 report. Although the report encompassed broader strategies for policy and legislative changes, it differentiated between health promotion, health protection, and preventive health services. Thus, within the *Healthy People* framework, health promotion focused primarily on individual behavior and lifestyle and largely neglected social and economic factors that can contribute to poor health. It was not until the third iteration, *Healthy People 2000*, that people with disabilities were included as a population of interest. The health promotion goals for these individuals are included in Box 18-1.

In the decades after the Lalonde (1974) Report was published, critiques of the behavioral approach to health promotion emerged from both ends of the political spectrum (MacDonald, 2002). Conservatives claimed that the state had no business interfering with the private lives of its citizens, even to promote healthy behavior. Liberals criticized the approach for neglecting structural influences on health and contributing to victim blaming (Labonté, 1994). Despite these critiques, much of the American health promotion literature in the decades after the Lalonde Report continued to reflect the uniquely American value of rugged individualism (Williams, 1989). Globally, however, the structural critique of the behavioral and lifestyle modification approach to health promotion began to shift the manner in which health promotion was theorized and implemented. Specifically, the WHO conceptualized a new social model of health promotion that integrated a systems perspective with an individual perspective of health promotion (Kickbush, 1994). In 1986, the WHO European office, Health and Welfare Canada, and the Canadian Public Health Association produced the Ottawa Charter on Health Promotion, which defined health promotion as "... the process of enabling people to increase control over and improve their health." Within the Ottawa Charter, advocating, enabling, and mediating were identified as the fundamental processes for health promotion practice. These core processes enable simultaneous health promotion practices at multiple levels by engaging in the five major strategies identified in the report: building healthy public policy, creating supportive environments, strengthening community action, developing personal skills, and reorienting health services.

Because of federal policy and the national objectives outlined in the *Healthy People* reports, the adoption of the socioecological perspective of health promotion outlined in the Ottawa Charter by the nursing profession in the United States has been slower than in other countries (MacDonald, 2002). Nevertheless, nursing practice in the United States is beginning to reflect an expanded conceptualization of health promotion. The American Nurses Association (ANA) includes the promotion of health in its definition of nursing, and the ANA (1995) social policy statement reflects a broad understanding of health promotion by its claim that nursing involves policy, advocacy, and empowerment. Whitehead (2006) has called on nurses to extend their health promotion

BOX 18-1 Healthy People 2020 Goals for People with Disabilities

Increase the number of population-based data systems used to monitor Healthy People 2020 objectives that include in their core a standardized set of questions that identify people with disabilities.

Increase the number of state and the District of Columbia health departments that have at least one health promotion program aimed at improving the health and well-being of people with disabilities.

Increase the proportion of all occupied homes and residential buildings that have features without barriers.

Reduce the number of people with disabilities living in congregate-care residences.

Increase the proportion of youth with special health-care needs whose health-care provider has discussed transition planning from pediatric to adult health care.

Increase the proportion of people with epilepsy and uncontrolled seizures who receive appropriate medical care.

Reduce the proportion of adults with disabilities aged 18 years and older who experience delays in receiving primary and periodic preventive care due to specific barriers.

practices into the legislative arena, paying attention to economic disparities, facilitating public consciousness raising, and influencing health-related policy development. Accordingly, APRNs are being called on to adopt an active role in promoting the health of individuals, families, and communities by "empowering individuals and communities, facilitating public awareness of health disparities, advocating for the underserved, enhancing access to care, involving patients in their care... and engaging in health policy work" (Raingruber, 2016, p. xii).

Disability and Health Promotion

In 1973, when Canadians were proposing health promotion as a means to action for better health, the United States legislature passed the Rehabilitation Act (1973). During a time when many Americans began demanding their civil liberties, people who had disabilities began to ask for access to federal buildings with their wheelchairs and other physical accommodations such as ramps and curb cuts. They also sought increased access to services, structures, and activities that provide health, excluding expanded housing and employment opportunities. When segments of the Rehabilitation Act (1973), sections 503 and 504b, made it illegal for a federal agency to discriminate based on perceived disability, leaders of this movement knew they were making positive strides to change the way people with disabilities lived their lives.

Fifteen years later, the Americans with Disabilities Act of 1990 significantly improved access and quality of life for those who have disabilities. Through this legislation, people with disabilities were finally given a portal to self-reliance through interdependence. A national focus on accommodations to enhance access and job performance began to surface. For instance, finding a brace for a person with carpal tunnel syndrome to diminish pain and enhance blood flow to the digits could keep a person working longer. Examples also include the use of a portable lift for picking up equipment that might be too heavy or a lift or a brace for people who have difficulty moving heavy or awkward items.

The steps to accomplishing an accessible and healthier society make health promotion for people with disabilities a clear goal. The process is formidable, and what works to improve health promotion for one type of disabling condition might not work for another. The actual application of health promotion interventions with evidence for outcomes is where we hope to see new possibilities and ideas emerge to improve quality of life for these populations.

PATIENT, INTERVENTION, CONTROL, OBSERVATION, AND TIME (PICOT) QUESTION

Among people with disabilities, how does health promotion compared to not engaging in health promotion activities influence health over a five-year period?

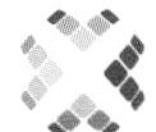

Case Study

The home health nurse is conducting an initial assessment visit for a 60 y/o woman who was discharged from the hospital yesterday with a diagnosis of Type 2 diabetes. The patient works full-time as an administrative assistant and is scheduled to return to work in 6-weeks. She lives with her seven month old Labrador Retriever in a ranch style home. The patient is able to perform activities of daily living, but has a 10 pound weight-lift restriction secondary to having a total hysterectomy. She is able to tether the dog outside for short bathroom breaks. Her grown children live over an hour away and visit her every 3 to 4 days to assist with buying groceries, filling prescriptions, and yardwork. The home health agency received a referral from the surgeon for follow up assessment, diabetes self-management, and education.

During the intake assessment interview, the home health nurse noticed the patient was squinting to read printed and online diabetic materials and the measurement scale on the insulin syringe. The nurse saw a glass case on the kitchen table and asked the patient if she wears glasses. The patient replied "Yes, I have glasses, but my dog chewed on them and they are broken. I have an appointment with my optometrist in 4-days. I am dependent on my children for transportation. Until then, I will have to make the best of the situation."

The nurse assessed the patient's overall knowledge of diabetes and self-care, performed a physical assessment, and surveyed the home for potential safety issues for an individual with low vision. In providing patient-centered care, the nurse employed universal design interventions to assist the patient in accessing health information and managing her diabetes:

1. Called the provider and asked if an insulin pen can be ordered until the patient is able to obtain new glasses. If the request is denied, the nurse will provide and demonstrate to the patient how to use an insulin syringe magnifier to enlarge the measurement scale on the syringe.

2. Discussed with the patient the use of an audio blood glucose monitoring system to check blood sugars.
3. Demonstrated to the patient how to enlarge the print on her laptop computer screen by using the zoom icon feature.
4. Located online audio links on health promotion and maintenance information for diabetics sponsored by the home health agency. The patient can access and listen to the information when desired. The audio link is available and accessible to patients based on their learning needs and preference The National Federations for the Blind website (https://nfb.org/diabetics) provides a vast amount of resources and support for diabetic patients with low or no vision.
5. Provided the patient with a magnifier card to read food labels and other printed materials using less than 12-point fonts.
6. Based on the home safety inspection, the nurse suggested the use of plastic cutting utensils (no sharp knifes) until an eye exam is performed and glasses are obtained. The nurse made sure that all medications were accessible to the patient, but not the dog. A referral was also made to Meals on Wheels for meal delivery for 1-week.
7. Scheduled a morning and evening nurse visit for the first week to assess patient's diabetes self-management and education. The nurse also scheduled an in-home visit with a dietitian regarding healthy food choices and preparation using educational materials in large print.
8. Verified future in-home visits (nurse and dietitian) and those with the provider. The nurse wrote the dates/times using large print on white paper with black ink.

Review of Literature on Health Promotion and Disability

A systematic review of the literature was performed to investigate the frequency of randomized control trials in the current (2013–2018) literature that address health promotion interventions with those with disability. The search was conducted using PUBMED, Cumulative Index to Nursing and Allied Health Literature (CINAHL), and Academic Search Complete. Keywords used in the search were *health promotion intervention*, *with disability*, and *randomized controlled trials*. Exclusion criteria included meta-analyses, future study protocols, studies that only addressed risk for disability or focused on outcomes of health-care providers of disability, and those did not study disability. Twenty-three articles were retrieved.

Initially, we found only a few studies that met the search criteria, so a second wider search was conducted to investigate the frequency of randomized control trials in the current (2013–2018) literature that address health promotion interventions with those who have disability or those with disability. The search was conducted using PUBMED, CINAHL, and Academic Search Complete. Keywords used in the search were *health promotion* (to reach a wider number of studies), *with disability*, and *randomized controlled trials*. Exclusion criteria included meta-analyses, future study protocols, studies that only addressed risk for disability or studies focused on the health-care provider, and those that did not study disability. This search retrieved 109 articles.

After applying the exclusion criteria, 24 studies remained for analysis. When considering countries that studied disability and health promotion with randomized controlled trials, the United States represented 10 of the total studies, or 41.6%. Countries represented in more than one study included Sweden with three studies (or 12.5%) and Australia with two studies (or 8.3%). Other countries represented in this analysis were Norway, Canada, the United Kingdom, Greece, Iran, the Netherlands, Switzerland, Belgium, and Hong Kong. These are found in Table 18-1.

Disabilities of Focus

The conditions identified as disabilities in these studies were (1) chronic conditions (subcategorized into a chronic campaign that included type 2 diabetes, coronary artery disease, asthma, and chronic obstructive pulmonary disease [COPD]; heart failure campaign; mental health campaign, which included chronic depression and schizophrenia), (2) intellectual disabilities, (3) sedentary older adults, (4) mental disorders, and (5) cancer. Some conditions were represented in more than one category; for example, chronic conditions included depression and schizophrenia, as did mental illnesses. The focus of each health promotion study intervention varied between and within these disability categories.

Countries of Origin and Focus

Countries that did research on disabilities in the past 5 years that were identified in this search included (1) the United States (two studies), (2) Belgium, (3) Germany, and (4) Scotland. Disability of focus in the U.S. studies included sedentary older adults and cancer survivors. The Belgium researchers' focus of study was adults with mental disorders. Researchers studied chronic conditions in Germany (Harter et al., 2016), and the Scotland researchers studied adults with intellectual disabilities (Matthews et al., 2016).

Table 18-1 Health Promotion Interventions

Search terms: *health promotion*, *with disabilities*, and *random control trials*
Time frame: March 2013 to March 2018

Author/Date	Disability	Country	Intervention/Purpose	Outcome
Bergström et al. (2013). A multicomponent universal intervention to improve diet and physical activity among adults with intellectual disabilities in community residences: A cluster randomised controlled trial.	Adults with intellectual disabilities n = 130; 74 females Ages: 20–66 years	Sweden	Investigation of an intervention (12–16 months) to improve diet and physical activity in people with ID by targeting both residents as well as caregivers using a clustered randomized controlled trial.	Primary outcome was physical activity, which was measured by a pedometer. A positive intervention effect was reported for physical activity in the intervention group ($p = 0.045$).
Brendbekken et al. (2016). Multidisciplinary intervention in patients with musculoskeletal pain: A randomized clinical trial.	Patients with musculoskeletal pain n = 284 adults Ages:18–60	Norway	This study compared a multidisciplinary intervention using a visual education tool and a structured interdisciplinary interview with a brief interview to examine effects on physical and mental symptoms, use of health services, functioning ability, and coping.	The multidisciplinary intervention (MI) group had significantly less use of health services at 3 and 12 months ($p < 0.05$). The MI group also reported better coping with complaints ($p < 0.001$) at 12 months. The MI group members also took better care of their health ($p < 0.001$), when compared to the brief intervention (BI) group.
Feldman et al. (2016). Randomized control trial of the 3Rs Health Knowledge Training Program for persons with intellectual disabilities.	Persons with intellectual disabilities (n = 22) Mean age: 50.9 (6.4) IG 5 males/7 females IG Mean age: 53.4 (14.1) CG 6 males/4 females CG	Canada	Health knowledge training to promote first steps toward health self-efficacy. Health training covered topics such as health maintenance, illnesses, body organs, and body systems. Controls received no training. Both groups received pre- and posttests.	Intervention group had significantly higher posttest scores related to health knowledge compared to the control group.
Fraser et al. (2015). PACES in epilepsy: Results of a self-management randomized controlled trial.	Adults with chronic epilepsy (n = 83) Mean age: 44.9 (12.5) Intervention Group (IG) Females 56% Control Group (CG) Mean age: 45.4 (12.6) CG Females 55% CG	United States (Seattle, Washington)	Eight-week groups meeting 75 minutes (led by a psychologist and trained peer) per week to discuss epilepsy self-management and medical, social, and cognitive aspects of epilepsy. Control group received treatment as usual.	When compared to controls, significant improvements remained in intervention group when considering epilepsy self-efficacy ($p = 0.004$) and medication effects ($p = 0.005$) at 6-month follow-up.

(*continued*)

Table 18-1 Health Promotion Interventions—cont'd

Author/Date	Disability	Country	Intervention/Purpose	Outcome
Froehlich-Grobe et al. (2014). Exercise for everyone: A randomized controlled trial of project workout on wheels in promoting exercise among wheelchair users.	Wheelchair users (stable, episodic, or progressive disability) (n = 128) 64 females Mean age: 45 years Mean time with impairment: 22 years	United States (Kansas)	Home-based exercise interventions were administered to IG and CG. IG received intensive staff exercise support; CG received minimal staff support with the intervention.	Over the year, the intervention group reported significantly more exercise time (approx. 17 min/week) compared to the self-guided control group.
Granbom et al. (2017). Effects on leisure activities and social participation of a case management intervention for frail older people living at home: A randomized controlled trial.	Frail elderly living at home who were over 65 years old, needed long-term care often and needing help to accomplish 2 activities of daily living (e.g. dressing, toileting, moving) (n = 153) Mean age: 81.4 (5.9) IG; Females 52% CG Mean age: 81.6 (6.8) CG; Females 50% CG	Sweden	To examine a one-year case management intervention (monthly home visits by case managers) as it affects leisure activities and social participation. The intervention included information sharing regarding social activities and exercises, information as needed specific to the person (e.g. medication), and reminder that the case manager would be available by phone.	A statistically significant proportion of members of the IG had either an unchanged number or the same number of social leisure activities from baseline period to 3 months (93.2% versus 75.4%, OR = 4.48, 95% CI: 1.37 - 14.58). There were no significant differences between groups with regard to social participation.
Harris et al. (2017). A cluster randomised control trial of a multicomponent weight management program for adults with intellectual disabilities and obesity.	Adults with intellectual disabilities and obesity (n = 50) Mean age: 40.6 (5.9) IG; Females 69.2% CG Mean age: 43.6 (6.8) CG; Females 58.3% CG	United Kingdom	IG received a multicomponent weight management program. CG received a health education program.	No significant difference was noted in the percentage of weight change when comparing the two groups.
Harter et al. (2016). To examine the effectiveness of telephone-based health coaching in chronically ill patients.	Eighteen years or older who had one or more of the following chronic conditions: ***Chronic campaign:*** diabetes type 2, hypertension, coronary artery disease, asthma, COPD (IG: 2,713; CG 2,596 = 5,309) ***Heart failure campaign:*** Heart failure (IG: 338; CG 322 = 660).	Germany	Telephone coaching (averaging 12.9 calls per participant), including establishing goals using shared decision making and motivational interviewing. Symptoms and adherence to medications were discussed as well as information regarding exercise and diet management. ***Control group:*** Received usual health care but no telephone coaching.	No significant differences were found between IG and CG in time until readmitted to hospital. In the chronic campaign, the probability of being hospital readmitted was higher in the IG compared to the CG (OR = 1.13; p = 0.045). In the chronic campaign, those in the IG demonstrated a significant increase in daily defined doses of medication.

Table 18-1 Health Promotion Interventions—cont'd

Author/Date	Disability	Country	Intervention/Purpose	Outcome
	Mental health campaign: Chronic depression and schizophrenia (IG: 101; CG: 138 = 239).			***Conclusions:*** In both the chronic and heart campaigns participants, there was a significantly reduced likelihood of dying in the IG compared to the CG in a 2-year period (chronic campaign: OR = 0.64; p = 0.005 and heart failure campaign: OR = 0.44; p = 0.001).
Hausmann et al. (2017). Testing a positive psychological intervention for osteoarthritis.	Patients who were older than 50 years and had hip or knee osteoarthritis with pain ratings of 4 or higher. (n = 42) Mean age: 69.2 (11.3) IG; Females 19.1% CG Mean age: 65.7 (9.1) CG; Females 14.3% CG	United States (Pennsylvania)	Six-week program; IG contained positive skill-building exercises such as writing positive experiences from the day. CG had neutral activities such as writing down events that occurred during the day.	Patients in the IG reported significant improvement in symptom severity (p = 0.02; Cohen's d = 0.86), life satisfaction (p = 0.02; Cohen's d = 0.36), and negative affect (p = 0.03; Cohen's d = 0.50) compared with the CG.
Lennox et al. (2016). A health advocacy intervention for adolescents with intellectual disability: A cluster randomized controlled trial.	Adolescents with intellectual disability (n = 435) Mean age: 15.4 (1.7) IG; Males 53.9% CG Mean age: 15.8 (1.5) CG; Males 55.5% CG	Australia	The intervention included classroom health education. The IG received a handheld record that was personalized to promote health advocacy and went to a health check.	Participants in the IG were more likely to have their hearing tested (OR 2.7; 95% CI 1.0–7.3) their vision tested (OR 3.3; 95% CI 1.8–6.1), and to have had their blood pressure checked (OR 2.4; 95% CI 1.6–3.7). No differences were noted in the identification of new diseases between the IG and the CG.
Luger et al. (2016). Effects of a home-based and volunteer-administered physical training, nutritional, and social support program on malnutrition and frailty in older persons: A randomized controlled trial.	Frail and pre-frail older individuals who are community dwelling and 65 years or older. (n = 80) Mean age: 83.0 (8.1) IG; Females 85% CG Mean age: 82.5 (8.0) CG; Females 83% CG	Australia	IG was administered physical training and nutritional topic discussion intervention. CG participated in a social support group with cognitive training. Both groups were visited 2 times a week by "buddies" who were trained volunteers.	There was a significant decrease of impaired nutritional status (25% IG and 23% CG) as well as frailty (17% IG and 16% CG) in both groups over time.

(*continued*)

Table 18-1 Health Promotion Interventions—cont'd

Author/Date	Disability	Country	Intervention/Purpose	Outcome
Matthews et al. (2016). To explore the delivery of a community based walking intervention for adults with intellectual disabilities.	Adults with intellectual disabilities. IG = 54; CG = 48 (n = 102) Female = 46% Mean age = 45 years Intellectual disabilities: Mild = 70% Moderate = 21% Severe = 9%	Scotland	Three consultations included goal setting, self-efficacy development, social support mobilization, and self-monitoring. Participants were encouraged to increase walking by 30 minutes per day at least 5 days of the week. Outcome measures included average steps walked per day, time spent doing varying levels of activity, waist circumference, BMI, measures of well-being. ***Control Group:*** Wait listed	No significant differences were noted between the IG and CG using mean difference in a 12-week period in percentage sedentary time, BMI, or subjective well-being.
Meraviglia et al. (2013). Health promotion for cancer survivors: Adaptation and implementation of an intervention.	Cancer survivors (n = 35) (IG = 14; CG = 20). Mean age = 50.37, SD = 8.07) 63% female, 40% White, 35% Hispanic, 11% African American, 11% Asian. Cancers were 40% breast, 14% colorectal, 11% lymphoma.	United States (Texas)	"The purpose of this feasibility study was to adapt, refine, and implement a holistic intervention to promote the use of health-promoting behaviors of cancer survivors after their initial therapy" (Meraviglia et al., 2013, pp. 141–142). Intervention: a. support relationships; b. health promotion classes weekly for 6 weeks, which included topics such as improving health for cancer survivors, smoking cessation and cancer survivorship; c. follow-up telephone support to encourage health promotion. CG: Completed a questionnaire at enrollment and at 3- and 6-month periods.	Changes over three time periods (enrollment, 3 months, 6 months) were examined: Self-rated abilities for health practices changed over time for both the intervention and control group (F 2, 66 = 3.43, $p < .05$). Health promoting behaviors assessed with Health-Promoting Lifestyle Profile II had significant change over time (F 2, 1.68 = 6.84, $p < .01$). Quality of life measured by FACIT had changes over time for both CG and IG (F 2, 66 = 0.63, $p < .10$). Conclusions: Health promotion interventions may improve the use of health-promoting behaviors and self-efficacy in cancer survivors.
Metikaridis et al. (2017). Effect of a stress management program on subjects with neck pain: A pilot randomized controlled trial.	Chronic neck pain (n = 53) Mean age: 56.5 (11.44) IG Females 92.9% CG Mean age: 55.0 (11.55) CG Females 96% CG	Greece	Eight-week program of stress management (including progressive muscle relaxation and breathing techniques) to examine its effects on neck pain. CG received no intervention.	The IG showed a significant reduction in stress (p = 0.03) as well as anxiety (p = 0.01) as well as a significant reduction in percentage of disability due to their neck pain (p = 0.000) and stress-related symptoms.

Table 18-1 Health Promotion Interventions—cont'd

Author/Date	Disability	Country	Intervention/Purpose	Outcome
Natale et al. (2017). Promoting healthy weight among children with developmental delays.	Children with developmental delays (DD) (n = 71) Mean age: 49.18 months (7.69) IG Females 46% CG Mean age: 35.9 months (15.40) CG Females 40% CG	United States (Florida)	Randomized child-care centers received a role modeling program and curriculum focused on obesity prevention. Control care centers received training in safety curriculum.	IG children decreased their junk food consumption slightly. CG increased their junk food consumption. Changes in consumption of vegetables and fruits by parents had a significant effect on the consumption of these foods in the preschool-age child with DD. If the parents ate more junk food, the child would also eat more junk food.
Osei et al. (2013). Effects of an online support group for prostate cancer survivors: A randomized trial.	Prostate cancer survivors (n = 40) Ages of CG and IG: 53–87 years (SD 7.6) with no significant difference in age.	United States (California)	The study purpose was to determine the effects of an online support group system on quality of life of men who had been diagnosed with prostate cancer.	Improvement in quality of life was noted in IG over time but then returned to baseline at 8 weeks.
Park et al. (2017). A pilot randomized controlled trial of the effects of chair yoga on pain and physical function among community-dwelling older adults with lower extremity osteoarthritis.	Community-dwelling older adults with lower extremity osteoarthritis (OA) (n = 112) Mean age: 75.9 (8.2) IG; Males 30.2% CG Mean age: 74.5 (6.5) CG; Males 16.5% CG	United States (Florida)	To determine if "Sit and Fit" chair yoga had an effect on pain and physical functioning in older adults with lower extremity OA when compared with a health education intervention.	The 8-week "Sit and Fit" program was associated with reduced pain during the intervention (p =.01) that was sustained for 3 months. Pain (using the WOMAC pain scale) (p =.048) and fatigue interference (p =.037) as well as gait speed (p =.024) improved during the yoga intervention (p =.048). However, these improvements did not continue postintervention.
Rejeski et al. (2017). Community weight loss to combat obesity and **disability** in at-risk older adults.	Older overweight obese adults with cardiovascular disease or metabolic syndrome (n = 249) Mean age combined: 66.8 (4.7) Females combined: 71.1%	United States (North Carolina)	3 groups: Weight loss Weight loss + aerobic training Weight loss + resistance training Purpose was to examine if a community-based program could affect weight reduction in older obese adults	All groups lost weight when compared to baseline.

(*continued*)

Table 18-1 Health Promotion Interventions—cont'd

Author/Date	Disability	Country	Intervention/Purpose	Outcome
Rimmer et al. (2013). Telehealth weight management intervention for adults with physical **disabilities**.	Adults with physical disabilities, which included multiple sclerosis, stroke, lupus, spinal cord injury, spina bifida, cerebral palsy. (n = 91) Mean age combined: 46.5 (12.7) Females combined 75.8%	United States (Chicago, Illinois)	Nine-month telephone-based weight management program for individuals with disabilities. Participants were randomized into (1) physical activity toolkit group with coaching telephone calls, (2) physical activity toolkit group + nutritional information with coaching phone calls, and (3) control group.	Intervention groups had a greater reduction in body weight when compared to the control group.
Robinson-Whelen et al. (2014). A safety awareness program for women with diverse disabilities: A **randomized controlled trial**.	Women with diverse disabilities who had experienced differing levels of abuse (n = 213) Mean age combined: 47.79 (13.69) Mean of duration of primary disability in years 19.83 (16.01)	United States (Houston, Texas)	The purpose of this study was to determine if participation in an eight-week peer-led personal safety awareness program will increase awareness of abuse, safety skills knowledge, social support, and safety-promoting behavior in women with disabilities when compared to controls.	The differences between the groups' safety knowledge scores at 6-month follow-up reached significance, (t(135) = 2.41, p = 0.17), with the IG scoring higher than the CG.
Sangelaji et al. (2014). Effect of combination exercise therapy on walking distance, postural balance, fatigue and quality of life in multiple sclerosis patients: A clinical **trial** study.	Multiple sclerosis patients (n = 59) IG (n = 39) CG (n = 20)	Iran	IG had 10 weeks of aerobic, stretching, and balancing exercises.	Exercise had a significant effect on improvement of multiple sclerosis symptoms. Symptom return in multiple sclerosis may have been related to exercise cessation.
van Schijndel-Speet et al. (2017). A structured physical activity and fitness program for older adults with intellectual disabilities: Results of a cluster-randomized clinical trial.	Older adults with intellectual disabilities (n = 151) Mean age: 58.2 (range 44–83) IG; Males 42% CG Mean age: 57.9 (range 42–78) CG; Males 47.7% CG	Netherlands	To determine if a physical activity program (including an educational program) will improve or maintain adequate levels of physical activity (steps per day) in older adults with intellectual disabilities when compared to a care-as-usual control program.	Significant findings were reported related to physical activity and muscle strength, blood pressure, serum cholesterol levels as well as cognitive functioning in participants of a physical activity program compared to controls.

Table 18-1 Health Promotion Interventions—cont'd

Author/Date	Disability	Country	Intervention/Purpose	Outcome
Stuck et al. (2015). Effect of health risk assessment and counselling on health behavior and survival in older people: A pragmatic randomised trial.	Adults 65 or older registered with primary-care physicians in Switzerland (n = 2284) Mean age: 74.5 (5.8) IG Females 56.9% CG Mean age: 74.5 (6.1) CG Females 56.5% CG	Switzerland	Two-year intervention including health risk assessment and counseling with older adults regarding preventative care, health behaviors, and long-term survival.	At 2 years, use of preventative care behaviors and health behaviors were reported to be more frequent in IG compared to CG. In the IG at 2 years, 70% were physically active compared to 62% in the CG (OR 1.43, 95% CI 1.16–1.77, $p = 0.001$). At 2 years, 66% of the IG had received their flu vaccine (in the last year) compared to 59% in the CG (OR 1.35, 95% CI 1.09– 1.66, $p = 0.005$).
Tao et al. (2015). A nurse-led case management program on home exercise training for hemodialysis patients: A randomized controlled trial.	Patients on maintenance hemodialysis (stable condition for 3 months) (n = 113) Mean age: 53.02 (11.62) IG; Males 50.9% CG Mean age: 56.68 (9.67) CG; Males 56.68% CG	Hong Kong, China	Twelve-week nurse-led case management program to facilitate home exercise for hemodialysis patients.	Quality-of-life improvements were noted across 3 time points only in the IG. Greater increases in normal gait speed were noted in the IG [$F(1,111) = 4.42$, $p = 0.038$].
Verhaeghe et al. (2013). Health promotion in individuals with mental disorders: A cluster preference randomized controlled trial.	Adults with mental disorders (n = 284) Mean age: 46.2 (12.5) IG; Females 40.8% CG Mean age: 46.6 (11.9) CG; Females 33.7% CG	Belgium	Psychoeducation groups and exercise, changes in body weight, BMI, waist circumference, and fat mass.	Significant differences were found between the IG and the CG in BMI (−0.12 versus +0.08 kg/m2; $p = 0.04$), body weight (−0.35 versus +0.22 kg; $p = 0.04$), waist circumference (−0.29 versus + 0.55 cm; $p < 0.01$), and fat mass (−0.99 versus −0.12%; $p < 0.01$) that disappeared at follow-up.
Zidén et al. (2014). Physical function and fear of falling 2 years after the health-promoting randomized controlled trial: Elderly persons in the risk zone.	Elderly persons (n = 459) Mean sge of all groups was 85 with a median of 85.	Sweden	The purpose was to study the effects of two health-promoting interventions (one home visit with health promotion information, and 4 weekly group meetings focusing on health strategies as well as peer learning) on fear of falling and physical functioning at 3 months and at 1- and 2-year follow-ups compared to controls.	A significantly larger proportion of participants in the IG maintained walking speed and reported higher falls efficacy compared with controls. At 1 and 2 years, a significantly higher proportion of participants in the IG performed regular physical activities compared with the CG.

The findings are discussed in detail as they relate to their country of origin. Given that different laws apply and the cultural views on disability drive variations in those laws with resultant expectations, we thought it best to discuss the findings within these countries.

In the U.S. study on cancer survivors, significant changes in health promotion behaviors were measured over time. Sedentary older adults in the other U.S. study did not have improvements in global or domain-specific cognitive functioning when compared to a health education program control group (CG) at postintervention (Park, McCaffrey, Newman, Liehr, & Ouslander, 2017).

The intervention group (IG) reported small significant improvements in body weight, body mass index (BMI), waist circumference, and fat mass at the end of the 10-week intervention (IG) when compared to the CG. At the 6-month follow-up, only fat mass remained decreased in the IG. However, a significant difference in steps per day was noted in the IG when compared to the CG. In the IG, mean steps per day increased, while in the CG, mean steps per day decreased (Verhaeghe et al., 2013).

The intervention was a telephone-based health coaching for patients who had chronic conditions in Germany. When considering time until being readmitted to the hospital, nonsignificant differences were found between the IG (n = 2,713) and CG (n = 2,596). In the chronic campaign (type 2 diabetes, hypertension, coronary artery disease, asthma, COPD), the probability of being hospital readmitted was higher in the IG when compared to the CG (OR = 1.13; p = .045). In the chronic campaign, those in the IG demonstrated a significant increase in daily defined doses of medication. In both the chronic and heart campaigns participants, there was a significantly reduced likelihood of dying in the IG when compared to the CG in a 2-year period (chronic campaign: OR = 0.64; p = .005; heart failure campaign: OR = 0.44; p = .001) (Harter et al., 2016).

Scotland's intervention was not effective in improving health outcomes or the increase in physical activity in adults with intellectual disabilities. No significant differences were noted between the IG and CG using mean difference in a 12-week period in percentage sedentary time, BMI, or subjective well-being (Matthews et al., 2016).

Health promotion interventions in the U.S. studies included health promotion classes, physical activity programs, and the use of support systems. In Belgium, health promotion interventions included exercise and educational groups as well as the use of support systems. In the German telephone coaching health promotion intervention, motivational interviewing and shared decision making were used (Harter et al., 2016). Scotland researchers used consultations to encourage participants to set goals and to increase walking time per day (Matthews et al., 2016).

Chronic Illness and Health Promotion

The researcher's portrayal or understanding of illness versus a limitation as a targeted disabling condition for health promotion varied. One study (4.2%) focused on psychiatric diagnoses as disability. Six studies, or 25% of studies, examined intellectual disabilities. Seven studies, or 29% of studies, focused on disabilities related to the function of our elderly. Pain was included in the description or title of a disability study in three studies (12.5%). Individuals with a diagnosis of cancer were classified as having a disability in two studies (8.3%). Muscle limitations as disabilities were examined in seven (29%) studies. This is important when dissecting the study. If the study is focused on a medical illness, then the approach might be to improve overall disease management, but when working on health promotion for the person with a disability, the focus is not on changing the person but perhaps on improving his or her ability to access and function while living a healthy lifestyle. These two approaches can be used hand in hand provided that the person who has a disability can take advantage of health promotion in his or her current body.

This concept can be illustrated through a discussion of how mental illness was approached. Randomized controlled trial studies that investigated health promotion interventions for those with mental illness as a disability were encountered in two countries, Belgium (Verhaeghe et al., 2013) and the United States (Robinson-Whelen et al., 2014). In the Belgium study (40.8% female IG; 33.7% female CG; n = 284) the mental disorders of focus were schizophrenia (41.2% IG; 30.1% CG), mood disorders (22.7% IG; 28.9% CG), substance use (15.5% IG; 16.9% CG), personality disorders (14.9% IG; 13.3% CG), and other (5.7% IG; 10.8% CG).

The U.S. study (100% women, n = 213) focused on health promotion for individuals with mental health disorders, implying something was functionally different in the processing of information that needed unique intervention for accessing information on abuse. These were labeled as (1) mental health disabilities, including 23.5% of total study participants; other disorders in processing that were included in the study were (2) physical disabilities or health conditions, (3) cognitive or learning disabilities, and (4) visual disabilities. They delineated in the study the types of abuse that were suffered by the participants, which included: sexual abuse (45.1%,; physical abuse (66.5%), being refused essential care (16.4%), and being refused an assistive device (5.6%). This approach to disability and health promotion was unique. The authors were working with the knowledge that those who have disabilities are at increased risk for abuse, and they targeted those with mental disorders as defined within the United States. They provided tools for overcoming abuse that were designed for individuals with mental health disorders.

Discussion of Evidence

These articles investigate the focus of different countries on promoting the health of people with disabilities. We also reviewed the conditions each study characterized as disabilities, including problems with movement (Park et al., 2017; Tao, Chow, & Wong, 2015), more specifically, falling (Zidén, Häggblom-Kronlöf, Gustafsson, Lundin-Olsson, & Dahlin-Ivanoff, 2014) and exercise (Bergström,Hagströmer, Hagberg, & Elinder, 2013; Froehlich-Grobe et al., 2014; van Schijndel-Speet, Evenhuis, van Wijck, van Montfort, & Echteld, 2017). Health promotion studies also included problems with coping (Brendbekken, Harris, Ursin, Eriksen, & Tangen, 2016), social support (Luger et al., 2016), and socialization (Granbom, Kristensson, & Sandberg, 2017). Some authors worked on problems with weight management (Rejeski, Ambrosius, Burdette, Walkup, & Marsh, 2017; Rimmer, Wang, Pellegrini, Lullo, & Gerber, 2013; Verhaeghe et al., 2013), including problems with nutrition (Bergström et al., 2013; Luger et al., 2016; Natale et al., 2017). Other researchers focused on theoretical problems, such as assisting with health self-efficacy (Feldman et al., 2016; Meraviglia, Stuifbergen, Parsons, & Morgan, 2013), which influenced how patients communicated their needs to health-care professionals (Lennox et al., 2016). Other researchers took a health promotion focus when working with problems related to the management or the ramifications of having disabilities (Feldman et al., 2016; Fraser et al., 2015; Sangelaji et al., 2014). Several health promotion studies worked on problems with pain (Hausmann et al., 2017; Metikaridis, Hadjipavlou, Artemiadis, Chrousos, & Darviri, 2017; Park et al., 2017), safety awareness knowledge (Robinson-Whelen et al., 2014), and self-care as a related concept to health promotion (Granbom et al., 2017). One author focused on problems with using preventive health-care services as a facet of health promotion (Stuck et al., 2015). As a collective, the work is quite varied and the underlying approaches vary as well.

Obesity may occur in conjunction with mental health disorders due to the use of second-generation antipsychotics and decreased physical activity (Verhaeghe et al., 2013). In the Belgium study (participants' age: 18–75 years; $n = 284$), this problem was addressed with a ten-week health promotion intervention, including weekly educational classes on healthy eating and exercise as well as supervised walks and follow-up support by mental health nurses. The purpose of this study was to determine if this educational intervention would influence changes in body weight, BMI, waist circumference, and fat mass. Although significant differences were discovered after the intervention between the IG and the CG BMI (−0.12 versus +0.08 kg/m2; $p = .04$), body weight (−0.35 versus +0.22 kg; $p = .04$), waist circumference (−0.29 versus + 0.55 cm; $p < .01$), and fat mass (−0.99 versus −0.12%; $p < .01$), these changes disappeared at follow-up.

Interpersonal violence is more likely to be experienced by women with disabilities than by women who do not have disabilities (Robinson-Whelen et al., 2014). In the U.S. study of adult women, a planned intervention for this issue offered eight weeks of safety awareness classes. The purpose of the study was to determine if taking these classes would lead to increased awareness of abuse, safety skills knowledge, social support, and safety-promoting behavior in women when compared to controls. Significant differences were noted between the IG and CG in safety knowledge scores at 6-month follow up ($t\ (135) = 2.41$, $p = .17$), with the IG scoring higher than the CG.

The Belgium study focused on the negative ramifications of medications that are widely used by individuals with mental disorders. It sought to find a solution to weight gain prevalent among individuals who take certain antipsychotics. However, education about proper eating and physical activity did not promote successful long-term change for those in this study. Although outcomes improved when researchers guided and supported the IGs, these improvements disappeared at 6-month follow-up when participants were required to continue the health promotion intervention independently (Verhaeghe et al., 2013).

The U.S. study (Robinson-Whelen, et al., 2014) sought to educate women regarding ways to be more aware of safety to promote protective behaviors. The participants in the study were women who had already experienced some form of abuse and were thus at higher risk for future abuse. Similarly, the findings of increased knowledge scores in the U.S. study participants might be considered promising but actually hold no assurance for future protection against abuse encounters.

The Belgium study and the U.S. study sought to improve the lives of those with mental illness in unique ways. Although their efficacy might be questioned by some, it cannot be doubted that these health promotion interventions show respect and hope for the mentally ill. Studies such as these demonstrate a hope that those who have a mental disorder as a disability can progress and acquire tools that may improve their quality of life as well as their protective factors.

UNIVERSAL DESIGN (UD) AND HEALTH EDUCATION

Since the enactment of the Americans with Disabilities Act (1990) and its subsequent amendments in 2008 (Americans with Disabilities Act Amendments Act, 2008), a collaborative effort between government agencies, professional health-care providers, advocacy groups, sports organizations, and researchers is raising awareness of health and health promotion through accessible education for individuals with disabilities to reduce health disparities and inequalities (Centers for Disease Control and Prevention [CDC], 2018; Krahn et al., 2015; Marks & Sisirak, 2017; Special Olympics, 2018). Individuals with disabilities have a right to participate fully in society and partake in health promotion and behavior change strategies to maintain and promote good health. As such, stakeholders must refocus efforts to consider accessible information and instructional practices to support health promotion education for everyone. Designing an accessible learning environment promotes universal opportunities for everyone, including those with disabilities, to obtain and utilize health information to achieve personal wellness.

Applying UD approaches to health promotion instruction aligns with health literacy initiatives to provide all individuals with easily accessible, navigable, and comprehensible basic health information and services to make appropriate health-care decisions (Björk, 2015; DeWalt et al., 2011; Levey, 2015; Möller, 2015). Health literacy is a predictor of health outcomes in the general population, and it is likely that lack of accessible knowledge has an impact on the health behavior risks, knowledge of disease self-management, use of preventive services, health-care costs, and rates of hospitalization and mortality for individuals with disabilities (Berkman, Sheridan, Donahue, Halperin, & Crotty, 2011; Havercamp & Scott, 2015; Parnell, McCulloch, Mieres, & Edwards, 2014; Sand-Jecklin, Daniels, & Lucke-Wold, 2017; Scott & Havercamp, 2016). From the health literacy perspective, universally designed health promotion programs consider the hidden barriers in obtaining, comprehending, evaluating, and utilizing health information for the making of educated choices to reduce health risks and improve health outcomes.

Background of UD

The concept of UD has a rich historical connection with the barrier-free movement and key legislation for architectural accessibility design (Architectural Barriers Act [1968], Rehabilitation Act [1973], Education of the Handicapped Act [1975], Fair Housing Amendments Act [1988], Americans with Disabilities Act [ADA; 1990], and Telecommunications Act [1996]). Grassroots advocates and architects recognized the legal, economic, and social justice implications of environment changes necessary to address the common needs of individuals, with and without disabilities (Center for Applied Special Technology [CAST], 2018; Krahn et al., 2015).

In the 1970s, architect Michael Bednar (1977) pioneered the idea that an individual's functional capacity is enhanced when environmental barriers are removed. He suggested moving beyond the accessibility concept to something broader and more *universal* for increasing access to physical environments, for example, curb cutouts that everyone can use (Institute for Human Centered Designed, 2016). Ron Mace, an architect, product developer, and educator of the late 1970s, coined the term *universal design* to describe the concept of "designing all products and the built environment to be aesthetic and usable to the greatest extent possible by everyone, regardless of their age, ability, or status in life" (Center for Universal Design, 2018).

Over time, the concept of UD diffused to academic learning environments. UD in education proactively creates inclusive learning environments for all learners, with and without disabilities (Black, Weinberg, & Brodwin, 2014; Burgstahler, 2017; Levey, 2018; McGuire, 2014; Scott & McGuire, 2017). The practice of UD in education focuses on promoting maximum usability and accessibility of curriculum content, materials, activities, resources, educational products, and environments during the planning, delivering, and evaluation of instruction (Burgstahler, 2017; Dallas & Sprong, 2015; Levey, 2015, 2016, 2017, 2018; Lombardi, Murray, & Gerdes, 2011). UD is applicable across learning environments and modalities (e.g., traditional, online, hybrid, and simulated classroom and clinical settings) and is flexible in meeting the learning needs of all individuals (Levey, 2014, 2016, 2018; Rao, Ok, & Bryant, 2014). Learning and participating in health promotion activities must be about the content and not about how to obtain and navigate around it.

Universal design for instruction (UDI) is a framework specifically for teaching methods. This pedagogical approach "consists of the proactive design and use of inclusive instructional strategies that benefit a broad range of learners including students with disabilities" (Scott, McGuire, & Embry, 2002). The framework comprises nine principles for consideration when creating and planning lessons, materials, and assessments, and selecting instructional methods for diverse adult learners (Scott, McGuire, & Shaw, 2001) (Table 18-2). The implementation of UD-based instruction is not a one-size-fits-all approach, accommodation, or modification of standards;

Table 18-2 Principles of Universal Design for Instruction

Principle	Definition	Example(s)
Principle 1: Equitable use	Instruction is designed to be useful to and accessible by people with diverse abilities. Provide the same means of use for all students: identical whenever possible, equivalent when not.	Provision of class notes online. Comprehensive notes can be accessed in the same manner by all students, regardless of hearing ability, English proficiency, learning or attention disorders, or note-taking skill level. In an electronic format, students can utilize whatever individual assistive technology is needed to read, hear, or study the class notes.
Principle 2: Flexibility in use	Instruction is designed to accommodate a wide range of individual abilities. Provide choice in methods of use.	Use of varied instructional methods (lecture with a visual outline, group activities, use of stories, or web-based discussions) to provide different ways of learning and experiencing knowledge.
Principle 3: Simple and intuitive	Instruction is designed in a straightforward and predictable manner, regardless of the student's experience, knowledge, language skills, or current concentration level. Eliminate unnecessary complexity.	Provision of a grading rubric that clearly lays out expectations for exam performance, papers, and/or projects; a syllabus with comprehensive and accurate information; a handbook guiding students through difficult homework assignments.
Principle 4: Perceptible information	Instruction is designed so that necessary information is communicated effectively to the student, regardless of ambient conditions or the student's sensory abilities.	Selection of textbooks, reading materials, and other instructional supports in digital format or online so students with diverse needs (e.g., vision, learning, attention, English language learners) can access materials through traditional hard copy or with the use of various technological supports (e.g., screen reader, text enlarger, online dictionary).
Principle 5: Tolerance for error	Instruction anticipates variation in individual student learning pace and prerequisite skills.	Structuring a long-term course project so that students have the option of turning in individual project components separately for constructive feedback and for integration into the final product; provision of online "practice" exercises that supplement classroom instruction.
Principle 6: Low physical effort	Instruction is designed to minimize nonessential physical effort in order to allow maximum attention to learning. *Note:* This principle does not apply when physical effort is integral to essential requirements of a course.	Allowing students to use a word processor for writing and editing papers or essay exams. This facilitates editing of the document without the additional physical exertion of rewriting portions of text (helpful for students with fine motor or handwriting difficulties or extreme organization weaknesses while providing options for those who are more adept and comfortable composing on the computer).
Principle 7: Size and space for approach and use	Instruction is designed with consideration for appropriate size and space for approach, reach, manipulations, and use regardless of a student's body size, posture, mobility, and communication needs.	In small class settings, use of a circular seating arrangement to allow students to see and face speakers during discussion—important for students with attention deficit disorder or who are deaf or hard of hearing.
Principle 8: A community of learners	The instructional environment promotes interaction and communication among students and between students and faculty members.	Fostering communication among students in and out of class by structuring study groups, discussion groups, e-mail lists, or chat rooms; making a personal connection with students and incorporating motivational strategies to encourage student performance through learning students' names or individually acknowledging excellent performance.

(*continued*)

Table 18-2 Principles of Universal Design for Instruction—cont'd

Principle	Definition	Example(s)
Principle 9: Instructional climate	Instruction is designed to be welcoming and inclusive. High expectations are espoused for all students.	A statement in the class syllabus affirming the need for class members to respect diversity in order to establish the expectation of tolerance as well as to encourage students to discuss any special learning needs with the instructor; highlight diverse thinkers who have made significant contributions to the field or share innovative approaches developed by students in the class.

Source: From *Principles of Universal Design for Instruction* by Sally S. Scott, Joan M. McGuire, and Stan F. Shaw, Center on Postsecondary Education and Disability, University of Connecticut. Copyright 2001. Reprinted with permission.

BOX 18-2 Resources for Universal Design

Center for Applied Special Technology (CAST): www.cast.org/
National Center for Accessible Media: http://ncam.wgbh.org
National Center on Universal Design for Learning: http://www.udlcenter.org/
National Service Inclusion Project: http://www.serviceandinclusion.org
North Carolina State University Center for Universal Design: https://projects.ncsu.edu/ncsu/design/cud/
The Do It Web site: https://www.washington.edu/doit/equal-access-universal-design-instruction
Universal Design for Learning in Higher Education: http://udloncampus.cast.org/home
Universal Design Resources Amara: Subtitling Platforms: https://amara.org/en/
University of Connecticut's Center on Postsecondary Education and Disability: UDI Online Project: http://udi.uconn.edu/index.php?q=content/universal-design-instruction-postsecondary-education
University of Washington's Disabilities, Opportunities, Internetworking, and Technology (DOIT) Center: https://www.washington.edu/doit/
University of Wisconsin–Milwaukee's Rehabilitation Research Design & Disability (R2D2) Center: Access-Ed: http://access-ed.r2d2.uwm.edu/
Web Accessibility Initiative (W3C): http://www.w3.org/WAI/intro/accessibility.php
Web Accessibility in Mind (WebAIM): https://webaim.org/

it is a holistic and accessible solution to prepare and disseminate curriculum in a learner-ready format (Levey, 2015; Scott & McGuire, 2017).

UD can be a useful guide for implementing and executing inclusive instructions, materials, and programs benefiting the maximum number of individuals, including English as a second language (ESL) learners, learning preferences (read/write, auditory, visual, and kinesthetic), abilities, and disabilities of learners (Capp, 2017; Levey, 2017, 2018; Roberts, Park, Brown, & Cook, 2011), especially in health promotion education. As a participatory design approach, the UD concept minimizes unnecessary barriers and reduces the need to accommodate or retrofit curriculum (Levey, 2015, 2018; Lombardi & Murray, 2011; Scott & McGuire, 2017). The adoption of UD inclusive teaching practices moves beyond the legal mandate of accessible physical environments to accessible educational encounters without compromising curriculum objectives, standards, or measurements (Gradel & Edson, 2010; Levey, 2014, McGuire, 2011; Shaw, 2011). See Box 18-2 for list of UD-based instruction resources.

UD and Health Promotion

For almost 40 years, health promotion efforts focused on improving health and well-being to avoid disability and inadvertently overlooked appropriate accessible interventions to health education programs for individuals who were already disabled (Anderson et al., 2013; de Vries McClintock et al., 2016; Havercamp & Scott, 2015; Krahn et al., 2015; Marrocco & Krouse, 2017; Sharby, Martire, & Iversen, 2015). The publications *Closing the Gap: A National Blueprint to Improve the Health of People with Mental Retardation* (USDHHS, 2002); *The Surgeon General's Call to Action to Improve the Health and*

Wellness of People with Disabilities (USDHHS, 2005), and *The Future of Disability in America* (Institute of Medicine [IOM], 2007) illuminated the existing state of disabilities and health promotion disparity between individuals with disabilities and those without. The overall themes from these reports identified a greater need not only to improve access to health services and health promotion activities for individuals with disabilities but also to increase disability awareness, sensitivity, and skills training in professional health-care curriculum. Due to the lack of professional development training, "inadequately prepared health-care professionals" was the reason cited most often as a barrier to care and preventive health and health promotion services for individuals with disabilities (Anderson et al., 2013; Bolland, 2017; de Vries McClintock et al., 2016; Havercamp & Scott, 2015; Krahn et al., 2015; Marks & Sisirak, 2017; Marrocco & Krouse, 2017; Scott & Havercamp, 2016; Sharby, Martire, & Iversen, 2015). Given the high rate of health risks and poor health outcomes for individuals with disabilities, health-care stakeholders should make every effort to promote accessible health education for this population (Havercamp & Scott, 2015).

UD in health promotion and self-management education is appearing in the health-care literature as an effective approach for education and practice across disciplines (Björk, 2015; Levey, 2014, 2015, 2016, 2017, 2018; Marks & Sisirak, 2017; Möller, 2015; Nápoles, Santoyo-Olsson, & Stewart, 2013; Williams & Moore, 2011). The rate of adoption of UD teaching practices depends on support for professional development training and resources from administration and leadership (Levey, 2015, 2016, 2017; McGuire, 2011; Scott & McGuire, 2017). Organizations willing to design accessible and inclusive health programs have the potential of reaching more underserved populations and reducing the health disparities and inequalities experienced by individuals with disabilities (Levey, 2015, 2016, 2017).

Research on universally designed teaching practices and programs is woefully needed to address the national health-care initiative of "closing the gaps" in health promotion education and services between those with and without a disability (Agency for Healthcare Research and Quality [AHRQ], 2004). A relevant and timely measurement known as Universal Design in Healthcare Education (UDinHE) examines health-care professionals' perceptions toward and willingness to adopt UD-based teaching concepts (Levey & Montenegro-Montenegro, 2018; Levey, Burgstahler, Montenegro-Montenegro, & Webb, in press). The UDinHE instrument can be used to measure the impact of professional development training. The UDinHE instrument (33 items; a 5-point Likert scale) is a three-concept model (Knowledge of UD, System Support for UD, and Perceptions of UD) structured on Rogers' (2003) Diffusion of Innovation Theory. The UDinHE has established face and content validity (scale content validity index was .98). Internal consistency analysis (test-retest; sample 22 paired surveys) revealed all subscales had a reliability coefficient (Cronbach's alpha) greater than 0.70, except for the social system at 0.62. Overall, there were no significant differences between Time 1 (M = 2.56, SD = 0.51) and Time 2 (M = 2.57, SD = 0.52) ($t = -0.26$, $p = .79$, $d = -0.06$) meaning the UDinHE has stable reliability over time. A strong relationship between the constructs was revealed when the correlations between subscales were statistically significant at $p < .001$ (two-tailed) and ranged from .53 to .83. The UDinHE is undergoing further statistical analysis, but it is showing promising results in identifying factors contributing to health-care professionals' perceptions of and willingness to adopt accessible and inclusive teaching/learning strategies.

For the advancement of translational research, further studies are required to enhance robust UD health promotion teaching practices and evaluate interventions. Addressing factors that facilitate change in health-care professionals' teaching methods is critical for sustainable adoption of UD in health promotion education for all learners. Advance practice nurses and educators have an essential role in promoting evidence-based accessible health education design that achieves this goal.

The Healthy People 2020 Connection

Healthy People 2020 articulates the importance of health promotion at the individual and community levels to achieve health equity, eliminate disparities, and improve the health of all groups. An objective for this national health initiative is to "reduce the proportion of adults with disabilities aged 18 and older who experience physical or program barriers that limit or prevent them from using available local health and wellness programs" (Healthy People 2020, Health and Disability, Objective DH-8). A barrier to a wellness program can be any obstacle to the learning environment and includes the instructional method(s) and formats learners must navigate to obtain, comprehend, and evaluate information to make appropriate health decisions. The objective is similar to the initiative for health literacy. UD instruction and health literacy concepts provide guidelines for the delivery of health information and interventions to reduce health risks, and improve health outcomes and quality of life for individuals with disabilities (Björk, 2015; Brach et al., 2012; Hollar & Rowland, 2015; Levey, 2014, 2015, 2016,

2017, 2018; Levey & Montenegro-Montenegro, 2018; Möller, 2015; Nápoles et al., 2013; Parnell et al., 2014).

To address the emerging health and disability issues from a UD and health literacy perspective, Healthy People 2020 Health and Disability (Overview) recommends: (1) removing barriers in the physical environment and public infrastructure by employing UD concepts and changing operational policies to improve health equality for individuals with disabilities; (2) ensuring technology is accessible, including health information technology tools and systems, electronic health records and personal health records, wearable technologies, and home-monitoring systems; (3) including disability status across the life span in public health data surveillance efforts to assist with program planning and management to reduce health disparities and improve health equity; (4) translating and implementing effective evidence-based interventions and health and wellness programs for individuals with disabilities from the clinical setting to community outreach programs; and (5) increasing awareness of disability and health training for all public health workers and health-care professionals at the employer and academic levels.

Educators and advance practice nurses have an essential role in meeting the Healthy People 2020 objectives by delivering universally accessible health promotion education to achieve health equity, eliminate disparities, and improve health for everyone. Through critical appraisal of teaching practices, educators and nurse practitioners can advocate for inclusive teaching practices and policies to promote quality of life, healthy development, and healthy behaviors across the life span. It is imperative that nurses in advanced roles lead multidisciplinary teams in translating robust UD teaching strategies in clinical and community settings to promote good health practices for all groups. Accessible health promotion education based in UD provides a way to improve health outcomes for individuals with and without disabilities and is congruent with the Healthy People 2020 objectives for the nation.

The variety of ways in which disability was defined and the associated problems experienced leave a need for tailored, person-centered approaches to health promotion. Krahn and Fox (2016) point out that disability diversity can create a multi-numeral variation in need, with disparities in disability and inequities in care highly prevalent in developed countries. The literature reviewed in this chapter demonstrates that chronic and disabling conditions range from intellectual impairment to sensory and mental illness. The problems experienced by persons with disabilities ranged from falling, obesity, and movement to socialization and nutrition. For a health-care provider to offer to personalize health promotion is an admission that what a person with a disability needs for health promotion is a very personal decision requiring careful individualized attention. The obvious approach is to plan based on careful listening to an individual's needs.

Person-centered care for everyone who has a disability would be a prohibitively costly approach. Creating and implementing UD interventions is a public health measure that can remove this barrier to health promotion and improved quality of life, with individualized attention and care limited to those who need assistance beyond what is available through targeted health promotion initiatives.

KEY POINTS

- Health promotion strategies enhance the environment, resources, and personal insights of an individual through efforts applied at the individual, community, and societal levels.
- The Americans with Disabilities Act allowed society to reimagine people with disabilities as having an entryway to health through self-reliance, regardless of their level of interdependence needed to achieve it.
- Health promotion for people with disabilities is about doing what each individual can with her or his body as it is today, not changing the body in order to be healthy.
- Research on health promotion is scattered across different countries.
- As a participatory design approach, the UD concept minimizes unnecessary barriers and reduces the need to accommodate or retrofit health promotion approaches.
- UD is a proactive approach for creating accessible materials and environments for learners, including individuals with disabilities.
- Incorporating UD and health literacy concepts into health promotion educational interventions provides a means for creating accessible health information and services to facilitate health decisions.
- The use of UD supports the Healthy People 2020 goal of promoting the inclusion, choice, health equity, quality of life, and health outcomes among individuals with disabilities across the life span.
- Instruments to measure health professionals' perceptions and adoption of UD and accessible education practices will help to guide this evolution in health promotion.
- Creating a society where person-centered care works with UD may decrease disability-related costs and provide the best outreach possible.

Check Your Understanding

1. Which group of patients would benefit from health promotion education based in UD principles? (Select all that apply.)
   A. People who speak English as a second language
   B. Individuals with disabilities
   C. People with diverse learning preferences
   D. Individuals without disabilities
2. Which of the following are important considerations when developing health information and interventions? (Select all that apply.)
   A. UD approaches
   B. Health literacy concepts
   C. Criminal background of the patient
   D. Educators' compensation for teaching
3. UD can be applied to which of the following learning environments? (Select all that apply.)
   A. Classrooms
   B. Online environments
   C. Hospitals
   D. Clinics
   E. Blended environments (classroom and online)
4. Which of the following are Healthy People 2020 objectives for health and disability? (Select all that apply.)
   A. Removing barriers in the physical environment and public infrastructure by employing UD concepts and changing operational policies to improve health equality for individuals with disabilities
   B. Ensuring that technology is accessible, including health information technology tools and systems, electronic health records and personal health records, wearable technologies, and home-monitoring systems
   C. Including disability status across the life span in public health data surveillance efforts to assist with program planning and management to reduce health disparities and improve health equity
   D. Translating and implementing effective evidence-based interventions and health and wellness programs for individuals with disabilities from the clinical setting to community outreach programs
   E. Decreasing access for individuals with disabilities to health promotion education as a way to achieve personal wellness
   F. Increasing awareness of disability and health training for all public health workers and health-care professionals at the employer and academic levels

See "Reflections on Check Your Understanding" at the end of the book for answers.

REFERENCES

Agency for Healthcare Research and Quality. (2004). *Closing the quality gap: A critical analysis of quality improvement strategies* [Fact sheet]. Rockville, MD: Author. Retrieved from https://permanent.access.gpo.gov/LPS110179/LPS110179/www.ahrq.gov/clinic/epc/qgapfact.pdf

American Nurses Association. (1995). *Nursing's social policy statement*. Washington, DC: American Nurses Publishing.

Americans with Disabilities Act. (1990). Pub. L. No. 101-336, 42 U.S.C. 12. 101–12, 213.

Americans with Disabilities Act Amendments Act. (2008). Pub. L. No. 110–325.

Anderson, L. L., Humphries, K., McDermott, S. Marks, B. Sisarak, J., & Larson, S. (2013). The state of the science of health and wellness for adults with intellectual and developmental disabilities. *Intellectual and Developmental Disabilities*, *51*(5), 385–398. https://doi.org/10.1352/1934-9556-51.5.385

Architectural Barriers Act. (1968). Pub. L. No. 90-480, 42 U.S.C. §§4151 et seq.

Becker, H. (1996). Measuring health among people with disabilities. *Family and Community Health*, *29*(1), 70S–77S.

Bednar, M. J. (1977). *Barrier-free environments*. Stroudsburg, PA: Dowden, Hutchinson & Ross.

Bergström, H., Hagströmer, M. Hagberg, J., & Elinder, L. S. (2013). A multi-component universal intervention to improve diet and physical activity among adults with intellectual disabilities in community residences: A cluster randomised controlled trial. *Research in Developmental Disabilities*, *34*(11), 3847–3857. https://doi.org/10.1016/j.ridd.2013.07.019

Berkman, N. D., Sheridan, S. L., Donahue, K. E., Halpern, D. J., & Crotty, K. (2011). Low health literacy and health outcomes: An updated systematic review. *Annals of Internal Medicine*, *155*(2), 97–107. https://doi.org/10.7326/0003-4819-155-2-201107190-00005

Björk (2015). A new theme within public health sciences for increased life quality. *Scandinavian Journal of Public Health*, *43*(Suppl. 16), 85–89. https://doi.org/10.1177/1403494814568602

Black, R. D., Weinberg, L. A., & Brodwin, M. G. (2014). Universal design for instruction and learning: A pilot study of faculty instructional methods and attitudes related to students with disabilities in higher education. *Exceptionality Education International*, *24*(1), 48–64. Retrieved from https://ir.lib.uwo.ca/eei/vol24/iss1/5

Bolland, M. (2017). Health promotion and intellectual disability: Listening to men. *Health and Social Care in the Community*, *25*(1), 185–193. https://doi.org/10.1111/hsc.12291

Brach, C., Keller, D., Hernandez, L. M., Baur, C., Parker, R., Dreyer, B.,... Schillinger, D. (2012). *Ten attributes of health literate health care organizations*. Washington, DC: Institute of Medicine. Retrieved from https://nam.edu/wp-content/uploads/2015/06/BPH_Ten_HLit_Attributes.pdf

Brendbekken, R., Harris, A., Ursin, H., Eriksen, H. R., & Tangen, T. (2016). Multidisciplinary intervention in patients with musculoskeletal pain: A randomized clinical trial. *International Journal of Behavioral Medicine*, *23*(1), 1–11. https://doi.org/10.1007/s12529-015-9486-y

Burgstahler, S. (2017). *Equal access: Universal design of instruction*. Seattle, WA: University of Washington. Retrieved from https://www.washington.edu/doit/sites/default/files/atoms/files/EA_Instruction.pdf

Capp, M. J. (2017). The effectiveness of universal design for learning: A meta-analysis of literature between 2013 and 2016. *International Journal of Inclusive Education*, *21*(8), 791–807. https://doi.org/10.1080/13603116.2017.1325074

Center for Applied Special Technology. (2018). About CAST. Retrieved from http://www.cast.org/about/timeline.html#.Wpr0wOjwbIU

Center for Universal Design (2018). About the center: History. Raleigh, NC: North Carolina State University. Retrieved from https://projects.ncsu.edu/design/cud/about_us/usronmace.htm

Centers for Disease Control and Prevention. (2018). *Disability and health*. Retrieved from https://www.cdc.gov/ncbddd/disabilityandhealth/index.html

Clark, J. M. (1993). From sick nursing to health nursing: Evolution or revolution? In J. Wilson Barnett & J. M. Clark (Eds.), *Research in health promotion and nursing* (pp. 256–270). Basingstoke, UK: MacMillan.

Dallas, B. K., & Sprong, M. E. (2015). Assessing faculty attitudes toward universal design instructional techniques. *Journal of Applied Rehabilitation Counseling*, *46*(4), 18–28.

de Vries McClintock, H. F, Barg, F. K., Katz, S. P., Stineman, M. G., Krueger, A., Colletti, P. M.,... Bogner, H. R. (2016). Health care experiences and perceptions among people with and without disabilities. *Disability and Health Journal*, *9*(1), 74–82. https://doi.org/10.1016/j.dhjo.2015.08.007

DeWalt, D. A., Broucksou, K. A., Hawk, V., Brach, C., Hink, A., Rudd, R., & Callahan, L. (2011). Developing and testing the health literacy universal precautions toolkit. *Nursing Outlook*, *59*(2), 85–94. https://doi.org/10.1016/j.outlook.2010.12.002

Education of the Handicapped Act. (1975). Pub. L. No. 94–142.

Ewles, L., & Simnet, I. (1999). *Promoting health: A practical guide* (4th ed.). Edinburgh, UK: Ballière Tindall.

Fair Housing Amendments Act. (1988). Pub. L. No. 100-430.

Feldman, M. A., Owen, F., Andrews, A. E., Tahir, M., Barber, R., & Griffiths, D. (2016). Randomized control trial of the 3Rs Health Knowledge Training Program for persons with intellectual disabilities. *Journal of Applied Research in Intellectual Disabilities*, *29*(3), 278–288. https://doi.org/10.1111/jar.12186

Fraser, R. T., Johnson, E. K., Lashley, S., Barber, J., Chaytor, N., Miller, J. W.,... Caylor, L. (2015). PACES in epilepsy: Results of a self-management randomized controlled trial. *Epilepsia*, *56*(8), 1264–1274. https://doi.org/10.1111/epi.13052

Froehlich-Grobe, K., Lee, J., Aaronson, L., Nary D. E., Washburn, R. A., & Little, T D. (2014). Exercise for everyone: A randomized controlled trial of project workout on wheels in promoting exercise among wheelchair users. *Archives of Physical Medicine and Rehabilitation*, *95*(1), 20–28. https://doi.org/10.1016/j.apmr.2013.07.006

Gradel, K., & Edson, A. J. (2010). Putting universal design for learning on the higher ed agenda. *Journal of Educational Technology Systems*, *38*(2), 111–121. https://doi.org/10.2190/ET.38.2.d

Granbom, M., Kristensson, J., & Sandberg, M. (2017). Effects on leisure activities and social participation of a case management intervention for frail older people living at home: A randomised controlled trial. *Health and Social Care in the Community*, *25*(4), 1416–1429. https://doi.org/10.1111/hsc.12442

Harris, L., Hankey, C., Jones, N., Pert, C., Murray, H., Tobin, J.,... Melville, C. (2017). A cluster randomised control trial of a multi-component weight management programme for adults with intellectual disabilities and obesity. *British Journal of Nutrition*, *118*(3), 229–240. https://doi.org/10.1017/S0007114517001933

Harter, M., Dirmaler, J., Swinger, S., Kriston, L., Herbarth, L., Siegmund-Schultze, E.,... Kong, H. (2016). Effectiveness of telephone-based health coaching for patients with chronic conditions: A randomized controlled trial. *PLoS One*, 11, e0161269. doi:10.1371/journal.pone.0161269

Hausmann, L. R. M., Youk, A., Kwoh, K., Ibrahim, S. A., Hannon, M. J., Weiner, D. K.,... Parks, A. (2017). Testing a positive psychological intervention for osteoarthritis. *Pain Medicine*, *18*(10), 1908–1920. https://doi.org/10.1093/pm/pnx141

Havercamp, S. M., & Scott, H. M. (2015). National health surveillance of adults with disabilities, adults with intellectual and developmental disabilities, and adults with no disabilities. *Disability and Health Journal*, *8*(2), 165–172. https://doi.org/10.1016/j.dhjo.2014.11.002

Healthy People 2020. Retrieved from https://www.healthypeople.gov

Hollar, D. W., Jr., & Rowland, J. (2015). Promoting literacy for people with disabilities and clinicians through a teamwork model. *Journal of Family Strengths*, *15*(2), Article 5. Retrieved from http://digitalcommons.library.tmc.edu/cgi/viewcontent.cgi?article=1286&context=jfs

Institute for Human Centered Design. (2016). *Universal design, human-centered design for the 21st century*. Retrieved from https://humancentereddesign.org/inclusive-design/library/barrier-free-environments

Institute of Medicine. (2007). Committee on disability in America board on health science policy. In M. Field & A. Jetta (Eds). *The future of disability in America*. Washington, DC: The National Academies Press. https://doi.org/10.17226/11898

Kickbush, I. (1994). Introduction: Tell me a story. In A. Pederson, M. O'Neill, & I. Rootman (Eds.), *Health promotion in Canada: Provincial, national and international perspectives* (pp. 8–17). Toronto, ON: W. B. Saunders.

Krahn, G.L., & Fox, M. H. (2016). Public health perspectives on intellectual and developmental disabilities. *Health Care for People with Intellectual and Developmental Disabilities across the Lifespan*, 395–408. doi:10.1007/978-3-319-18096-0_33

Krahn, G. L., Walker, D. K., & Correa-de-Araujo, R. (2015). Persons with disabilities as an unrecognized health disparity population. *American Journal of Public Health, 105*(Suppl. 2), S198–S206. https://doi.org/10.2105/AJPH.2014.302182

Labonté, R. (1994). Death of program, birth of metaphor: The development of health promotion in Canada. In A. Pederson, M. O'Neill, & I. Rootman (Eds.), *Health promotion in Canada: Provincial, national and international perspectives* (pp. 72–90). Toronto, ON: W. B. Saunders.

Lalonde, M. (1974). *A new perspective on the health of Canadians.* Ottawa, ON: Health and Welfare Canada.

Lennox N., McPherson, L., Bain, C., O'Callaghan, M., Carrington, S., & Ware, R. S. (2016). A health advocacy intervention for adolescents with intellectual disability: A cluster randomized controlled trial. *Developmental Medicine & Child Neurology, 58*(12), 1265–1272. https://doi.org/10.1111/dmcn.13174

Levey, J. A. (2014). Attitudes of nursing faculty towards nursing students with disabilities: An integrative review. *Journal of Postsecondary Education and Disability, 27*(3), 321–322. Retrieved from https://eric.ed.gov/?id=EJ1048784

Levey, J. A. (2015). *Diffusion of inclusion: Measuring willingness* (Doctoral dissertation). Retrieved from https://epublications.marquette.edu/cgi/viewcontent.cgi?article=1473&context=dissertations_mu

Levey, J. A. (2016). Measuring nurse educators' willingness to adopt inclusive teaching strategies. *Nursing Education Perspectives, 37*(4), 215–220. https://doi.org/10.1097/01.NEP.0000000000000021

Levey, J. A. (2017). Development and psychometric examination of the inclusive teaching strategies in a nursing education instrument. *Journal of Nursing Measurement, 25*(2), 130E–151E. https://doi.org/10.1891/1061-3749.25.2.E130

Levey, J. A. (2018). Universal design for instruction in nursing education: An integrative review. *Nursing Education Perspectives, 39*(3), 156–161. https://doi.org/10.1097/01.NEP.0000000000000249

Levey, J. A., Burgstahler, S., Montenegro-Montenegro, E. & Webb, A. (in press). The psychometric properties of the universal design in healthcare education (UDinHE) instrument. *Journal of Nursing Measurement.*

Levey, J. A., & Montenegro-Montenegro, E. (2018). *Evaluation of the validity and reliability of the revised universal design in healthcare education instrument.* Presentation at the Sigma Theta Tau 29th International Research Congress, Melbourne, Australia. Retrieved from https://sigma.nursingrepository.org/bitstream/handle/10755/624182/Levey_90700_Info.pdf?sequence=2&isAllowed=y

Lombardi, A. R., & Murray, C. (2011). Measuring university faculty attitudes toward disability: Willingness to accommodate and adopt universal design principles. *Journal of Vocational Rehabilitation, 34*(1), 43–56. https://doi.org/10.3233/jvr-2010-0533

Lombardi, A. R., Murray, C., & Gerdes, H. (2011). College faculty and inclusive instruction: Self-reported attitudes and actions pertaining to universal design. *Journal of Diversity in Higher Education, 4*(4), 250–261. https://doi.org/10.1037/a0024961

Luger, E., Dorner, T. E., Haider, S., Kapan, A., Lackinger, C., & Schindler, K. (2016). Effects of a home-based and volunteer-administered physical training, nutritional, and social support program on malnutrition and frailty in older persons: A randomized controlled trial. *Journal of the American Medical Directors Association, 17*(7), e9-671.e16. https://doi.org/10.1016/j.jamda.2016.04.018

Maben, J., & Clark, J. M. (1995). Health promotion: A concept analysis. *Journal of Advanced Nursing, 22*(6), 1158–1165. https://doi.org/10.1111/j.1365-2648.1995.tb03118.x

MacDonald, M. M. (2002). Health promotion: Historical, philosophical, and theoretical perspectives. In L. E. Young & V. E. Hayes (Eds.), *Transforming health promotion practice: Concepts, issues, and applications* (pp. 22–45). Philadelphia, PA: F. A. Davis.

Marks, B., & Sisirak, J. (2017). Nurse practitioners promoting physical activity: People with intellectual and developmental disabilities. *The Journal for Nurse Practitioners, 13*(1), e1–e5. https://doi.org/10.1016/j.nurpra.2016.10.023

Marrocco, A., & Krouse, H. J. (2017). Obstacles to preventive care for individuals with disability: Implications for nurse practitioners. *Journal of the American Association of Nurse Practitioners, 29*(5), 282–293. https://doi.org/10.1002/2327-6924.12449

Matthews, L., Mitchell, F., Stalker, K., McConnachie, A., Murray, H., Melling, C.,... Melville, C. (2016). Process evaluation of the Walk Well study: A cluster-randomised controlled trial of a community based walking programme for adults with disabilities. *BMC Public Health*, 16, 1–11. doi: 10.1186/x12889-016-3179-6

Maville, J. A., & C. G. Huerta (2002). *Health promotion in nursing.* Albany, NY: Delmar.

McGuire, J. M. (2011). Inclusive college teaching; Universal design for instruction and diverse learners. *Journal of Accessibility and Design for All, 1*(1), 38–54. https://doi.org/10.17411/jacces.v1i1.80

McGuire, J. M. (2014). Universally accessible instruction: Oxymoron or opportunity? *Journal of Postsecondary Education and Disability, 27*(4), 387–398. Retrieved from https://eric.ed.gov/?id=EJ1060009

Meraviglia, M., Stuifbergen, A., Parsons, D., & Morgan, S. (2013). Holistic promotion for cancer survivors: Adaptation and implementation of an intervention. *Holistic Nursing Practice, 27*(3), 140–147. https://doi.org/10.1097/HNP.0b013e31828a0988

Metikaridis, D. T., Hadjipavlou, A., Artemiadis, A., Chrousos G. P., & Darviri, C. (2017). Effect of a stress management program on subjects with neck pain: A pilot randomized controlled trial. *Journal of Back and Musculoskeletal Rehabilitation, 30*(1), 23–33. https://doi.org/10.3233/BMR-160709

Möller, A. (2015). Disability from a public health perspective. *Scandinavian Journal of Public Health, 43*(Suppl. 16), 81–84. https://doi.org/10.1177/1403494814568601

Nápoles, A. M., Santoyo-Olsson, J., & Stewart, A. L. (2013). Methods for translating evidence-based behavioral interventions for health-disparity communities. *Preventing Chronic Disease, 10*, 130133. https://doi.org/10.5888/pcd10.130133

Natale, R. R., Camejo, S. T., Asfour, L., Uhihorn, S. B., Delamater, A., & Messiah, S. E. (2017). Promoting healthy weight among children with developmental delays. *Journal of Early Intervention, 39*(1), 51–65. https://doi.org/10.1177/1053815116689060

National Federation for the Blind. (2018). *Diabetes action network.* Retrieved from https://nfb.org/diabetics

Osie, D. K., Lee, J. W., Modest, N. N., & Pothier, P. K. T. (2013). Effects on an online support group for prostate cancer survivors: A randomized trial. *Urol Nurse*, 33(3), 123–133.

Park, J., McCaffrey, R., Newman, D., Liehr, P., & Ouslander, J. G. (2017). A pilot randomized controlled trial of the effects of chair yoga on pain and physical function among community-dwelling older adults with lower extremity osteoarthritis. *Journal of the American Geriatrics Society*, *65*(3), 592–597. https://doi.org/10.1111/jgs.14717

Parnell, T. A., McCulloch, E. C., Mieres, J. H., & Edwards, F. (2014). *Health literacy as an essential component to achieving excellent patient outcomes* [Discussion paper]. Washington, DC: National Academy of Medicine. https://doi.org/10.31478/201401b

Piper, S. (2009). *Health promotion for nurses: Theory and practice*. New York: Routledge.

Raingruber, B. (2016). *Contemporary health promotion in nursing practice* (2nd ed.). Burlington, MA: Jones & Bartlett Learning.

Rao, K., Ok, M. W., Bryant, B. R. (2014). A review of research on universal design educational models. *Remedial and Special Education*, *35*(3), 153–156. https://doi.org/10.1177/0741932513518980

Rehabilitation Act (1973). 29 U.S.C. §§ 701 et seq.

Rejeski, W. J., Ambrosius, W. T., Burdette, J H., Walkup, M. P., & Marsh, A. P. (2017). Community weight loss to combat obesity and disability in at-risk older adults. *Journals of Gerontology: Series A*, *72*(11), 1547–1553. https://doi.org/10.1093/gerona/glw252

Rimmer, J. H., Wang, E., Pellegrini, C. A., Lullo, C., & Gerber, B. S. (2013). Telehealth weight management intervention for adults with physical disabilities: A randomized controlled trial. *American Journal of Physical Medicine & Rehabilitation*, *92*(12), 1084–1094. https://doi.org/10.1097/PHM.0b013e31829e780e

Roberts, K. D., Park, H. J., Brown, S., Cook, B. (2011). Universal design for instruction in postsecondary education: A systematic review of empirically based articles. *Journal of Postsecondary Education and Disability*, *24*(1), 5–15. Retrieved from https://eric.ed.gov/?id=EJ941728

Robinson-Whelen, S., Hughes, R. B., Gabrielli, J., Lund, E. M., Abramson, W., & Swank, P. R. (2014). A safety awareness program for women with diverse disabilities: A randomized controlled trial. *Violence Against Women*, *20*(7), 846–868. https://doi.org/10.1177/1077801214543387

Rogers, E. M. (2003). *Diffusion of innovations* (5th ed.). New York: Free Press.

Sand-Jecklin, K., Daniels, C. S., & Lucke-Wold, N. (2017). Incorporating health literacy screening into patients' health assessment. *Clinical Nursing Research*, *26*(2), 176–190. https://doi.org/10.1177/1054773815619592

Sangelaji, B., Nabavi, S. M., Estebsari, F., Banshi, M. R., Rashidian, H., Jamshidi, E., & Dastoorpour, M. (2014). Effect of combination exercise therapy on walking distance, postural balance, fatigue and quality of life in multiple sclerosis patients: A clinical trial study. *Iran Red Crescent Medical Journal*, *16*(6), e17173. https://doi.org/10.5812/ircmj.17173

Scott, H. M., & Havercamp, S. M. (2016). Systematic review of health promotion programs focused on behavioral changes for people with intellectual disability. *Intellectual and Developmental Disabilities*, *54*(1), 63–76. https://doi.org/10.1352/1934-9556-54.1.63

Scott, S., & McGuire, J. (2017). Using diffusion of innovation theory to promote universally designed college instruction. *International Journal of Teaching and Learning in Higher Education*, *29*(1), 119–128. Retrieved from https://files.eric.ed.gov/fulltext/EJ1135837.pdf

Scott, S., McGuire, J. M., & Embry, P. (2002). *Universal design for instruction fact sheet*. Storrs, CT: University of Connecticut, Center on Postsecondary Education and Disability.

Scott, S. S., McGuire, J. M., & Shaw, S. F. (2001). *Principles of universal design for instruction*. Storrs, CT: University of Connecticut, Center on Postsecondary Education and Disability.

Sharby, N., Martire, K., & Iversen, M. D. (2015). Decreasing health disparities for people with disabilities through improved communication strategies and awareness. *International Journal of Environmental Research and Public Health*, *12*(3), 3301–3316. https://doi.org/10.3390/ijerph120303301 10.3390/ijerph120303301

Shaw, R. A. (2011). Employing universal design for instruction. *New Directions for Student Services*, *2011*(134), 21–33. https://doi.org/10.1002/ss.392

Smith, M. C. (1990). Nursing's unique focus on health promotion. *Nursing Science Quarterly*, *3*(1), 105–106. https://doi.org/10.1177/089431849000300304

Special Olympics. (2018). Retrieved from https://www.specialolympics.org

Stuck, A. E., Moser, A., Morf, U., Wirz, U., Wyser, J., Gillmann, G.,... Egger, M. (2015). Effect of health risk assessment and counselling on health behaviour and survival in older people: A pragmatic randomised trial. *PLoS Medicine*, *12*(10), e1001889. https://doi.org/10.1371/journal.pmed.1001889

Tao, X., Chow, S. K. Y., & Wong, F. K. Y. (2015). A nurse-led case management program on home exercise training for hemodialysis patients: A randomized controlled trial. *International Journal of Nursing Studies*, *52*(6), 1029–1041. https://doi.org/10.1016/j.ijnurstu.2015.03.013

Telecommunications Act. (1996). Pub. L. No. 104-104.

University of Washington. (2018). Do it: Disabilities, opportunities, internetworking, and technology. Retrieved from https://www.washington.edu/doit/equal-access-universal-design-instruction

U.S. Department of Health and Human Services. (2002). *Closing the gap: A national blueprint to improve the health of persons with mental retardation: Report of the Surgeon General's Conference on Health Disparities and Mental Retardation*. Washington, DC: U.S. Department of Health and Human Services, Office of the Surgeon General.

U.S. Department of Health and Human Services (2005). *The Surgeon General's call to action to improve the health and wellness of people with disabilities*. Washington, DC: U.S. Department of Health and Human Services, Office of the Surgeon General.

U.S. Department of Health and Human Services. (2018). *Healthy People 2020 health and disability objectives*. Retrieved from https://www.healthypeople.gov/2020/topics-objectives/topic/disability-and-health/objectives

U.S. Department of Health, Education, and Welfare. (1976). *Forward plan for health, FY 1978–82* (DHEW Publication No. OS 76-50046). Washington, DC: U.S. Public Health Service.

U.S. Department of Health, Education, and Welfare. (1979). *Healthy People: The Surgeon General's report on health promotion and disease prevention* (DHEW Publication No. 79-55071). Washington, DC: U.S. Government Printing Office.

van Schijndel-Speet, M., Evenhuis, H. M., van Wijck, R., van Montfort, K. C. A. G. M., & Echteld, M. A. (2017). A structured physical activity and fitness programme for older adults with intellectual disabilities: Results of a cluster-randomised clinical trial. *Journal of Intellectual Disability Research*, *61*(1), 16–29. https://doi.org/10.1111/jir.12267

Verhaeghe, N., Clays, E., Vereecken, C., De Maeseneer, J., Maes, L., Van Heeringen, C.,... Annemans, L. (2013). Health promotion in individuals with mental disorders: A cluster preference randomized controlled trial. *BMC Public Health*, *13*, 657. https://doi.org/10.1186/1471-2458-13-657

Whitehead, D. (2006). Health promotion in the practice setting: Findings from a review of clinical issues. *Worldviews on Evidence-Based Nursing*, *3*(4), 165–184. https://doi.org/10.1111/j.1741-6787.2006.00068.x

Whitehead, D. (2008). An international Delphi study examining health promotion and health education in nursing practice, education and policy. *Journal of Clinical Nursing*, *17*(7), 891–900. https://doi.org/10.1111/j.1365-2702.2007.02079.x

Williams, A. S., & Moore, S. M. (2011). Universal design of research: Inclusion of persons with disabilities in mainstream biomedical studies. *Science Translational Medicine*, *3*(82), 82cm12. https://doi.org/10.1126/scitranslmed.3002133

Williams, D. M. (1989). Political theory and individualistic health promotion. *Advances in Nursing Science*, *12*(1), 14–25.

World Health Organization. (1974). Constitution of the World Health Organization. *Chronicle of the World Health Organization*, *1*, 29–43.

World Health Organization. (1986). *Ottawa Charter for health promotion*. Ottawa, ON: Canadian Public Health Association & Health and Welfare Canada.

Young, L. E. (2002). Transforming health promotion practice: Moving towards holistic care. In L. E. Young & V. E. Hayes (Eds.), *Transforming health promotion practice: Concepts, issues, and applications, 3–21*. Philadelphia, PA: F. A. Davis.

Zidén, L., Häggblom-Kronlöf, G., Gustafsson, S., Lundin-Olsson, L., & Dahlin-Ivanoff, S. (2014). Physical function and fear of falling 2 years after the health-promoting randomized controlled trial: Elderly persons in the risk zone. *The Gerontologist*, *54*(3), 387–397. https://doi.org/10.1093/geront/gnt078

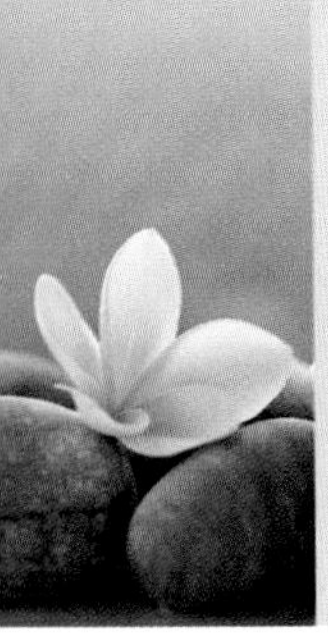

Chapter 19

Patients Experiencing Homelessness

April Bigelow and Chin Hwa (Gina) Yi Dahlem

LEARNING OBJECTIVES

After completing this chapter, the student will be able to:

1. Describe the federal definition of homelessness.
2. Discuss factors that affect health promotion in people experiencing homelessness.
3. Describe the impact of homelessness on health promotion.
4. Identify useful resources for health promotion in people experiencing homelessness.
5. Discuss strategies for practice in homeless populations.

INTRODUCTION

The relationship between homelessness and health is profound and complicated, underscoring the need for strong health promotion efforts in this population. Severe illness can lead to homelessness because of job loss and the high cost of health-care services, and lacking a stable home increases risk for certain diseases and conditions. The 2017 national estimate of homelessness in the United States identified 553,742 people. Between 2016 and 2017, the rate of homelessness increased nationally by 0.7%, with the largest increases among unaccompanied children and young adults. Thirty-four percent of those individuals lived in a place not meant for human habitation (street or abandoned building), while the majority of homeless lived in transitional housing. The overall homeless numbers are trending downward, but 20 states experienced increases in homelessness in 2017 (National Alliance to End Homelessness, 2018).

This issue is further complicated by the current health-care climate and the struggle of patients, especially those who are homeless, to obtain timely health care with a primary-care provider to ensure proper preventive measures and health promotion. Most homeless individuals receive disjointed, uncoordinated care from local emergency departments and urgent-care centers. Maintaining the health of all community members, including homelessness, is necessary to decrease the burden on our health-care systems.

This chapter will present the current federal definition of homelessness, discuss health promotion and homelessness across the life span, describe the relationship of being homeless to overall health, provide examples of specific epidemiology to people experiencing homelessness, and present gaps in the present literature and current guidelines. Finally, resources for health-care providers and recommendations for practice will be presented.

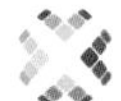

Case Illustration

Consider the case of Mr. S, a 53-year-old man who is in and out of housing. He was forced out of his job because of a history with alcoholism. He is currently experiencing homelessness. He has no income, is sleeping on the streets, and has no known past medical history or disease. He is a current smoker and consumes alcohol, both of which depend on the amount of money he is able to collect and earn doing odd jobs around town. He has no insurance, is not eligible for public assistance, and has not had a primary-care provider for over 10 years.

DEFINITION OF HOMELESSNESS

Homelessness is a complex social problem in the United States and around the world, and it is influenced by a variety of variables, policies, and cultures. In the United States, the federal definition of *homeless* changes as the rates of homelessness fluctuate over the years. Federal funding agencies also have an impact on the definition of homelessness. The U.S. Department of Housing and Urban Development (HUD) and the U.S. Department of Health and Human Services (USDHHS) have slightly different definitions of homelessness (National Healthcare for the Homeless Council, 2017).

In 2009, President Obama signed the Homeless Emergency and Rapid Transition to Housing (HEARTH) Act, reauthorizing prior language from the McKinney-Vento Homeless Act from 1987 (Oliva, 2011). Not only did the HEARTH Act consolidate the different programs for homeless assistance in the United States, but it also formally redefined homelessness into four categories: (1) individuals and families who lack regular or fixed nighttime housing; (2) individuals and families who are at high risk of losing their nighttime housing; (3) unaccompanied youth and families with children who defined as homeless elsewhere but do not meet the above two definitions; and (4) individuals and families that are attempting to flee violent situations including, but not limited to, domestic violence, sexual assault, stalking, or any life-threatening conditions (Oliva, 2011).

In practice, a variety of other terms may be used to describe people experiencing homelessness. Patients may be part of a "doubled-up" family in which two families share one home or residence, or they may be "precariously housed" or "transient," or "hard sleepers" who reside outdoors due to preference or no formal shelter options. While not official federal definitions, these terms may be used in practice to describe a patient's living situation.

HEALTH PROMOTION FOR HOMELESS PATIENTS ACROSS THE LIFE SPAN

Traditional health promotion often happens in the primary-care setting, through preventive health-care visits, or through community screening efforts. These methods provide limited access to people experiencing homelessness. Thus, traditional programs aimed at health promotion and health screenings need to be tailored to the patient's current situation, insurance status, and competing demands. Further complicating health promotion in the homeless population is the higher risk of being underinsured or uninsured. Most adults younger than age 65 are insured through programs offered through their employers, which is not the case for someone who is homeless and unemployed (Hellander & Bhargavan, 2012), placing a larger burden for health promotion on safety-net clinics, emergency departments, urgent-care centers, and the public health departments through community outreach.

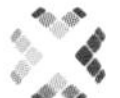

Case Illustration

Mr. S. obtains the majority of his health care through a local homeless shelter clinic, where he goes for most meals. At this clinic, he has been able to obtain blood pressure screening, depression screening, the influenza vaccine, and occasional medications and treatments for acute issues or concerns. Due to limited resources, however, the clinic has not been able to offer him access to more expensive, but recommended, age-appropriate screening such as colonoscopy or screening for abdominal aortic aneurysm.

In 2010, the Affordable Care Act (ACA) was signed in an attempt to fill the gaps in insurance coverage. The ACA increased the number of poor Americans who were eligible for Medicaid (Democrats.senate, 2017). While a number of provisions improve access to care for a variety of Americans, several provisions are particularly helpful for people experiencing homelessness. Most important, the ACA promotes the concept of prevention and offers reimbursement and incentives for wellness and public health programs at the local, state, and federal levels (Democrats.senate, 2017). In an effort to prevent and manage chronic disease, the ACA has identified several target areas:

1. Preventive obesity services that promote coverage for children and adults seeking to prevent or reduce obesity through screening programs, education programs, and research-based treatment strategies.
2. Tobacco cessation services for pregnant women, including counseling and pharmacologic interventions offered at no cost to the patient.
3. Prevention of chronic diseases programs offering incentives to patients of all ages when they identify a prevention goal and engage in an approved prevention program. (Democrats.senate, 2017)

The ACA not only shifted the focus of health care to preventive care and health promotion, but it also planned for expansion of community and home supports in an effort ultimately to improve overall access to health care. Strengthening existing centers, providing funding or subsidies for new community centers, and providing select services for patients with disabilities all improved access to health care for the most vulnerable and poor patients, including those experiencing homelessness. Finally, the ACA allowed individuals with preexisting conditions access to fair and quality insurance options (Centers for Medicare and Medicaid Services, 2017).

Ultimately, however, certain aspects of Medicaid expansion vary by state. Thus, a person experiencing homelessness in Michigan may have very different resources than one residing in Georgia. The full benefit of the ACA is also complicated by low health literacy rates, inability to apply for Medicaid expansion if available in the patients' area, and long waits to establish care and obtain screening with primary-care providers in some areas.

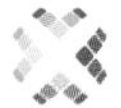

Case Illustration

Under the ACA, Mr. S was able to apply for Medicaid expansion through his state. Unfortunately, his assigned primary-care provider had a wait-list of 9 months for new patients. While waiting for an initial visit with his provider, Mr. S developed abdominal pain and noted he had blood in his stool. These concerning symptoms forced him to seek care in the local emergency department. While his visit was technically covered from a health insurance standpoint, his symptoms could have been prevented with access to routine screening and a primary-care provider.

While the future of the ACA is unclear, it has been successful in educating both the American people and providers about the importance of health promotion and disease prevention. In addition to specific allowances from ACA, federal and state funding exists for preventive care and health promotion for women and children. While the specifics of the program may vary from state to state, the Children's Health Insurance Program (CHIP) and the Women, Infants, and Children (WIC) program ensure that services, including education, vaccines, health care, specialty referrals, and preventive care, will be offered to children and pregnant or lactating women (United States Department of Agriculture [USDA], 2017). Currently, persons must qualify for Medicaid by meeting low-income criteria and predetermined criteria: children, pregnant women, parents of dependent children, seniors, and those with severe disabilities (USDA, 2017). Because of this, a homeless adult may not meet eligibility criteria and may not have access to affordable health care, further increasing his or her risk for preventable disease or illness.

Another aspect of health promotion focuses on lifestyle changes, such as increased physical activity, proper nutrition, and decreased use of alcohol and cigarettes to decrease risk for preventable disease. In the homeless population, however, it is difficult to talk to patients about increased fruit and vegetable intake when a food pantry, homeless shelter, or charity is providing meals. It is also difficult for health-care providers to prescribe specific amounts of daily physical activity to patients when they have many competing demands for their time. Due to transportation challenges, people experiencing homelessness often walk more than their housed counterparts. Although this amount of physical activity can be protective for some cardiovascular diseases, homeless people may be carrying large bags that strain joints and muscles.

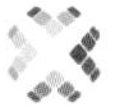

Case Illustration

After a brief hospital stay and resolution of his lower gastrointestinal bleed, Mr. S was released back to the streets of his community without stable housing. On his discharge instructions, he was told to consume more fruits and vegetables and to follow up with his primary-care provider. As he consumes his meals at the local church and homeless shelter, he is less able to increase produce intake as prescribed. And when he calls his provider for a follow-up visit, he still cannot be seen for some time because he has not officially established care with the office. Mr. S begins to worry if he is destined to be sick because of his homelessness.

Relationship of Homelessness to Overall Health

Just as complications from illness or disease can lead a person toward homelessness, homelessness itself is associated with an increased risk for communicable disease, chronic illness, and other preventable conditions. Lack of shelter, poor nutrition, inadequate hygiene, and no access to basic first aid complicate the health of the homeless at the most fundamental level. The lack of access to these basic elements is more complex when a patient has a chronic condition. In fact, even one chronic diagnosis in a person experiencing homelessness puts him or her at greater risk for morbidity and mortality than their housed counterparts (Maness & Kahn, 2014). People experiencing homelessness who also have complicated medical histories that require regular follow-up or uninterrupted treatment are at particular risk for devastating consequences (O'Connell, 2005).

While people experiencing homelessness tend to have the same medical conditions as the general population, they are at greater risk for specific diseases due to close living quarters, exposure to the elements, and access to recreational substances. Common diagnoses in people experiencing homelessness are (1) cardiovascular diseases such as hypertension, coronary artery disease, and hyperlipidemia; (2) dual diagnoses, meaning that a person has a mental illness in combination with a substance abuse disorder; (3) cognitive disorders and traumatic brain injury; and (4) illness related to injuries or violence (Maness & Kahn, 2014). Unfortunately, these common diagnoses are complicated by lack of timely treatment, inability to obtain pharmacologic intervention, and exposure to the risk factors listed above.

Although few deaths are directly linked to exposure illnesses, such as frostbite or hypothermia, the risk of death is significantly increased in those with a history of those conditions. Other factors that tend to complicate the health of homeless patients are sleep deprivation, risk of violence, and physical and emotional trauma (Maness & Kahn, 2014). Finally, limited access to screening, vaccinations, and community supports is a challenge to maintaining optimum health in the homeless population.

Case Illustration

While Mr. S is continuing to wait on his follow-up from his hospitalization and his initial visit to establish care with his provider, he continues to seek intermittent care at the local safety-net clinic. At one of his visits, his blood pressure is elevated, and Mr. S admits to an increase in stress related to concerns for safety while sleeping on the streets. He states that he has had thoughts of suicide and occasionally hears voices. This potential for violence coupled with a newly developing psychiatric illness and possible diagnosis of hypertension complicate his case. Seeing a care provider is now an urgent matter.

Challenges to Health Promotion in Homeless Patients

Unfortunately, many people experiencing homelessness have limited access or lack the tools to seek basic health care, including health promotion. Barriers to care have been identified as lack of knowledge of where to seek care, limited transportation, and inability to produce identification if asked (Nickasch & Marnocha, 2009). In addition to these physical barriers, people experiencing homelessness have expressed concerns over health literacy, limited ability to communicate with health-care providers, self-consciousness about hygiene and dress, and mistrust of the health-care system. The largest barrier to seeking timely appropriate health care was cost (Nickasch & Marnocha 2009).

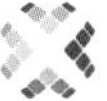

Case Illustration

After a consultation from the safety-net clinic provider, Mr. S's primary-care provider agrees to see him sooner. Mr. S expresses concern about the copayment cost and states that he is worried that he will be judged by the provider as well as the other patients in the waiting room. He has not been able to bathe in four days, is missing many teeth due to poor access to dental services, and needs to carry a large backpack of belongings with him. He worries that these factors will influence the type of care he receives and he expresses a desire to "just stay at the safety-net clinic."

Despite Medicaid expansion and the push for preventive services and health promotion, low health literacy plays a big role in use of the health-care system. Health literacy depends on both patient and provider factors, but it has a direct impact on a patient's ability to navigate the health-care system, engage in self-care management of disease and health, and understand risk regarding her or his health status (USDHHS, 2017b). Low health literacy and limited access to screening, vaccinations, and community supports are challenges to maintaining optimum health in the homeless population.

GAPS IN LITERATURE AND GUIDELINES

People experiencing homelessness have higher rates of chronic and mental health conditions, report far worse health status, and die 10-15 years earlier than the general population (Baggett et al., 2013; Fazel, Geddes, & Kushel, 2014; Gambatese et al., 2013). The unique contextual factors surrounding homelessness bring forth challenges to implementing, sustaining, and disseminating health promotion initiatives. For instance, the homeless population is a highly transient and heterogeneous group with varying needs. The health-care needs of a homeless adult male with substance abuse history sleeping on the streets of Los Angeles are different than those of homeless youth living in transitional housing in Michigan. Thus, health promotion initiatives need to be tailored with a wide range of health promotion strategies to meet the needs of the heterogeneous homeless population. In addition, the immediate needs for housing, warmth, and food often supersede health-care needs. People experiencing homelessness seek medical care in emergency departments at much higher rates than the general population (Niska, Bhulya, & Xu, 2010). Thus, disease prevention and screening, which is often provided in primary-care clinics for the general population, is not the standard for the homeless.

Nevertheless, we should not view these challenges as barriers to provision of health promotion but instead as special considerations that should be recognized in designing and conducting research. In fact, in a recent mixed-method review investigating community-based health and health promotion for the homeless, the authors found that the use of and having close relationships with case workers were of fundamental importance in encouraging the homeless to access health care and partake in health promotion activities (Coles, Themessl-Huber, & Freeman, 2012).

Intensive case management that includes provision of housing has improved mental health outcomes among homeless persons with substance abuse and HIV (Kirst, Zerger, Misir, Hwang, & Stergiopoulos, 2015; Whittaker & Burns, 2015). Another key element in engagement is to consider the contextual factors such as social determinants of health in designing interventions and allow those who are experiencing homelessness to set the health promotion priorities (Coles et al., 2012). Needs assessment of the community must be completed as a priority, with inputs from all parties involved, including those experiencing homelessness. Thus, adopting a tailored approach by involving homeless clients to define their health needs that are important to them, building trusting relationships through the use of case workers to increase interaction with health-care systems and professionals, and incorporating psychosocial and life circumstances when developing health promotion interventions are foundational elements to engage and sustain health promotion initiatives effectively for the homeless.

The U.S. Interagency Council on Housing (USICH) promotion of the Housing First model across homeless programs has resulted in substantial evidence on the effectiveness of permanent support housing. The Housing First approach urges federal, state, and local agencies to provide housing to people experiencing homelessness as quickly as possible and then provide additional service supports to maintain housing (USICH, 2010). Studies using the Housing First model have shown that participants had longer housing stability and lower supportive housing and service costs than the comparison group assigned to traditional programs, and higher utilization of supportive services by clients (USICH, 2010). The population that has benefitted most from permanent housing are those experiencing comorbid conditions such as substance abuse problems and serious mental illness.

Results indicate that provision of housing was significantly associated with greater length of drug abstinence, lower costs on use of public services, and longer housing tenure than those with no housing (Larimer et al., 2009; Whittaker & Burns, 2015). Specifically, abstinence-contingent housing was more effective on drug abstinence than non-abstinence-contingent housing. Overall, whether the housing is abstinence-contingent or not, research continues to show the beneficial effects of housing on lowering substance use, increasing the number of days abstinent, and reducing medical service use (Fitzpatrick-Lewis et al., 2011). Provision of housing also has an impact on HIV prevention and treatment by improving adherence to medications and reducing risky behaviors (Leaver, Bargh, Dunn, & Hwang, 2007). A gap in the available evidence is whether permanent supportive housing improves physical health outcomes across different subpopulations of people experiencing homelessness and if housing affects health-related perceptions and behaviors positively or negatively (Henwood et al., 2013). For instance, will housing influence health promotion behaviors and thus lead to healthier lifestyles choices and improved health, or will it lead to a more sedentary, isolated lifestyle?

Although significant advances have been made in homelessness research to inform policy and programming, more is needed to improve the overall health status and outcomes for people experiencing homelessness. In a rapid systematic review conducted by Fitzpatrick-Lewis et al. (2011) on the effectiveness of interventions to improve the health of the homeless, the authors recommend more methodological and rigorous studies of stronger quality in relationship to their study design and statistical analyses. Study designs must consider threats to external validity such as selection bias of clients included in the studies and increasing statistical power through adequate sample sizes (Fitzpatrick-Lewis et al., 2011). The transient nature of the homeless population continues to be a challenge when recruiting clients and conducting follow-ups.

Other knowledge gaps in homelessness research pertain to studies on specific subpopulations of the homeless, such as women, children, and families; the lesbian, gay, bisexual, transgender, and queer (LGBTQ+) community; and the elderly. In a review of the last 25 years, family homelessness has increased in prevalence, but there has been a paucity of research studies, public awareness, and government reports that have addressed family homelessness (Grant, Gracy, Goldsmith, Shapiro, & Redlener, 2013). Research aimed at effective screening and assessment, the relationship between housing subsidies and housing options on family outcomes, and the cost-effectiveness of integrated housing and service models need to be examined for homeless families (Bassuk, DeCandia, Tsertsvadze, & Richard, 2014).

Another subpopulation of homelessness that requires more attention is improving the care for the LGBTQ+ youth and adults who are homeless (Keuroghlian, Shtasel, & Bassuk, 2014). A disproportionate number of LGBTQ+ youth are homeless, comprising about 30% to 43% of clients being served in drop-in centers, street outreach programs, and housing programs (Durso & Gates, 2012). Research needs to examine the effects of social isolation and homelessness on mental health outcomes, develop interventions in reducing risks of chronic homelessness into adulthood for homeless youth, and assess how homelessness affects life milestones and options for the future for LBGTQ+ homeless youth (Keuroghlian, Shtasel, & Bassuk, 2014).

Homelessness varies between Europe and the United States. In Europe, the population is comprised of mostly women, families, migrants, and young people. In the United States, the homeless population has a median age of 50, leading to the need for increased management of chronic diseases and geriatric conditions such as cognitive, visual, and functional impairments; depression; frailty; and end-of-life issues (Christensen, 2015; Fazel, Geddes, & Kushel, 2014).Thus, research should investigate the effectiveness of integrated geriatric programs for the elderly experiencing homelessness, such as specialized integrated psychiatric clinics and the effect of permanent supportive housing on reducing medical costs and institutional care (Christensen, 2015; Kushel, 2012).

Among all homeless populations, research studies should focus on interventions on identification and management of infectious and chronic medical conditions such as HIV/AIDS, tuberculosis, skin disorders such as scabies/lice, podiatry care, hypertension/diabetes, traumatic brain injuries, and substance abuse treatments. Evidence-based practices are needed to manage effectively for co-occurring mental health and substance abuse disorders. Promising interventions integrating primary and behavioral care services with intensive case management and supportive housing need to be further evaluated in rigorous, randomized controlled trials.

Research should investigate how to tailor specific health promotion activities such as smoking cessation, weight loss management, exercise, nutrition, oral health, stress management, and foot care, and the provision of health maintenance services (e.g., vaccinations and preventive screening examinations). Researchers should be aware of the unique contextual factors surrounding homelessness when designing interventions such as access to basic physiological and safety needs, lack of access to health care, lack of transportation, and varying health literacy levels.

For instance, many people experiencing homelessness use local food banks and free meal programs, which limits their ability to make healthier choices and adhere to medical recommendations. Health promotion research should investigate the nutrient content of meals; identify low-cost, nutrient-dense meals that are easy to prepare; and examine the impact of these factors on health outcomes for the homeless. The delivery of health promotion education should be written at appropriate health literacy levels and be accompanied by practical assistance. For example, encouraging oral hygiene optimally should be delivered with provision of oral hygiene products such as toothpaste and toothbrushes. Practical provision of toiletries, clean socks, sunscreen, clothing, and shoes also facilitates health promotion behaviors. Many similar health promotion strategies apply to managing chronic illnesses; thus, effective, evidence-based programs such as the Stanford Chronic Disease Self-Management program should be implemented and tested for effectiveness for people experiencing homelessness.

Many clinical guidelines are available to guide providers in the care for specific diseases. Lack of current specific literature that is geared toward homelessness makes it difficult for clinicians and health-care providers to decipher and interpret guidelines for children, adults, and specific disease states. Providers may often feel overwhelmed because people experiencing homelessness tend to present with more advanced disease, competing demands, and/or limited resources. The patient, intervention, control, observation, and time (PICOT) statement below identifies a research question based on the discussion above.

PICOT Statement: Are patients experiencing homelessness at higher risk for lack of health promotion services than their stably housed counterparts?

P: homeless patients
I: health promotion services
C: stably housed patients
O: less health promotion activities
T: one calendar year

Refer to Table 19-1 for evidence addressing this question.

Table 19-1 Review of Evidence

What is your PICOT question? Are patients experiencing homelessness at higher risk for lack of health promotion services than their stably housed counterparts?

What database(s), years, and keywords will be searched? CINAHL: *Homeless*, *homelessness* and as keywords; limited to English and research

Citation*	Subjects	Method	Results	Rigor of Evidence	Applicable	Cost
Brown et al. (2015)	250 older homeless adults.	Prospective cohort study.	Those who obtained housing had improved depressive symptoms and reduced acute-care utilization compared with those who remained homeless.	High: Instruments with acceptable estimates of reliability and validity were used along with hospital records.	Yes.	Housing older adults may be especially cost-effective given higher morbidity in this age group. Costs not measured.
Palar et al. (2015)	346 people with HIV who were homeless or marginally housed for a median of 28 months.	Descriptive, based on quarterly assessments.	Severe food insecurity in the previous period was associated with increased depressive symptom severity ($b = 1.22$; $p = 0.001$)	High: Instruments had acceptable estimates of reliability and had been validated with homeless people.	Yes.	Policy options to address food insecurity were discussed. Costs not measured.
Wenzel et al. (2017)	421 homeless adults before they moved into public housing.	Qualitative.	Interviews show that homeless adults with HIV have significant risk for HIV transmission. Entering public housing is a period of transition and services that integrate HIV prevention services are needed to ensure the health of other residents.	Although qualitative research, the population ($n = 421$) was significant.	Yes.	Cost not addressed.
Kirst et al. (2015)	575 individuals placed in a Housing First program.	RCT.	After 24 months, participants in the Housing First program had significantly greater reductions in days with alcohol problems than did participants in a treatment-as-usual group.	High: Use of standardized measures of substance use problems.	Yes.	Costs not discussed.

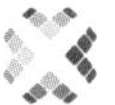

Case Illustration

After a long discussion with Mr. S, he agreed to be comanaged for a time by the safety-net clinic and his primary-care provider. A transition plan was put in place so that he would move all of his care to the primary-care provider within a few months. He was able to obtain treatment for his mental illness and begin medication for his elevated blood pressure (and be monitored at the safety-net clinic), and he was brought up to date on routine recommended screenings. Despite the many challenges of being homeless and having comorbid conditions and competing demands, Mr. S was able to work with his safety-net provider as an advocate to assist him in navigating the health-care system. He is now an established patient within the health-care system and is able to participate in routine screenings and prevention programs, despite his homelessness.

See Box 19-1 for a listing of Healthy People 2020 objectives related to those experiencing homelessness.

USEFUL RESOURCES ON HOMELESSNESS

Many resources are available for health-care providers who are working with homeless populations. One key organization is the National Health Care for the Homeless Council. This network of interdisciplinary professionals, advocates, and clients strives to eliminate homelessness through education, training, research, and political advocacy to secure housing and comprehensive health care for all. It is a comprehensive one-stop resource for service providers working with the homeless, including adapted practice guidelines and patient education materials. For those that are involved in academia, Caring with Compassion offers a formal, online, interactive curriculum for students and for providers working with the homeless (see Table 19-2). For health-care providers, screening for substance abuse, mental health, and trauma are key components of conducting a comprehensive assessment for those experiencing homelessness (see Table 19-3 for assessment tools).

BOX 19–1 Healthy People 2020 Objectives Related to Those Experiencing Homelessness

MHMD-12: Increase the proportion of homeless adults with mental health problems who receive mental health services.

AHS-1: Increase the proportion of persons with health insurance.

AHS-5: Increase the proportion of persons who have a specific source of ongoing care.

AHS-6: Reduce the proportion of persons who are unable to obtain or who experience a delay in obtaining necessary medical care, dental care, or prescription medicines.

Source: United States Department of Health and Human Services (2017a), Office of Disease Prevention and Health Promotion.

Table 19-2 Web Site Resources on Homelessness

Name	Description	Web Site
National Health Care for the Homeless Council (NHCHC)	Provides comprehensive clinical and advocacy resources to interdisciplinary professionals who are committed to eliminating homelessness.	https://www.nhchc.org/
Homelessness Resource Center	As a division of the Substance Abuse and Mental Health Administration, it provides a broad range of resources, best practices, and facts on homelessness.	http://homeless.samhsa.gov/

(*continued*)

Table 19-2 Web Site Resources on Homelessness—cont'd

Name	Description	Web Site
Caring with Compassion	Supports health-care professionals working with at-risk populations through online, interactive curriculum.	https://caringwithcompassion.org/
Homeless Resource Exchange	HUD provides federal resources on shelter, food, health care for service providers who are working with the homeless.	https://www.hudexchange.info/homelessness-assistance/
National Alliance to End Homelessness	Informs policy makers and elected officials on the latest data and research on preventing and ending homelessness.	http://www.endhomelessness.org/
Homeless Veterans	Help for veterans who are homeless.	http://va.gov/homeless/
National Center on Family Homelessness	Comprehensive resources for those working with families who are homeless.	http://www.familyhomelessness.org/
Family & Youth Services Bureau	Works with the National Clearinghouse on Families & Youth to support organizations and communities that are focused on youth homelessness, adolescent pregnancy, and domestic violence.	http://www.acf.hhs.gov/programs/fysb
National Coalition for the Homeless	Provides information on advocacy, projects, facts about homelessness.	http://nationalhomeless.org/

Table 19-3 Assessment Tools for Addressing Substance Abuse, Mental Health, and Trauma

Topic	Description	Web Site
Substance Abuse		
Drug Abuse Screening (DAST-10)	10-item brief screening tool of yes or no response to screen for drug use.	https://www.drugabuse.gov/sites/default/files/files/DAST-10.pdf
Alcohol Use Disorders Identification Test (AUDIT-10)	0-item screening tool for hazardous or harmful alcohol consumption. Shorter 3-item screening AUDIT-C is also available	https://www.drugabuse.gov/sites/default/files/files/AUDIT.pdf http://www.integration.samhsa.gov/images/res/tool_auditc.pdf
Tobacco Cessation	National Tobacco Cessation Collaborative provides a broad range of resources for smoking cessation and aids.	http://www.tobacco-cessation.org/resources/tools.html
Mental Health		
Patient Health Questionnaire (PHQ-9)	Most common screening tool to identify depression.	http://www.integration.samhsa.gov/images/res/MDQ.pdf

Table 19-3 Assessment Tools for Addressing Substance Abuse, Mental Health, and Trauma—cont'd

Topic	Description	Web Site
Mood Disorder Questionnaire (MDQ)	13-item screening for bipolar disorder.	http://www.integration.samhsa.gov/clinical-practice/GAD708.19.08Cartwright.pdf
Generalized Anxiety Disorder (GAD-7)	7-item screening tool for generalized anxiety disorder.	http://www.integration.samhsa.gov/images/res/SBQ.pdf
Suicide Behaviors Questionnaire	Screens for suicide-related thoughts and behaviors.	http://www.integration.samhsa.gov/clinical-practice/PC-PTSD.pdf
Trauma		
Primary Care Post-traumatic Stress Disorder Screen (PC-PTSD)	4-item screen for PTSD used for veterans.	http://www.integration.samhsa.gov/clinical-practice/SAMSA_TIP_Trauma.pdf
SAMHSA's TIP on Trauma-Informed Care in Behavioral Health Services	Comprehensive resource on screening and assessment tools for trauma.	http://www.getdomesticviolencehelp.com/hits-screening-tool.html
Domestic Violence Screening Tool	Hurt-Insult-Threaten-Scream (HITS) screens for risk of intimate partner violence.	https://www.nhchc.org/forms-hch-projects/
General Medical and Housing Assessment		
Sample Forms from Health Care for the Homeless Projects	Clinical practice examples of forms used to assess medical and mental health needs of the homeless for clinicians.	http://www.endhomelessness.org/library/entry/alliance-coordinated-assessment-tool-set
Comprehensive Assessment Tool	Helps organizations prioritize and assess housing needs for those experiencing homelessness.	https://nhchc.org/clinical-practice/homeless-services/assessment-intake/

RECOMMENDATIONS FOR PRACTICE

Working with people experiencing homelessness requires interpersonal skills including the ability to display compassion, respect, patience, and quality patient-provider communication. Trust is a key component of this patient-provider relationship. Many people experiencing homelessness have often been mistreated and misunderstood due to their social and personal life circumstances. As a result, they often have a deep-rooted feeling of mistrust with health-care systems and providers (Nickasch & Marnocha, 2009; Wen, Hudak, & Hwang, 2007). To overcome the mistrust, health-care systems and organizations who serve the homeless should consider adopting concepts of trauma-informed care (TIC) into their organizations. According to Hopper, Bassuk, and Olivet (2010), a consensus-based definition of TIC has been established: Trauma-Informed Care is a framework that is grounded in an understanding of and responsiveness to the impact of trauma. It incorperates physical, psychological, and emotional safety for providers and survivors, ultimately creating opportunities for survivors to rebuild a sense of control and empowerment. Specifically, health-care practice organizations that serve the homeless should assess the strengths and resources of all clients; screen for trauma histories; integrate substance abuse, mental health, and trauma services; avoid practices that may retraumatize the client; be culturally and linguistically competent; and involve clients in their own care (Hopper et al., 2010).

Health-care providers should be informed of federal, state, and local resources for people who are homeless. They should incorporate adapted clinical guidelines that are available through the National Health Care Council for the Homeless (www.nhchc.org) to better meet the needs of these clients. Clinics should utilize case management through trained peer advocates, supporters, or navigators to help clients who are homeless gain access and navigate through the complex healthcare system (Corrigan et al., 2017). Whether through peer supporters or the health-care team, *engaging* with the client is an essential component to developing quality patient-provider relationships.

Finally, collaboration between professionals across areas of the health-care spectrum is essential. Interdisciplinary team care utilizes expertise from different professions and settings to coordinate care for especially complex patients. The best model of care involves "an integrated, multidisciplinary approach by a team of health care personnel knowledgeable about the unique challenges faced by homeless persons, utilizing a patient-centered... model in association with outreach services at multiple sites with ready access to secondary/tertiary care, convalescent and respite care, community resources and local agencies for housing, employment, and legal assistance" (Mannes & Kahn, 2014, p. 638). Ensuring that team members have clear roles, demonstrate mutual respect and trust for other team members, and are effective communicators increases the likelihood of success. When the team works with people experiencing homelessness to create mutually shared goals and measurable processes and outcomes, they are more likely to be effective, and they are driving to improve health literacy and overall health as well.

KEY POINTS

- Homelessness is both a risk for and a result of chronic disease and poor health.
- Homelessness is a complex social problem that is influenced by social, medical, political, and cultural factors.
- Individuals and families who have no nighttime housing, are at high risk to lose nighttime housing, or attempting to flee violence meet the federal definition of homelessness.
- ACA expanded Medicaid services, increased eligibility, and shifted health focus to prevention and health promotion.
- Barriers to health promotion in people experiencing homelessness are lack of knowledge, limited transportation, lower health literacy, self-consciousness, mistrust of the health-care system and providers, and overall cost.
- Health promotion should be tailored to the needs of people experiencing homelessness and should incorporate their unique psychosocial and life circumstances.
- Permanent housing results in lower rates of substance use, better management of chronic illness, and reduced medical service use.
- Excellent interpersonal skills and trauma-informed care help to ensure a trusting patient-provider relationship.
- An integrated, multidisciplinary team approach utilizing the expertise of the team's members and working toward mutual goals with the patient increases the chance for successful outcomes in people experiencing homelessness.

Check Your Understanding

1. The nurse practitioner working with the person experiencing homelessness knows that:
   A. All homeless patients are substance users and seek care to obtain narcotic medications.
   B. Homeless patients often present with complex histories and competing demands.
   C. Homeless patients often require immediate psychiatric evaluation to determine competency.
   D. Homeless patients have the same rates of chronic disease as the general population.
2. Barriers to effective health promotion efforts in people experiencing homelessness have been identified as:
   A. Illiteracy, mistrust, substance use, and psychotic behavior
   B. Limited time, inability to navigate public transportation, and mistrust
   C. Low health literacy, limited transportation, and cost
   D. Low health literacy, history of incarceration, and mistrust of the health-care system
3. Qualities of effective multidisciplinary teams aimed at improved outcomes in people experiencing homelessness include all of the following EXCEPT:
   A. Effective communication
   B. Clear roles of team members
   C. Imposed goals upon the patient or other team members
   D. Measurable processes and outcomes
4. The nurse practitioner knows that health promotion interventions in people experiencing homelessness should:
   A. Incorporate the patient's unique psychosocial and life circumstances

B. Be based on extensive research in the homeless population
C. Address the underlying cause of the homelessness prior to intervention
D. Be addressed at later visits when the patient is more likely to have established housing

5. Challenges to research and development of health promotion guidelines in the homeless are related to:
   A. Multiple comorbid conditions that make it difficult to utilize homeless subjects
   B. The fact that people are often unreliable and lost to follow-up
   C. The inability to recruit participants who are sober
   D. Threats to external validity and the transient nature of the homeless population

See "Reflections on Check Your Understanding" at the end of the book for answers.

REFERENCES

Baggett, T. P., Hwang, S. W., O'Connell, J. J., Porneala, B. C., Stringfellow, E. J., Orav, E. J.,... Rigotti, N. A. (2013). Mortality among homeless adults in Boston: Shifts in causes of death over a 15-year period. *JAMA Internal Medicine*, *173*(3), 189–195.

Bassuk, E. L., DeCandia, C. J., Tsertsvadze, A., & Richard, M. K. (2014). The effectiveness of housing interventions and housing and service interventions on ending family homelessness: A systematic review. *American Journal of Orthopsychiatry*, *84*(5), 457–474.

Brown, R. T., Yinghui, M., Mitchell, S. L., Bharel, M., Patel, M., Ard, K. L.,... Steinman, M. A. (2015). Health outcomes of obtaining housing among older homeless adults. *American Journal of Public Health*, *105*(7), 1482–1488. doi:10.2105/AJPH.2014.302539

Centers for Medicare and Medicaid Services. Pre Existing Condition Insurance Plan (2017). Retrieved from https://www.cms.gov/CCIIO/Programs-and-Initiatives/Insurance-Programs/Pre-Existing-Condition-Insurance-Plan.html

Christensen, R. C. (2015). Caring for the invisible and the forgotten. *Pharos*, (2015). 49.

Coles, E., Themessl-Huber, M., & Freeman, R. (2012). Investigating community-based health and health promotion for homeless people: A mixed methods review. *Health Eeducation Research*, *27*(4), 624–644.

Corrigan, P. W., Kraus, D. J., Pickett, S. A., Schmidt, A., Stellon, E., Hantke, E., & Lara, J. L. (2017). Using peer navigators to address the integrated health care needs of homeless African Americans with serious mental illness. *Psychiatric Services*, *68*(3), 264–270.

Democrats. senate (2017). The Patient Protection and Affordable Care Act: Detailed summary. Retrieved from https://www.dpc.senate.gov/healthreformbill/healthbill04.pdf

Durso, L. E, & Gates, G. J. (2012). Serving Our Youth: Findings from a National Survey of Services Providers Working with Lesbian, Gay, Bisexual and Transgender Youth Who Are Homeless or At Risk of Becoming Homeless. *UCLA: The Williams Institute*. Retrieved from https://escholarship.org/uc/item/80x75033

Fazel, S., Geddes, J. R., & Kushel, M. (2014). The health of homeless people in high-income countries: Descriptive epidemiology, health consequences, and clinical and policy recommendations. *The Lancet*, *384*(9953), 1529–1540.

Fitzpatrick-Lewis, D., Ganann, R., Krishnaratne, S., Ciliska, D., Kouyoumdjian, F., & Hwang, S. W. (2011). Effectiveness of interventions to improve the health and housing status of homeless people: A rapid systematic review. *BMC Public Health*, *11*(1), 638.

Gambatese, M., Marder, D., Begier, E., Gutkovich, A., Mos, R., Griffin, A.,... Madsen, A. (2013). Programmatic impact of 5 years of mortality surveillance of New York City homeless populations. *American Journal of Public Health*, *103*(S2), S193–S198.

Grant, R., Gracy, D., Goldsmith, G., Shapiro, A., & Redlener, I. E. (2013). Twenty-five years of child and family homelessness: Where are we now? *American Journal of Public Health*, *103*(S2), e1–e10.

Hellander, I., & Bhargavan, R. (2012). Report from the United States: The U.S. health crisis deepens amid rising inequality—A review of data, fall 2011. *International Journal of Health Services*, *42*(2), 161–175.

Henwood, B. F., Hsu, H. T., Dent, D., Winetrobe, H., Carranza, A., & Wenzel, S. (2013). Transitioning from homelessness: A "fresh-start" event. *Journal of the Society for Social Work and Research*, *4*(1), 47–57.

Hopper, E. K., Bassuk, E. L., & Olivet, J. (2010). Shelter from the storm: Trauma-informed care in homelessness services settings. *The Open Health Services and Policy Journal*, *3*(2), 80–100.

Keuroghlian, A. S., Shtasel, D., & Bassuk, E. L. (2014). Out on the street: A public health and policy agenda for lesbian, gay, bisexual, and transgender youth who are homeless. *American Journal of Orthopsychiatry*, *84*(1), 66.

Kirst, M., Zerger, S., Misir, V., Hwang, S., & Stergiopoulos, V. (2015). The impact of a Housing First randomized controlled trial on substance use problems among homeless individuals with mental illness. *Drug and Alcohol Dependence*, *146*, 24–29.

Kushel, M. (2012). Older homeless adults: Can we do more? *Journal of General Internal Medicine*, *27*(1), 5–6.

Larimer, M. E., Malone, D. K., Garner, M. D., Atkins, D. C., Burlingham, B., Lonczak, H. S.,... Marlatt, G. A. (2009). Health care and public service use and costs before and after provision of housing for chronically homeless persons with severe alcohol problems. *JAMA*, *301*(13), 1349–1357.

Leaver, C. A., Bargh, G., Dunn, J. R., & Hwang, S. W. (2007). The effects of housing status on health-related outcomes in people living with HIV: A systematic review of the literature. *AIDS and Behavior*, *11*(2), 85–100.

Maness, D. L., & Khan, M. (2014). Care of the homeless: An overview. *American Family Physician*, *89*(8).

National Healthcare for the Homeless Council. (2017). Retrieved from https://www.nhchc.org/faq/official-definition-homelessness/

National Alliance to End Homelessness. (2018). *State of homelessness*. Retrieved from https://endhomelessness.org/homelessness-in-america/homelessness-statistics/state-of-homelessness-report/

Nickasch, B., & Marnocha, S. K. (2009). Healthcare experiences of the homeless. *Journal of the American Association of Nurse Practitioners*, *21*(1), 39–46.

Niska, R., Bhuiya, F., & Xu, J. (2010). National Hospital Ambulatory Medical Care Survey: 2007 emergency department summary. *National Health Statistics Report*, *26*(26), 1–31.

O'Connell, J. J. (2005). Premature mortality in homeless populations: A review of the literature. Nashville, TN: National Health Care for the Homeless Council.

Oliva, M. (2011). HEARTH Act. Federal Register, 76(233), Washington, DC: US Government Printing Office.

Palar, K., Kushel, M., Frongillo, E., Riley, E., Grede, N., Bangsberg, D., & Weiser, S. (2015). Food insecurity is longitudinally associated with depressive symptoms among homeless and marginally-housed individuals living with HIV. *AIDS & Behavior*, *19*(8), 1527–1534. doi:10.1007/s10461-014-0922-9

Substance Abuse and Mental Health Services Administration. (2018). *Key substance use and mental health indicators in the United States: Results from the 2017 National Survey on Drug Use and Health* (HHS Publication No. SMA 18-5068, NSDUH Series H-53). Rockville, MD: Center for Behavioral Health Statistics and Quality, Substance Abuse and Mental Health Services Administration. Retrieved from https://www.samhsa.gov/data/United States Department of Agriculture. (2017). Special Supplemental Nutrition Program for Women, Infants, and Children Fact Sheet. Retrieved from https://www.fns.usda.gov/fns-101-wicU.S, Department of Health and Human Services. (2017a). *Access to health services.* Office of Disease Prevention and Health Promotion. Retrieved from https://www.healthypeople.gov/node/3495/objectives#3965

United States Interagency Council on Homelessness (2010). Opening Doors: Federal strategic plan to prevent and end homelessness. Retrieved from https://www.usich.gov/resources/uploads/asset_library/Opening%20Doors%202010%20FINAL%20FSP%20Prevent%20End%20Homeless.pdf

U.S. Department of Health and Human Services. (2017b). Health literacy basics. Retrieved from https://health.gov/communication/literacy/quickguide/factsbasic.htm

Wen, C. K., Hudak, P. L., & Hwang, S. W. (2007). Homeless people's perceptions of welcomeness and unwelcomeness in healthcare encounters. *Journal of General Internal Medicine*, *22*(7), 1011–1017.

Wenzel, S. L., Rhoades, H., Harris, T., Winetrobe, H., Rice, E., Henwood, B. (2017). Risk behavior and access to HIV/AIDS prevention services in a community sample of homeless persons entering permanent supportive housing. *AIDS Care*. 2017;29(5):570–574. doi:10.1080/09540121.2016.1234690

Whittaker, E & Burns, L. (2015). Stable housing, stable substance use? Evaluation of two 'Housing First' programs for homeless individuals. *Drug and Alcohol Dependence, 156: e239.* DOI: 10.1016/j.drugalcdep.2015.07.643

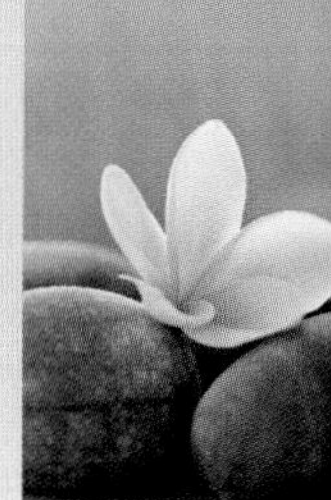

Chapter 20

Health Promotion for Patients Who Are Lesbian, Gay, Bisexual, Transgender, or Queer

Michele J. Eliason

LEARNING OBJECTIVES

After completing this chapter, the student will be able to:

1. Define terms related to sexual orientation and gender identity.
2. Explain the process by which stigma causes or contributes to health problems.
3. Describe the most common health problems associated with the LGBTQ+ stigma.
4. Apply cultural humility as a framework for working with LGBTQ+ patients.
5. Identify five action steps that will improve the quality of care of LGBTQ+ patients and their families.
6. Identify resources that will foster continued education about LGBTQ+ health issues.

INTRODUCTION

Individuals and families with lesbian, gay, bisexual, transgender, queer/questioning plus other less commonly used sexual/gender minority identifications (LGBTQ+) often face barriers to health-care access. Only recently have LGBTQ+ people been recognized as having unique health disparities because the major health surveillance instruments previously excluded questions about sexual orientation and gender identity. In the 2020 version of Healthy People, LGBTQ+ health disparity reduction goals were outlined for the first time. Societal stigma has created a climate of hostility, ignorance, and/or invisibility for LGBTQ+ people. Even in the absence of blatant discrimination or violence, LGBTQ+ people encounter multiple daily instances of verbal snubs and insults called microaggressions. Some of the most devastating are the microaggressions that occur in health-care settings and from health-care providers, including behaviors and language that erases, trivializes, or stereotypes people based on their sexual/gender identities (Eliason & Dibble, 2015).

This chapter begins with a brief history, followed by basic terminology for nurses, a summary of the most common health disparities of LGBTQ+ populations, a critique of the literature on health-care quality for LGBTQ+ clients, and recommendations for nursing practice grounded in the concept of cultural humility. The acronym LGBTQ+ is used as shorthand, but readers should keep in mind that not all people use the terms that these letters stand for and that each term in the acronym represents a subgroup with unique characteristics. This chapter focuses primarily on the shared experiences of stigma that create conditions of stress for these populations.

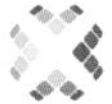

Case Illustration

Kari is a 42-year-old white woman and her partner Jan is a 37-year-old Latina woman. They have been together for 14 years, but they were only able to marry in the summer of 2015 when the Supreme Court ruling made same-sex marriage legal in all states of the United States. Although they are both female-identified now, Kari was born and raised as male. She always felt different and began transitioning to a female role and appearance in young adulthood. She has had several surgeries to alter her physical body to align with her gender identity. She met Jan, who was born female and has always been comfortable in her female body, at a bisexual women's support group. They both identify as bisexual. They have two children, ages 10 and 7. Jan was inseminated with sperm that Kari banked prior to surgery 18 years ago. In effect, Kari is both mother and father to her children. Kari works as a radiology technician but is not "out" about her gender, sexual orientation, or relationship at the Catholic hospital where she works. For about 10 years, Kari identified as transgender, but for the past 10, she just thinks of herself as female, so she rarely shares her history with others. Jan is an accountant in a large firm, and she is out only to close friends there. Recently, Jan was diagnosed with multiple sclerosis, putting the family into more frequent contact with health-care systems and providers.

NURSE KNOWLEDGE ABOUT LGBTQ+ ISSUES

What do nurses know about LGBTQ+ issues? What information comes from nursing education? The answer to both questions is: very little. A recent study of more than 1,200 nurse educators' knowledge of LGBTQ+ issues and experience teaching about LGBTQ+ health revealed 43% had limited knowledge of LGBTQ+ health issues, 70% had never or seldom read anything related to LGBTQ+ health in their professional journals, and 80% said that faculty meetings or committees they attended never mentioned LGBTQ+ topics for the curriculum. When asked how much time in the curriculum was devoted to LGBTQ+ health, the mean was two hours (range of 0 to 10 hours), with 17% reporting none at all (Lim, Johnson, & Eliason, 2015).

This lack of LGBTQ+ knowledge in nursing education extends to nursing practice. A study by Carabez et al. (2015) of practicing nurses found an astounding lack of knowledge of terminology as well as lack of knowledge of LGBTQ+ health concerns. Some thought that the main health problem for all LGBTQ+ people was HIV, and others had no idea what the health problems were. For these clients, health-care experiences can be stressful when nurses rely on stereotypes or do not consider health concerns specific to the LGBTQ+ population (Rondahl, Innala, & Carlsson, 2006; Rounds, McGrath, & Walsh, 2013). For example, a nurse may assume that same-sex partners are friends or siblings. The gaps in knowledge are even greater for transgender health issues, with nurses reporting many misconceptions, a lot of confusion, and uncertainty about how to care for transgender clients (Carabez, Eliason, & Martinson, 2016).

LGBTQ+ nurses also report many challenges in the workplace, with some not feeling safe to disclose to coworkers and others experiencing awkward, uncomfortable, or overtly discriminatory behaviors in the workplace (Eliason, DeJoseph, Dibble, Deevey, & Chinn, 2011). Nursing has trailed other health-care professions in conducting research on LGBTQ+ client-care issues, adding LGBTQ+ content to the curriculum, and addressing LGBTQ+ issues in professional advocacy organizations (Eliason, Dibble, & DeJoseph, 2010).

HISTORICAL OVERVIEW

Grouping people based on their sexuality or gender identity is a relatively new phenomenon and has its roots in the classification systems developed by the early sexologists in the late 1800s. Of course, people had same-sex experiences and expressed gender differently prior to this, but these were considered behaviors rather than defining characteristics. The new labeling of sexual and gender identities had both positive and negative consequences. People banded together and formed supportive communities based on the shared identity. LGBTQ+ culture arose because of the shared identity and the need for support to survive the stigma. This culture spawned a wide variety of cultural institutions and support systems, from bars to bookstores, to community nonprofit agencies, as well as creative productions such as art, theater, music, and books. However, LGBTQ+ people were also stigmatized as sinners by many religions, as sick by the psychiatric institutions of medicine, and as criminals in the legal system by laws prohibiting same-sex behaviors.

The Diagnostic and Statistical Manual of Mental Disorders included homosexuality as a diagnostic category in its first issue in 1952, but it was removed in 1973 after activists forced the psychiatric community to reexamine the research on sexual orientation and mental health. Gender identity disorder was added as a diagnosis in 1980. Changing societal attitudes in the 1970s that resulted from the social liberation movements of the 1960s started to improve attitudes, and from the experiences of civil rights movements, antiwar protests, and women's liberation, the "gay liberation" movement was born.

The onset of the HIV/AIDS epidemic in the early to mid-1980s created some backlash against the progress made in the 1970s, but it also led to a new emphasis on health within LGBTQ+ communities. At the time of this writing, at least in the United States and Canada, laws that had criminalized adult consensual same-sex behavior have been eradicated. In June 2015, the U.S. Supreme Court legalized same-sex marriage and in June of 2020, banned employment discrimination on the basis of sexual orientation and gender identity. On the other hand, in October 2017, a draconian religious freedom bill was implemented in Mississippi that allows health-care providers to refuse care to LGBTQ+ people on the basis of their religious beliefs (among many other forms of discrimination). In addition, many states still allow discrimination in housing and public services. Updated information about these laws and policies is available from the National LGBTQ Task Force.

Many religions have changed their doctrines to become welcoming and inclusive of LGBTQ+ people, and some even ordain openly LGBTQ+ ministers; however, many still preach a message of exclusion or even hatred. Even less progress has been made in full inclusion of transgender people, who are still exposed to high levels of harassment, discrimination, and violence. LGBTQ+ people still routinely face family rejection, employment discrimination, religious condemnation, bullying, and other forms of invalidation and harassment. The chronic levels of everyday stress affect the health of LGBTQ+ people in myriad ways, which are outlined in a later section of this chapter.

Before reviewing health outcomes and issues, understanding the ever-evolving terminology about sexuality and gender is necessary. The definitions are drawn from Eliason and Chinn (2015) unless otherwise noted.

LGBTQ+ TERMINOLOGY

Oppressed minority groups commonly develop their own language to describe their experiences, sometimes in reaction to the terms that were coined by oppressive systems (for example, terms developed by psychiatry such as *homosexuality* and *transsexual*). This language can be specific to communities based on geographic location, age, race/ethnicity, country of origin, and many other factors. This section reviews terminology drawn from the research literature, not slang or highly specific terms to one subgroup. Nevertheless, nurses who work with many LGBTQ+ people should learn the local slang and common language of the specific populations they serve.

The language reviewed in this chapter is divided into three sections based on sexual orientation, gender, and stigma. Sometimes people are accused of being "too sensitive," but many clients feel offended if nurses use language that is offensive to one's religion or to one's ethnicity. Words have great power to hurt or to include and heal; words matter to LGBTQ+ people as much as to other subgroups of the general population.

Sexual Orientation

Sexual orientation refers to patterns of attraction, behavior, and identity related to one's preferred sexual and romantic partners. Some research finds that sexual orientation is relatively fixed and stable for most people, although efforts to find a "gay gene" or biological marker have not been successful. Most people report recognizing that they were different from an early age, lending support to theories that sexual orientation may have a biological underpinning. Lisa Diamond (2009) described the "FBI" of sexual orientation, including three components of fantasy, behavior, and identity:

- Fantasy (attraction): Some people are attracted to those of the same sex but may not act on these feelings. They may endorse categories on research surveys like "not completely heterosexual." This category includes people who are early in their coming-out process and may eventually identify as LGB+, or they may always consider themselves as entirely heterosexual. A large portion of the population has experienced a same-sex attraction at some time in their lives.
- Behavior (same-sex experiences): A significant number of people may experiment with their sexuality and have one, a few, or even many same-sex experiences in their lifetimes, but they do not identify as lesbian, gay, or bisexual.
- Identity (self-labeling): A smaller number of people who have consistent same-sex attractions and behaviors declare themselves to be lesbian, gay, bisexual (or queer, fluid, or another preferred term). Recent studies suggest that between 3% and 4% of the U.S. population labels themselves as lesbian, gay, or bisexual (Gates & Newport, 2012).

Sexual Preference

Often used by opponents of LGBTQ+ rights, the term *sexual preference* suggests that sexuality is a choice and can be changed. Proponents of this term may suggest that LGBTQ+ individuals should make different choices about partners or receive reparative or conversion therapies to change their sexuality to heterosexual. All respected professional associations in the western world have denounced reparative therapies not only as ineffective but also as potentially harmful; examples include the American Psychiatric Association, the American Psychological Association, the National Association of Social Workers, and the American Academy of Nursing's LGBTQ Expert Panel.

Nurses should avoid using the term *sexual preference.*

Sexual Identity

This neutral term indicates an individual's preferred self-identification, similar to other personal self-identifications such as terms related to gender, racial, ethnic, national origin, and religious or spiritual identity. This term is acceptable and widely used. Whether nurses use *sexual orientation* or *sexual identity*, they should understand that these labels indicate only the type of person an individual is attracted to and not preferred sexual behavior or number of partners. Some of the most common terms used to describe specific sexual identities include:

- *Lesbian:* women who are attracted to other women
- *Gay:* men who are attracted to other men
- *Bisexual:* people who are attracted to both men and women
- *Asexual:* people who experience romantic and emotional attachments to others but who have little or no sexual desire
- *Queer:* preferred term by some, meaning not completely heterosexual. It is used as an umbrella term for LGBTQ+. Nurses should not use the term *queer* to refer to individuals unless they work closely with LGBTQ+ populations where the term is widely used.

Nurses can determine the information they need about a client's sexuality depending on the context of the clinical encounter. If the setting addresses sexually transmitted infections (STIs), then it is critical to ask about sexual behavior. If the client will be involved in ongoing care, then identities and relationships are important to know.

Terms Related to Sex and Gender

Sex can refer to the behaviors that lead to reproduction, pleasure, or intimacy and also to the biological differences that we label as male and female. This chapter discusses the second definition. Many scientists have tried to sort out the effects of the small genetic and anatomical differences between men and women and the differences created by socialization. There seem to be very few truly biological differences because genetic codes are nearly identical, with the exception of a handful of genes that govern genital development and hormones (Jordan-Young, 2010).

Nearly 3% of the population is born with a genetic or other biological difference that puts their bodies somewhere between the categories of male and female, and many with no identifiable genetic difference have a naturally more androgynous body type (Mouriquand, Caldamone, Malone, Frank, & Hoebeke, 2014). Those with genetic and biological differences may be diagnosed with a disorder of sexual development (DSD) or an intersex condition. Examples include genetic differences such as Klinefelter's syndrome and hormonal differences related to congenital adrenal hyperplasia and androgen insufficiency syndrome. These conditions can sometimes be identified at birth, when they cause ambiguous genitalia.

Differences in sexual development can create a crisis at the time of birth, not because they are life-threatening conditions or carry serious health risks but because no one can say clearly, "It's a girl," or "It's a boy." Usually a rush occurs to find treatments to make the baby more clearly female or male, but advocates for people with intersex or DSD differences urge parents and medical professionals to slow down, let the child develop, and make decisions when the child is old enough to have a say in their own care (Diamond & Garland, 2013).

Nurses can model acceptance, openness, and compassion for the child with DSD and encourage parents not to feel shame or guilt or try to hide their child's differences from others. Most DSD differences are not life-threatening, so there is no need for families to make a treatment decision before they have had time to consider all options. There are too many diverse causes of DSD to make any reliable recommendations for health-care needs, so each case must be taken as a unique combination of medical condition, family reactions, and child needs.

Gender refers to an individual's psychological interpretation of his or her biological sex, and *gender identity* describes a person's sense of how well he or she fits the cultural categories of male or female. *Cisgender* is a relatively new term used to describe people whose current gender is consistent with their sex assigned at birth; for example, a person who was assigned a female sex at birth and now identifies as a woman may be called a ciswoman (Schilt & Westbrook, 2009).

The term *transgender* refers to people who currently have a gender identity that is not consistent with their sex assigned at birth and who identify using terms such as *transgender*, *gender queer*, *gender nonconforming*, or *gender nonbinary*. *Gender identity* and *sexual orientation* are independent terms, and people on the transgender spectrum can be of any sexual orientation. Some experience a change in their sexual identity after they transition. Transgender women are assigned male at birth and transition to a female identity; transgender men are assigned female at birth and transition to a male identity. *Transsexual* is an outdated term created by the medical profession to label people who seek to change their sex through hormonal and surgical means, and some older people may still use that term as a self-identification.

The term *transition* refers to the many possible processes and procedures that a person may choose to undergo to align their physical bodies and psychological gender. A person changing from male to female may have genital surgery to remove the penis and create a vaginal opening (vaginoplasty); cosmetic surgeries to feminize the body, such as removal of the Adam's apple and breast implants; hormone therapy to block testosterone and introduce more estrogen; electrolysis to remove facial hair; speech therapy to change the timbre of the voice; and counseling/guidance on female behavior patterns of communicating, walking, sitting, dressing, and accessorizing. A person changing from female to male may have genital surgery to create a penis (phalloplasty), breast reduction or removal, and hormone therapy to increase testosterone. Testosterone lowers the voice and increases facial hair, so speech therapy and other therapies might not be necessary. Some people who identify on the transgender spectrum are not interested in any medical or surgical treatments.

Individuals on the transgender spectrum often experience legal and social issues related to changing their names and gender identifications on legal documents such as driver's licenses, Social Security records, and health records. This process can be time-consuming and expensive. Each state has different laws about the process of changing sex, although name changes are relatively easy, and the process is similar in most places. Some states require that the person have completed genital surgeries before changing their sex on official records, putting some people in an awkward position of having an official sexual identity that is inconsistent with their appearance. This discrepancy may increase the risk for harassment and violence and prevent individuals from being recognized by their chosen names and pronouns. As a sign of respect, nurses should always use their clients' chosen names and pronouns regardless of the gender stated on their legal documents.

Social issues related to transition include the challenges of disclosing one's gender identity to family, friends, coworkers and health-care providers. The deep-seated stigma against transgender people has led to high rates of unemployment, housing, and discrimination, and contributes to high rates of violence against people who are gender nonconforming.

Terminology Related to Stigma

In the 1970s, a psychologist-coined term, *homophobia*, started to catch on because it put the blame on people with negative attitudes about lesbian and gay people rather than on LGBTQ+ people themselves for societal attitudes. Similar terms were created to describe attitudes about bisexual people (*biphobia*) and transgender people (*transphobia*). Technically, the attitudes about LGBTQ+ people rarely fit the definition for a phobia (a powerful irrational fear that creates a physiological response of fight or flight). Often the negative attitudes are not fear-based but come from anger or strongly held prejudices that are based in ignorance or hatred. But these terms are still found in the research literature as well as in the media and popular press.

Heterosexism/Heteronormativity

The terms *heterosexism* and *heteronormativity*, technically more accurate than *homophobia*, refer to institutionalized oppression based on the assumption that heterosexuality is the only normal option for human relationships. This assumption is imbedded in all systems of society, from medicine to education, to law, and much of it stems from fundamentalist religious beliefs (Clarke, Ellis, Peel, & Riggs, 2010).

Gender Normativity

The term *gender normativity* refers to the myth that each person is born as either a man or a woman and that sex is biologically fixed at birth. Gender stereotypes severely restrict the behaviors and appearance of individuals and force conformity to the gender norm. In many communities, individuals who deviate from assigned birth sex and/or the associated gender stereotypes may risk rejection, bullying, harassment, discrimination, and even violence. Gender normativity is built into all the systems and structures of society, although the nuances vary across cultures.

Revealing Identities

Two terms are used to refer to the processes of adopting and sharing information about one's sexual and gender identities. *Coming out* refers to a lifelong process of self-acknowledgment; acceptance; and adopting of labels such as *lesbian*, *gay*, *bisexual*, or *transgender*. The step of revealing to others is called disclosure in the research literature, and there is a small body of knowledge about disclosure to health-care providers. This disclosure can be challenging when providers never ask the question about sexual and gender identity. An LGBTQ+ person must find the right opening in the interaction to disclose, and this can be stressful and challenging. Some people may choose not to disclose because of fears of being treated poorly by health-care providers (Durso & Meyer, 2012). Nurses can create the opening for LGBTQ+ clients to disclose by asking questions about sexual and gender identities, and modeling inclusive language, which takes much stress off the client.

Minority Stress

This theory stems from the study of people of color and proposes that minority status subjects individuals to an additional load of stress above and beyond the stressors of daily life related to finances, health, relationships/family, work, and others. Minority stress operates through two processes: external and internal. The external sources of discrimination stem from actual or perceived bullying; family rejection; work discrimination; harassment in public spaces; rejection by religious or spiritual groups; hateful political campaigns; and many events that threaten the life, livelihood, or well-being of the individual. Internalized stigma occurs when individuals believe the negative stereotypes about the groups with whom they identify; it results in a sense of shame, guilt, doubt, and/or self-hatred (Meyer, 2013).

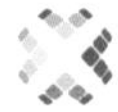

Case Illustration

Jan was raised Catholic, and in her adolescence and early adult years, she experienced intense feelings of shame and guilt over her attractions to women. When she came out as bisexual, she was afraid she would have to give up religion, but she found a welcoming and inclusive religious community in her city that helped her with self-acceptance.

Microaggressions

As negative attitudes about the LGBTQ+ community have become less overt, some authors suggest that many of these individuals still experience common microaggressions, which are described as less hostile and subtle forms of discrimination and invalidation. For example, even well-intentioned people might behave or respond according to stereotypes or dismiss concerns of LGBTQ+ people as invalid, such as saying that there is no more anti-LGBTQ+ sentiment because same-sex couples can marry in many states. Microaggressions tend to render LGBTQ+ people and issues invisible or see demands for LGBTQ+ civil rights as trivial or as wanting "special treatment" (Nadal, 2013). Because microaggressions are far more common than more overt types of discrimination, nurses need to be aware of them to avoid enacting them in health-care settings (Eliason & Dibble, 2015).

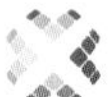

Case Illustration

Kari and Jan's 10-year-old daughter, Maya, had a parent's day at school. The teacher made Maya decide which parent should sit at the "mothers" table and which one should sit at the "fathers" table. This request made everyone uncomfortable. It was not overt discrimination or harassment, but it was a microaggression that followed the stereotype that one member of a same-sex couple must play the male role and one the female role.

HEALTH DISPARITIES AMONG LGBTQ+ POPULATIONS

Figure 20–1 shows the relationship between stigma, the two components of minority stress (external sources of discrimination and internalized stigma), stress, and illness. This model draws from decades of research on the impact of stress on health. Frequent stress reactions result in damage to organ systems and increase vulnerability to illness, injury, and disease. Chronic stress can lead to hypervigilance, a condition in which the body is constantly on high alert. The individual may feel overwhelmed, helpless, or traumatized. In the case of LGBTQ+ people, stress can begin before coming out and persist throughout life because of the uncertainty of the attitudes of nearly every new person they meet. It is impossible to know if each person will be accepting, tolerant, rejecting, or even violent, and that uncertainty is stressful. Stress and stigma increase the health vulnerability of the individual, making them more susceptible to both chronic and acute health problems. Little was known about the specific impact of COVID-19 on LGBTQ+ people at the time of this book, but it is likely that there may be disproportionate adverse consequences for this community (Human Rights Campaign, 2020).

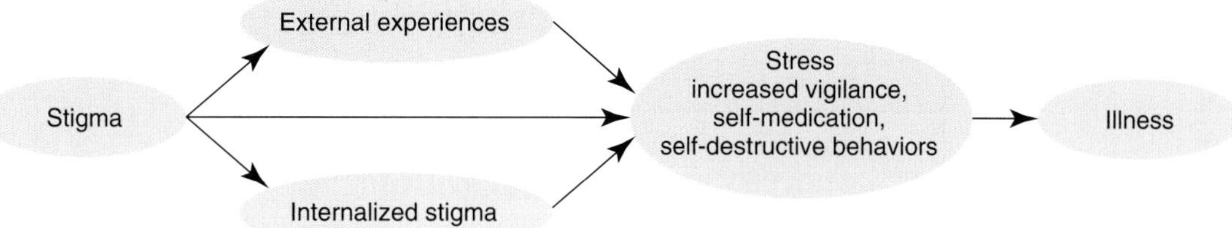

FIGURE 20–1 Effects of Stigma on Health.

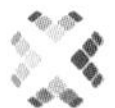

Case Illustration

Jan has experienced minority stress all her life as a Latina woman, and she experiences it in her adulthood as a bisexual person and partner of a transgender woman. That stress may have contributed to her multiple sclerosis, an autoimmune disorder. Minority stress certainly has affected her health-care experiences from the stress of receiving care in the hospital/clinic setting where Kari works.

The most thoroughly studied and documented health disparities of LGBTQ+ individuals include mental health disorders and suicide, substance use and abuse, and access to and quality of health care (Institute on Medicine, 2011). Other issues are particular to one or more of the subgroups under LGBTQ+, such as HIV/AIDS and other sexually transmitted infections that predominantly affect men who have sex with men and transgender women; breast cancer, pap testing, and obesity in lesbian/bisexual women; bullying of LGBTQ+ youth; and transition needs of transgender clients. A growing body of literature addresses parenting issues common to this community.

This review will focus on the three most common issues outlined above because they cut across LGBTQ+ populations. It is also important to keep in mind that most LGBTQ+ individuals are healthy and resilient (Kwon, 2013). However, all LGBTQ+ people are at risk for discrimination or poor-quality treatment when they enter health-care settings, regardless of whether they are receiving care for a problem related to societal stigma. For example, in some states, a female partner of a woman admitted to the emergency department following a car accident may be denied visitation rights, even if they are legally married or have legal documents such as power of attorney for health care. A transgender youth with polycystic ovaries may be treated with derision or even refused care in an ob/gyn clinic because of his masculine appearance.

Mental Health and Suicide Risks

Some of the earliest research on LGBTQ+ populations focused on mental health, and the findings are consistent even across the diversity of research designs that have been used. This research finds elevations in several types of mental health disorders and symptoms, most notably depression and PTSD. Table 20-1 shows the data for past month diagnoses of depression and anxiety disorders by sexual identity (Bostwick, Boyd, Hughes, & McCabe, 2010). Some studies find that mental health disorders are linked to discrimination, with higher rates of depression and anxiety disorders found in LGBTQ+ people who experience a greater number of discrimination experiences (Bostwick, Boyd, Hughes, West, & McCabe, 2014).

Table 20-1 Mental Health and Substance Use Disparities by Sexual Orientation and Gender

Diagnosis	Heterosexual Woman	Lesbians	Bisexual Women	Heterosexual Men	Gay Men	Bisexual Men
Major depression	27%	42%	52%	15%	38%	36%
Any anxiety disorder	38%	41%	58%	19%	41%	39%
Binge drinking in the past year	14%	26%	34%	31%	39%	52%
Marijuana use in the past year	3%	17%	22%	9%	25%	13%

Source: Data from Bostwick et al. (2010) and McCabe et al. (2009).

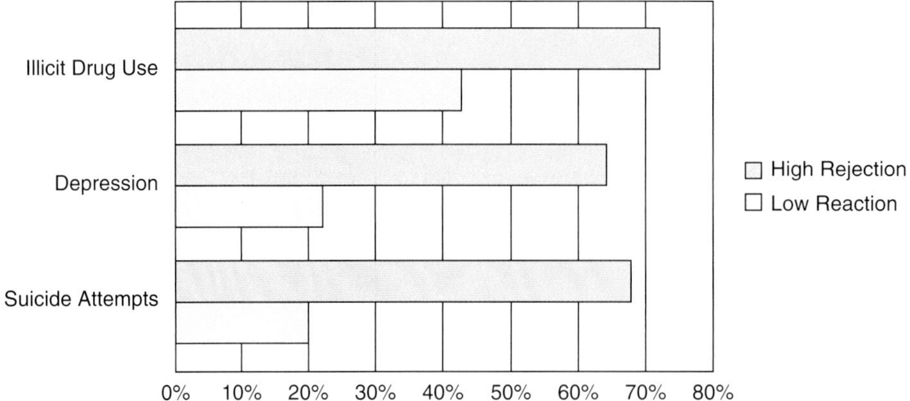

FIGURE 20–2 Relationship Between Parental-Rejecting Behaviors and Mental Health/Substance Abuse Outcomes in Young Adulthood *Source: Data from Ryan et al., 2009.*

Studies of suicide behaviors show a few consistent findings. LGBTQ+ people are more likely to report suicide ideation and make suicide attempts than comparable heterosexual people. These attempts are more severe in nature and more likely to result in hospitalizations, suggesting that they are not an attempt to get attention but a true desire to take one's own life. Less can be said about completed suicide because coroner's reports and psychological autopsy studies have rarely assessed the sexual or gender identity of the deceased. Suicide attempts may peak during the months or years before coming out (disclosing one's sexual or gender identity), so other people in the deceased person's life may not be aware of the inner turmoil that led to the suicide (Meyer, 2013).

Among LGBTQ+ youth, family rejection and bullying by peers are strongly predictive of depression, substance abuse, and suicide. Ryan, Huebner, Diaz, and Sanchez (2009) studied the characteristics of family rejection of LGBTQ+ children and found behaviors such as verbal and physical abuse, not allowing LGBTQ+ friends in the house, kicking the youth out of the house, and sending them to counseling. When the authors divided the sample into youth who had experienced low, moderate, or high rejection from parents, the results were startling. Figure 20–2 shows just how much parental rejection has an impact on mental health outcomes.

Suicide risk is often associated with a fear of rejection. Nurses can reduce this fear by openly expressing acceptance for people of all sexual and gender minority identities, correcting or challenging coworkers on uninformed or biased comments, and including partners and families of choice in discharge planning. If the nurse is silent about LGBTQ+ issues, clients may feel anxiety and stress about disclosure. You can ask your client to tell you about his or her family members and loved ones or inquire about what pronouns he or she prefers.

Substance Use and Abuse

Another consistent finding for several decades relates to higher use and higher levels of abuse of and dependence on drugs, alcohol, and tobacco. Refer back to Table 20-1 for data on marijuana use and binge drinking. LGBTQ+ people are approximately three times more likely to use illicit drugs and have a diagnosed alcohol dependency in the past year than heterosexual people (McCabe, Hughes, Bostwick, West, & Boyd., 2009). Other studies show that LGBTQ+ people are more likely to be in recovery from alcohol or drug use than heterosexual people (Matthews, Lorah, & Fenton, 2005). Most of the population-based studies have not included questions on gender identity, but the few convenience sample studies of transgender individuals also identify high risk for alcohol and drug use (e.g., Clement-Nolle, Marx, Guzman, & Katz, 2001).

In addition, many studies find that LGBTQ+ people are more likely to smoke (Ward, Dahlhamer, Galinsky & Joestl, 2014), and some subgroups are more likely to be exposed to secondhand smoke at home or in the workplace (Cochran, Bandiera, & Mays, 2013). The few studies of smoking cessation programs specific to LGBTQ+ populations generally show encouraging results (Eliason, Dibble, Gordon, & Soliz, 2012; Matthews, Li, Kuhns, Tasker, & Cesario, 2013). All clients should be asked about their alcohol, drug, and tobacco use because these factors can affect medication effectiveness, medication side effects, and treatment outcomes for a number of disorders. LGBTQ+ clients may benefit most from culturally sensitive treatment options and LGBTQ+ mentors/sponsors to address their substance use disorders.

Many have speculated that one factor in the higher rates of substance use is related to the prevalence of gay bars as a main social outlet for the LGBTQ+ population in many communities (Drabble & Eliason, 2012). Of course, it is too simplistic to blame bars entirely for the higher rates of substance abuse. People who do most of their socializing in bars often have distorted community norms about use of drugs and alcohol and are more permissive in their attitudes about drug use (Cochran, Grella, & Mays, 2012). Societal stigma is the main force that drove people to socialize in bars, and that contributes to the shame, guilt, and fear that people seek to self-medicate to reduce those unpleasant feelings (Meyer, 2013). In a society where socialization about same-sex dating and relationships is nonexistent, some felt a need for alcohol or drugs to release inhibitions enough to be sexual with someone of the same sex. Finally, others started socializing in bars and subsequently met partners and best friends there. Making friends in bars often means that one's social network consists of substance users, who influence the peer norms about substance use. Over time, by mere exposure, some people develop substance abuse problems.

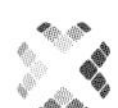

Case Illustration

Kari is in recovery from alcohol and marijuana abuse, stemming from her anxieties as an adolescent and young adult about transitioning. She was brutally beaten after leaving a gay bar intoxicated, so she entered treatment and sobered up before starting her transition. She did not come out as transgender during treatment because on the first day in the agency, she heard anti-LGBTQ+ comments from both staff members and other clients and never felt safe to reveal herself.

Health-Care Access and Quality of Care

Health-care access is a complicated issue related to economics, politics, and attitudes about health care in general or specific health-care practices, such as pap tests or prostate screening. More LGBTQ+ people live in poverty compared to heterosexual people because stigma can limit educational and employment opportunities, and/or many LGBTQ+ people choose to work in lower-paying nonprofits or human service careers where they are more likely to be accepted if they are out. In addition, many LGBTQ+ youth ran away or were thrown out of homes when parents rejected them for their sexual or gender identities. As a result, homeless populations contain disproportionately more LGBTQ+ individuals (Keuroghlian, Shtasel, & Bassuk, 2014). One good example of how poverty affects health is recent data on food insecurity. Almost one in three LGBTQ+ Americans experiences food insecurity (Gates, 2014).

Health-Care Microaggressions

Eliason and Dibble (2015) explored how the concept of microaggressions played out in health-care settings and suggested that LGBTQ+ clients might experience differences in three areas that have been outlined in the literature (e.g., Nadal, 2013). Microassaults are the more obvious examples, and they may include refusal to touch a client, using a derogatory name, making anti-LGBTQ+ comments, referring a client to reparative therapy, refusing to treat the client, and physically rough treatment. Microinsults consist of rude, insensitive, or condescending comments or behaviors, such as refusing to use the chosen name or pronoun of a transgender client, insisting that all gay men must have HIV, being rude to partners and families of LGBTQ+ patients, or treating LGBTQ+ clients as "less than" others. Finally, microinvalidations are dismissals of the pain experienced by LGBTQ+ people because of stigma, such as telling someone that they are being "too sensitive" when the admissions, intake, and medical history forms do not allow them to disclose their family structures or telling an LGBTQ+ person that their sexual or gender identity is irrelevant to their care ("you are here for cancer treatment—we treat everyone the same").

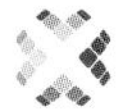

Case Illustration

Kari and Jan's experiences with health-care providers and systems since Jan's diagnosis have been riddled with microaggressions as well as more overt discrimination. Jan's medical records were the source of discussion in the nurses' station, and information about Kari's transgender identity was revealed to her coworkers. On another occasion, Jan had to explain four different times that they were legally married, and her annoyance showed in her tone of voice the last time. Her physician said, "Well, you don't have to be so sensitive about it." On another visit, when their children were present, a nurse said, "I don't care what consenting adults do, but I don't think it's fair to the children to raise them in such an unconventional family."

DISCUSSION OF THE EVIDENCE

Early studies of LGBTQ+ health relied on convenience and thus reported on nonrepresentative samples of people who were mostly out and open about their sexuality. It took several decades of researcher-activist work to get sexual orientation questions into some of the large-scale health surveillance instruments used in the United States, and most of them still do not have questions that would identify transgender individuals. However, questions about the representativeness of samples remain even on more rigorous population-based surveys. Given the high levels of societal stigma even today, how often do LGBTQ+ people reply honestly on health surveys? Another problem is that sexuality is measured in several different ways in health studies. Sometimes the questions are about identity; sometimes they are about behavior; and, on rare occasions (mostly studies of youth), they are about attraction only. No data indicate whether those different questions actually measure the same thing. Measures of gender identity are also varied. Most experts agree that at least two questions are needed to identify the transgender population: one about sex assigned at birth and one about current gender identification (GenIUSS Group, 2014). The few population-based health surveys that measure gender identity have used one or two questions.

Another problem is the focus on the individual rather than on the structural and systemic influences on health. This individualistic focus can sometimes lead to victim-blaming. Focus on health problems and differences rather than resilience, good health, and similarities can also skew nurses' perceptions of LGBTQ+ clients, who are receiving health-care services most of the time for problems unrelated to their sexuality or gender identity. Finally, very few studies have focused on nurses' experiences with LGBTQ+ care or on LGBTQ+ nurses, limiting what we can conclude about these issues. It is challenging to develop evidence-based practices for LGBTQ+ health care when the literature on LGBTQ+ issues in nursing is so scant.

Client Differences

This chapter did not review specific health issues for subgroups within the LGBTQ+ population, and these are substantial. Nurses will need education on the issues and populations that are most relevant to their own practice. For those who work in HIV/STI settings, understanding the needs of men who have sex with men and transgender women will be critical. Nurses who work in pediatric settings may need information about same-sex parenting and the early coming-out process. Oncology nurses need to know about rates of cancer in this population and experiences of LGBTQ+ clients in cancer-care settings. In addition to differences by sexual or gender identity labels, LGBTQ+ people are diverse in terms of race/ethnicity, age, religion, educational level, geographic region, disability status, and many other factors that may affect health as much as, or more than, sexual orientation and gender identity. Further research is needed on the health impacts of intersecting oppressed minority identities. Recall that all three groups (gay/bisexual men, lesbian/bisexual women, and transgender people) have higher rates of substance abuse, mental health disorders, and suicide behaviors than the general population—those differences cut across all sexual and gender identity groups.

Recommendations for Nursing Practice

The recommendations are divided into two interrelated sections: systems change and individual nurses' knowledge, attitudes, and behavior. Both are critical for the improvement of care for LGBTQ+ clients.

Systems Change

LGBTQ+ people are often hypervigilant in health-care settings because of bad experiences, and they look for clues that the clinic, hospital, or practice is safe (see Figure 20–3). Health-care settings can help create this sense of safety with small changes, such as updating written forms to ask explicitly for sexual orientation and gender identity information and ensuring that prominently displayed clients' or patient's rights statements include sexual orientation and gender identity. Choose some educational materials such as posters, brochures, and magazines that depict or focus on LGBTQ+ people or issues to increase visibility. The Joint Commission's Field Guide regarding LGBTQ+ care (2011) offers suggestions for changing the systems of health care to be more open and inclusive. Although less visible to clients, the practice should review all policies and procedures to make sure that they are inclusive of LGBTQ+ people, including but not limited to visitation policies, employee sexual harassment policies, benefits packages, hiring and retention practices, and staff continuing education (Eliason & Chinn, 2015).

In nursing education, efforts are needed to integrate LGBTQ+ content into the curriculum; support LGBTQ+ students, staff members, and faculty members; and encourage LGBTQ+-related research.

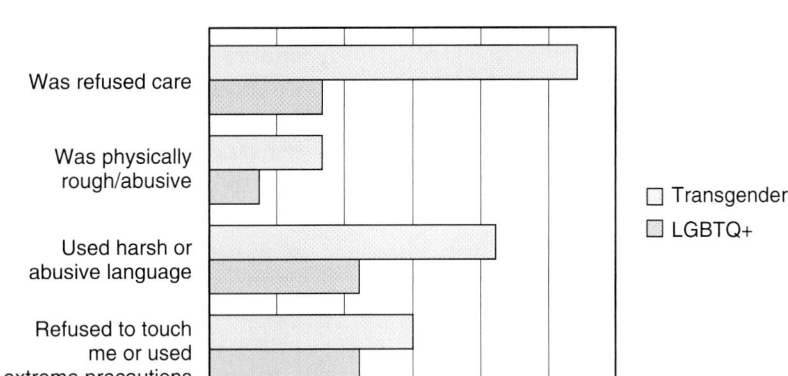

FIGURE 20–3 Experiences of LGB and T People in Health-Care Settings *Source: Data from Lambda Legal (2010). When health care isn't caring: Lambda Legal's survey of discrimination against LGBT people and people with HIV, New York, NY. Retrieved from www.lambdalegal .org/health-care-report*

Before the content can be fully integrated, nurse educators need training on these issues. Too often, it falls to the one or two openly LGBTQ+ faculty members to teach the LGBTQ+ content in the curriculum, and this content is lost if they leave the program. Sustainable education practices are necessary, and every nurse educator should be comfortable teaching some basic elements of LGBTQ+ health just as they need to be competent to discuss racial/ethnic differences in health. Nondiscrimination policies that protect employees, and partner benefits for states that do not have legal marriage options, also support LGBTQ+ nurses. In addition, nursing education needs systems that encourage students and junior faculty members to conduct LGBTQ+ research (Eliason, Dibble, & DeJoseph, 2010).

Individual Nurse Responsibilities

Nurses can easily feel information overload when it comes to addressing the vast diversity of client populations. One promising model for addressing LGBTQ+ issues in nursing is to use the concept of cultural humility (Tervalon & Murray-Garcia, 1998). This model is a process for using introspection to consider how client and provider differences may have an impact on nursing care. Cultural humility is a lifelong learning process that involves deep listening and creating a provider-client relationship that reduces some of the power dynamic and allows for co-learning; that is, nurses can be open to learning from clients as much as imparting information and skills to clients and families. Four suggestions for practicing nurses include:

1. Examine one's personal biases. Everyone has biases and many of them stem from childhood experiences. Questions such as the following may prompt a productive introspection:
   a. What is the first thing you remember about becoming aware of LGBTQ+ people: Was it on the playground, in your religious community, from parents?
   b. What did you learn about LGBTQ+ issues in nursing school? Did this information come from the formal curriculum, incidents in clinical settings, comments of other students and faculty members, or elsewhere?
   c. What do you need to know to be a more effective nurse to LGBTQ+ clients?
2. Educate yourself about LGBTQ+ issues. Nurses can consider continuing education programs, reading articles in professional journals in their specialty area, or having discussions with other nurses about LGBTQ+ nursing care. See the Client Education materials below for some starting points.
3. Find out what local resources for LGBTQ+ people are available. Is there an LGBTQ+ community center? LGBTQ+ Alcoholics Anonymous groups? Clinics that specialize in gender transition? Parents and Friends of Lesbians and Gays (PFLAG) groups? Gay-straight alliances at schools?
4. Become an ally or advocate at work. Model acceptance and professional conduct, start conversations to break the silence, use inclusive language, and encourage changes in the systems level.

HEALTHY PEOPLE 2020

The 2020 version of Healthy People included LGBTQ+ goals and objectives for the first time in its history, with a goal that states: "Improve the health, safety, and well-being of lesbian, gay, bisexual, and transgender (LGBTQ) individuals." In Healthy People 2020, one overarching objective is specifically related to LGBTQ+ populations, and several secondary objectives outline health concerns that are more prevalent in LGBTQ+ populations. The specific objective includes several subcomponents related to data collection systems:

> LGBTQ-1 (Developmental) Increase the number of population-based data systems used to monitor Healthy People 2020 objectives that include in their core a standardized set of questions that identify lesbian, gay, bisexual, and transgender populations.

In nursing settings, these data collection systems might include agency and/or unit intake forms, student admissions forms, and procedure for taking oral histories. Secondary objectives were identified by an LGBTQ+ workgroup and noted as particularly of interest in LGBTQ+ health (although the objectives do not parcel out individuals by sexuality or gender identity). These secondary objectives include several that relate to the three main areas discussed in this chapter:

- Mental health: Bullying among adolescents, mental health, and mental illness.
- Substance abuse: Binge drinking and alcohol use, illicit drug use, tobacco use.
- Health-care access: Breast cancer screening, cervical cancer screening, usual source of care, health insurance coverage.

Other secondary objectives include condom use, HIV testing, educational achievement, and nutrition and weight status.

Assessment

One critical issue, as noted in Healthy People 2020, is to add questions about sexual orientation and gender identity to admissions forms, procedures for taking oral histories, and research instruments. The current state of assessment is rather poor, with only a handful of health surveillance instruments and institutional data collection systems gathering this information. Examples of sexual orientation questions are:

1. Based on identities: These questions ask for the label that a person uses for their sexuality. The National Health Interview Survey uses this question: "Which of these best describes you?" The options are "lesbian or gay; bisexual; straight, that is, not gay; or something else." Other questions use options such as "entirely heterosexual, mostly heterosexual, bisexual, mostly lesbian/gay, entirely lesbian/gay." In less formal clinical interviews or history taking, questions such as "Can you tell me what words you use to describe your sexual orientation" can open the door to disclosures.
2. Based on behavior: These questions ask whether a person has sexual relationships primarily with men, women, both, or neither. They take many forms, with some questions time limited (the past year versus lifetime), some are one question (exclusively men, mostly men, men and women equally, mostly women, exclusively women), while some ask about actual numbers (how many men have you had sex with in the past month, how many women?).

Few surveys assess attraction, although some youth surveys or intake forms, sensitive about asking questions about actual sexual behavior in underage children, will ask about attraction. It is important to remember that it takes at least two questions to identify people on the transgender spectrum: sex assigned at birth (male, female, other) and current gender identification (male, female, transgender, other) (GenIUSS Group, 2014).

Client Education Materials

Unfortunately, availability of pamphlets or flyers for all the health topics that concern LGBTQ+ clients may be limited. Some topics, like Human Immunodeficiency Virus (HIV) among men who have sex with men (MSM), are well-covered and much information can be downloaded from the Centers for Disease Control and Prevention (CDC) and other government sites. The Web sites and written information below may provide more guidance:

- Fenway Health (http://fenwayhealth.org/): This LGBTQ+ health center in Boston has extensive information available about LGBTQ+ health care, mostly directed at provider education. Fenway Health also has a textbook on LGBTQ+ health that addresses particular health concerns for each subset of the LGBTQ+ population.
- Health Professionals Advancing LGBT Health (GLMA) (www.glma.org): This professional organization includes all health-care providers and has a nursing section dedicated to understanding and improving LGBTQ+ health. The Web site also includes a provider directory that allows visitors

to search for LGBTQ+ affirmative providers in locations across the United States.

- Various federal government sites (e.g., http://www.cdc.gov/lgbthealth/ and http://www.hrsa.gov/lgbt/): The CDC, the Health Resources and Services Administration (HRSA), Substance Abuse and Mental Health Services Administration (SAMHSA), and National Institutes of Health (NIH) all have dedicated Web pages on LGBTQ+ health that are updated frequently.
- The Joint Commission (http://www.jointcommission.org/lgbt/): This detailed report addresses quality inclusive care of LGBTQ+ clients.
- Lavender Health (http://lavenderhealth.org): This nurse-administrated educational and information site includes an "LGBTQ-101" PowerPoint presentation as well as a packet of case studies, classroom activities, and discussion questions that can be used in many nursing settings.
- Center of Excellence for Transgender Health (http://www.transhealth.ucsf.edu/): This center at the University of California, San Francisco, includes detailed information about transition health services as well as legal and social issues facing transgender populations.
- World Professional Association of Transgender Health (http://www.wpath.org/): This is an international resource on standards of care for transgender populations.

KEY POINTS

- Nursing education, research, and practice have lagged behind many other health professions in developing standards for LGBTQ+ nursing care, encouraging students and faculty to conduct LGBTQ+-related research, and integrating the nursing curriculum.
- Policies and procedures in both education and practice settings may render LGBTQ+ clients, students, and employees invisible.
- Some practicing nurses, beyond lack of knowledge, harbor negative attitudes stemming from religious or familial/cultural socialization, and these attitudes may interfere with the provision of quality health-care services. More nurses are well-intentioned but lack the information needed to provide quality care.
- LGBTQ+ clients still experience microaggressions. When these insults, oversights, or slights occur in health-care settings, they compromise the quality of care and potentially lead to avoidance or delay in seeking necessary health care.
- Nurses, as members of the frontline health-care profession, can do much to improve quality of care for LGBTQ+ people and their families.
- Three types of health disparities cut across the LGBTQ+ spectrum: mental health, substance abuse, and health-care access and quality of care.

Check Your Understanding

1. The health disparities of LGBTQ+ clients are predominantly related to:
   A. Genetic differences that cause diversity in sexuality/gender and contribute to disease
   B. Coming out as LGBTQ+ at a younger age
   C. Inability to accept one's own sexuality or gender identity
   D. Higher rates of minority stress
2. Healthy People 2020 has one objective related to LGBTQ+ health, calling for:
   A. Federal approval of same-sex marriage
   B. Better systems of data collection.
   C. Reduction in rates of internalized homophobia/transphobia
   D. Addressing the stigma of HIV
3. Which statement about the *Diagnostic and Statistical Manual of Mental Disorders* is correct?
   A. Lesbian, gay, bisexual, and transgender have all been labeled as disorders since the first edition.
   B. Lesbian, gay, bisexual, and transgender were all once disorders, but they were removed in 1973.
   C. Homosexuality was a disorder until 1973; gender identity disorder was added in 1980.
   D. The DSM has never addressed sexual orientation or gender identity.
4. When referring to a client's sexuality, which term is the most appropriate for nurses to use?
   A. Sexual orientation
   B. Homosexual
   C. Sexual preference
   D. Sexual deviation
5. A person who was assigned male at birth and has identified as a man and masculine all his life is considered:
   A. Heterosexual
   B. Transgender
   C. Cisgender
   D. Intersex

6. Minority stress has two main components:
   A. Internal and external
   B. Gender normative and homophobia
   C. Heterosexism and stigma
   D. Discrimination and hormone differences

7. One major factor in the higher rates of suicide among LGBTQ+ people is:
   A. Rejection by parents
   B. Genetic susceptibility to suicide
   C. Rejection by romantic partners
   D. Brain-based differences in cognitive processing

8. A person who was born male and transitions to female is often referred to as a:
   A. Transgender woman
   B. Transgender man
   C. Cisgender woman
   D. Cisgender man

See "Reflections on Check Your Understanding" at the end of the book for answers.

REFERENCES

Bostwick, W. B., Boyd, C. J., Hughes, T. L., & McCabe, S. E. (2010). Dimensions of sexual orientation and the prevalence of mood and anxiety disorders in the United States. *American Journal of Public Health, 100*(3), 468–475.

Bostwick, W. B., Boyd, C. J., Hughes, T. L., West, B. T., & McCabe, S. E. (2014). Discrimination and mental health among LGB adults in the U.S. *American Journal of Orthopsychiatry, 84*(1), 35–45.

Carabez, R., Eliason, M., & Martinson, M. (2016). Nurses' knowledge about transgender care: A qualitative study. *Advances in Nursing Science*, 39(3), 257–271

Carabez, R., Pelligrini, M., Mankovitz, A., Eliason, M., Ciano, M., & Scott, M. (2015). "Never in all my years...": Nurses' education about LGBT health. *Journal of Professional Nursing, 31*(4), 323–329.

Clarke, V., Ellis, S. J., Peel, E., & Riggs, D. W. (2010). *Lesbian, gay, bisexual, transgender, and queer psychology: An introduction.* London, UK: Cambridge University Press.

Clements-Nolle, K., Marx, R., Guzman, R., & Katz, M. (2001). HIV prevalence, risk behaviors, health care use, and mental health status of transgender persons. *American Journal of Public Health, 91*(6), 915–921.

Cochran, S. D., Bandiera, F. C., & Mays, V. M. (2013). Sexual orientation-related differences in tobacco use and second-hand smoke exposure among U.S. adults age 20–59: 2003–2010 NHANES. *American Journal of Public Health, 103*, 1837–1844.

Cochran, S. D., Grella, C. E., & Mays, V. M. (2012). Do substance use norms and perceived drug availability mediate sexual orientation differences in patterns of substance use? Results from the California Quality of Life Survey II. *Journal of Studies on Alcohol and Drugs, 73*(3), 675–685.

Diamond, L. (2009). *Sexual fluidity: Understanding women's love and desire*. Boston, MA: Harvard University Press.

Diamond, M., & Garland, J. (2013). Evidence regarding cosmetic and medically unnecessary surgery on infants. *Journal of Pediatric Urology, 10*(1), 2–6.

Drabble, L. & Eliason, M.J. (2012). Sexual minority women and treatment for substance use disorders: A review of literature. *Journal of LGBT Counseling: Special Issue on Addictions in LGBTQ Communities, 6*(4), 274-292.

Durso, L. E., & Meyer, I. (2012). Patterns and predictors of disclosure of sexual orientation to healthcare providers among lesbians, gay men, and bisexuals. *Sexuality Research and Social Policy, 10*(1), 35–42.

Eaklor, V. L. (2008). *Queer America: A people's GLBT history of the United States*. New York, NY: The New Press.

Eliason, M. J., & Chinn, P. (2015). LGBTQ cultures: What healthcare professionals need to know about sexual and gender diversity (2nd ed.). Philadelphia, PA: LWW Press.

Eliason, M. J., DeJoseph, J, Dibble, S., Deevey, S., & Chinn, P. (2011). Lesbian, gay, bisexual, transgender and queer /questioning (LGBTQ) nurses' experiences in the workplace. *Journal of Professional Nursing, 27*(4), 237–244.

Eliason, M. J., & Dibble, S. L. (2015). Patient-provider interactions for LGBT people with cancer. In U. Boehmer. & R. Elk (Eds)., *Cancer and the LGBT Community: Unique perspectives from risk to survivorship* (pp. 187–202). New York, NY: Springer.

Eliason, M. J., Dibble, S., & DeJoseph, J. (2010). Nursing's silence on lesbian, gay, bisexual, and transgender issues: The need for emancipatory efforts. *Advances in Nursing Science, 33*(3), 206–218.

Eliason, M. J., Dibble, S. L., Gordon, R., & Soliz, G. (2012). The Last Drag: A smoking cessation group intervention for lesbian, gay, bisexual, and transgender individuals. *Journal of Homosexuality, 59*(6), 864–878.

Gates, G. J. (2014). *Food insecurity and SNAP (food stamps) participation in LGBT communities.* Los Angeles, CA: The Williams Institute.

Gates, G. J., & Newport, F. (2012, Oct 18). *Special report: 3.4% of U.S. adults identify as LGBT.* Retrieved from www.gallup.com/poll/158066

The GenIUSS Group. (2014). *Best practices for asking questions to identify transgender and other gender minority respondents on population-based surveys*. J. L.Herman, (Ed.), Los Angeles, CA: The Williams Institute.

Healthy People 2020 (2020). Lesbian, gay, bisexual, and transgender health. https://www.healthypeople.gov/2020/topics-objectives/topic/lesbian-gay-bisexual-and-transgender-health

Human Rights Campaign (2020). The lives and livelihoods of many in the LGBTQ community are at risk amidst COVID 19 crisis. Policy Brief, https://assets2.hrc.org/files/assets/resources/COVID19-IssueBrief-032020-FINAL.pdf?_ga=2.247645959.1045528366.1592940975-1056293096.1590597378

Institute of Medicine. (2011). *The health of LGBT people: Building a foundation for better understanding.* New York: National Academies Press.

Jordan-Young, R. M. (2010). *Brainstorm: The flaws in the science of sex differences.* Cambridge, MA: Harvard University Press.

Keuroghlian, A. S., Shtasel, D., & Bassuk, E. L. (2014). Out on the street: A public health and policy agenda for lesbian, gay, bisexual, and transgender youth who are homeless. *American Journal of Orthopsychiatry*, *84*(1), 66.

Kwon, P. (2013). Resilience in lesbian, gay, and bisexual individuals. *Personality and Social Psychology Review*, *17*(4), 371–383.

Lambda Legal. (2010). When health care isn't caring: Lambda Legal's survey of discrimination against LGBT people and people with HIV, New York, NY. Retrieved from www.lambdalegal.org/health-care-report

Lim, F., Johnson, M., & Eliason, M.J. (2015). A national survey of faculty knowledge, experience, and readiness for teaching LGBT health in baccalaureate nursing programs. *Nursing Education Perspectives*, *36*(3), 144–152.

Matthews, A. K., Li, C. C., Kuhns, L. M., Tasker, T. B., & Cesario, J. A. (2013). Results from a community-based smoking cessation treatment program for LGBT smokers. *Journal of Environmental and Public Health*, epub. doi: 10.1155/2013/984508

Matthews, C. R., Lorah, P., & Fenton, J. (2005). Toward a grounded theory of lesbians' recovery from addiction. *Journal of Lesbian Studies*, *9*(3), 57–68.

McCabe, S. E., Hughes, T. L., Bostwick, W. B., West, B. T., & Boyd, C. J. (2009). Sexual orientation, substance use behaviors, and substance dependence in the U.S. *Addiction*, *104*(8), 1333–1345.

Meyer, I. (2013). Prejudice, social stress and mental health in lesbian, gay, and bisexual populations: Conceptual issues and research evidence. *Psychology of Sexual Orientation and Gender Diversity*, *1*(S), 3–26.

Mouriquand, P., Caldamone, A., Malone, P., Frank, J. D., & Hoebeke, P. (2014). The ESPU/SPU standpoint on the surgical management of disorders of sex development. *Journal of Pediatric Urology*, *10*(1), 8–10.

Nadal, K. L. (2013). *That's so gay! Microaggressions and the lesbian, gay, bisexual, and transgender community.* Washington DC: American Psychological Association.

Röndahl, G., Innala, S., & Carlsson, M. (2006). Heterosexual assumptions in verbal and non-verbal communication in nursing. *Journal of Advanced Nursing*, *56*(40), 373–381.

Rounds, L. E., McGrath, B. B., & Walsh, E. (2013). Perspectives on provider behaviors: A qualitative study of sexual and gender minorities regarding quality of care. *Contemporary Nurse*, *44*, 99–110.

Ryan, C., Huebner, D., Diaz, R. M., & Sanchez, J. (2009). Family rejection as a predictor of negative health outcomes in White and Latino LGB young adults. *Pediatrics*, *123*, 346–352.

Schilt, K., & Westbrook, L. (2009). Doing gender, doing heteronormativity: "Gender normal," transgender people, and the social maintenance of heterosexuality. *Gender and Society*, *23*(4), 440–464.

Tervalon, M., & Murray-Garcia, J. (1998). Cultural humility versus cultural competence: A critical distinction in defining physician training outcomes in multicultural education. *Journal of Health Care for the Poor and Underserved*, *9*(2), 117–125.

The Joint Commission (2011). Advancing effective communication, cultural competence, and patient- and family-centered care for the lesbian, gay, bisexual, and transgender (LGBT) community: A field guide. Oak Brook, IL, Oct. 2011, LGBTFieldGuide.pdf.

Ward, B. W., Dahlhamer, J. M., Galinsky, A. M., & Joestl, S. S. (2014). Sexual orientation and health among U.S. adults: National Health Interview Survey, 2013. *National Health Statistics Reports*, 77. Hyattsville, MD: National Center for Health Statistics.

Substance Use

Carolyn Baird

LEARNING OBJECTIVES

After completing this chapter, the student will be able to:

1. State an evidence-based definition for substance use disorder.
2. Identify the major health and wellness risks associated with substance use.
3. Identify the role of nursing practice in addressing major risks to health and wellness.
4. Apply an evidence-based approach to acquiring nursing skills and knowledge for the prevention, intervention, and treatment of substance use and substance use disorders.
5. Identify pertinent sources for current information on health promotion initiatives for substance abuse.
6. Identify resources for knowledge and skill areas required for professional specialty area credentials.

INTRODUCTION

The use of psychoactive substances and the behaviors associated with it occurs along a continuum of use, abuse, dependence, and addiction. While the term *misuse* is often used interchangeably with *abuse*, it is important to differentiate between the two. *Misuse* refers to the improper use of medications when seeking therapeutic results; *abuse* is repeated and willful substance use for the purpose of pleasure, euphoria, and ecstasy. The appropriate term to be used in the continuum is *abuse*.

The American Society for Addiction Medicine (ASAM) defines addiction as "a primary, chronic disease of brain reward, motivation, memory and related circuitry" (ASAM, 2011, p.1). This disease is particularly concerning because disability and death can happen at any time along the continuum; in fact, drug poisoning, more commonly known as overdose, is currently identified as the leading cause of injury-related accidental death (Hedegaard, Chen, & Warner, 2015). Many overdose deaths today are caused by opioid prescription medications and heroin (Cicero & Ellis, 2015; Hedegaard, Chen, & Warner, 2015).

Healthy People: The Surgeon General's Report on Health Promotion and Disease Prevention first identified that prevention and early intervention through health education and health promotion could reduce the loss of human potential caused by addiction (Public Health Service, 1979). This national public health agenda established five measurable goals for improving the health of all Americans and provided a rationale for the use of disease prevention and health promotion in achieving these goals (Public Health Service, 1980). Succeeding goals and objectives have been included in Healthy People 2000, Healthy People 2010, and Healthy People 2020, including those that address health risks associated with the misuse and abuse of licit and illicit drugs (Green & Allegrante, 2011).. A focus group is already holding meetings to identify the leading health indicators for Healthy People 2030.

The U.S. Census Bureau (2019) reported that approximately 328 million people were living in the United States on July 1, 2019, 1.6 more than 2018 (USAFacts,

2020). The Substance Abuse and Mental Health Services Administration (SAMHSA) conducts an annual survey for data related to trends for substance use and mental health. Known as the National Survey on Drug Use and Health (NSDUH), it asks individuals 12 and older about the prior month and lifetime experiences. According to the data from the 2018 survey of the 327 million living in the United States approximately 164.8 million of them 12 and older had used some type of substance (alcohol, tobacco, or illicit drugs) in the prior month (SAMHSA, 2019).

Of the 138.9 million drinking alcohol 16.6 million drank heavily and 67.1 million were binge drinkers. There were 2.2 million adolescents (12 to 17) who used alcohol and 1.2 million of them were binge drinkers. Of the 58.8 million that had used tobacco in the past month 47 million smoked cigarettes. There were 27.3 million who smoked daily and 10.8 million of them smoked a pack or more a day (SAMHSA, 2019). There has been a decline over the past years. In 2013 sixty-seven million used tobacco in some form (SAMHSA, 2014a). The decrease has been attributed to the increasing use of vaporizing devices such as electronic nicotine delivery systems (ENDS) frequently referred to as e-cigarettes, vape pens, juuls, ans so on (SAMHSA, 2019). Questions about the use of these devices have not been included in the survey.

The NSDUH presents illicit drug use according to the past year rather than past month. In 2013 almost 25 million individuals ages 12 and older used one or more illicit substances, most commonly marijuana (20 million) (SAMHSA, 2014a), compared to 53.2 million individuals 12 and older in 2018. Marijuana was still the most frequently used substance with 43.5 million compared to 20 million in 2013. Although many states have legalized marijuana for both medical and recreational use it is still a Schedule 1 drug federally. The 2018 NSDUH marijuana section asked about marijuana and hashish as one substance, combined all methods of using together, and asked about age of first use, month and year of use, how many days used, and length of time since last use (SAMHSA, 2019.

The second most frequent substance was opioids at 10.3 million (9.9 million prescription opioids, 808,000 heroin, and 506,000 both) (SAMHSA, 2019). In addition, 22 million individuals (8%) were diagnosed with substance abuse or dependence in 2013 (SAMHSA, 2014a) compared to 20.3 million (7.8%) in 2018 (SAMHSA, 2019). Only 2 million (2013) and 3 million (2018) of these identified individuals received treatment for their substance use disorder. The most common reason reported for foregoing treatment in both surveys was lack of insurance and/or financial resources (SAMHSA, 2014a; 2019).

This chapter will discuss current and emerging concerns about substance use disorders from a health promotion perspective. An evidence-based approach is used to consider what we know about prescription drug abuse and opioid dependency, which treatments are most effective, areas where more research is needed, and how nurses can prepare to care for clients whose lives have been affected by substance use and addictive disorders. An overview of the credentials available to nurses in the specialty area of addictions nursing or tobacco dependency is also included.

Although the chapter covers multiple substances, opioids are a primary focus because opioid dependency was identified in 2011 as an epidemic and is now a national crisis. In the twelve-month period from February 2017 to January 2018, 69,703 overdose deaths were reported in the United States—roughly 191 overdose deaths per day (Ahmad, Rossen, Spencer, Warner, & Sutton, 2018). In 2018 there were approximately 47,000 overdose deaths specifically attributed to opioids (National Institute on Drug Abuse [NIDA], 2020b).

The COVID-19 pandemic in 2020 exacerbated challenges for those with substance use disorders (NIDA, 2020a). Preexisting risks such as homelessness, housing instability, lack of access to care, incarceration, and stigma put individuals with substance use disorders (SUDs) in situations and settings that expose them to the transmission of the coronavirus. As to the disease itself, little is known about all the ways COVID-19 affects the body. Individuals with SUDs have compromised immune systems and a greater risk for respiratory, lung, and cardiac disorders (NIDA, 2020a). Individuals who smoke are especially at risk for respiratory infections leading to increased risk of contracting COVID-19 or have more severe complications if they contract the disease. Using e-cigarettes or vapes expose the lungs to toxic chemicals. Whether their use increases the risk of contracting the coronavirus is unknown but since most users are former cigarette smokers there are concerns the complications could be more severe (NIDA, 2020a).

Individuals with opioid use disorders (OUDs) also seem to be at great risk due to the negative impact that opioids have on the cardiac and pulmonary systems. High doses of opioids affect the brain stem and cause suppression of the respiratory system. This is often the cause of fatal overdoses. It also results in diminished lung capacity, which is a risk factor in the severity of Covid-19 (NIDA, 2020a). Methamphetamine is another drug that impacts the pulmonary system causing lung damage and pulmonary hypertension. This may be a risk factor in contracting COVID-19 and determining its severity (NIDA, 2020a). Access to medication and social supports systems increased the stress for individuals during times of social distancing and additional support is needed (NIDA, 2020a).

SCREENING, BRIEF INTERVENTION, REFERRAL TO TREATMENT (SBIRT)

Increased insurance opportunities and federal funding are insufficient to address the prevalence and depth of substance abuse and associated issues. The intervention must occur at the beginning of the substance use continuum, an assertion supported by the results of the annual NSDUH. Reviewing the trends reveals that substance use is a public health problem, and health-care providers need a comprehensive approach to deliver an intervention to individuals who might be at risk for developing a substance use disorder or to identify and refer to treatment individuals who already have a substance use disorder (Office of National Drug Control Policy [ONDCP], 2012; SAMHSA, 2014b). SBIRT is an approach consisting of four steps. which are reviewed in Table 21-1.

All health and human services professionals are encouraged to be competent at conducting SBIRT. The federal government has designated the Institute for Research, Education and Training in Addictions (IRETA) as the national SBIRT Addiction Technology Transfer Center (ATTC). IRETA offers an SBIRT suite of services to assist providers in using SBIRT. The largest group of health-care professionals comprises 4 million registered nurses (National Council of State Boards of Nursing [NCSBN], 2018). With these numbers, and the fact that registered nurses are present in most settings across the field of health care, they are often the first person encountered by the client (Strobbe & Broyles, 2013).

Nurses, both generalist and advanced, and regardless of specialty or practice setting, should have the knowledge and skill to use SBIRT to identify clients across the life span who have or are at risk for substance use disorders and respond effectively with interventions and referrals (Strobbe & Broyles, 2013). Advanced practice nurses have a role to play in ensuring that research into the application, feasibility, and effectiveness of SBIRT across client populations and health-care settings related to the use of alcohol, tobacco, and other substances is ongoing (Mitchell et al., 2015). Nursing leadership must advocate for the inclusion of knowledge and skill content pertaining to SBIRT in undergraduate, graduate, and continuing education curricula. In addition, nurse educators and others need to advocate for the inclusion of information on the use of psychoactive substances, substance use disorders, neurobiology of addiction, and treatment of substance use disorders in all educational curricula (Mitchell et al., 2013). All nurses need to have the requisite knowledge and competencies to provide high-quality, cost-effective, comprehensive care to any client, in any setting, who may be affected by alcohol or other psychoactive substances (Kane et al., 2014).

BACKGROUND AND SCOPE OF THE PROBLEM

In 2004, the Surgeon General's Report estimated a cost to this country of $559 billion a year for drug abuse and addiction related to alcohol, tobacco, and other drugs (National Institute on Drug Abuse [NIDA], 2017). This includes costs for health care; lost productivity; crime;

Table 21-1 Screening, Brief Intervention, and Referral to Treatment

STEP 1	Screening	Screen clients using any of a number of evidence-based prescreening questions to assess level and severity of substance use. SAMHSA has a number of them available at http://www.samhsa.gov/sbirt/resources. The National Institute on Drug Abuse (NIDA) has an online tool called the NIDA Quick Screen, which is available at http://www.drugabuse.gov/nmassist/?q=nida_questionnaire The National Institute on Alcohol Abuse and Alcoholism (NIAAA) has several site-specific interventions available at http://pubs.niaaa.nih.gov/publications/arh28-2/55-56.htm
STEP 2	Brief intervention	Clients whose screening reveals moderate risk receive an intervention to raise their awareness of the potential consequences of their use. Providers may use motivational interviewing techniques to encourage behavioral change.
STEP 3	Brief therapy	In cases in which more than a brief intervention is needed, additional assessment and a more comprehensive approach to education and problem solving are required. Clients may be taught coping mechanisms and assisted in building a supportive social environment.
STEP 4	Referral to treatment	Clients who are revealed to be at high risk are given a referral to specialty treatment providers deemed appropriate for their type and severity of need.

incarceration; and enforcement of laws related to getting, having, and using drugs. The amount has since risen to $740 billion a year (NIDA, 2017). The societal costs calculated for prescription opioid abuse alone were $11 billion in 2001 and rose to $55.7 billion by 2007 (Birnbaum et al., 2011; National Center for Injury Control and Prevention, 2011). In 2010, overdoses associated with prescription opioid abuse were responsible for 16,000 deaths, and the number has increased significantly since then. When calculated by deaths per 100,000 population, the rate rose from 12.3 in 2010 to 16.3 in 2015. Statistics are available in some cases for types of opioids, but not all death certificates specify the drug involved. Heroin and synthetics other than methadone are responsible for most of the increase. From 2014 to 2015, the death rate for natural/semisynthetic opioids increased only 2.6%. During this same period, heroin deaths increased by 20%, and deaths from synthetic opioids other than methadone increased by 72.2% (Rudd, Seth, David, & Scholl, 2016) with 46 individuals dying each day from opioid or heroin overdose (Hedegaard, Chen, & Warner, 2015). Based on data from the 2019 Annual Surveillance Report of Drug-related Risks and Outcomes the current daily death rate associated with fatal opioid overdoses is approximately 130 (CDC, 2019a).

This initial decrease in deaths was attributed to natural/semisynthetic opioid overdoses as a result of the Executive Office of the President of the United States (2011) plan for addressing what it called a "national epidemic of prescription drug abuse." The four-pronged plan of education, tracking and monitoring, proper medication disposal, and enforcement was based on a collaborative effort of policy, programming, and community and agency initiatives. The proposed approaches were based on best advice because evidence-based best practice information was not yet available. The approaches were judged effective after an immediate drop of 12% of those abusing these drugs between 2011 and 2012 (Baird, 2014; Executive Office of the President of the United States, 2011; National Center for Injury Control and Prevention, 2014; Trust for America's Health, 2013). That decrease has been turned around by the rise in the manufacturing of fentanyl analogues as one of the NPSs (New Psychotropic Substances) (Ventura, Carvalho, & Dinis-Oliveira, 2018).

Evolution of the Disease to a Public Health Problem

One of the challenges in addressing substance misuse and abuse is the evolution of patterns in the use of licit and illicit psychoactive substances. Over the years, public health concerns have changed from a focus on alcohol, marijuana, and tobacco to prescription drug abuse and heroin (Furek, 2008). Tobacco has been a problem across many generations; it accounts for nearly $300 billion in smoking-related illness and causes 480,000 deaths (Centers for Disease Control and Prevention [CDC], 2018) each year in the United States alone. The cost of direct medical care for associated comorbidities accounts for $176 billion of this; even more concerning, however, are the associated public health issues from secondhand smoke. This is one substance whose use by one party can directly affect the health of another, costing this country $5.6 billion a year in lost productivity (CDC, 2019c).

Law enforcement, health-care providers, health educators, and lawmakers are forced to stay ahead of this evolution (U.S. Department of Health and Human Services, 2014). Programs have been developed to address the global issue of nicotine dependence and smoking-related comorbidities from the use of tobacco products. Organizations like the American Lung Association provide education and support for community health programs, and the Association for the Treatment of Tobacco Use and Dependence (ATTUD) supports providers through resources, competencies for treatment, credentialing of programs, and certification as a tobacco treatment specialist (TTS). Although comprehensive tobacco control policies in the United States have resulted in an overall decrease in tobacco use for most population groups (CDC, 2019b), the problem has begun to grow around the world according to the World Health Organization (WHO).

Many agencies and organizations have been founded to control opioid use and educate the community. SAMHSA is one of these agencies; it manages the funding for treatment and education. ONDCP advises the president on issues around drug-control; manages funding related to drug-control activities; coordinates drug-control activities under a federal umbrella; and produces the annual National Drug Control Strategy, an outline of what is being done to reduce illicit drug use, manufacturing and trafficking, drug-related crime and violence, and drug-related health consequences.

We have learned that addiction is a primary, chronic disease of brain reward, motivation, memory, and related circuitry, which means that reducing the availability of psychoactive substances by controlling manufacturing and trafficking is not sufficient to control its far-reaching effects. Opioid pain medications and heroin share a high risk for relapse and death. External cues such as certain people, places, things, smells, sounds, and tasks trigger a persistent risk of relapse (NIDA).

Medication-assisted treatment with opioid agonists such as methadone, buprenorphine, and naltrexone has long been the therapy of choice. A medication that reverses an opioid overdose, naloxone (Narcan®), is a pure opioid antagonist and can be used to reverse opioid depression partially until medical attention can be obtained. Its use is highly controversial and, until recently, laws controlling its use made it difficult to obtain and meant that it was unavailable to the individuals who would need to administer it. The current epidemic and increasing death rate have given support to laws that decriminalize the use of naloxone by friends, family members, Good Samaritans, police officers, and emergency responders (Davis, 2015). Protection is provided to those calling for help and to the individuals overdosing (SAMHSA, 2013).

New Psychotropic Substances and Synthetics

Even as the efforts to address opioid substance abuse begin to bear fruit, another epidemic is on its way. Synthetic analogs for controlled illicit substances are making their way onto the market internationally. These designer drugs fall into one of three categories: synthetic cathinones ("bath salts," "flakka"), synthetic cannabinoids ("spice"), and synthetic hallucinogens ("N-bomb") and have been given the name new psychotropic substances (NPSs). They are safe to manufacture and distribute because no current drug laws govern their sale. The growing international concern is due to the acute toxicity and severe physical and psychological effects from these NPSs. They have many serious side effects, and deaths have been reported. The primary users are young adults who seldom come in contact with health-care providers unless they present for treatment at the emergency department with severe neuropsychiatric symptoms (Weaver, Hopper, & Gunderson, 2015). These drugs can take a variety of forms, from capsules and pills to liquids, crystals, and powder. They can be taken orally by swallowing or held under the tongue or in the cheek. They can also be vaporized for inhaling or snorting, or injected intravenously.

Synthetic Cathinones

Cathinones contain one or more amphetamine-like chemicals related to the stimulant cathinone found in the khat plant. They are usually a white or brown crystalline powder sold in a small plastic or foil package labeled "not for human consumption." Although initially known as "bath salts," this drug may be labeled as plant food, screen cleaner, or jewelry cleaner to avoid detection by authorities. The user may ingest, inhale, or inject them. Once they enter the body, they travel to the brain and cause the release of the neurotransmitters dopamine, norepinephrine, and serotonin. The effects may be similar to those of stimulants such as amphetamines and cocaine, including increased alertness, euphoria, sociability, and sex drive. Adverse effects may include tachycardia, paranoia, agitation, violent behavior, hallucinatory delirium, psychosis, and death (Marusich, Antonazzo, Wiley, Blough, Partilla, & Baumann, 2014; Weaver, Hopper, & Gunderson, 2015).

The cathinone known as flakka, or α-pyrrolidinopentiophenone (alpha-PVP), is a white or pink crystal with a foul smell that can be taken orally, snorted, or injected. After the drug is ingested, it takes about 30 minutes to start seeing the effect, compared to seeing the effect in about 10 seconds after vaporizing. Because the drug gets into the system so quickly, overdosing is easier. The usual effect is an "excited delirium," with hyperstimulation, paranoia, and hallucinations that can lead to self-injury, suicide, and violent behavior toward others. Death may result from a heart attack, or the body's temperature may rise causing hyperthermia, kidney damage, and renal failure.

Synthetic Cannabinoids

Chemically related to delta-9-tetrahydrocannabinol (THC), synthetic cannabinoids mirror the psychoactive ingredient in cannabis. Although called synthetic marijuana, this drug is actually a chemical that can be added to vegetable material and then smoked. Because this substance is much more powerful than naturally occurring THC, it has a much stronger and more dangerous impact on the cannabinoid receptors in the central nervous system. Some of the potential effects for users include anxiety and agitation, difficulty thinking clearly, nausea and vomiting, high blood pressure, shaking and seizures, hallucinations, delusions, and paranoia. Incidences of violence and acute psychosis have also occurred. Individuals who have genetic vulnerabilities are at high risk and may experience psychotic symptoms that last from 1 week to 5 months (Weaver, Hopper, & Gunderson, 2015).

Synthetic Hallucinogens

This class of drugs distorts the perception of reality and includes two categories: (1) classic hallucinogens, which are alkaloids extracted from certain plants and mushrooms, some of which have been used in religious rituals for many centuries, and (2) dissociatives, which cause users to feel disconnected from their bodies and out of control. Their chemical structure is very similar to that of the naturally occurring neurotransmitters acetylcholine, serotonin, and catecholamine. They are believed to interfere with the binding action of the receptor sites in the brain. The earliest hallucinogens are peyote (active ingredient is mescaline) and psilocybin. In 1938, D-lysergic acid diethylamide (LSD) was synthesized from the lysergic acid in ergot, a fungus found on grain. In 1950, the first dissociative, phencyclidine (PCP), was developed as a surgical anesthetic, but it was discontinued because it proved too dangerous for use. It was followed by ketamine (K, special K, or cat valium), a dissociative anesthetic used for animals and humans. The effects of these drugs include the inability to think clearly, communicate, or recognize reality; violent or bizarre behavior; rapid heart rate; and psychotic symptoms and episodes (flashbacks) that continue from beyond the time of use (NIDA, 2015).

The annual Monitoring the Future survey shows a decrease in the use of older hallucinogens, but concern is growing about so-called designer or club drugs, like 3,4-methylenedioxy-methamphetamine (MDMA), better known as Ecstasy and Molly), and other synthetic hallucinogens, such as 251-NBOMe and N-bomb. Both of the latter are based on phenethylamine, which has effects similar to both amphetamine and mescaline (Johnston, O'Malley, Miech, Bachman, & Schulenberg, 2015).

The new N-bomb drugs are very dangerous because of their potency—users need only a few grains to feel the effects. At first the user might feel an enhanced mood with more energy, and alterations in perception with visual and auditory hallucinations may occur. Serotonin toxicity with tachycardia, hypertension, diarrhea, and vomiting, or even an excited delirium with severe agitation, dysphoria, severe confusion, paranoia, aggression, and violence is possible. Hyperthermia and renal failure, prolonged psychoactive states, flashbacks, self-harm, and death are also possible. The N-bomb drugs are quickly becoming a source of public health concern because they are readily available, are sold online, and are frequently presented as legal lysergic acid (Schifano, Orsolini, Papanti, & Corkery, 2015; Weaver, Hopper, & Gunderson, 2015).

Vaporizing

Vaporizers, sometimes called electronic cigarettes or e-cigarettes, have three primary components: a battery, an atomizing or vaporizing unit, and a cartridge for the vaping solution. The solution is composed of a humectant, usually propylene glycol or glycerin; flavoring; and nicotine or another psychoactive substance. Using an e-cigarette is called vaping, users are vapers, and the e-cigarettes are vapes. First-generation e-cigarettes had prefilled cartridges, but second-generation e-cigarettes have stronger batteries and reservoirs for users to fill with their solution of choice. Nicotine is the most common psychoactive ingredient in vaping solutions, but vaporizers that deliver tetrahydrocannabinol (THC) and cannabidiol (CBD) (the active chemicals in marijuana) are also available.

The use of e-cigarettes is growing. They are no longer used just for smoking cessation but also by many individuals who prefer vaping to smoking because of the lack of smoke and associated odor. The 2014 Monitoring the Future survey found that twice as many adolescents in grades 8 and 10 use e-cigarettes than any other form of tobacco, while 12th graders have converted to e-cigarettes in smaller numbers (Johnston et al., 2015).

The increasing prevalence of vaping devices and the increasing availability of solutions with various psychoactive substances have led to an entirely new set of public health problems. The use of and dependency on psychoactive substances, accidental poisonings due to ingestion or absorption of the solutions, overdoses and deaths, and burns from the misuse of the devices are all increasing.

Concern is growing that the use of e-cigarettes is just as damaging to the lungs as smoking regular cigarettes and that the vaporized solutions have just as many carcinogenic substances. So far, only limited evidence supports that concern, and all current research has been conducted with nicotine. However, too many people believe e-cigarettes to be a "safe way to smoke," so they are switching rather than quitting, or they are even starting to use because of the perceived safety of this method. This includes adolescents, who may quickly find illicit substances in solutions that they use (Farsalinos & Polosa, 2014; Sussan et al., 2015).

Personal and Societal Cost

Regardless of the substance used and how it is ingested, the impact of the use, misuse, and abuse of psychoactive substances often affects friends, family members, and community members as much as it does the individual using the substance. United States Department of Justice conducts an annual *National Drug Threat Assessment* (National Drug Intelligence Center, 2014) and the United Nations Office on Drugs and Crime (UNODC) monitors trends in the use and impact of psychoactive substances. Its 2012 World Drug Report (UNODC, 2012) found that substance abuse–related illnesses and death are costly, productivity is lost, criminal activity increases, and health-care costs for treatment are increasing. The 2017 World Drug Report identified the cost as the loss of 28 million "healthy" years of life (UNODC, 2017). More of an issue is the fact that, of all illicit drug users, an average of 12% become dependent. This percentage varies widely among the drugs used, however, with a low of 10% for cannabis and a high of 50% for heroin.

The percentage of individuals who become dependent is reflective of the impact on the neurotransmitters in the area of the brain known as the pleasure center or reward pathway. As the abuse progresses to dependency and addiction, the dysfunction in the neurocircuitry controlling brain reward, motivation, and memory increases, demonstrating specific biological, psychological, social, and spiritual characteristics; a pathological pursuit of reward and relief; and impairment in behavior, emotions, and interpersonal relationships. These negative effects generate substantial discomfort in the people around the user and lead to stigma toward the individuals who suffer from this disease.

Unfortunately, at the global level, fewer than one in every five individuals needing treatment in 2010 received it (UNODC, 2012), and, by 2015, that number had improved to only one in every six (UNODC, 2017). Barriers to seeking treatment for substance abuse and addiction include a lack of treatment facilities; the high cost of treatment; and the stigma surrounding addiction, including the opinions of friends and family members. Often, medication-assisted treatment is still considered substance use by friends and family members. Treatment for substance dependence can be a source of stigma even without medication.

Health promotion programs cannot focus only on educating the public about prevention, intervention, and treatment for the disease of addiction—they must also present the information in a manner that will decrease or eliminate stigma. For this reason, health promotion professionals need to understand the disease and the evidence-based best practices for treating substance dependence.

Although this chapter provides general coverage of substance abuse, the following content focuses on the ever-worsening national emergency of opioid dependency.

PATIENT, INTERVENTION, CONTROL, OBSERVATION, AND TIME (PICOT) STATEMENT: EVIDENCE TABLES

Medication-assisted treatment (MAT), especially with methadone, is a source of stigma for opioid-dependent individuals. For health promotion professionals to understand the differences between MAT and psychotherapy, the following PICOT question is proposed.

In clients with an opioid dependency, does MAT rather than psychotherapy provide better long-term (more than 2 years) recovery?

Population: Clients with opioid dependency
Intervention: MAT
Comparison: Psychotherapy
Outcome: Recovery
Time: Long term (more than 2 years)

See Table 21-2.

Opioid Dependency

Opioid dependency has been a costly issue in U.S. society since the Civil War. At that time, opioid drugs were widely available without legal constraints on their use. As use became more prevalent, however, society became less accepting. Immigration brought new waves of users, and the Harrison Act of 1914 curtailed the availability by legal means. Clinics opened in which dependent individuals could be treated with small doses of short-acting morphine to help manage withdrawal (SAMHSA, 2011a). All psychoactive substances have withdrawal symptoms when use is discontinued. Because opioids are highly psychoactive, withdrawal is very difficult. The symptoms of any withdrawal are the opposite of the effect the substance has on the body. Opioid withdrawal usually starts within 12 hours after the last dose, although agitation can start earlier. Aches and pains are accompanied by rhinorrhea (running nose), lacrimation (excessive tear formation), chills, gooseflesh, and sweating. After 24 to 48 hours, abdominal cramping and diarrhea begin. Symptoms mostly resolve by day 6, but the drug-seeking behavior continues and relapse is possible even years later.

Opioid Replacement Therapy

Opioid replacement therapy has been used historically to maintain or detoxify individuals who are dependent on an opioid substance. One of the drawbacks to using short-acting opioids is the euphoric side effect and blurring of cognition. During World War II, German scientists developed the long-acting opioid methadone hydrochloride (SAMHSA, 2011b). Because of its longer action, it has a slower onset and does not cause euphoria. The United States acquired the rights to this drug after the war and, because the rate of relapse and potential for death from an opioid overdose is so high, began using it for pain management and for detoxification and maintenance in opioid dependency (SAMHSA, 2011b).

Because many view methadone as a replacement opioid, individuals treated with methadone have been

Table 21-2 PICOT Exemplar

What is your PICOT question?
In clients with an opioid dependency does medication assisted treatment (MAT) rather than psychotherapy provide better long-term (more than two years) recovery?

What database(s), years, and keywords were searched?
Databases searched included PubMed, CINAHL Complete, Medline with Full Text, Cochrane Central Register of Controlled Trials, Cochrane Database of Systematic Reviews, Cochrane Methodology Register, Health Business FullTEXT, Health Technology Assessments, PsycARTICLES, PsycINFO, Database of Abstracts of Reviews of Effects, Legal Collections, eBook Collection (EBSCOhost), Academic Search Premier, AHFC Consumer Medication Information, PsycTESTS, and ERIC. They were searched for the years 2010 through 2015 for the following keywords: *opioid dependency, opiate dependency, substance abuse*, and *addiction modified by medication-assisted treatment, psychopharmacology, and recovery*.

Citation	Subjects	Methods	Results	Rigor of Evidence	Applicable?	Cost?
Rapeli, Fabritius, Kalska, & Alho (2012)	Opioid- dependent individuals ages 18–50 on opioid substitution therapy (OST) for 6 months or more.	Volunteer. Cognitive tests for visual and verbal memory three hours after dose of methadone or buprenorphine.	Individuals taking buprenorphine had better results than those taking methadone. Methadone group was older. Some subjects in both groups taking other psychoactive drugs.	Moderate.	Yes, measured MAT effect on cognitive function.	Subjects paid for completion.
Fox et al. (2015)	Opioid- dependent individuals, history of incarceration, abstinent-based treatment setting.	Qualitative. Attitude toward buprenorphine maintenance treatment (BMT). One hour semistructured interview based on social cognitive theory.	Reentry to society is difficult. Relapse is frequent. It is important to offer BMT.	Small convenience sample.	Yes, measured attitude toward and benefit of MAT.	No mention.
Hser et al. (2014)	1,267 opioid- dependent individuals from nine separate treatment sites receiving methadone (MET) or buprenorphine (BUP).	Randomized control trial. Random assignment to MET or BUP. Participant characteristics and outcomes. Comparison to Cochrane review of similar trials.	Retention is higher with MET; retention is higher with higher doses of both; higher doses result is less use of other opioid drugs, BUP more than MET.	High.	Yes, measured effect of MAT on retention.	No mention.
Dennis et al. (2014)	Opioid- dependent individuals on some form of MAT.	Systematic review of articles about the various medication protocols.	None at this time.	Will be high for completed review.	No, only explains how they conducted their review.	No mention.
Mannelli, Peindl, Lee, Bhatia, & Wu (2012)	26 studies of opioid-dependent individuals switched from MET to BUP.	PubMed search of clinical investigations and conference papers.	Individuals can safely be switched from MET to BUP or MET to BUP to naltrexone (NAL).	Moderate.	Yes, availability of new psychotherapeutics requires new knowledge.	No mention.
Diaper, Law, & Melichar (2014)	Individuals undergoing detoxification from various psychoactive substances, including opioids.	Systematic review of articles about detoxification studies.	Psychosocial therapies along with the pharmacologic therapies are essential.	Evidence is limited by a lack of robust controlled trials.	Yes, detox occurs in all forms of opioid dependency treatment.	No mention.

(continued)

Table 21-2 PICOT Exemplar—cont'd

Citation	Subjects	Methods	Results	Rigor of Evidence	Applicable?	Cost?
Blum et al. (2014)	2,919 opioid-dependent individuals using at least one prescribed medication.	Retrospective quantitative analysis of urine drug screen (UDS) data from 6 eastern U.S. states.	Random UDSs are a crucial component for successful treatment.	High due to strong objective evidence.	Yes, speaks to adherence and treatment outcomes.	No mention.
Mauger, Fraser, & Gill (2014)	Studies dealing with opioid- dependent individuals receiving treatment with buprenorphine.	Systematic review using Medline and Cochrane database of systematic reviews.	BUP effective for short- and long-term use, decreases abuse, risk of health-related problems.	High, level 1 evidence.	Yes.	No mention.
Quest, Merrill, Roll, Saxon, & Rosenblatt, (2012)	Physicians in the first cohort to prescribe buprenorphine in rural Washington state.	Survey to determine volume of clients, efficacy of treatment, and perceived barriers.	24 of the 33 replied, 20 still prescribing, averaged 23 active clients, total of 125 treated, felt efficacy high with 95% recommendation for peers to prescribe. Barriers were lack of funding, local behavioral health providers, consultants to manage complex patients, and other physicians prescribing.	Self-report.	Yes.	No mention.
Harlow, Roman, Happell, & Browne (2013)	Policies on opioid replacement therapy (ORT) from the United States, Australia, and the United Kingdom	Hand search for articles on how ORT or MAT is accessed, who provides it, length of treatment need for more providers, and so on.	Australia ahead of the United States and the United Kingdom in some areas, no measure of quality, individuals wait for treatment.	Low.	No.	No mention.
O'Conner, Collett, Alto, & O'Brien (2013)	Infants born to opioid-dependent women.	Retrospective chart review breastfeeding and NAS.	Initially three-quarter of the women breastfed; at 6–8 weeks, two-thirds were breastfeeding. NAS less severe and less medication used.	Not statistically significant.	Yes.	No mention.
Wesson & Smith (2010)	Opioid-dependent individuals in clinical trials using placebo, methadone, or buprenorphine.	Systematic review of Cochrane reviews.	Buprenorphine effective but not more effective than methadone; best for initial treatment experience and those needing less structure.	High.	Yes.	No mention.

(continued)

Table 21-2 PICOT Exemplar—cont'd

Citation	Subjects	Methods	Results	Rigor of Evidence	Applicable?	Cost?
Tanner, Bordon, Conroy, & Best (2011)	Opioid-dependent individuals on buprenorphine or who had switched from methadone to buprenorphine.	Structured interviews.	Buprenorphine offers greater "clarity of thought" (seen as both positive and negative), switching can be the first step for detoxing from MAT, part of reintegration, will require additional support services.	Low, opportunistic data.	Yes.	No mention.
Saber-Tehrani, Bruce, & Altice (2011)	Opioid-dependent individuals receiving MAT and psychotropics.	Systematic review using 60 studies.	Array of interactions. Most serious, QT prolongation with methadone. More study indicated.	High.	Yes, many opioid-dependent individuals have comorbid psychiatric problems.	No mention.
Albizu-García, Caraballo, Caraballo-Correa, Hernández-Viver, & Román-Badenas (2012)	10,849 sentenced inmates from prisons in Puerto Rico, midyear 2004	Random selection of 1,331 inmates for computer-assisted personal interview (CAPI), Composite International Diagnostic Interview (CIDI), symptom scales for ADHD and PTSD, and Stages of Change Readiness and Treatment (SOCRATES)	80% of chosen completed. 308 were ready for treatment with only 44 slots available. High comorbidity of depression and ADHD.	High.	Yes, supports needed for treatment within criminal justice population.	No funding so self-report used for HIV rather than serologic testing.
Feelemyer, Jarlais, Arasteh, Abdul-Quader, & Hagan (2013)	Opioid-dependent individuals in MAT programs using methadone and buprenorphine in low- and middle-income countries.	International systematic review using systematic reviews and meta-analyses.	Average of 50% retention after 12 months with wide variation across programs but little difference between methadone and buprenorphine.	High.	Yes.	No mention.
D'Onofrio, et al. (2015)	329 opioid-dependent individuals treated at an urban teaching hospital emergency department (ED).	Randomized clinical trial. Three groups: referral, brief intervention, buprenorphine.	ED-initiated buprenorphine significantly increased engagement in treatment and decreased illicit opioid use.	High.	Yes, measured MAT versus brief intervention and referral.	No mention.

stigmatized. The Institute of Medicine (2001) report, *Crossing the Quality Chasm: A New Health System for the 21st Century*, and the designation of addiction as a brain disorder changed some of the approaches to treatment. Interest grew in developing other long-acting opioid medications that could be used to treat dependency and withdrawal. Three medications—methadone, buprenorphine, and naltrexone—are now available and have U.S. Federal Drug Administration (FDA) approval for use in MAT for opioid dependency.

Discussion of the Evidence

The results of a literature search showed that all three of these medications—methadone, buprenorphine, and naltrexone—are used for withdrawal symptoms and that individuals can be switched between medications as needed (Beheshti, 2014). Clients are less apt to relapse when supported pharmacologically as well as psychologically. Individuals coming from the criminal justice system have a particularly difficult time with reentry to society and have an easier time when on MAT. All three medications are appropriate for detox and short- and long-term use. Treatment programs must have structure, include psychotherapy and other recovery-oriented services, use urine drug screens, and match the needs of the client with the characteristic of the medication and the program.

Strengths and Limitations of the Body of Evidence

Much of the literature was composed of systematic reviews and meta-analyses; however, the data varied between randomized control trials (RCTs) and convenience studies. Some included volunteer populations, and one had clients who were paid to participate. Very little information is available regarding quality control within the programs. Several sources demonstrated that the field needed to do a better job of monitoring the quality of the programs.

Important Client Differences to Consider in Applying the Evidence in Practice

All the subjects involved were individuals with opioid dependency. Providers must consider the individual characteristics that would determine which medication or program would be the best fit. For example, does the client need a lot of or a little structure? Does he or she have an underlying physical problem that would make one medication a better fit than another? Does the client want or need to stay on MAT, or would he or she rather be weaned to an abstinence program? Is the client a pregnant female who needs to be on MAT to protect the fetus?

Areas Where Further Research Is Needed

Any research will add to the body of knowledge within the field and improve the expertise of health-care providers. Considerable research still needs to be conducted on optimum doses for retention and discontinuation of illicit substances. Programs continue to have their own internal stigma and commonly focus on getting clients off the medication before they have stabilized. No research has been conducted so far to support how long MAT should be continued, and internal quality improvement efforts are scant. Programs need to focus more on quality and patient safety for best outcomes.

Recommendations for Practice

The evidence supports MAT as best practice, and this knowledge must be disseminated as such within the entire health-care field. Clinical training should be held on the action and use of the medications used in MAT. Community education should be provided to disseminate information about addiction, dependency, and treatment with MAT to decrease stigma.

Risk, Costs, and Benefits of Applying the Evidence

Applying the evidence confers zero risk. The only cost is that of funding treatment. But because this would be a cost either way and because MAT could decrease recidivism, it is actually a cost-benefit. Other benefits include better treatment outcomes, lower disability and death rates, and increased productivity.

Feasibility and System Issues to Consider in Applying the Evidence

As mentioned, only one in five individuals needing treatment is able to receive it. Lack of funding and stigma are partially responsible, but the lack of facilities available for those needing and agreeing to go to treatment compounds the problem. Once individuals are in treatment, keeping them in long enough to receive adequate help may be difficult due to lack of funding and arbitrary limits on length of stay. More effort must be put into developing providers along a continuum of care, acknowledging that funding is needed for longer treatment experiences, recognizing that addiction is a chronic disease, and applying a recovery orientation to the system of care.

Key Stakeholders in Making Evidence-Based Practice Changes

The key stakeholders are the funding sources, opioid treatment staff members and administrators, policy makers, and community leaders. People in recovery also have much to add to this discussion.

Safe and Effective Care Planning Implications

Care planning must start with a complete assessment, integrate pharmacology and psychotherapy, add ancillary services as needed, and provide a continuum of care. Treatment must be adjusted to the needs of the clients and their progression in recovery.

Interprofessional Health Education Implications

All health-care providers need to be knowledgeable about the neurobiology of the disease of addiction, screening and brief intervention skills, and an understanding of all treatment modalities including MAT. Counselors may cover substance abuse in their undergraduate curriculum, but for nurses, this topic is most frequently part of graduate education, where it is included as an elective or a certificate program.

SUBSTANCE USE IN HEALTHY PEOPLE 2020

Since the first set of national Healthy People 2020 goals and objectives was introduced in 1979, few new topics have been added, although objectives have been revised and reviewed. From the beginning, the substance abuse and tobacco use topic areas have been separate (Fielding, Kumanyika, & Manderscheid, 2014). The stated goal for substance abuse is to reduce substance abuse to protect the health, safety, and quality of life for all, especially children. The specific objectives for the decade 2011 to 2020 can be found in Table 21-3. The goal for tobacco use is to reduce illness, disability, and death related to tobacco use and secondhand smoke. The specific objectives for the decade 2011 to 2020 can be found in Table 21-4.

Table 21-3 Healthy People 2020 Substance Abuse

Policy and Prevention	
SA-1 Reduce the proportion of adolescents who report that they rode, during the previous 30 days, with a driver who had been drinking alcohol.	
SA-2 Increase the proportion of adolescents never using substances.	SA-2.1 Increase the proportion of at-risk adolescents aged 12 to 17 years who, in the past year, refrained from using alcohol for the first time. SA-2.2 Increase the proportion of at-risk adolescents aged 12 to 17 years who, in the past year, refrained from using marijuana for the first time. SA-2.3 Increase the proportion of high school seniors never using substances—alcoholic beverages. SA-2.4 Increase the proportion of high school seniors never using substances—illicit drugs.
SA-3 Increase the proportion of adolescents who disapprove of substance abuse.	SA-3.1 Increase the proportion of adolescents who disapprove of having one or two alcoholic drinks nearly every day—8th graders. SA-3.2 Increase the proportion of adolescents who disapprove of having one or two alcoholic drinks nearly every day—10th graders. SA-3.3 Increase the proportion of adolescents who disapprove of having one or two alcoholic drinks nearly every day—12th graders. SA-3.4 Increase the proportion of adolescents who disapprove of trying marijuana or hashish once or twice—8th graders. SA-3.5 Increase the proportion of adolescents who disapprove of trying marijuana or hashish once or twice—10th graders. SA-3.6 Increase the proportion of adolescents who disapprove of trying marijuana or hashish once or twice—12th graders.
SA-4 Increase the proportion of adolescents who perceive great risk associated with substance abuse.	SA-4.1 Increase the proportion of adolescents aged 12 to 17 years perceiving great risk associated with substance abuse—consuming five or more alcoholic drinks at a single occasion once or twice a week. SA-4.2 Increase the proportion of adolescents aged 12 to 17 years perceiving great risk associated with substance abuse—smoking marijuana once per month. SA-4.3 Increase the proportion of adolescents aged 12 to 17 years perceiving great risk associated with substance abuse—using cocaine once per month.

(*continued*)

Table 21-3 Healthy People 2020 Substance Abuse—cont'd

SA-5 (Developmental) Increase the number of drug, driving while impaired (DWI), and other specialty courts in the United States.	
SA-6 Increase the number of states with mandatory ignition interlock laws for first and repeat impaired driving offenders in the United States.	
Screening and Treatment	
SA-7 Increase the number of admissions to substance abuse treatment for injection drug use.	
SA-8 Increase the proportion of persons who need alcohol and/or illicit drug treatment and received specialty treatment for abuse or dependence in the past year.	SA-8.1 Increase the proportion of persons who need illicit drug treatment and received specialty treatment for abuse or dependence in the past year. SA-8.2 Increase the proportion of persons who need alcohol and/or illicit drug treatment and received specialty treatment for abuse or dependence in the past year. SA-8.3 Increase the proportion of persons who need alcohol abuse or dependence treatment and received specialty treatment for abuse or dependence in the past year.
SA-9 (Developmental) Increase the proportion of persons who are referred for follow-up care for alcohol problems, drug problems after diagnosis, or treatment for one of these conditions in a hospital emergency department (ED).	
SA-10 Increase the number of Level I and Level II trauma centers and primary-care settings that implement evidence-based alcohol screening and brief intervention (SBI).	
Epidemiology and Surveillance	
SA-11 Reduce cirrhosis deaths.	
SA-12 Reduce drug-induced deaths.	
SA-13 Reduce past-month use of illicit substances.	SA-13.1 Reduce the proportion of adolescents reporting use of alcohol or any illicit drugs during the past 30 days. SA-13.2 Reduce the proportion of adolescents reporting use of marijuana during the past 30 days. SA-13.3 Reduce the proportion of adults reporting use of any illicit drug during the past 30 days.
SA-14 Reduce the proportion of persons engaging in binge drinking of alcoholic beverages.	SA-14.1 Reduce the proportion of students engaging in binge drinking during the past 2 weeks—high school seniors. SA-14.2 Reduce the proportion of students engaging in binge drinking during the past 2 weeks—college students. SA-14.3 Reduce the proportion of persons engaging in binge drinking during the past 30 days—adults aged 18 years and older. SA-14.4 Reduce the proportion of persons engaging in binge drinking during the past month—adolescents aged 12 to 17 years.
SA-15 Reduce the proportion of adults who drank excessively in the previous 30 days.	

Table 21-3 Healthy People 2020 Substance Abuse—cont'd

SA-16 Reduce average annual alcohol consumption.	
SA-17 Decrease the rate of alcohol-impaired driving (.08+ blood alcohol content [BAC]) fatalities.	
SA-18 Reduce steroid use among adolescents.	SA-18.1 Reduce steroid use among 8th graders. SA-18.2 Reduce steroid use among 10th graders. SA-18.3 Reduce steroid use among 12th graders.
SA-19 Reduce the past-year nonmedical use of prescription drugs.	SA-19.1 Reduce the past-year nonmedical use of pain relievers. SA-19.2 Reduce the past-year nonmedical use of tranquilizers. SA-19.3 Reduce the past-year nonmedical use of stimulants. SA-19.4 Reduce the past-year nonmedical use of sedatives. SA-19.5 Reduce the past-year nonmedical use of any psychotherapeutic drug (including pain relievers, tranquilizers, stimulants, and sedatives).
SA-20 Reduce the number of deaths attributable to alcohol.	
SA-21 Reduce the proportion of adolescents who use inhalants.	

Source: Office of Disease Prevention and Health Promotion (2016a).

Table 21-4 Healthy People 2020 Tobacco Use

	Tobacco Use
TU-1 Reduce tobacco use by adults.	TU-1.1 Reduce cigarette smoking by adults. TU-1.2 Reduce use of smokeless tobacco products by adults. TU-1.3 Reduce use of cigars by adults.
TU-2 Reduce tobacco use by adolescents.	TU-2.1 Reduce use of tobacco products by adolescents (past month). TU-2.2 Reduce use of cigarettes by adolescents (past month). TU-2.3 Reduce use of smokeless tobacco products by adolescents (past month). TU-2.4 Reduce use of cigars by adolescents (past month).
TU-3 Reduce the initiation of tobacco use among children, adolescents, and young adults.	TU-3.1 Reduce the initiation of the use of tobacco products among children and adolescents aged 12 to 17 years. TU-3.2 Reduce the initiation of the use of cigarettes among children and adolescents aged 12 to 17 years. TU-3.3 Reduce the initiation of the use of smokeless tobacco products by children and adolescents aged 12 to 17 years. TU-3.4 Reduce the initiation of the use of cigars by children and adolescents aged 12 to 17 years. TU-3.5 Reduce the initiation of the use of tobacco products by young adults aged 18 to 25 years. TU-3.6 Reduce the initiation of the use of cigarettes by young adults aged 18 to 25 years. TU-3.7 Reduce the initiation of the use of smokeless tobacco products by young adults aged 18 to 25 years. TU-3.8 Reduce the initiation of the use of cigars by young adults aged 18 to 25 years.
TU-4 Increase smoking cessation attempts by adult smokers.	TU-4.1 Increase smoking cessation attempts by adult smokers. TU-4.2 (Developmental) Increase smoking cessation attempts using evidence-based strategies by adult smokers.
TU-5 Increase recent smoking cessation success by adult smokers.	TU-5.1 Increase recent smoking cessation success by adult smokers. TU-5.2 (Developmental) Increase recent smoking cessation success by adult smokers using evidence-based strategies.

(continued)

Table 21-4 Healthy People 2020 Tobacco Use—cont'd

TU-6 Increase smoking cessation during pregnancy.	
TU-7 Increase smoking cessation attempts by adolescent smokers.	
	Health Systems Changes
TU-8 Increase comprehensive Medicaid insurance coverage of evidence-based treatment for nicotine dependency in the states and the District of Columbia.	
TU-9 Increase tobacco screening in health-care settings.	TU-9.1 Increase tobacco screening in office-based ambulatory-care settings. TU-9.2 Increase tobacco screening in hospital ambulatory-care settings. TU-9.3 Increase tobacco screening in dental-care settings. TU-9.4 Increase tobacco screening in substance abuse care settings.
TU-10 Increase tobacco cessation counseling in health-care settings.	TU-10.1 Increase tobacco cessation counseling in office-based ambulatory-care settings. TU-10.2 Increase tobacco cessation counseling in hospital ambulatory-care settings. TU-10.3 Increase tobacco cessation counseling in dental-care settings. TU-10.4 Increase tobacco cessation counseling in substance abuse care settings.
	Social and Environmental Changes
TU-11 Reduce the proportion of nonsmokers exposed to secondhand smoke.	TU-11.1 Reduce the proportion of children aged 3 to 11 years exposed to secondhand smoke. TU-11.2 Reduce the proportion of adolescents aged 12 to 17 years exposed to secondhand smoke. TU-11.3 Reduce the proportion of adults aged 18 years and older exposed to secondhand smoke.
TU-12 Increase the proportion of persons covered by indoor worksite policies that prohibit smoking.	
TU-13 Establish laws in the states, District of Columbia, territories, and tribal lands on smoke-free indoor air that prohibit smoking in public places and worksites.	TU-13.1 Establish laws in the states and the District of Columbia on smoke-free indoor air that prohibit smoking in private worksites. TU-13.2 Establish laws in the states and the District of Columbia on smoke-free indoor air that prohibit smoking in public worksites. TU-13.3 Establish laws in the states and the District of Columbia on smoke-free indoor air that prohibit smoking in restaurants. TU-13.4 Establish laws in the states and the District of Columbia on smoke-free indoor air that prohibit smoking in bars. TU-13.5 Establish laws in the states and the District of Columbia on smoke-free indoor air that prohibit smoking in gaming halls. TU-13.6 Establish laws in the states and the District of Columbia on smoke-free indoor air that prohibit smoking in commercial day-care centers. TU-13.7 Establish laws in the states and the District of Columbia on smoke-free indoor air that prohibit smoking in home-based day-care centers. TU-13.8 Establish laws in the states and the District of Columbia on smoke-free indoor air that prohibit smoking in public transportation. TU-13.9 Establish laws in the states and the District of Columbia on smoke-free indoor air that prohibit smoking in hotels and motels.

Table 21-4 Healthy People 2020 Tobacco Use—cont'd

	TU-13.10 Establish laws in the states and the District of Columbia on smoke-free indoor air that prohibit smoking in multi-unit housing. TU-13.11 Establish laws in the states and the District of Columbia on smoke-free indoor air that prohibit smoking in vehicles with children. TU-13.12 Establish laws in the states and the District of Columbia on smoke-free indoor air that prohibit smoking in prisons and correctional facilities. TU-13.13 Establish laws in the states and the District of Columbia on smoke-free indoor air that prohibit smoking in substance abuse treatment facilities. TU-13.14 Establish laws in the states and the District of Columbia on smoke-free indoor air that prohibit smoking in mental health treatment facilities. TU-13.15 Establish laws in the states and the District of Columbia on smoke-free indoor air that prohibit smoking in entrances and exits of all public places. TU-13.16 Establish laws in the states and the District of Columbia on smoke-free indoor air that prohibit smoking on hospital campuses. TU-13.17 Establish laws in the states and the District of Columbia on smoke-free indoor air that prohibit smoking on college and university campuses.
TU-14 Increase the proportion of smoke-free homes.	
TU-15 Increase tobacco-free environments in schools, including all school facilities, property, vehicles, and school events.	TU-15.1 Increase tobacco-free environments in junior high schools, including all school facilities, property, vehicles, and school events. TU-15.2 Increase tobacco-free environments in middle schools, including all school facilities, property, vehicles, and school events. TU-15.3 Increase tobacco-free environments in high schools, including all school facilities, property, vehicles, and school events. TU-15.4 (Developmental) Increase tobacco-free environments in Head Start, including all school facilities, property, vehicles, and school events.
TU-16 Eliminate state laws that preempt stronger local tobacco control laws.	TU-16.1 Eliminate state laws that preempt stronger local tobacco control laws on smoke-free indoor air. TU-16.2 Eliminate state laws that preempt stronger local tobacco control laws on advertising. TU-16.3 Eliminate state laws that preempt stronger local tobacco control laws on youth access.
TU-17 Increase the federal and state taxes on tobacco products.	TU-17.1 Increase the federal and state taxes on cigarettes. TU-17.2 Increase the federal and state taxes on smokeless tobacco products. TU-17.3 (Developmental) Increase the federal and state taxes on other smoked tobacco products.
TU-18 Reduce the proportion of adolescents and young adults in grades 6 through 12 who are exposed to tobacco marketing.	TU-18.1 Reduce the proportion of adolescents and young adults in grades 6 through 12 who are exposed to tobacco marketing on the Internet. TU-18.2 Reduce the proportion of adolescents and young adults in grades 6 through 12 who are exposed to tobacco marketing in magazines and newspapers. TU-18.3 Reduce the proportion of adolescents and young adults in grades 6 through 12 who are exposed to tobacco marketing in movies and television. TU-18.4 Reduce the proportion of adolescents and young adults in grades 6 through 12 who are exposed to tobacco marketing at point of purchase (convenience store, supermarket, or gas station).
TU-19 Reduce the illegal sales rate to minors through enforcement of laws prohibiting the sale of tobacco products to minors.	TU-19.1 Reduce the illegal sales rate to minors through enforcement of laws prohibiting the sale of tobacco products to minors in the states and the District of Columbia. TU-19.2 Reduce the illegal sales rate to minors through enforcement of laws prohibiting the sale of tobacco products to minors in the territories.

(continued)

Table 21-4 Healthy People 2020 Tobacco Use—cont'd

TU-20 (Developmental) Increase the number of states, territories, and tribal lands with sustainable and comprehensive evidence-based tobacco control programs, and include the District of Columbia.	TU-20.1 (Developmental) Increase the number of states, and include the District of Columbia, with sustainable and comprehensive evidence-based tobacco control programs. TU-20.2 (Developmental) Increase the number of territories with sustainable and comprehensive evidence-based tobacco control programs. TU-20.3 (Developmental) Increase the number of Tribal lands with sustainable and comprehensive evidence-based tobacco control programs.

Source: Office of Disease Prevention and Health Promotion (2016b).

National Guidelines

As the Healthy People initiative has evolved, expanded knowledge about the social determinants of health has increased the awareness of health disparities. The Institute of Medicine (2001) report *Crossing the Quality Chasm: A New Health System for the 21st Century* drew even more attention to health disparities, the failure of the current health-care system, and the lack of consistency in treatment approaches. Clearly, to improve the quality of care, an evidence-based approach to health promotion, disease prevention, and treatment is needed (Mayberry, Nicewander, Qin, & Ballard, 2006). Performance and outcome measurements are being developed, and national guidelines are being established (NIDA, 2012).

The SAMHSA Center for Substance Abuse Treatment (CSAT) has been providing best practice guidelines through a series of publications known as Treatment Improvement Protocols (TIPs) since the early 1990s. They are developed by expert panels composed of subject matter experts in the treatment of substance use disorders, frontline clinical staff working directly with individuals in a variety of substance-related settings, and researchers who are studying the disease of addiction (CSAT, n. d.). All of the TIPs in this series can be ordered or downloaded in electronic format from the SAMHSA store, National Center for Biotechnology Information, U.S. National Library of Medicine, and National Institutes of Health.

In 2005, SAMHSA's Center for the Application of Prevention Technologies (CAPT) implemented a Service to Science initiative. Although it was focused on SAMHSA priorities, the Service to Science initiative was beneficial in raising the awareness of the community about the importance of the evidence, providing expected performance and outcome measurements, and acknowledging evidence-based programs. This effort grew into additional change initiatives for SAMHSA and more of a focus on evidence-based practice (SAMHSA, 2011a. As a result, SAMHSA established the National Registry of Evidence-Based Programs and Practices (NREPP). Although not a complete inventory, it offers a searchable database (at http://www.nrepp.samhsa.gov/) of more than 340 evidence-based mental health and substance abuse interventions.

NIDA has a number of publications. One of the most comprehensive is the *Principles of Drug Addiction Treatment: A Research Based Guide*. It was last reviewed in late 2012 and is currently in its third edition (NIDA, 2018).

Many other organizations have also developed guidelines for the treatment of substance abuse disorders and libraries of treatment resources, including.

- ASAM: http://www.asam.org/for-the-public/treatment
- American Psychological Association (APA): http://apa.org/practice/guidelines/index.aspx
- American Psychiatric Association: http://psychiatryonline.org/guidelines

USEFUL RESOURCES

Clinicians have many demands on their time and frequently find it difficult to stay up-to-date in the field. The following information takes the guesswork out of searching for the latest diagnostic tools, recent information, and assistance in meeting criteria as a treatment provider.

Assessment Tools

Many sources for screening and assessment tools are in the public domain, so purchase is not necessary. Making your own tool is also feasible if you know what your regulatory agency requires. SAMHSA is one of the best sources for assessment tools. The SAMHSA-Health Resources and Services Administration (HRSA) Center for Integrated Solutions offers an entire Web page (http://www.integration.samhsa.gov/clinical-practice/screening-tools) devoted to resources; sample screening forms; and screening tools for depression, drug and alcohol use, bipolar disorder, suicide risk, anxiety disorders, and trauma. For example, a TIP publication discusses screening and assessment for adolescents with substance use disorders. TIPs for specific populations include screening and assessment tools for those populations, co-occurring disorders, opioid dependency, and women, to name a few.

NIDA's NIDAMED is specifically for medical and health professionals. This section includes many tools and resources. A mini-section titled Screening, Assessment, and Drug Testing Resources (http://www.drugabuse.gov/nidamed-medical-health-professionals/tool-resources-your-practice/additional-screening-resources) includes a chart of evidence-based screening tools. This section has links to all the resources and documents.

No resource list for screening and assessment would be complete without mention of the ATTC SBIRT Web site (http://www.attcnetwork.org/national-focus-areas/?rc=sbirt), which is sponsored by SAMHSA. This site contains links to lists of qualified trainers, webinars, online resources, and downloadable products, and a toolkit. The ATTC SBIRT Web site is staffed by IRETA (ireta.org). Additional resources are available on the IRETA Web site (http://ireta.org/improve-practice/health-and-human-service-professionals/screening-brief-intervention-and-referral-to-treatment/sbirt-suite-of-services/).

Client Education Materials

One of the sources of provider and client education resources is NIDA, whose Web site contains sections devoted to medical professionals, clients and families, parents and educators, researchers, and children and teens. Within those sections, the general information pages, like Drugs of Abuse, Related Topics, Funding, and Publications are refined to meet the audience. The Drugs of Abuse section has a breakdown for each drug and an emerging trends section that includes the National Drug Early Warning System (NDEWS) Network (http://www.drugabuse.gov/related-topics/trends-statistics/national-drug-early-warning-system-ndews), where anyone can sign up to be notified about the specific trends in drug use for their area. Fact sheets and publications on the site are directed toward the medical professional, the media, the client's family and friends, and the client. They are easy to find and download.

The SAMHSA Web site (http://www.samhsa.gov and http://www.samhsa.gov/atod) is another comprehensive source of information related to alcohol, tobacco, and other drugs with links to annual surveys, publications, fact sheets, and treatment providers. One page has a listing with active links to every program and campaign SAMHSA is involved with, and each of the pages or sections for those programs and campaigns gives additional information and links. Several downloadable apps have also been developed.

SPECIALTY CERTIFICATION CRITERIA

Professionals who possess the specialty knowledge, skills, and abilities to provide effective, evidence-based interventions and treatments to clients affected by substance use or abuse often choose, or are required, to become certified or credentialed in addiction. Specialty nursing certification for addictions nursing practice is available at the generalist level as a Certified Addictions Registered Nurse (CARN) and at the advanced level as a Certified Addictions Registered Nurse–Advanced Practice (CARN-AP). These certifications are available through the Addictions Nursing Certification Board (ANCB) at http://www.intnsa.org/certification/ancb_board for nurses who work in the substance use and abuse treatment field or who work in other settings with clients and families affected by the disease of addiction. Exams are administered by the Center for Nursing Education and Testing (C-Net). These exams were accredited by the Accreditation Board for Specialty Nursing Certification (ABSNC) in 2018.

Certification as a TTS is available for individuals providing services to clients who may be using, abusing, or dependent on tobacco. Like other substance abuse professionals, TTSs may come from a variety of disciplines and professional affiliations, may work in a variety of settings, or may be educators or researchers. ATTUD is a professional organization supporting the establishment of standards and competencies to be used in determining how best to deliver effective, evidence-based interventions for tobacco dependency. ATTUD is not a certifying body, nor does it promote certification, but it does provide a set of competencies to guide states working on certification criteria, agencies developing treatment programs, and individuals seeking to be certified and work in this field. Some of the core competencies may also be used to guide the development of health promotion programs.

KEY POINTS

- Substance misuse refers to the improper use of medications when seeking therapeutic results; abuse is repeated and willful substance use for the purpose of pleasure, euphoria, and ecstasy.
- Nurses and health-care providers should be familiar with the SBIRT framework to intervene with clients seeking help with substance abuse.
- Addiction to heroin and prescription opiates is a major public health issue leading to significant loss of life and financial cost to society.
- Research on MAT shows that many successfully overcome opioid addiction with a combination of pharmaceutical opioid replacement and psychological support.
- National organizations such as SAMHSA CSAT provide guidelines on best practices and treatment modalities for busy practitioners who see individuals suffering from addiction.
- Specialty certifications are available for nurses and health-care professionals who want to focus on caring for individuals who struggle with addiction.

Check Your Understanding

1. Addiction is a:
   A. Moral failing
   B. Disease
   C. Choice
   D. Social disorder

2. Dependency is possible:
   A. With any substance
   B. If there is a preexisting mental health disorder
   C. With any psychoactive drug
   D. Only after a brain injury

3. Synthetic substances ________________ the substances they mimic.
   A. Have the same properties as
   B. Are regulated the same way as
   C. Are safer to use than
   D. Are more dangerous than

4. Drugs are considered psychoactive when they:
   A. Affect the neurotransmitters in the brain
   B. Cause a mental health disorder
   C. Trigger psychosis
   D. Affect someone only if she or he is exercising

5. ____________ is the costliest drug as far as loss of life and productivity.
   A. Heroin
   B. Tobacco
   C. Marijuana
   D. Xanax

6. The costs related to drug use and abuse, including health care, lost productivity, crime, incarceration, and enforcement of laws, were over _______ in 2014.
   A. $1 million
   B. $1 billion
   C. $700 billion
   D. $500 million

7. Only one-_____ of individuals diagnosed as needing substance abuse treatment receive it.
   A. Fifth
   B. Half
   C. Third
   D. Tenth

8. The national initiative for early intervention is:
   A. The Intervention Project
   B. SBIRT
   C. National Screening Day
   D. Community Outreach

9. The medication used to treat an opioid overdose is __________.
   A. Methadone
   B. Buprenorphin
   C. Naloxone
   D. Naltrexone

10. Evidence-based practice for treating an opioid dependency supports the use of medication and ____________.
    A. Psychotherapy
    B. Incarceration
    C. Inpatient treatment
    D. House arrest

See "Reflections on Check Your Understanding" at the end of the book for answers.

REFERENCES

Ahmad, F. B., Rossen, L. M., Spencer, M. R., Warner, M., & Sutton, P. (2018). Provisional drug overdose death counts. National Center for Health Statistics. Retrieved from https://www.cdc.gov/nchs/nvss/vsrr/drug-overdose-data.htm

Albizu-García, C. E., Caraballo, J. N., Caraballo-Correa, G., Hernández-Viver, A., & Román-Badenas, L. (2012). Assessing need for medication-assisted treatment for opiate-dependent prison inmates. *Substance Abuse*, *33*, 60–69.

American Society of Addiction Medicine. (2011). *ASAMNews* 26(3), 1–23.

American Society of Addiction Medicine. (2011, August 15). *Public policy statement: definition of addiction*. Retrieved from http://www.asam.org/for-the-public/definition-of-addiction

Baird, C. (2014). Guest editorial: Prescription drugs or heroin: The overdoses continue. *Journal of Addictions Nursing (JAN)* 25(2), (63)–(65).

Beheshti, S. (2014, Nov 9). Controversies of Using Buprenorphine for Maintenance in Opioid Dependency. Published on Psychiatric Times 3 pages (http://www.psychiatrictimes.com).

Birnbaum, H. G., White, A. G., Schiller, M., Waldman, T., Cleveland, J. M., & Roland, C. L. (2011). Societal Costs of Prescription Opioid Abuse, Dependence, and Misuse in the United States. *Pain medicine*, *12*, 657–667. Retrieved from http://www.asam.org/docs/advocacy/societal-costs-of-prescription-opioid-abuse-dependence-and-misuse-in-the-united-states.pdf

Blum, K., Han, D., Femino, J., Smith, D. E., Saunders, S., Simpatico, T., . . . Gold, M. S. (2014, September 23). Systematic evaluation of "compliance" to prescribed treatment medications and "abstinence" from psychoactive drug abuse in chemical dependence programs: Data from the comprehensive analysis of reported drugs. *PLoS One*, *9*(9), e104275.

Center for Substance Abuse Treatment. (n.d.). *Treatment improvement protocol (TIP) series*. Substance Abuse and Mental Health Services Administration (SAMHSA), U.S. Department of Health and Human Services. Retrieved from http://www.ncbi.nlm.nih.gov/books/NBK82999/ and http://store.samhsa.gov/list/series?name=TIP-Series-Treatment-Improvement-Protocols-TIPs

Centers for Disease Control and Prevention. (2018). Tobacco-related mortality. Retrieved from https://www.cdc.gov/tobacco/data_statistics/fact_sheets/health_effects/tobacco_related_mortality/

Centers for Disease Control and Prevention. (2019a, Nov 1). 2019 Annual Surveillance Report of Drug-Related Risks and Outcomes — United States Surveillance Special Report. Centers for Disease Control and Prevention, U.S. Department of Health and Human Services. Accessed June 6, 2020 from https://www. cdc.gov/drugoverdose/pdf/ pubs/2019-cdc-drug-surveillancereport.pdf.

Centers for Disease Control and Prevention. (2019b). Burden of tobacco use in the U.S. Retrieved from https://www.cdc.gov/tobacco/campaign/tips/resources/data/cigarette-smoking-in-united-states.html

Centers for Disease Control and Prevention. (2019c). Economic trends in tobacco. Retrieved from https://www.cdc.gov/tobacco/data_statistics/fact_sheets/economics/econ_facts/

Cicero, T. J., & Ellis, M. S. (2015, March). Abuse-deterrent formulations and the prescription opioid abuse epidemic in the United States. *JAMA Psychiatry*, 2015; 72(5):424–430. doi:10.1001/jamapsychiatry.2014.3043

Davis, C. (2015, March). *Legal interventions to reduce overdose mortality: Naloxone Good Samaritan laws*. Network for Public Health Law. Robert Wood Johnson Foundation. Retrieved from https://www.networkforphl.org/_asset/qz5pvn/legal-interventions-to-reduce-overdose.pdf

Dennis, B. B., Naji, L., Bawor, M., Bonner, A., Varenbut, M., Daiter, J., . . . Thabane, L. (2014, September 18). The effectiveness of opioid substitution treatments for patients with opioid dependence: A systematic review and multiple treatment comparison protocol. *Systematic Reviews*, *3*, 105.

Diaper, A. M., Law, F. D., & Melichar, J. K. (2014, February). Pharmacological strategies for detoxification. *British Journal of Clinical Pharmacology*, 77(2), 302–314.

D'Onofrio, G., O'Connor, P. G., Pantalon, M. V., Chawarski, M. C. Busch, S. H., Owens, P. H., . . . Fiellin, D. A. (2015). Emergency department–initiated buprenorphine/naloxone treatment for opioid dependence: A randomized clinical trial. *JAMA*, 313(16), 1636–1644. doi:10.1001/jama.2015.3474

Executive Office of the President of the United States. (2011). *Epidemic: Responding to America's prescription drug abuse crisis*. Retrieved from http://www.whitehouse.gov/sites/default/files/ondcp/issues-content/prescription-drugs/rx_abuse_plan.pdf

Farsalinos, K. E., & Polosa, R. (2014). Safety evaluation and risk assessment of electronic cigarettes as tobacco cigarette substitutes: A systematic review. *Therapeutic Advances in Drug Safety*, *5*(2), 67–86. doi:10.1177/2042098614524430

Feelemyer, J., Jarlais, D. D., Arasteh, K., Abdul-Quader, A. S., & Hagan, H. (2013). Retention of participants in medication-assisted programs in low- and middle-income countries: an international systematic review. *Addiction*, *109*, 20–32.

Fielding, J. E., Kumanyika, S., & Manderscheid, R. W. (2014). A perspective on the development of the Healthy People 2020 framework for improving U.S. population health. *Public Health Reviews*, *35(1)*, 1–24. Retrieved from http://www.publichealthreviews.eu/upload/pdf_files/13/00_Fielding.pdf

Fox, A. D., Maradiaga, J., Weiss, L., Sanchez, J., Starrels, J. L., & Cunningham, C. O. (2015, January 16). Release from incarceration, relapse to opioid use and the potential for buprenorphine maintenance treatment: A qualitative study of the perceptions of former inmates with opioid use disorder. *Addiction Science and Clinical Practice*, *10*(1), 2.

Furek, M. W. (2008). *The death proclamation of Generation X: A self-fulfilling prophecy of goth, grunge, and heroin*. New York: Universe, Inc.

Green, L. W., & Allegrante, J. P. (2011). *Healthy People* 1980–2020: Raising the ante decennially or just the name from public health education to health promotion to social determinants? *Health Education & Behavior*, *38*(6), 558–562. Retrieved from http://www.healthedpartners.org/ceu/lhi/hp1980-2020.pdf

Harlow, W., Roman, M. W., Happell, B., & Browne, G. (2013). Accessibility versus quality of care plus retention: The formula for service delivery in Australian opioid replacement therapy? *Issues in Mental Health Nursing*, *34*, 706–714.

Hedegaard, H., Chen, L. H., & Warner, M. (2015). Drug-poisoning deaths involving heroin: United States, 2000–2013. NCHS Data Brief, no 190. Hyattsville, MD:

National Center for Health Statistics. Retrieved from http://www.cdc.gov/nchs/products/databriefs.htm

Hser, Y-I., Saxon, A. J., Huang, D., Hasson, A., Thomas, C., Hillhouse, M., . . . Ling, W. (2014, January). Treatment retention among patients randomized to buprenorphine /naloxone compared to methadone in a multi-site trial. *Addiction,109*(1), 79–87.

Institute of Medicine. (2001). *Crossing the quality chasm: A new health system for the 21st century.* Washington, DC National Academy Press.

Johnston, L. D., O'Malley, P. M., Miech, R. A., Bachman, J. G., & Schulenberg, J. E. (2015). *Monitoring the Future national survey results on drug use:1975–2014: Overview, key findings on adolescent drug use*. Ann Arbor, MI: Institute for Social Research.

Kane, I., Mitchell, A. M., Puskar, K. R., Hagle, H., Talcott, K., Fioravanti, M, . . . Lindsay, D. (2014). Identifying at risk individuals for drug and alcohol dependence: Teaching the competency to students in classroom and clinical settings. *Nurse Educator, 39*(3), 126–134.

Mannelli, P., Peindl, K. S., Lee, T., Bhatia, K. S., & Wu, L-T. (2012, March). Buprenorphine-mediated transition from opioid agonist to antagonist treatment: State of the art and new perspectives. *Current Drug Abuse Review, 5*(1), 52–63.

Marusich, J. A., Antonazzo, K. R., Wiley, J. L., Blough, B. E., Partilla, J. S., & Baumann, M. H. (2014). Pharmacology of novel synthetic stimulants structurally related to the "bath salts" constituent 3,4-methylenedioxypyrovalerone (MDPV). *Neuropharmacology*, 87, 206–213. http://dx.doi .org/10.1016/j.neuropharm.2014.02.016

Mauger, S., Fraser, R., & Gill, K. (2014). Utilizing buprenorphine–naloxone to treat illicit and prescription-opioid dependence. *Neuropsychiatric Disorders Treatment, 10*, 587–598.

Mayberry, R. M., Nicewander, D. A., Qin, H., & Ballard, D. J. (2006). Improving quality and reducing inequities: A challenge in achieving best care. *Proceedings (Baylor University. Medical Center), 19*(2), 103–118.

Mitchell, A. M., Hagle, H., Puskar, K., Kane, I., Lindsay, D., Talcott, K., . . . Goplerud, E. (2015). Alcohol and other drug use screenings by nurse practitioners: Clinical issues and costs. *The Journal for Nurse Practitioners, 11*(3), 347–355.

Mitchell, A. M., Puskar, K., Hagle, H., Gotham, H. J., Talcott, K. S., Terhorst, L., . . . Burns, H. K. (2013). Screening, brief intervention, and referral to treatment: Overview of and student satisfaction with an undergraduate addiction training program for nurses. *Journal of Psychosocial Nursing and Mental Health Services, 51*(10), 29–37.

National Center for Injury Control and Prevention. (2011, November). *Policy impact: Prescription pain killer overdoses.* Centers for Disease Control. Retrieved from http://www .cdc.gov/homeandrecreationalsafety/rxbrief/

National Center for Injury Control and Prevention. (2014, January). *Drug overdose.* Centers for Disease Control. Retrieved from http://www.cdc.gov/homeandrecreational safety/overdose/

National Council State Boards of Nursing. (2018). *A profile of nursing licensure in the US.* Retrieved from https://www .ncsbn.org/6161.htm

National Drug Intelligence Center. (2014). *National drug threat assessment.* Washington, DC: United States Department of Justice. Retrieved from http://www.justice .gov/archive/ndic/pubs44/44849/44849p.pdf

National Institute on Drug Abuse. (2012). *Principles of drug addiction treatment: A research based guide* (3rd ed.). NIH Publication No. 12–4180. Retrieved from http://www .drugabuse.gov/sites/default/files/podat_1.pdf

National Institute on Drug Abuse. (2014). A media guide. Public Information and Liaison Branch. Office of Science Policy and Communications. The National Institute on Drug Abuse. Retrieved from http://www.drugabuse.gov/publications /media-guide/science-drug-abuse-addiction-basics

National Institute on Drug Abuse. (2015, February). Hallucinogens and dissociative drugs including LSD, psilocybin, peyote, DMT, ayahuasca, PCP, ketamine, dextromethorphan, and salvia. National Institutes of Health Publication Number 15-4209.

National Institute on Drug Abuse. (2017, April 24). Trends & statistics. Retrieved from https://www.drugabuse.gov /related-topics/trends-statistics

National Institute on Drug Abuse. (2018, January 17). Principles of drug addiction treatment: A research-based guide (3rd ed.). Retrieved from https://www.drugabuse .gov/publications/principles-drug-addiction-treatment -research-based-guide-third-edition

National Institute on Drug Abuse. (2020a, May 11). COVID-19 Resources. Retrieved from https://www .drugabuse.gov/related-topics/covid-19-resources on 2020, June 6

National Institute on Drug Abuse. (2020b, March 10). Overdose Death Rates. Retrieved from https://www .drugabuse.gov/related-topics/trends-statistics/overdose -death-rates on 2020, June 6.

O'Conner, A. B., Collett, A., Alto, W. A., & O'Brien, L. M. (2013, July–August). Breastfeeding rates and the relationship between breastfeeding and neonatal abstinence syndrome in women maintained on buprenorphine during pregnancy. *Journal of Midwifery & Women's Health, 58*(4), 383–388.

Office of Disease Prevention and Health Promotion. (2016a). Heart disease and stroke: Substance abuse. In *Healthy People 2020.* Retrieved from https://www.healthypeople .gov/2020/leading-health-indicators/2020-lhi-topics /Substance-Abuse

Office of Disease Prevention and Health Promotion. (2016b). Heart disease and stroke: Tobacco. In *Healthy People 2020.* Retrieved from https://www.healthypeople.gov/2020 /leading-health-indicators/2020-lhi-topics/Tobacco

Office of National Drug Control Policy. (2012, July). *Screening, brief intervention, and referral to treatment (SBIRT): A fact sheet.* Substance Abuse Mental Health Services Administration. Retrieved from www .WhiteHouse.gov/ONDCP

Public Health Service. (1979). Healthy people: The Surgeon General's report on health promotion and disease prevention. Washington, DC: US Department of Health, Education, and Welfare. Public Health Service, DHEW publication no. (PHS)79-55071.

Public Health Service. (1980). Promoting health/preventing disease: Objectives for the nation. Washington, DC: US

Department of Health and Human Services, Public Health Service.

Quest, T. L., Merrill, J. O., Roll, J., Saxon, A. J., &. Rosenblatt, R. A. (2012, January–February). Buprenorphine therapy for opioid addiction in rural Washington: The experience of the early adopters. *Journal of Opioid Management, 8*(1), 29–38.

Rapeli, P., Fabritius, C., Kalska, H., & Alho, H. (2012). Do drug treatment variables predict cognitive performance in multidrug-treated opioid-dependent patients? A regression analysis study. *Substance Abuse Treatment Prevention Policy,* 7(45), https://doi.org/10.1186/1747-597X-7-45

Rudd, R. A., Seth, P., David, F., & Scholl, D. (2016, December 30). Mortality and morbidity weekly report: Increases in drug and opioid-involved overdose deaths—United States, 2010–2015. *US Department of Health and Human Services /Centers for Disease Control and Prevention 65*(50 & 51), 144–152.

Saber-Tehrani, A. S., Bruce, R. D., & Altice, F. L. (2011). Pharmacokinetic drug interactions and adverse consequences between psychotropic medications and pharmacotherapy for the treatment of opioid dependence. *The American Journal of Drug and Alcohol Abuse, 37*, 1–11.

Schifano, F., Orsolini, L., Papanti, G. D., & Corkery, J. M. (2015). Novel psychoactive substances of interest for psychiatry. *World Psychiatry, 14*, 15–26.

Strobbe, S., & Broyles, L. M. (2013, May). *Expanded roles and responsibilities for nurses in screening, brief intervention, and referral to treatment (SBIRT) for alcohol use: A joint position statement.* International Nurses Society on Addictions (IntNSA) and the Emergency Nurses Association (ENA). Retrieved from http://www.intnsa.org/resources/publications/position_may_2013.pdf

Substance Abuse and Mental Health Services Administration. (2011a). *Leading change: A plan for SAMHSA's roles and actions 2011–2014.* HHS Publication No. (SMA) 11-4629. Rockville, MD: Author.

Substance Abuse and Mental Health Services Administration. (2011b). *Medication-assisted treatment for opioid addiction.* Knowledge Application Program (KAP), a Joint Venture of The CDM Group, Inc., and JBS International, Inc., under contract number 270-04-7049, with SAMHSA, U.S. Department of Health and Human Services (HHS).

Substance Abuse and Mental Health Services Administration. (2013). *Opioid overdose prevention toolkit.* HHS Publication No. (SMA) 13-4742. Rockville, MD: Author.

Substance Abuse and Mental Health Services Administration. (2014a). *Results from the 2013 National Survey on Drug Use and Health: Summary of national findings*, NSDUH Series H-48, HHS Publication No. (SMA) 14-4863. Rockville, MD: Author. Retrieved from http://www.samhsa.gov/data/sites/default/files/NSDUHresultsPDFWHTML2013/Web/NSDUHresults2013.pdf

Substance Abuse and Mental Health Services Administration. (2014b). *Screening, brief intervention, and referral to treatment (SBIRT).* Retrieved from http://www.samhsa.gov/sbirt

Substance Abuse and Mental Health Services Administration. (2019). *Key substance use and mental health indicators in the United States: Results from the 2018 National Survey on Drug Use and Health* (HHS Publication No. PEP19-5068, NSDUH Series H-54). Rockville, MD: Center for Behavioral Health Statistics and Quality, Substance Abuse and Mental Health Services Administration. Retrieved from https://www.samhsa.gov/data/

Sussan, T. E., Gajghate, S., Thimmulappa, R. K., Ma, J., Kim, J-H., Sudini, K., . . . Biswal, S. (2015). Exposure to electronic cigarettes impairs pulmonary anti-bacterial and anti-viral defenses in a mouse model. *PLoS ONE 10*(2): e0116861. doi:10.1371/journal.pone.0116861

Tanner, G. R., Bordon, N., Conroy, S., & Best, D. (2011, June). Comparing methadone and suboxone in applied treatment settings: The experiences of maintenance patients in Lanarkshire. *Journal of Substance Use, 16*(3), 171–178.

Trust for America's Health. (2013, October). *Prescription drug abuse: Strategies to stop the epidemic.* Robert Wood Johnson Foundation. Retrieved from www.healthyamericans.org/reports/drugabuse2013/

United Nations Office on Drugs and Crime. (2012, June). *World drug report 2012.* United Nations publication, Sales No. E.12.XI.1. Retrieved from http://www.unodc.org/documents/data-and-analysis/WDR2012/WDR_2012_web_small.pdf

United Nations Office on Drugs and Crime. (2017, June). *World drug report 2017.* United Nations publication, Sales No. E.17.XI.6. Retrieved from https://www.unodc.org/wdr2017/field/Booklet_1_EXSUM.pdf

United States Census Bureau. (2019). State and county quick facts. Retrieved from https://www.census.gov/quickfacts/fact/table/US/PST045219.

USAFacts. (2020). *Population: How is the population changing*? Penn Wharton Budget Model and the Stanford Institute for Economic Policy Research (SIEPR). https://usafacts.org/state-of-the-union/population/

U.S. Department of Health and Human Services. (2014). *The health consequences of smoking—50 years of progress.* A Report of the Surgeon General. Atlanta, GA: U.S. Department of Health and Human Services, Centers for Disease Control and Prevention, National Center for Chronic Disease Prevention and Health Promotion, Office on Smoking and Health.

Ventura, L., Carvalho, F., & Dinis-Oliveira, R. J. (2018). Opioids in the frame of new psychoactive substances network: A complex pharmacological and toxicological issue. *Current Molecular Pharmacology*. 11(2):97–108. edoi: 10.2174/1874467210666170704110146

Weaver, M. F., Hopper, J. A., & Gunderson, E. W. (2015). Designer drugs 2015: Assessment and management. *Addiction Science & Clinical Practice, 10*(8). doi:10.1186/s13722-015-0024-7

Wesson, D. R., & Smith, D. E. (2010, June). Buprenorphine in the treatment of opiate dependence. *Journal of Psychoactive Drugs,42*(2), 161–175.

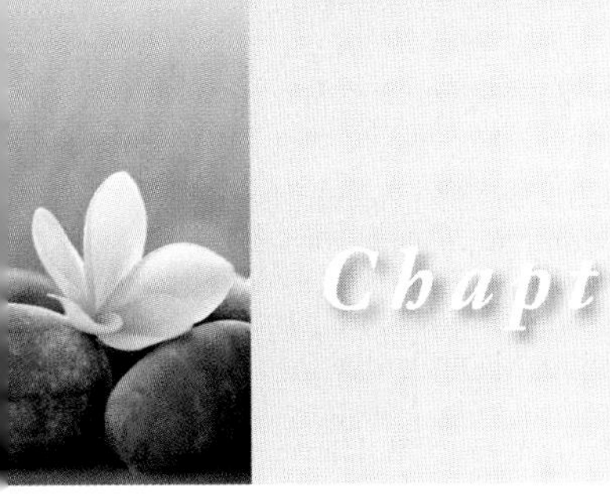

Chapter 22

Health Promotion and Palliative Care

Susan Breakwell

LEARNING OBJECTIVES

After completing this chapter, the student will be able to:

1. Describe the relationship between palliative care, hospice, and end-of-life care within the context of current health-care issues.
2. Distinguish between primary and specialty palliative care.
3. Discuss palliative care in relationship to health promotion.
4. Identify opportunities for incorporating primary palliative care, including advance-care planning, into health promotion endeavors.

INTRODUCTION

The limited attention to palliative and end-of-life care in health promotion is increasing as the rise in the number of individuals affected by serious, chronic, or terminal illness continues to outpace the number of palliative-care specialists. Although palliative-care, hospice, and end-of-life care are related, palliative care is the broadest of the three because it is both a philosophy and system of the whole person and family-focused care that can be applied at any time along the health–illness continuum. It encompasses an array of services: some begin before diagnosis or early in the course of a serious illness; some center around hospice and end-of-life services and are typically provided during the last months or days of life and extend into the family's bereavement period. The continued growth of palliative care presents new, untapped health promotion opportunities for nurses and health-care providers.

Recent figures show that the daily functional abilities and quality of life of 49.8% of individuals in the United States are directly affected by at least one serious or chronic condition; 20% of individuals have multiple chronic conditions (Ward, Schiller, & Goodman, 2014). More than 90% of individuals die of chronic diseases, including cancer and cardiovascular, pulmonary, and neurologic disease, often with an extended and unpredictable trajectory. A staggering 80% of U.S. health-care spending is concentrated in the last months of life, often on individuals with one or more chronic conditions (Institute of Medicine [IOM], 2015; Morrison, Deitrich, & Meier, 2008). These chronic diseases and serious illnesses are often complex, associated with multiple disease and treatment-related symptoms, costly to manage, and likely to benefit from earlier integration of a palliative approach to care.

The impact of serious illness and chronic disease is not limited to the United States. According to global figures for 2011 from the Worldwide Palliative Care Alliance (WPCA) and World Health Organization (WHO), approximately 29 million people (94% adults and 6% children) died from a disease that would have benefitted from inclusion of palliative care (WPCA & WHO, 2014). In the United States, 10 of the 15 leading causes of death are due to chronic cardiovascular, respiratory, renal, liver, or neurological diseases (Xu, Murphy, Kochanek, Bastiana, & Arias, 2018). With the impact of serious, chronic, and terminal illness on individuals, families, communities, and health-care systems, the need to incorporate palliation into multiple levels of care, including individuals of all ages, families, communities, and systems, could not be more pressing (IOM, 2015; WHO, 2017). A study of palliative care needs in 12 countries, including the United States and Canada, revealed that from 34% to 76% (38% to 76% in the United States) of individuals who had died would likely have benefitted from having a generalist or specialist palliative approach incorporated into their care (Morin et al., 2017). Only 30% of individuals have any understanding of palliative care and its potential contribution to their health care and quality of life (Center to Advance Palliative Care [CAPC] & American Cancer Society Cancer Action Network [ACS CAN], 2011).

As a holistic person- and family-centered approach, palliative care is part of the essence of nursing. Florence Nightingale's work with Crimean War soldiers at the end of life set the foundation for this care in the mid- to late 1800s. A century later, early leaders in nursing, medicine, and other disciplines established the foundations on which palliative, hospice, and end-of-life care continues to grow. Dame Cicely Saunders, who was a nurse, social worker, and physician over the course of her career, established St. Christopher's Hospice in Great Britain in the 1960s to provide end-of-life care for individuals with advanced terminal illness. It continues to serve as a model for hospice and palliative-care services around the globe. In *On Death and Dying* (Kübler-Ross, 1969) author-psychiatrist Dr. Elisabeth Kübler-Ross laid the groundwork for decades of improvements in care of the terminally ill. Dr. Florence Wald, nurse and dean of the Yale School of Nursing, and physician Dr. Balfour Mount of Canada's Royal Victoria Hospital were instrumental in studying the needs of the dying and establishing programs in their respective countries: Connecticut Hospice in the United States and St. Bonafice and Victoria Hospice in Canada. (American Nurses Association [ANA] & Hospice and Palliative Nurses Association [HPNA], 2014; Hospice Society of the Columbia Valley, n.d.). In the early 2000s, the lack of palliative-care education of nursing and other health-care students was recognized (Ferrell, Virani, Grant, & Juarez, 2000), and programs to ameliorate this knowledge gap were established.

Initiatives of the End of Life Nursing Education Consortium (ELNEC) and its constituents have been effective in educating over 730,000 nurses and others in health-care disciplines across many health-care and academic settings in 100 countries, including the United States and Canada. The American Association of Colleges of Nursing (AACN) has recognized palliative care as a basic human right and endorsed primary palliative-care competencies that should be addressed in all undergraduate and graduate nursing programs (AACN, 2016; AACN & ELNEC–City of Hope, 2019). Palliative-care education is increasingly incorporated into all areas of nursing curricula, from prelicensure to graduate and postgraduate programs (ELNEC, 2019; Fennimore et al., 2018; Wholihan & Tilly, 2016).

Coverage of palliative care varies widely. It is a defined benefit under the U.S. Medicare system and may also be covered through Medicaid and private insurance plans. Health insurance coverage for palliative-care services is more limited and inconsistent than for hospice care. Coverage and reimbursement for advance-care planning and advance directives conversations falls behind coverage for other palliative-care services. In Canada, coverage is available through a variety of provincial, territorial, and private health plans (MyHealth.Alberta.ca, n.d.; U.S. Centers for Medicare & Medicaid Services, n.d.).

The National Consensus Project (NCP) for Quality Palliative Care, an interdisciplinary group of palliative-care providers, educators, researchers, and supporters, convened first in the early 2000s and developed the evidence-informed document detailing eight palliative-care domains (NCP, 2018). The document, now in its fourth edition, continues to serve as a guide for the emerging field of palliative care, detailing the structures and processes of care, holistic aspects of care (physical, psychological, social, spiritual, cultural, and end-of-life), and ethical and legal aspects of palliative care (NCP, 2018). Incorporated into the fourth edition of the guidelines are updates on the current state and need for further development of health promotion palliative care, particularly in primary care (NCP, 2018).

Palliative care is provided through primary-, secondary-, and tertiary-level health services to address communication about values and goals of care between patient and health-care providers and relief of serious illness or treatment-associated symptoms and stress (NCP, 2018; Quill & Abernethy, 2013; Weissman & Meier, 2011; WPCA & WHO, 2014). It is whole-person, family-centered care that strives to reduce physical, psychosocial, and existential suffering. It is concordant with and supportive of an individual's goals, priorities, and values for care. It can be incorporated into care in varying degrees along the health–illness continuum, such as during an early prediagnosis encounter with a primary-care provider, when serious illness is diagnosed, and during end of life and bereavement.

DEFINITIONS

The term *palliative care* was not commonly used to describe care for individuals with serious or terminal illness prior to the 1990s. However, its precepts have historically been an important part of nursing care, woven into the fabric of hospice and end-of-life care since the 1960s. Palliative care is a philosophy, a health-care specialty for nursing and varied disciplines, and an organized system of whole-person-focused care for individuals with serious or life-limiting illness and their families. It can be provided at any time during a disease trajectory, from the time of diagnosis onward, for patients of any age and in any setting of care, including in communities, homes, and varied health-care settings. Palliative, hospice, and end-of-life care are related, but they have some distinct differences. *Palliative care*, the broadest of the three terms, will be used in this chapter.

Palliative care focuses on fostering quality of life and well-being for individuals and their families facing serious illness regardless of the diagnosis, stage of illness (including before time of diagnosis as well as through end of life and into bereavement), age of the individual, or setting of care. It is an extra layer of holistic care and support often provided by an interdisciplinary team. It is a philosophy as well as a structured system of care that is necessary across primary, secondary, and tertiary palliative levels. It can be provided either as the sole focus of care or in conjunction with curatively focused care (ANA & HPNA, 2014; Canadian Virtual Hospice, 2015; CAPC, 2011; IOM, 2015; NCP, 2018; WPCA & WHO, 2014). Over the past 15 years, the major growth in U.S. palliative care has been at the specialty level (secondary and tertiary) and with the inpatient population in large hospitals and academic medical centers (CAPC & NPCRC, 2015).

Currently the terms *hospice* and *end-of-life care* are most familiar to the public and are used most often in health-care settings in the United States. In Canada, the term *hospice palliative care* is more common. Terms such as *comfort care* and *supportive care* are also used to describe palliative care. Hospice and end-of-life care are part of palliative care. Hospice is care for patients and families whose goals are for supportive care of advanced, serious, terminal illness. It is whole-person care focused on improving quality of life, not quantity (extension) of life, but it does continue through and beyond the death of an individual in the form of bereavement support for the family.

Primary, Secondary, and Tertiary Palliative Care

Primary palliative care is a generalist-level of holistic care integrated into an individual's health care at any time, regardless of a serious illness diagnosis. It can occur in a variety of settings, including during health promotion and primary-care encounters. Nurses and other health professionals providing this care are not palliative-care specialists, but they provide care using the skills and competencies expected of all clinicians. Primary palliative care may also be referred to as basic or integrated palliative care (NCP, 2018).

Secondary and tertiary specialty levels of palliative care focus on individuals with serious illness and with complex needs for care, coordination, and support, as well as on more complex team or organization palliative concerns. This specialty level of palliative care is provided most often in inpatient and hospice settings and sometimes in specialty palliative care or hospice units. Secondary and tertiary palliative care are provided by clinicians with specialized preparation, often with certification in palliative care (Gorman & Wholihan, 2016; Weissman & Meier, 2011; WPCA & WHO, 2014). Secondary palliative care providers are of various disciplines with specialty training for addressing complex issues through consultation, coordination, and direct care provision. Tertiary palliative care is delivered by specialty trained providers in academic medical centers and focuses on complex palliative care issues and research (Quill & Abernethy, 2013; Weissman & Meier, 2011; WPCA & WHO, 2014).

DEVELOPMENTS IN PALLIATIVE CARE

Building on early calls to expand palliative and end-of-life care (AACN, 1998; IOM, 1997), new reports highlight the evolution of palliative care and make recommendations for further efforts. The growth in many areas of palliative care is promising. Education for health-care clinicians and the public continues to grow, and models and domains of care are becoming recognized. For clients and their families, palliative care specialty services that focus on care of serious, advanced, or terminal illness well after diagnosis continue to grow. In addition, nursing, medicine, and other palliative-care certifications recognize specialty-level practitioners. Research and policy initiatives are underpinning new understanding and acceptance of palliative care (Canadian Hospice Palliative Nurses Association, 2015; CAPC & National Palliative Care Reserch Center [NPCRC], 2015; IOM, 2015; NCP, 2018; WPCA & WHO, 2014). ELNEC is a nursing-centric, "train the trainer" program that has reached over 675,000 nurses and other health-care providers, faculty members, and students from the United States, Canada, and 95 other countries (AACN, n.d.).

While it is important to recognize these developments, it is also important to acknowledge that gaps and challenges remain. Too many consumers and health-care providers still have limited or erroneous information about palliative-care services; the number of accessible palliative-care specialists and services falls short of the growing need. Health-care services and systems are challenged to deliver care that aligns with what matters most to individuals who appropriately need palliative care and their families (CAPC & NPCRC, 2015; Gawande, 2014; Hawley, 2017; IOM, 2015; Pallium Canada, n.d.; Weissman & Meier, 2011). Palliative care and hospice are likely to be introduced late during an individual's illness, leaving little time to optimize impact on quality of life. Lack of understanding and discomfort with advance-care planning and advance directives discussions remain (Kim, Udow-Phillips, & Peters, 2016). Disparities in perceptions of, access to, preferences for, and satisfaction with palliative care exist across sociocultural groups and vulnerable populations. These disparities are also apparent regarding advance-care planning and advance directives (Evans & Ume, 2012; Jimenez et al., 2018; Johnstone & Kanitsaki, 2009; McHugh, Arnold, & Buschman, 2012; National Academies of Sciences, Engineering & Medicine [NASEM], 2017). More research and evidence-based initiatives, earlier integration of palliation into care, and understanding of the potential of palliative care to have a health promotion impact on quality of life and well-being are needed.

HEALTH PROMOTION AND PALLIATIVE CARE

The mismatch in growth between the number of people who would benefit from primary (basic) or secondary-tertiary (specialized) palliative care, as well as the availability and accessibility of such services, has been recognized as a public health crisis (Kellehear, 1999a, 1999b; McHugh, Arnold, & Buschman, 2012; WPCA & WHO, 2014). Health-promoting palliative care, which can be integrated into care even before the presence of a serious illness, has received little attention. Although palliative care is not specifically addressed in Healthy People 2020 (Office of Disease Prevention and Health Promotion [ODPHP], 2016), efforts that align palliative care and health promotion can contribute toward meaningful progress in the overarching goal of promoting quality of life and well-being across all life stages.

Palliative care "sorely needs" a health promotion perspective (Kellehear, 1999a, p. 17), and health promotion similarly needs to include a primary palliative approach. For too long, palliative care's public health and health-promotion aspects have remained underrecognized by health-care providers. Both palliative care and health promotion focus on promoting holistic care, quality of life, and well-being, so a public health approach to health-promoting palliative care is warranted (DeLima & Pastrana, 2016; Dempers & Gott, 2017; Huang et al., 2018; Kellehear, 1999a, 1999b; Rosenberg & Yates, 2010; Stjernswärd, Foley, & Ferris, 2007; WPCA & WHO, 2014). Actions recommended originally in the 1986 Ottawa Charter for Health Promotion (WHO, n.d.), and later by key advocates (Kellehear & O'Connor, 2008; Stjernswärd et al., 2007; WPCA & WHO, 2014), include the development of health-promoting palliative-care initiatives that support improving individuals' own health advocacy and engagement in services; advancing public policy; and fostering social and health-care environments that support health, community action, and personal health-care management and communication skills (WHO, 2017). The imperative for better and earlier integration of palliative care into health-care services for all individuals and populations across the health–illness continuum and at all levels of it is becoming more apparent (Casarett & Teno, 2016; Kellehear 1999b; Kellehear & O'Connor, 2008; Rosenberg & Yates, 2010; WPCA & WHO, 2014).

More nurses and health-care providers must integrate health-promoting primary palliative care into their practice (AACN & ELNEC–City of Hope, 2019; McHugh, Arnold & Buschman, 2012; NCP, 2018; Quill & Abernethy, 2013; WPCA & WHO, 2014). Nurses can make significant contributions to this area (AACN, 2014; ANA Center for Ehtics and Human Rights, 2016; Canadian Hospice Palliative Care Association [CHPCA], 2009, 2015; HPNA, 2015, 2016; McHugh, Arnold & Buschman, 2012; WPCA & WHO, 2014) as early responders to the increasing impact of serious and chronic illness on clients, including individuals, families, populations, and communities.

Advance-Care Planning and Advance Directives

Since the enactment of the U.S. Patient Self-Determination Act (1990) to allow individuals to establish advance directives for care, acknowledgment of the importance of these documents and the associated planning decisions has slowly increased. A variety of consensus-building, education, community engagement, research, and policy initiatives have furthered the understanding of advance-care planning and utilization of advance directives. However, too few individuals communicate their advance-care planning wishes or complete an advance directive (IOM, 2015; Schüklenk et al., 2011). Based on findings by Rao, Anderson, Lin, and Laux (2014), only 26.3% of the U. S. population has an advance directive in place.

Advance-care planning is a foundational part of the process of formulating a personally meaningful advance directive. Advance-care planning, as defined by a multidisciplinary Delphi panel with representatives from the United States, Canada, and the Netherlands, is a process to ensure that individuals' values, wishes, and goals for care are communicated and honored. It includes three key elements (Sudore et al., 2017):

1. Advance-care planning is a process that supports adults at any age or stage of health in understanding and sharing their personal values, life goals, and preferences regarding future medical care.
2. The goal of advance-care planning is to help ensure that people receive medical care that is consistent with their values, goals, and preferences during serious and chronic illness.
3. For many people, this process may include choosing and preparing another trusted person or persons to make medical decisions in the event the person can no longer make his or her own decisions (Sudore et al., 2017)

Nurses and other health-care providers who have limited knowledge, skill, confidence, or support for engaging in advance-care planning and advance directives conversations may be reticent to open a dialogue about the subject in their encounters with patients (Ke, Huang, O'Connor, & Lee, 2017; Rietze, Heale, Roles, & Hill, 2018). As recognized by Johnstone and Kanitsaki (2009), additional complexities have an impact on advance-care planning in multicultural environments, with their broad range of values, decision making, and family structures.

It is all too common for decisions about advance directives and orders for care—including living will, health-care power of attorney, surrogate decision maker, do not resuscitate (DNR), allow natural death (AND), and physician orders for life-sustaining treatment (POLST)—to occur without prior discussion or forethought, when an individual is in an advanced stage of illness (IOM, 2015). These decisions, often made in a time of crisis, are unlikely to align with the individual's values and preferences for care. Barriers contributing to the lateness of advance-care planning and advance directives conversations include lack of knowledge about advance directives and associated resources, discomfort in talking about the topic, fear of saying the wrong thing, and entrenched beliefs about when such conversations should occur and who should be involved in them. Consequently, these important conversations between an individual, their loved ones, caregivers, and their health-care providers happen too infrequently and too late. Compounding these difficulties are the disparities in understanding of advance-care planning and completion of advance directives among vulnerable and underrepresented groups (Braun, Beyth, Ford, & McCullough, 2008; Breakwell, Callahan, & Hughes, 2014; Evans & Ume, 2012; IOM, 2015).

Understanding and completion of advance-care planning and advance directives is limited. Results of a mail survey representative of the U.S. population revealed that 26.3% of respondents had an advance directive. Factors affecting whether or not one had an advance directive included awareness, age, racial identity, education, and income. Those who had an advance directive were more likely to be older, have a chronic health condition, and obtain regular health care, while those who did not were more nonwhite and with no known end-of-life concerns (Rao et al., 2014). The negative impact of late and limited advance-care planning on care has been recognized (NASEM, 2017; Schüklenk et al., 2011) and further identified as an urgent concern in public health (DeLima & Pastrana, 2016; Tilden et al., 2012).

Recommendations for further improvements from the American Academy of Nursing's Palliative and End of Life Care Expert Panel include: encouraging individuals to articulate their advance-care planning preferences, improving reimbursement for advance-care planning and directives, communicating information via centralized and electronic health records, and providing interprofessional health-care professional education and training (Tilden et al., 2012). Although recent scoping review of the advance directives literature reinforced substantive growth in understanding and utilization of advance directives, more research about their impact at individual, population, and systems levels is still needed to appreciate fully their potential influence on care (Jimenez et al., 2018).

In a health-promoting approach to palliative care, these life-changing advance-care planning conversations, including articulation of what matters most and decisions about an individual's wishes for care, are normalized and integrated in routine health encounters. These discussions are approached consistently and begin much earlier, including before diagnosis of serious illness has been made (HPNA, 2016; Kim, Udow-Phillips & Peters, 2016; Myers, Duthie, Denson, Denson, & Simpson, 2017). Recognizing barriers that can hamper effective advance-care planning discussions is important. Conversations about advance-care planning and end of life may be uncomfortable, and misperceptions about palliative care and advance directives often need to be addressed. In addition, values, decision-making style, and cultural practices unique to each client must be recognized and respected.

The Nurse Role in Health-Promoting Palliative Care

"Because palliative care is embedded in nursing practice, all nurses practice aspects of primary palliative care" (ANA & HPNA, 2014, p. 19). Nurses have the vital role of incorporating palliative care into their health promotion practices through education of self and others, practice, collaboration, community engagement, advocacy, and policy-focused activities. The need for evidence-based initiatives to guide advances in this area of care provides nurses with opportunities to conduct research (ANA, 2017).

Raising one's own and others' awareness about palliative care is particularly relevant in helping overcome continued misperceptions held by health-care providers, individuals seeking care, and the general public that the topic of palliative care should be introduced only well after a serious illness diagnosis has been made and subsequently provided only as the end of life is near. An informed nurse is better prepared to engage in meaningful conversations with a patient and incorporate aspects of palliative care into holistic care that aligns with the individual's values, decision-making preferences, and goals for health care. Providing information will also enable individuals to make more informed and better decisions about their care.

Results from a literature search about nurses' perceptions of whether they have information and support for engaging effectively in early advance-care planning and advance directives with their clients were limited (Table 22-1). This underscores the need for further study of inhibiting and enabling factors and practice exemplars. Based on the Johns Hopkins Nursing Evidence-Based Practice model, the studies were qualitative and mixed-method, well-designed (Level III), and of good quality (A/B) (Dang & Dearholt, 2017). Findings revealed that nurses recognize the importance and the complexities of advance-care planning but lack confidence in discussing them with their clients (Ke et al., 2015; Rietze et al., 2018; Seymour, Almack, & Kennedy, 2010). Rietze and colleagues (2018) found that nurses in nonacute care settings (such as within the

Table 22-1 Patient, Intervention, Control, and Observation (PICO) Question and Evidence Table

PICO Question: For nurses who will be engaging in early advance-care planning (ACP) and advance directives activities that are part of health-promoting palliative care, do they (compared with specialty palliative-care providers) have the information and support to work effectively with individuals?

Publication Citation; Level (I–Iv)* and Quality (A–C)† of Evidence	Purpose, Aims	Design, Methods, Sample	Findings	Critique of Study
Ke et al. (2015) Level III Quality A/B	To synthesize the literature about nurses' experiences and perceptions regarding ACP for older adults.	Qualitative meta-synthesis. A search of databases was conducted to find English language qualitative studies of nurses' experiences with or perceptions of ACP with older adults. Ultimately, 18 studies from seven countries, including the United States and Canada, were reviewed. An established critical appraisal program checklist (CASP) was used, and a three-stage meta-synthesis was performed to identify themes.	Findings included that nurses identified benefits associated with, and their roles in, ACP with older adults. Nurses recognized barriers, including the need for further educational preparation, organizational and policy support, and time for engaging in ACP. They also recognized family dynamics, culture, language, environment, and health-care teams and systems issues that had an impact on older adults' involvement in their ACP. Recommendations for development of education, supportive policies, and more formalization of nurses' role in ACP are discussed as well.	A well-designed meta-synthesis encompassing the literature about nurses' experiences and perceptions of ACP from seven countries.

(continued)

Table 22-1 Patient, Intervention, Control, and Observation (PICO) Question and Evidence Table—cont'd

Publication Citation; Level (I–Iv)* and Quality (A–C)† of Evidence	Purpose, Aims	Design, Methods, Sample	Findings	Critique of Study
Rietze et al. (2018) Level III Quality A/B	To ascertain nurses' engagement in and understanding of factors associated with ACP.	Cross-sectional descriptive survey design. RNs with willingness to participate in research as indicated as part of licensure renewal were randomly selected; of 1,000 RNs contacted, 125 RNs in varied settings in Ontario, Canada, participated. The mailed survey tool, developed by the research team from earlier studies and validated by expert ACP and palliative-care nurses, consisted of demographic questions and 35 questions related to ACP and factors that influence nurses' practice decisions. Quantitative analysis using descriptive statistics, Spearman correlation and X^2 , and inductive content analysis were performed. Qualitative responses went through three stages of categorization to arrive at main themes.	Respondents agreed that end-of-life decision making was important to their roles, but almost 60% did not participate in ACP with their patients. Non-acute-care nurses were less likely to participate in ACP than their acute-care counterparts. Barriers to their participation in ACP included limited education about ACP, limited expectations that they engage in ACP, limited organizational policy or support, and perception that patients and families were not ready to participate in ACP discussions..	A well-designed study, reporting adequate power (0.8) with moderate effect size (X^2 analysis) that provides new insights about nurses and ACP. Limitations include a low response rate and participation from nurses in one country (Canada).
Seymour, Almack, & Kennedy (2010) Level III Quality A/B	To understand English community nurses' understanding and views of, roles in, and education needs for ACP.	Qualitative study of 23 nurses who participated in one of six focus groups and three follow-up collaborative interpretation discussion workshops to interpret focus group findings and identify themes and ideas for education resources.	Nurses were knowledgeable about the meaning of ACP and related policy and resources. They lacked confidence in the complexities and timing of ACP. Barriers to implementing ACP included inadequate resources, services, education, and support.	Generalizability limited due to small sample size of nurses in England who were invited by a gatekeeper/supervisor to participate. A strength was participants' involvement in prefocus group session to help develop key objectives and postvalidation exercise to develop recommendations for future ACP.

Table 22-1 Patient, Intervention, Control, and Observation (PICO) Question and Evidence Table—cont'd

Publication Citation; Level (I–Iv)* and Quality (A–C)† of Evidence	Purpose, Aims	Design, Methods, Sample	Findings	Critique of Study
				education programs, which paved the way for actionable changes.

* Evidence Levels: *Level I* = experimental study, RCT, systematic review of RCT; *Level II* = non-experimental study, systematic review of RCTs plus quasi-experimental studies only; *Level III* = non-experimental study, systematic review of RCTs plus quasi-experimental studies only; qualitative study or systematic review including or not including meta-analysis; *Level IV* = expert opinion or consensus based on scientific evidence, clinical practice guidelines.

† Quality guides: *high quality* = consistent, generalizable results and recommendations based on comprehensive review of literature and scientific evidence, sufficient sample size, definitive conclusions; *good quality* = reasonably consistent results, sufficient sample size, reasonable consistent recommendations based on literature and scientific evidence; *low quality* = insufficient evidence or sample size, inconsistent results, unable to draw conclusions (Dang & Dearholt, 2017, Appendix D).

community) were less likely to participate in advance-care planning with clients than the nurses in acute care. Nurses in these studies reported the need for additional education, support from their organizations (including time for client interactions), and resources (Ke et al., 2015; Rietze et al., 2018; Seymour et al., 2010).

To address nurses' need for personal education and professional development about palliative care, resources are available through professional organizations, programs, conferences, and Web sites. In providing health-promoting palliative care, nurses must also be aware of type, range, and availability of palliative-care resources in the community. Information about palliative, hospice, and end-of-life care; advance-care planning; and advance directives resources is growing and is readily accessible for health-care providers and the general public.

Beginning with the first encounter with clients, communication skills are key to establishing trust and to ensuring that their values, decision-making style, and goals and wishes for health care can be integrated into their advance-care planning and into their care. Findings from a comprehensive assessment encompassing the physical, psychological, social, cultural, existential/spiritual, and family concerns of the individual contribute to a plan of care that aligns with the individual's needs, values, and preferences.

Case Illustration

Jennifer is an advanced practice nurse working in a primary-care practice. In addition to working at the clinic, she has been active in advance-care planning, advance directives, and palliative-care awareness initiatives in the health system and in the local community. Jennifer is seeing a new client, 65-year-old Mrs. Sullivan, who has made an appointment for a checkup at her daughter's insistence. She has no diagnosed health problems and a family history of diabetes and heart disease. On her health history form, she indicates that she takes multivitamins and occasional non-steroidal anti-inflammatory drugs (NSAIDs) for arthritis. She acknowledges low energy, lack of motivation, and "feeling blue" in recent months. In talking further, Jennifer finds out that Mrs. Sullivan strongly values her family and her faith as sources of support. Following the unexpected death of her husband, she has recently moved from the home, church, and community of many years. She is now living in a new community, in the home of her daughter, son-in-law, and three school-age grandchildren.

Jennifer integrates elements of health-promoting palliative care into her initial visit with Mrs. Sullivan. She schedules enough time at the initial encounter to begin establishing a good rapport; discusses the client's questions and concerns related to her health, quality of life, and well-being; and begins the conversation about advance-care planning and directives. Prior to this conversation, Mrs. Sullivan's only understanding of advance directives occurred when her husband died unexpectedly of a stroke. She does not have an advance directive and is interested in learning more.

Nursing Role in Advance-Care Planning and Advance Directives

Perhaps the aspect of health-promoting palliative care with the most impact for nurses is advance-care planning and advance directives. As advocates for patients, nurses are engaged in actions that foster advance-care planning in individual encounters and communicate with other team members about the individual's decisions for care.

Incorporating the transtheoretical model's stages of change into an assessment can help ensure that advance-care planning is tailored meaningfully to a client's readiness and needs. As described by Fried et al. (2010), the transtheoretical model is a useful tool to understand a client's stage of readiness for change in relation to advance-care planning, first by gauging willingness to take in new information about one's health status in relationship to advance-care planning (precontemplation), next in thinking and talking about values and preferences (contemplation and preparation for change) related to advance-care planning, and then by developing and sharing one's advance-care planning decisions with health-care providers and loved ones such as through an advance directive (action and maintenance).

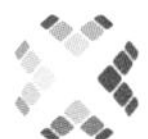

Case Illustration

Mrs. Sullivan. has returned for a routine follow-up visit. Jennifer has included some extra time during the visit to provide her client with resource information about advance-care planning and advance directives. Jennifer recognizes that her role is to provide information and address questions; she cannot help Mrs. Sullivan complete her advance directive. Therefore, Jennifer has also explored local advance-care planning and advance directives resources and encourages her client to participate in an upcoming informational event at the community senior center. At this event, Mrs. Sullivan will receive information about talking with her family about her wishes for the future, identifying an individual she trusts to be her health-care decision maker, incorporating the information into a recognized and accepted advance directive document, and sharing the information with her loved ones and health-care providers. In the event that Mrs. Sullivan is no longer able to speak for herself, her wishes and preferences for care will serve as a guide for her care.

An advance-care planning conversation can begin during a routine initial health-care visit with a client or at a community event. This initial discussion creates a foundation for the client to make decisions and convey his or her values and preferences for care and advance directives. These conversations can continue during subsequent interactions with family members and health-care providers. While advance-care planning discussion is important as part of good holistic care, whether these conversations translate into an advance directive document varies widely across individuals, communities, and cultures (Johnstone & Kanitsaki, 2009; Rao et al., 2014). Continued research and practice initiatives are needed to overcome remaining barriers to effective advance-care planning and advance directives (Jimenez et al., 2018).

Information and tools to foster reflection, discussion, and decisions about advance-care planning and advance directives are available to meet the varied learning styles and needs of health-care providers and the general public. Resources for documenting and communicating advance directives are available as well (see Box 22-1).

SPIKES is a recognized palliative-care communication tool used for sensitive conversations with patients and family members about a difficult prognosis, such as the worsening of a serious illness. This framework is also applicable to earlier advance-care planning discussions (Baile et al., 2000). Preparing in advance to *set up* for a conversation and arranging for a conducive *setting* (S) are key. The setting should be comfortable for listening and talking, allow for privacy, and include both the patient and provider as well as significant individuals as determined by the patient.

Anticipate if informational resources will be used in the conversation and have them readily available. Find out the individual's *perceptions* (P) about advance-care planning and advance directives. Obtain their *invitation* (I) for the kind of information they are willing to take in and share, which will help create a conversation that is meaningful to the client.

Provide *knowledge* (K) and information that is aligned with the client's invitation to learn more and conveyed in understandable language. Give the client time to process the information. Recognize that conversations about what is important to an individual may be uncomfortable or spark an emotional response, and prepare to respond to *emotions* with compassion and *empathy* (E). Close the conversation with a *summary* and identify a *strategy* (S) for next steps. These steps might include continuing the conversation at a next visit, making some beginning decisions about a surrogate health-care decision maker, or conveying one's values and wishes in the form of an advance directive.

BOX 22–1 Palliative Care Information and Education Resources

GENERAL RESOURCES

Canadian Hospice Palliative Care Organization: http://www.chpca.net/professionals/nurses.aspx
Center to Advance Palliative Care (CAPC): https://www.capc.org/
End of Life Nursing Education Consortium (ELNEC): http://www.aacnnursing.org/ELNEC/About
Fast Facts and Concepts, Palliative Care Network of Wisconsin (PCNOW): https://www.mypcnow.org/fast-facts
Hospice and Palliative Nurses Association (HPNA): https://advancingexpertcare.org/
National Hospice and Palliative Care Organization (NHPCO): https://www.nhpco.org/

ADVANCE-CARE PLANNING AND ADVANCE DIRECTIVES RESOURCES

American Bar Association, Advance Care Planning Tool Kit: https://www.americanbar.org/groups/law_aging/resources/health_care_decision_making/consumer_s_toolkit_for_health_care_advance_planning.html
Canadian Hospice Palliative Care Organization: http://www.chpca.net/
The Conversation Project: http://theconversationproject.org/resources/
National Healthcare Decisions Day: https://www.nhdd.org/#welcome
Primary Toolkit–National (Canada), Speak Up: http://www.advancecareplanning.ca/resource/primary-care-toolkit/

THINKING AND TALKING WITH OTHERS ABOUT ADVANCE-CARE PLANNING

Five Wishes, Aging with Dignity: http://www.agingwithdignity.org/index.php
Go Wish, Coda Alliance: http://www.gowish.org/staticpages/index.php/thegame
Hello (formerly My Gift of Grace), The Action Mill: http://mygiftofgrace.com
My Directives and My Directives Mobile (version 2016.0913): https://mydirectives.com/
PREPARE for Your Care: https://www.prepareforyourcare.org/

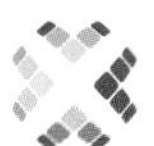

Case Illustration

As part of the next routine visit, Jennifer asks Mrs. Sullivan if she has taken any new steps toward creating an advance directive. Mrs. Sullivan states that she has completed the document and provides the nurse a copy for her records. Jennifer and Mrs. Sullivan review it together, so the nurse is updated on Mrs. Sullivan's wishes and her designated decision maker. They make some corresponding updates to Mrs. Sullivan's care plan. After the visit, Jennifer ensures that the advance directive is added to Mrs. Sullivan's health record so it can be accessed by her other care providers.

Nursing has traditionally espoused a whole-person approach to care of clients at the individual, group, and community levels across the health continuum. This approach aligns strongly with health-promoting palliative care; thus, nurses will remain instrumental advocates, providers, leaders, educators, and researchers in this increasingly recognized area.

KEY POINTS

- Primary palliative care can be integrated into care early, even before a serious illness diagnosis has been made.
- Advance-care planning and advance directives are important aspects of health-promoting palliative care.
- Resources are available to meet a wide range of learning styles and needs.
- More research is needed to strengthen the evidence of the potential influence of health-promoting palliative care on quality of life and well being.

Check Your Understanding

1. An advance practice nurse is preparing for the initial visit with a new client. Which statement about advance-care planning and advance directives is most accurate?
   A. By the end of the visit, the client must have an advance directive completed.
   B. Advance-care planning should be the main focus of the initial visit.

C. The nurse is responsible for completing the client's advance directive.

D. The client's interest and comfort in discussing advance-care planning will guide the nurse-client interaction.

2. To provide primary palliative care, a nurse must meet which criterion?

A. Be certified in specialty palliative care

B. Have at least 1 year of experience in hospice care

C. Have core knowledge of palliative care principles and precepts

D. Be certified in advance directives

3. During part of a routine visit, a client reveals the recent death of his only sibling. What primary palliative care action should the nurse take next?

A. Make an immediate referral to a palliative-care specialist for further follow-up with the client.

B. Invite the client to say more about this loss, including its meaning and impact.

C. Redirect the client's attention to the reason for the routine appointment so it can be completed in the allotted time.

D. Provide written information about area hospice services.

4. Which of the activities by an advance practice nurse exemplifies health-promoting palliative care?

A. Participation in an event about advance directives at a local community center

B. Attending a service of remembrance for staff of recently deceased hospitalized clients

C. Completing an advance directive on behalf of a client

D. Providing tertiary palliative care services in a trauma unit

5. Which statement about advance-care planning is most accurate?

A. Establishing medical orders such as POLST is a required component of advance-care planning.

B. Normalizing advance-care planning discussions into routine provider-client health-care encounters can lay important groundwork for future client-centered care decisions.

C. Advance-care planning conversations must be led by a specialty-level palliative-care provider.

D. The best time to make advance-care planning decisions is during a life-or-death health crisis.

See "Reflections on Check Your Understanding" at the end of the book for answers.

REFERENCES

American Association of Colleges of Nursing. (n.d.). *About ELNEC*. Retrieved from http://www.aacnnursing.org/ELNEC/About

American Association of Colleges of Nursing. (1998, February). *Peaceful death: Recommended competencies and curricular guidelines for end-of-life nursing care.* Retrieved from http://www.aacn.nche.edu/elnec/publications/peaceful-death

American Association of Colleges of Nursing. (2014). *Primary vs. specialty palliative nursing*. PowerPoint presentation. Retrieved from http://www.aacn.nche.edu/search-results?cx=004745212939755731071%3A9ffni8oukg8&cof=FORID%3A11&ie=UTF-8&q=primary+vs+specialty+palliataive+nursing&siteurl=www.aacn.nche.edu%2F&ref=www.bing.com%2F&ss=11259j3733475j51&sa.x=0&sa.y=0

American Association of Colleges of Nursing. (2016). *CARES: Competencies and recommendations for educating undergraduate nursing students: Preparing nurses to care for the seriously ill and their families*. Retrieved from http://www.aacn.nche.edu/elnec/New-Palliative-Care-Competencies.pdf

American Association of Colleges of Nursing & ELNEC–City of Hope. (2019). *Preparing graduate nursing students to ensure quality palliative care for the seriously ill & their families.* Retrieved from https://www.aacnnursing.org/Portals/42/ELNEC/PDF/Graduate-CARES.pdf?ver=2019-01-29-141816-073

American Nurses Association. (2017, March 13). *Call for action: Nurses lead and transform palliative care*. ANA & HPNA, Professional Issues Panel. Retrieved from http://nursingworld.org/CallforAction-NursesLeadTransformPalliativeCare

American Nurses Association & Hospice and Palliative Nurses Association. (2014). *Scope and standards of practice: Palliative nursing: An essential resource for hospice and palliative nurses.* Silver Spring, MD: ANA.

ANA Center for Ethics and Human Rights. (2016). *Nurses' roles and responsibilities in providing care and support at the end of life*. Revised position statement. Silver Spring, MD: ANA.

Baile, W. F., Buckman, R., Lenzi, R., Glober, G., Beale, E. A., Kudelka, A. P. (2000). SPIKES: A six-step protocol for delivering bad news: Application to the patient with cancer. *Oncologist*. *5*(4), 302–311. Retrieved from https://www.ncbi.nlm.nih.gov/pubmed/10964998

Braun, U. K., Beyth, R. J., Ford, M. E., & McCullough, L. B. (2008). Voices of African American, Caucasian, and Hispanic surrogates on the burdens of end-of-life decision making. *Journal of General Internal Medicine 23*(3), 2267–274. doi:10.1007/s11606-1007-0487-7

Breakwell, S., Callahan, M., & Hughes, R. (2014). *African Americans' perceptions and recommendations for palliative care in an urban community*. [PowerPoint presentation]. Singapore: Second Annual International Home Care Nurses Organization Conference. Retrieved from https://tsaofoundation.org/doc/ihcno/Breakout_Session/PCN_4.pdf

Canadian Hospice Palliative Care Association. (2015, March). *The Way Forward National Framework: A roadmap for an integrated palliative approach to care.* Retrieved from http://www.hpcintegration.ca/resources/the-national-framework.aspx

Canadian Hospice Palliative Care Association. (2009). *Canadian hospice palliative care nursing standards of practice* (2nd ed.). CHPCA, Nursing Standards Committee. Retrieved from http://www.chpca.net/media/7505/Canadian_Hospice_Palliative_Care_Nursing_Standards_2009.pdf

Canadian Nurses Association, Canadian Hospice Palliative Care Association, & CHPCA–Nurses Group. (2015, June). *Joint position statement: The palliative approach to care and the role of the nurse*. Ottawa, Canada: Canada Nurses Association. Retrieved from https://www.cna-aiic.ca/en/advocacy/policy-support-tools/cna-position-statements

Canadian Virtual Hospice. (2015). *What is palliative care?* Retrieved from http://www.virtualhospice.ca/en_US/Main+Site+Navigation/Home/Topics/Topics/What+Is+Palliative+Care_/What+Is+Palliative+Care_.aspx

Casarett, D., & Teno, J. (2016). Why population health and palliative care need each other. *JAMA, 316*(1), 27–28. doi:10.1001/jama2016.5961

Center to Advance Palliative Care. (2011). *About palliative care: Definition of palliative care.* Retrieved from https://www.capc.org/about/palliative-care/

Center to Advance Palliative Care & American Cancer Society Cancer Action Network. (2011). *2011 public opinion survey of palliative care: State-by-state report card on access to palliative care in our nation's hospitals.* Retrieved from https://www.acscan.org/sites/default/files/Palliative-Care-Consumer-Research-Findings-Summary.pdf

Center to Advance Palliative Care & National Palliative Care Research Center. (2015). *America's care of serious illness: 2015 state-by-state report card on access to palliative care in our nation's hospitals.* Retrieved from https://reportcard.capc.org/

Dang, D., & Dearholt, S. (2017). *Johns Hopkins nursing evidence-based practice: Model and guidelines* (3rd ed.). Indianapolis, IN: Sigma Theta Tau International. Retrieved from https://www.hopkinsmedicine.org/evidence-based-practice/ijhn_2017_ebp.html

De Lima, L., & Pastrana, T. (2017. Opportunities for palliative care in public health. *Annual Review of Public Health 37*, 357–374. Retrieved from https://www.annualreviews.org/doi/full/10.1146/annurev-publhealth-032315-021448

Dempers, C., & Gott, M. (2017). Which public health approach to palliative care? An integrative literature review. *Progress in Palliative Care 25*(1), 1–8.

End of Life Nursing Education Consortium. (2019). *End of Life Education Consortium (ELNEC) fact sheet*. Retrieved from https://www.aacnnursing.org/ELNEC/About

Evans, B. C., & Ume, E. (2012). Psychosocial, cultural, and spiritual health disparities in end-of-life and palliative care: Where we are and where we need to go. *Nursing Outlook, 60*, 370–375. Retrieved from http://www.ncbi.nlm.nih.gov/pmc/articles/PMC3496155/

Fennimore, L., Wholihan, D., Breakwell, S., Malloy, P., Virani, R., & Ferrell, B. (2018). A framework for integrating oncology palliative care in doctor of nursing practice (DNP) education. *Journal of Professional Nursing 34*, 444–448. doi:https://doi.org/10.1016/j.profnurs.2018.09.003

Ferrell, B., Virani, R., Grant, M., & Juarez, G. (2000). Analysis of palliative care content in nursing textbooks. *Journal of Palliative Care Montreal 16*(1), 39–47.

Fried, T. R., Redding, C. A., Robbins, M. L., Paive, A., O'Leary, J. R., & Iannone, L (2010). Stages of change for the component behaviors of advance care planning. *Journal of the American Geriatrics Society, 58*(12), 2329–2336.

Gawande, A. (2014). *Being mortal: Medicine and what matters in the end*. New York: Metropolitan Books.

Gorman, R., & Wholihan, D. (2016). The advanced practice registered nurse in primary care. In C. Dahlin, P. J. Coyne, & B. R. Ferrell (Eds.), *Advance practice palliative nursing* (pp. 133–140). New York: Oxford University Press.

Hawley, P. (2017). Barriers to access to palliative care. *Palliative Care Research & Treatment, 10*, 1–6. doi:10.1177/1178224216688887. Retrieved from https://journals.sagepub.com/doi/full/10.1177/1178224216688887

Hospice and Palliative Nurses Association. (2015). *HPNA standards for clinical education of hospice and palliative nurses* (2nd ed.). C. Dahlin (Ed.). Pittsburgh, PA: Author. Retrieved from http://hpna.advancingexpertcare.org/wp-content/uploads/2015/08/HPNA-Clinical-Education-Standards.pdf

Hospice and Palliative Nurses Association. (2016, May). *Position statement: The nurses' role in advance care planning* (rev. ed.). Pittsburgh, PA: Author. Retrieved from http://community.hpna.org/p/do/sd/sid=12&fid=183&req=direct

Hospice Society of the Columbia Valley. (n.d.). *International history of hospice*. Author. Retrieved from: https://hospicesocietycv.com/our-organization/history/

Huang, S., Huang, C., Woung, L., Lee, O. K., Chu, D., Huang, T., … & Curtis, R. (2018). The 2017 Taipei declaration for health-promoting palliative care. *Journal of Palliative Medicine, 21*(5), 581–582. doi:10.1089/jpm.2017.0708.

Institute of Medicine. (1997). *Approaching death: Improving care at the end of life.* Washington, DC: The National Academies Press. Retrieved from https://doi.org/10.17226/5801

Institute of Medicine. (2015). *Dying in America: Improving quality and honoring individual preferences near the end of life.* Washington, DC: The National Academies Press. Retrieved from https://doi.org/10.17226/18748

Jimenez, G., Tan, W. S., Virk, A. K., Low, C. K., Car, J., & Ho, A. H. Y. (2018). Overview of systematic reviews of advance care planning: Summary of evidence and global lessons. *Journal of Pain and Symptom Management, 56*(3), 436–459. doi:https://doi.org/10.1016/j.jpainsymman.2018.05.016

Johnstone, M. J., & Kanitsaki, O. (2009). Ethics and advance care planning in a culturally diverse society. *Journal of Transcultural Nursing, 20*(4), 405–416.

Ke, L. S., Huang, X., O'Connor, M., & Lee, S. (2015). Nurses' views regarding implementing advance care planning for older people: A systematic review and synthesis of qualitative studies. *Journal of Clinical Nursing, 24*, 2057–2073. doi:10.1111/jocn.1285

Kellehear, A. (1999a). *Health promoting palliative care*. South Melbourne, Australia: Oxford University Press.

Kellehear, A. (1999b). Health promoting palliative care: Developing a social model for practice. *Mortality, 4*(1), 75–82.

Kellehear, A., & O'Connor, D. (2008). Health promoting palliative care: A practice example. *Critical Public Health, 18*(1), 111–115.

Kim, O., Udow-Phillips, M., & Peters, C. (2016, August). *Advance care planning: Tying community perspective to the national conversation.* Retrieved from https://www.chrt.org/publication/advance-care-planning-tying-community-perspective-national-conversation/

Kübler-Ross, E. (1969). *On death and dying.* New York: The Macmillan Company.

McHugh, M. E., Arnold, J., & Buschman, P. R. (2012). Nurses leading the response to the crisis of palliative care for vulnerable populations. *Nursing Economics, 30*(3), 140–147.

Morin, L., Aubry, R., Frova, L., MacLeod, R., Wilson, D. M., Loucka, M., . . . Cohen, J. (2017). Estimating the need for palliative care at the population level: A cross-national study in 12 countries. *Palliative Medicine, 31*(6), 526–536.

Morrison, R. S., Deitrich, J., & Meier, D.(2008), *America's care of serious illness: A state-by-state report card on access to palliative care in our nation's hospitals.* Center to Advance Palliative Care. Retrieved from: https://www.capc.org/

Myers, J., Duthie, E., Denson, K., Denson, S., & Simpson, D. (2017). What can a primary care physician discuss with older patients to improve advance directive completion rates? A Clin-IQ. *Journal of Patient-Centered Research and Reviews, 4*(1), 42–45.

MyHealth.Alberta.ca (n.d.). *Palliative and end-of-life care.* Author. Available at: https://myhealth.alberta.ca/palliative-care

National Academies of Sciences, Engineering & Medicine. (2017). *Integrating the patient and caregiver voice into serious illness care: Proceedings of a workshop.* Washington, DC: The National Academies Press. doi:10.17226/24802

National Consensus Project for Quality Palliative Care (2018). *Clinical practice guidelines for quality palliative care* (4th ed.). Richmond, VA: National Coalition for Hospice and Palliative Care.

Office of Disease Prevention and Health Promotion. (2016). *Healthy people 2020.* Retrieved from https://www.cdc.gov/nchs/healthy_people/hp2020.htm

Pallium Canada. (n.d.). *Palliative care education for all care providers: Mobilizing compassionate communities.* Retrieved from http://development.pallium.ca/about-us/history-2/

Patient Self-Determination Act. (1990). 4206-4751. Pub L No. 101-508. Retrieved from https://www.congress.gov/bill/101st-congress/house-bill/4449

Quill, T. E., & Abernethy, A. P. (2013). Generalist plus specialist palliative care: Creating a more sustainable model. *New England Journal of Medicine, 368*(13), 1173–1175. Retrieved from https://www.nejm.org/doi/full/10.1056/NEJMp1215620

Rao, J. K., Anderson, L. A., Lin, F. C., & Laux, J. P. (2014). Completion of advance directives among U.S. consumers. *American Journal of Preventive Medicine, 46*(1), 65–70. doi:10.1016/j.amepre.2013.09.008

Rietze, L., Heale, R., Roles, S., & Hill, L. (2018). Identifying the factors associated with Canadian registered nurses' engagement in advance care planning. *Journal of Hospice and Palliative Nursing, 20*(3), 230–236. doi:10.1097/NJH.0000000000000423

Rosenberg, J. P., & Yates, P. M. (2010). Health promotion in palliative care: The case for conceptual congruence. *Critical Public Health, 20*(2), 201–210. doi:10.1080/09581590902897394

Schüklenk, U., Van Delden, J. J. M., Downie, J., Mclean, S. A. M., Upshur, R., & Weinstock, D. (2011). End-of-life decision-making in Canada: The report by the Royal Society of Canada Expert Panel on End-of-Life Decision-Making. *Bioethics, 25*(Suppl 1), 1–4. Retrieved from http://doi.org/10.1111/j.1467-8519.2011.01939.x

Seymour, J., Almack, K., & Kennedy, S. (2010). Implementing advance care planning: A qualitative study of community nurses' views and experiences. *BMC Palliative Care, 9*(4). Retrieved from https://www.ncbi.nlm.nih.gov/pmc/articles/PMC2854100/

Stjernswärd, J., Foley, K. M., & Ferris, F. D. (2007). The public health strategy for palliative care. *Journal of Pain and Symptom Management, 33*(5), 486–493. doi:10.1016/j.jpainsymman.2007.02.016

Sudore, R. L., Lunn, H. D., You, J. J., Hanson, L. C., Meier, D. E., Pantilat, S. Z., . . . Heyland, D. K. (2017) Defining advance care planning for adults: A consensus definition from a multidisciplinary delphi panel. *Journal of Pain & Symptom Management, 53*(5), 821–832.

Tilden, V., Corless, I., Dahlin, C., Ferrell, B., Gibson, R., & Lenz, J. (2012). Advance care planning as an urgent public health concern. *Nursing Outlook, 60*(6), 418–419. Retrieved from https://www.nursingoutlook.org/article/S0029-6554(12)00250-3/fulltext

Ward, B. W., Schiller, J. S., & Goodman, R. A. (2014) Multiple chronic conditions among US adults: A 2012 update. *Preventing Chronic Disease,11130389* http://dx.doi.org/10.5888/pcd11.130389. Retrieved from https://www.cdc.gov/pcd/issues/2014/13_0389.htm

Weissman, D., & Meier, D. (2011). Identifying patients in need of a palliative care assessment in the hospital setting: A consensus report from the Center to Advance Palliative Care. *Journal of Palliative Medicine, 14*(1), 17–23. doi:10.1089/jpm.2010.0347. Retrieved from http://www.ncbi.nlm.nih.gov/pubmed/21133809

Wholihan, D., & Tilly, C. (2016). Fundamental skills and education for the palliative advanced practice registered nurse. In C. Dahlin, P. J. Coyne, & B. R. Ferrell (Eds.), *Advance practice palliative nursing* (pp. 133–140). New York: Oxford University Press.

World Health Organization. (n.d.). The Ottawa charter for health promotion. First International Conference on Health Promotion, Ottawa, Canada, November 21, 1986. Retrieved from http://www.who.int/healthpromotion/conferences/previous/ottawa/en/

World Health Organization. (2017). Global strategy and action plan on aging and health. Geneva: Author.

Worldwide Palliative Care Alliance & World Health Organization. (2014, January). *Global atlas of palliative care at the end of life.* Retrieved from http://www.who.int/ncds/management/palliative-care/palliative-care-atlas/en/

Xu, J., Murphy, S. L., Kochanek, K. D., Bastian, B., & Arias, E. (2018). Deaths: Final data for 2016. *National Vital Statistics Report, 67*(5), pp. 5–9. Retrieved from https://www.cdc.gov/nchs/data/nvsr/nvsr67/nvsr67_05.pdf

Chapter 23

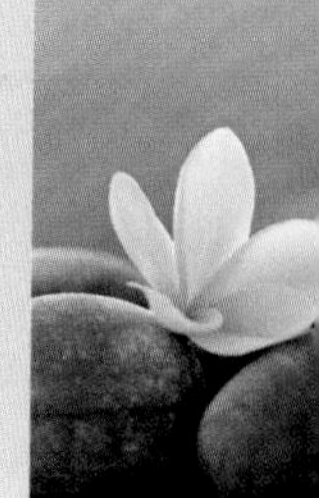

Synthesizing the Evidence and Using It in Health Promotion Practice

Diane Whitehead

LEARNING OBJECTIVES

After completing this chapter, the student will be able to:

1. Understand the process of grading evidence.
2. Develop a plan to translate evidence into practice using a selected model.
3. Develop a strategy to include stakeholders in incorporating evidence into practice.

INTRODUCTION

A 2018 editorial in the *American Journal of Health Promotion* (Terry, 2018) speaks to increased growth in health promotion activities over the past 40 years. Services once available only to high-level executives, such as breast cancer screenings, tobacco cessation initiatives, and HIV education, are now commonplace. Schools, community centers, workplaces, and churches are promoting healthy activities. If these increases in health promotion activities are true, why does the author of this editorial state the need for improved health promotion? Terry stresses the importance of expanding the use of evidence-based practice in health promotion far beyond the current level. The increased ability of primary-care nurse practitioners to manage chronic conditions outside the acute-care facility will address this question of increasing access to health promotion activities (Bodenheimer & Bauer, 2016). Knowing how to search for evidence and the ability to analyze best evidence are imperative to quality practice in promoting health.

SEARCHING FOR EVIDENCE

If you are fortunate enough to be connected to a university or an academic medical center, you probably have access to an extensive online library with databases such as Cumulative Index to Nursing and Allied Health Literature (CINAHL), MEDLINE, ProQuest Health and Medical Collection, ProQuest Nursing & Allied Health Source, and PubMed. These databases contain journals and e-books on an extensive variety of nursing, medicine, and allied health topics. However, many nurse practitioners no longer have access to the resources available to students. See Box 23-1 for a list of free and subscription-based research services.

Systemic Search Strategies

Searching for evidence often feels like searching for a needle in a haystack. A systematic approach to searching for evidence should be developed to ensure that you have done an exhaustive search. Melnyk, Gallagher-Ford, and

Fineout-Overholt (2017) describe a sequence of steps that will promote a systematic search:

1. Use your patient, intervention, control, observation, and time (PICOT) question to identify relevant search terms.
2. Identify at least two appropriate databases for searching.
3. Develop a search strategy. Both the Virginia Commonwealth University and the Johns Hopkins Nursing Evidence-Based Practice (JHNEBP) Web sites have resources available to practitioners that assist with developing PICOT questions and search strategies (Table 23-1).
4. Obtain your evidence.

BOX 23-1 Evidence-Based Practice Resources Databases

PubMed for Nurses: https://www.nlm.nih.gov/bsd/disted/nurses/cover.html. Provides free access to MEDLINE, the NLM database of indexed citations and abstracts.

CINAHL Complete: https://www.ebscohost.com/nursing/products/cinahl-databases/cinahl-complete. Cumulative index for nursing and allied health professionals. Available by subscription.

Joanna Briggs Institute: http://joannabriggs.org/. A repository for publications and guidelines for evidence-based practice.

Virginia Henderson Global Nursing e-Repository: http://www.nursinglibrary.org/vhl/. A resource of the Honor Society of Nursing, Sigma Theta Tau International.

Cochrane Library: http://www.cochranelibrary.com/. A resource for systematic reviews and clinical trials.

US National Library of Medicine: https://www.nlm.nih.gov/. Extensive resources that also include PubMed and MEDLINE PLUS.

Google Scholar: https://scholar.google.com/. An online resource for broad searches of scholarly literature. Publications include articles, theses, books, abstracts, and court opinions from a variety of sources. Not all literature is peer reviewed.

Table 23-1 Search Strategy Resources

Virginia Commonwealth University	Johns Hopkins Nursing Evidence-Based Practice (Jhnebp)
Searching Tips and Useful Web Resources Handout: https://guides.library.vcu.edu/ld.php?content_id=30249414	Question Development Tool PICO https://www.hopkinsmedicine.org/evidence-based-practice/_images/EBP%20Tool%20Samples/2017_Appendix%20B_Question%20Development%20Tool_Page_1.png
Basic Search Process Checklist: https://guides.library.vcu.edu/ld.php?content_id=1720920	Research Evidence Appraisal Tool https://www.hopkinsmedicine.org/evidence-based-practice/_images/EBP%20Tool%20Samples/2017_Appendix%20E_Research%20Appraisal%20Tool_Page_0.png
	Individual Evidence Summary Tool https://www.hopkinsmedicine.org/evidence-based-practice/_images/EBP%20Tool%20Samples/2017_Appendix%20G_Individual%20Evidence%20Tool_Page_1.png
	Evidence Synthesis and Recommendation Tool https://www.hopkinsmedicine.org/evidence-based-practice/_images/EBP%20Tool%20Samples/2017_Appendix%20H%20Evidence%20Synthesis%20and%20Recommendation%20Tool_Page_1.png
	Copyright permission https://www.ijhn-education.org/content/johns-hopkins-nursing-evidence-based-practice-model-and-tools

APPRAISING AND GRADING EVIDENCE

An important step in using evidence is evaluating its strength using one of two common scales: a level of evidence scale and a grading scale. Although numerous levels of evidence scales are found in the literature, most of these are quite similar to one another. The level of evidence scale rates the strength of the evidence based on the research design and/or the methodology. Although no common scale exists, ratings do have some consistency. Two of the most well-known scales used in nursing are the Johns Hopkins Evidence Level and Quality Guide and the Melynk, Gallagher-Ford, and Fineout-Overholt Levels of Evidence Scale. Table 23-2 compares the different rating systems (Melnyk, Gallagher-Ford, Fineout-Overholt, 2017; Thompson, 2017).

Besides appraising the level of evidence, practitioners may grade the evidence to ascertain its readiness to apply to practice. Grading asks whether the strength and quality of the evidence support the practice recommendation that has been proposed. The United States Preventive Services Task Force (USPSTF) began in 1964 as an independent volunteer panel of national experts in disease prevention and evidence-based medicine. USPSTF makes evidence-based recommendations about clinical preventive services and publishes them on its Web site at www.uspreventiveservicestaskforce.org and in peer-reviewed journals. USPSTF published new guidelines for grading the strength of recommendations in 2012 (USPSTF, 2017). Table 23-3 explains the grades and suggestions for practice.

Table 23-2 Levels of Evidence Comparison

Levels	Jhnebp Evidence Level and Quality Guide	Melnyk, Gallagher and Overholt Levels of Evidence
Level 1	Experimental study, RCT,* SR* of RCTs, with or without meta-analysis.	SRs or meta-analysis of all relevant RCTs.
Level II	Quasi-experimental study. SR of a combination of RCTs and quasi-experimental, or quasi-experimental studies only, with or without meta-analysis.	Well-designed RCTs.
Level III	Non-experimental study. SR of a combination of RCTs, quasi-experimental and non-experimental, or non-experimental studies only, with or without meta-analysis. Qualitative study or systematic review, with or without meta-analysis.	Well-designed non-randomized trials.
Level IV	Opinion of respected authorities and/or nationally recognized expert committees/consensus panels based on scientific evidence. Includes: • Clinical practice guidelines. • Consensus panels.	Well-designed case-control and cohort studies.
Level V	Based on experiential and nonresearch evidence. Includes: • Literature reviews. • Quality improvement, program or financial evaluation. • Case reports. • Opinion of nationally recognized expert(s) based on experiential evidence.	SR of descriptive and qualitative studies.
Level VI		Single descriptive or qualitative studies.
Level VII		Opinions of experts and/or authorities or reports of expert committees.

*SR = systematic review; RCT = randomized control trial.
Source: Adapted from: Melnyk, Gallagher-Ford, & Fineout-Overholt, 2017; Thompson, 2017.

Table 23-3 Definitions of USPSTF Grades Beginning 2012

Grade	Definition	Suggestions For Practice
A	Practice recommended with high certainty of substantial net benefit.	Offer or provide service.
B	Practice recommended. High certainty of moderate to substantial benefit.	Offer or provide service.
C	Use professional judgment and patient preferences in offering service to selected individuals. Moderate benefit certainty.	Offer or provide service to selected individuals.
D	Recommend against service. Moderate to high certainty of no benefit or harm to individuals.	Discourage use of service.
I	Current evidence insufficient to evaluate harm or benefit.	If service is offered, patients should understand the uncertainly related to harm or benefit.

Source: Adapted from USPSTF (2018). Retrieved from https://www.uspreventiveservicestaskforce.org/Page/Name/grade-definitions

TRANSLATING EVIDENCE INTO PRACTICE

The lack of translation of evidence into implementation contributes to poor health outcomes. Implementation and dissemination of evidence-based interventions can traditionally take up to two decades. This sizable gap has often caused insufficient evidence to guide public health policy and practice recommendations (Titler, LoBiondo-Wood, & Haber, 2018; Wolfenden et al., 2016).

Models for Translating Evidence

Translation science includes many published theories and models. The study by Birken and colleagues (2017) found more than 100 different theories used by 223 implementation scientists in multiple disciplines worldwide.

JHNEBP Model

The JHNEBP model involves a three-step process: practice question, evidence, and translation (PET). The model is user-friendly, with multiple tutorials and resources available online for professional use. Practitioners may seek permission to use the model and the tools in their practices. The PET process includes numerous subphases described on the Web site (Dang & Dearholt, 2017).

Advancing Research and Clinical Practice Through Close Collaboration (ARCC) Model

The ARCC Model supports system-wide implementation, evidence-based practice (EBP), beginning with an organizational assessment of the current EBP culture that identifies strengths and barriers to implementation. One distinct feature of the model is the identification and use of mentors to assist point-of-care clinicians. Numerous studies have demonstrated support for the use of this model in improving job satisfaction, decreasing turnover, and improving patient outcomes (Melnyk et al., 2017).

i-PARIHS Framework

The promoting action on research implementation in health services (PARIHS) framework has been revised and is now titled the i-PARIHS Framework. The framework was first introduced in 2008 and addressed the fact that successful implementation of evidence into practice was a function of the quality and type of evidence, the characteristics of the setting, and the way in which the evidence was put into practice. As social, political, economic, and policy issues became more complex, users of the framework recognized the need to put more emphasis on implementation (Harvey & Kitson, 2015).

IOWA Model

The IOWA Model has been used in nursing practice for almost two decades. More than 3,900 requests for permission to use the model are documented. The most recent revision and validation of the model occurred in 2015. Steps in the model include:

1. Identify triggering issues.
2. State question or purpose.
3. Form a team.
4. Synthesize relevant literature.
5. Design and pilot practice change.
6. Adopt change or consider alternatives.
7. Integrate practice change. (Iowa Model Collaborative, 2017)

ACE Star Model

Developed by Stevens in 2004, the ACE Star Model of Knowledge Transformation focuses on translation of evidence into practice. The five-step model is circular; after evaluation in the fifth step, discovery begins again (Stevens, 2013).

- Point 1: Discovery research
- Point 2: Evidence summary
- Point 3: Translation into guidelines
- Point 4: Practice integration
- Point 5: Process, outcome evaluation

Rosswurm and Larrabee (1999) Model

Colleagues at West Virginia University School of Nursing, Mary Ann Rosswurm and June Larrabee developed their EBP model in 1999, and the model continues to gain support. It includes the following six steps:

1. Assess the need for a practice change.
2. Link problem interventions and outcomes.
3. Synthesize best evidence.
4. Design practice change.
5. Implement and evaluate the change.
6. Integrate and maintain.

SQUIRE Guidelines

The Standards for Quality Improvement Reporting Excellence (SQUIRE) guidelines were developed in 2008 and updated in 2015. The purposes of the guidelines are to eliminate redundancy and promote standardization of quality improvement (QI) initiatives. SQUIRE begins with four questions: (a) Why did you start? (b) What do you do? (c) What did you find? and (d) What does it mean? (McQuellan & Wong, 2016). Subheadings under each question help the user report specific information. The guidelines and resources for using them are available at http://squire-statement.org/.

RE-AIM Framework

Originally developed as a framework for consistent reporting of research results in 1999, the reach, effectiveness, adoption, implementation, maintenance (RE-AIM) Framework is widely used in public health for health promotion and disease prevention. With this framework, users can focus on essential program elements, including external validity that can improve the sustainable adoption and implementation of effective, generalizable, evidence-based interventions (Harden et al., 2018; RE-AIM, 2018). Questions to ask when using this framework are:

- How do I reach the targeted population with the intervention? (*Reach*)
- How do I know my intervention is effective? (*Efficacy*)
- How do I develop organizational support to deliver my intervention? (*Adoption*)
- How do I ensure the intervention is delivered properly? (*Implementation*)
- How do I incorporate the intervention so that it is delivered over the long term? (*Maintenance*) (RE-AIM, 2018)

PRECEDE-PROCEED Model

The PRECEDE-PROCEED model is widely used in health promotion activities. The premise of this model is that stakeholders, or those whose behavior or actions you want to change, must be included in the process, not at the end but from the beginning. Health is considered a community issue and part of a constellation of factors, including economic, social, political, and ecological, that have an impact on health at the individual and community levels.

PRECEDE stands for predisposing, reinforcing, and enabling constructs in educational/environmental diagnoses and evaluation. At this point, we are doing the processes that precede the intervention. PROCEED, the intervention, represents policy, regulatory, and organizational constructs in educational and environmental development (Center for Community Health and Development, 2018). This model has eight phases; four in PRECEDE and four in PROCEED. Table 23-4 outlines the model phases.

A variety of models can be used for translating evidence into practice. Review the examples in Table 23-5; each example uses the model to support a practice change.

Working with Stakeholders

Think back to both personal and professional decisions that were made without your input or even input from your family, friends, or colleagues. Did those decisions always lead to sustained improved change and increased satisfaction? Especially in health promotion activities, which are often voluntary, stakeholder involvement is critical. Current evidence supports the importance of stakeholder participation using a variety of methods such as Delphi, a group of experts who anonymously reply to questionnaires. After receiving feedback on the group response, the process repeats until a group consensus is reached. Other methods include telephone interviews, focus groups, online surveys, and individual face-to face interviews (Boyko, Wathen, & Kothan, 2017; Morton et al., 2018; Mroz, Zhang, Williams, Conlon, & LaConte, 2017; O'Rourke, Higuchi, & Hogg, 2016; Pinto, Waldemore, & Rosen, 2015). Stakeholder involvement

Table 23-4 PRECEDE-PROCEED Model Phases

Precede	Proceed
Phase 1: Identify the desired result.	Phase 5: Implementation—the design and actual conducting of the intervention.
Phase 2: Identify and set priorities among health or community issues that might affect the result.	Phase 6: Implementation—the design and actual conducting of the intervention.
Phase 3: Identify predisposing, enabling, and reinforcing factors.	Phase 7: Impact evaluation—Is the intervention having the desired impact on the target population?
Phase 4: Identify administrative and policy influencing factors.	Phase 8: Outcome evaluation—Is the intervention leading to the outcome (the desired result) that was envisioned in Phase 1?

Source: Adapted from Green, L. W., & Marshall W. Kreuter. (1999). *Health promotion and planning: An educational and environmental approach* (4th ed.). Mountain View, CA: Mayfield Publishing Co.

Table 23-5 Examples of Translational Research Using Identified Models

JHNEBP Model	Egyud, A., Stephens, K., Swanson-Bierman, B., DiCuccio, M., & Whiteman, K. (2017). Practice improvement: Implementation of human trafficking education and treatment algorithm in the emergency department. *Journal of Emergency Nursing, 43*, 526–531.
ARCC Model	Melnyk, B. M., Fineout-Overholt, E., Giggleman, M., & Choy, K. (n.d.). A test of the ARCC (c) Model improves implementation of evidence-based practice, healthcare culture, and patient outcomes. *Worldviews on Evidence-Based Nursing, 14*(1), 5–9.
PARIHS Model	Harris, M., Jones, P., Heartfield, M., et al. (2015). Changing practice to support self-management and recovery in mental illness: Application of an implementation model. *Australian Journal of Primary Health, 21*(3):279–285. doi:10.1071/PY13103
IOWA Model	Buckwalter, K. C., Cullen, L., Hanrahan, K., Kleiber, C., McCarthy, A. M., Rakel, B.,& Tucker, S. (2017). Iowa Model of evidence-based practice: Revisions and validation. *Worldviews on Evidence-Based Nursing, 14*(3), 175–182.
ACE STAR Model	Gordon, J. M., Lauver, L. S., & Buck, H. G. (2018). Strict versus liberal insulin therapy in the cardiac surgery patient: An evidence-based practice development, implementation and evaluation project. *Applied Nursing Research, 39*, 265–269.
Rosswurm and Larrabee Model	Saunier, D. T. (2017). Creating an interprofessional team and discharge planning guide to decrease hospital readmissions for COPD. *MEDSURG Nursing, 26*(4), 258–262.
SQUIRE Guidelines	McQuillan, R. F., & Wong, B. M. (2016). The SQUIRE Guidelines: A scholarly approach to quality improvement. *Journal of Graduate Medical Education, 8*(5), 771–772.
RE-AIM Model	Trego, L. L., Steele, N. M., & Jordan, P. (2018). Using the RE-AIM Model of health promotion to implement a military women's health promotion program for austere settings. *Military Medicine, 183*(suppl. 1), 538–546.
PRECEDE-PROCEED Model	Sezgin, D., & Esin, M. N. (n.d.). Effects of a PRECEDE-PROCEED model based ergonomic risk management programme to reduce musculoskeletal symptoms of ICU nurses. *Intensive and Critical Care Nursing, 47*, 89–97.

builds trust and support, divides the responsibility for decision making among the participants, and leads to strong working relationships. Solutions are more likely to be implemented with strong stakeholder involvement. If stakeholder input is not used or valued, however, these individuals may feel that their time was wasted. Making sure that stakeholder input is recognized and added to the planning process is vital (MacPherson, Tonning, & Faalasli, 2018).

Who should be invited as a stakeholder? Four types of stakeholders are important to the process: (a) implementers, (b) decision makers, (c), participants, and (d) partners (Centers for Disease Control and Prevention [CDC], 2012):

- Implementers: Those directly involved in the program
- Decision makers: Those who can do something or decide something about the program
- Participants: Those directly affected by the program
- Partners: Those who already actively support the program, are invested in supporting the program, or are in the population served by your program

Once the stakeholder group is formed, develop a framework for stakeholder involvement. Decide how the group will be structured, how decisions will be made, and the roles and responsibilities of each member. Set program goals, ground rules, decision-making methods, and expected deliverables from the group. Above all, have an agenda for each meeting. Value the stakeholders' time!

Don't feel that consensus is needed for every decision. Decision making depends on a variety of factors such as time available, importance of the decision, available information related to the decision, and the ability of the group to make that decision (MacPherson et al., 2018).

Stakeholders are often a very important part of implementation and translation of evidence. Stakeholder groups will be different for each process, depending on the driving and restraining factors and the goals and objectives. However, stakeholder involvement is considered integral to most public health interventions (Morton et al., 2018).

USEFUL RESOURCES

In addition to the references and resources provided in the tables and the list of references at the end of the chapter, the following resources are useful in identifying health promotion issues and implementing evidence-based practices:

Ace Star Model of Knowledge Transformation, http://nursing.uthscsa.edu/onrs/starmodel/institute/su08/starmodel.html

Centers for Disease Control and Prevention, https://www.cdc.gov/

Community Tool Box, https://ctb.ku.edu/en/table-of-contents

Healthy People 2020, https://www.healthypeople.gov/

Johns Hopkins Nursing Evidence-Based Practice (JHNEBP) Model, https://www.hopkinsmedicine.org/evidence-based-practice/ijhn_2017_ebp.html

RE-AIM Framework Web site, http://www.re-aim.org

United States Preventive Services Task Force, https://www.uspreventiveservicestaskforce.org/

KEY POINTS

- Health-care resources are a valuable commodity. Only through using the best evidence, coupled with our clinical judgment and attention to our patients' preferences, can we continue to provide safe, quality care.
- The Quadruple Aim in health care of improving the patient experience, improving the health of populations, decreasing costs, and improving the work life of clinicians continues to be met through the translation of evidence into practice (Bodenheimer & Sinsky, 2014).
- Widely used evidence-based practice models that move us from identifying a practice problem to translating and evaluating evidence in practice are explored.
- There is no one size fits all. You will decide the model(s) that fit the practice issue, the stakeholders involved, and the time you have for implementation.
- Many books, Web sites, and online tools are available for you to use.
- Stay grounded in the commitment to search for evidence. It is there for you to find.

Check Your Understanding

1. In searching for evidence, the first step should be:
   A. Select a journal of your choice and look through it
   B. Ask a few colleagues what they feel is current in practice
   C. Develop a PICOT question
   D. Use only Google Scholar
2. Although scales are used to grade evidence, all of them are consistent in that the strongest evidence is found in studies done as:
   A. Cohort studies
   B. Randomized control trials
   C. Qualitative studies
   D. Quasi-experimental studies
3. The reason for grading evidence is to:
   A. Organize the literature review
   B. Support the strength of the practice recommendation
   C. Develop a time line for implementation
   D. Explore the cost of implementation

4. Evidence-based practice models are used to develop a process for:
   A. Grading the literature
   B. Implementation
   C. Searching the literature
   D. Managing patients

5. Stakeholder involvement includes different types of participants to do all of the following except:
   A. Implement the program
   B. Make decisions for the program
   C. Receive services from the program
   D. Grade the evidence supporting the program

See "Reflections on Check Your Understanding" at the end of the book for answers.

REFERENCES

Birken, S. A., Powell, B. J., Shea, C. M., Haines, E. R., Kirk, M. A., Leeman, J., & Presseau, J. (2017). Criteria for selecting implementation science theories and frameworks: Results from an international survey. *Implementation Science*, *12*(1) 124. doi:10.1186/s13012-017-0656

Bodenheimer, T., & Bauer, L. (2016). Rethinking the primary care workforce: An expanded role for nurses. *New England Journal of Medicine*, *375*, 1015–1017. doi:10.1056/NEJMp1606869

Bodenheimer, T., & Sinsky, C. (2014). From Triple to Quadruple Aim: Care of the patient requires care of the provider. *Annals of Family Medicine*, *12*, 573–576.

Boyko, J., Wathen, N., & Kothan, A. (2017). Effectively engaging stakeholders and the public in developing violence prevention messages. *BMC Women's Health*, *17*(35), 1–4. doi:10.1186/s12905-017-0390-2

Center for Community Health and Development. (2018). *Community Tool Box: Section 2: PRECEDE-PROCEED.* Retrieved from https://ctb.ku.edu/en/table-contents/overview/other-models-promoting-community-health-and-development/preceder-proceder/main

Centers for Disease Control and Prevention. (2012). Step 1: Engage stakeholders. Retrieved from https://www.cdc.gov/std/program/pupestd/Step-1-SPREADS.pdf

Dang, D., & Dearholt, S. (2017). *Johns Hopkins nursing evidence-based practice: model and guidelines.* 3rd ed. Indianapolis, IN: Sigma Theta Tau International

Green, L. W., & Kreuter, M. W. (1999). *Health promotion and planning: An educational and environmental approach*. Mountain View, CA: Mayfield Publishing.

Harden, S. M., Smith, M. L., Ory, M. G., Smith-Ray, R. L., Estabrooks, P. A., & Glasgow R. E. (2018). RE-AIM in clinical, community, and corporate settings: Perspectives, strategies, and recommendations to enhance public health impact. *Frontiers in Public Health*, 6,71 doi:10.3389/fpubh.2018.00071

Harvey, G., & Kitson, A. (2015). PARIHS revisited: From heuristic to integrated framework for the successful implementation of knowledge into practice. *Implementation science*, *11*(1), 33.

Iowa Model Collaborative. (2017). Iowa model of evidence-based practice: Revisions and validation. *Worldviews on Evidence-Based Nursing*, *14*(3), 175–182. doi:10.1111/wvn.12223

MacPherson, C., Tonning, B., & Faalasli, E. (2018). *Engaging and involving stakeholders in your watershed*. Washington, DC: U.S. Environmental Protection Agency.

McQuellin, R., & Wong, B. (2016, December 1). The SQUIRE guidelines: A scholarly approach to quality improvement. *Journal of Graduate Medical Education*, *8*(5), 771–772.

Melnyk, B., Gallagher-Ford, L., & Fineout-Overholt, E. (2017). *Evidence-based competencies in healthcare: A practical guide for improving quality, safety, & outcomes*. Indianapolis, IN: Sigma Theta Tau International.

Morton, K., Atkin, A., Corder, K., Suhrcke, M., Turner, D., & van Shuijs, E. (2018). Engaging stakeholders and target groups in prioritizing a public health intervention: The Creating Active School Environments (CASE) online Delphi study. *BMJ Open*, 7(e013340), 1–11. doi.org/10.1136/bmjopen-2016-013304

Mroz, S., Zhang, X., Williams, M., Conlon, A., & LaConte, N. (2017). Working to increase vaccination for human papillomavirus: A survey of Wisconsin stakeholders, 2015. *Preventing Chronic Disease*, *14* (E85), 1–9.

O'Rourke, T., Higuchi, K., & Hogg, W. (2016). Stakeholder participation in system change: A new conceptual model. *Worldviews on Evidence-Based Nursing*, *13*(4), 261–269.

Pinto, B., Waldemore, M., & Rosen, R. (2015). A community-based partnership to promote exercise among cancer survivors: Lessons learned. *Journal of Behavioral Medicine*, *22*, 328–335. doi10:1007/s12529-014-9395-5

RE-AIM. (2018). RE-AIM Workgroup. Retrieved from http://www.re-aim.org/

Rosswurm, M., & Larrabee, J. (1999). A model for change to evidence-based practice. *Image: Journal of Nursing Scholarship*, *31*(3), 317–348.

Stevens, K. (2013, May 31) The impact of evidence-based practice in nursing and the next big ideas. *OJIN: The Online Journal of Issues in Nursing*, *18*(2), Manuscript 4. doi:10.3912/OJIN.Vol18No02Man04

Terry, P. (2018). Why health promotion needs to change. *American Journal of Health Promotion*, *32*(1), 13–15. doi:10.1177/0890117117774544

Thompson, K. (2017). What does "grading the evidence" mean in evidence based practice? Retrieved from https://nursingeducationexpert.com/grading-evidence/

Titler, M., LoBiondo-Wood, G., & Haber, J. (2018). Overview of evidence-based practice. *Evidence-Based Practice for Nursing and Healthcare Quality Improvement*, 1.

United States Preventive Services Task Force. (2017). Retrieved from https://www.uspreventiveservicestaskforce.org/

Wolfenden, L., Jones, J., Williams, C. M., Finch, M., Wyse, R. J., Kingsland, M., & Small, T. (2016). Strategies to improve the implementation of healthy eating, physical activity and obesity prevention policies, practices or programmes within childcare services. *The Cochrane Library*.

Appendix A

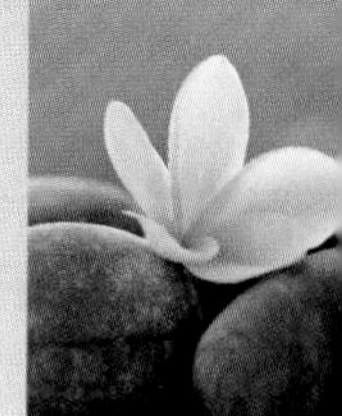

Reflections on Check Your Understanding Questions

Chapter 2

1. B
2. A
3. A
4. B
5. B

Chapter 3

1. A
2. C
3. A
4. D
5. C
6. B
7. B
8. D

Chapter 4

1. D
2. A
3. B
4. E
5. E

Chapter 5

1. B
2. D
3. D
4. A
5. C

Chapter 6

1. B
2. D
3. C
4. E
5. E
6. E
7. D
8. E
9. E
10. E

Chapter 7

1. D
2. A
3. D
4. C
5. A
6. D
7. A
8. False
9. C
10. A

Chapter 8

1. C
2. C
3. B
4. A
5. A
6. A
7. A
8. A
9. A
10. A

Chapter 9

1. A
2. D
3. C
4. B
5. D

Chapter 10

1. C
2. B
3. D
4. A
5. C
6. D
7. C
8. C

Chapter 11

1. D
2. E
3. A
4. C
5. E

Chapter 12

1. A
2. C
3. B
4. B
5. B
6. C
7. C
8. B

Chapter 13

1. D
2. D
3. B
4. A
5. D
6. D
7. A
8. C
9. A
10. D

Chapter 14

1. B
2. D
3. A
4. B
5. D
6. D

Chapter 15

1. B
2. C
3. C
4. A
5. D

Chapter 16

1. B
2. A
3. C
4. B

Chapter 17

1. C
2. B
3. D
4. A
5. B
6. C
7. A
8. C
9. D
10. A

Chapter 18

1. A, B, C, D
2. A, B
3. A, B, C, D, E
4. A, B, C, D, F

Chapter 19

1. B
2. C
3. C
4. A
5. D

Chapter 20

1. D
2. B
3. C
4. A
5. C
6. A
7. A
8. A

Chapter 21

1. B
2. C
3. D
4. A
5. B
6. C
7. D.
8. B
9. C
10. A

Chapter 22

1. D
2. C
3. B
4. A
5. B

Chapter 23

1. C
2. B
3. B
4. B
5. D

Chapter 24

1. D
2. A
3. C
4. B

Index

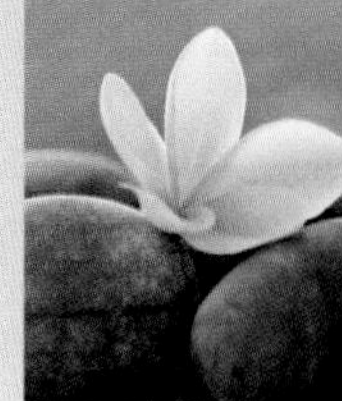

Page numbers followed by *f* denote figures; those followed by *t* denote tables; those followed by *b* denote boxes; those followed by *e* denote online chapters.